# CLINICAL
# ORTHOPAEDIC
# PHYSICAL
# THERAPY

# CLINICAL
# ORTHOPAEDIC
# PHYSICAL
# THERAPY

*Jan K. Richardson, PT, PhD, OCS*

Director and Professor
Graduate School of Physical Therapy
Slippery Rock University
Slippery Rock, Pennsylvania

*Z. Annette Iglarsh, PT, PhD*

President, Orthopaedic Section
American Physical Therapy Association
Adjunct Associate Professor
University of Delaware School of Life and Health Sciences
Department of Physical Therapy
Newark, Delaware

**W.B. SAUNDERS COMPANY**

*A Division of Harcourt Brace & Company*
Philadelphia ■ London ■ Toronto ■ Montreal ■ Sydney ■ Tokyo

**W.B. Saunders Company**
*A Division of Harcourt Brace & Company*

The Curtis Center
Independence Square West
Philadelphia, Pennsylvania 19106

### Library of Congress Cataloging-in-Publication Data

Richardson, Jan K.

    Clinical orthopaedic physical therapy / Jan K. Richardson,
Z. Annette Iglarsh.
      p.    cm.
    ISBN 0-7216-3257-2

    1. Orthopedics.  2. Physical therapy.  I.  Richardson, Jan K.  II.  Iglarsh, Z. Annette.
III. Title.
    [DNLM:  1.  Physical Therapy—methods.  2. Orthopedics—methods.
WB 460 R523c 1994]          RD736.P47R53 1994

    615.8′2—dc20
DNLM/DLC                                  93-7209

Clinical Orthopaedic Physical Therapy           ISBN 0-7216-3257-2

Last digit is the print number:    9    8    7    6    5    4    3

# *Dedication*

To Ryan, my special surprise, who came into this world on his own time schedule and has since made me accelerate just to keep one step ahead.

To Kara, my cherished princess, who brings me joy, happiness, and pride on a daily basis.

To Delores and Steve, my parents, who molded and solidified my values, drive, and sense of accomplishment.

To Bob, my husband, mentor emeritus and love of my life, who has encouraged, supported, led, and on occasion nudged me every step of the way throughout my professional career.

To Maddy, our administrative assistant, friend, and backup, who on a daily basis adjusted for our crisis management idiosyncrasies and executive decisional alterations.

To Gary, our photographer extraordinaire, whose professional expertise, talented vision, and tolerance has assisted in the artistic value of this scientific text.

Jan K. Richardson

To my daughter, Maggie, as she begins to discover the joys of writing and the pleasure of academic success.

To my husband, Gary, for his continued support, patience, and photographic talent.

To the readers of this text, since you provide the momentum and will perpetuate the speciality of orthopaedic physical therapy. It is my hope that this text contributes significantly to your efforts.

Z. Annette Iglarsh

# Contributors

**RICHARD W. BOWLING, PT, MS**
President, CORE Network, McKeesport, Pennsylvania
*Thoracic Spine*

**JILL G. BRASEL, PT**
Guest Lecturer, University of Tennessee, Memphis; Assistant Director, Center Coordinator of Clinical Education, Campbell Clinic, Physical Therapy Department, Memphis, Tennessee
*Elbow*

**CARL DeROSA, PT, PhD**
Associate Professor and Chairman, Physical Therapy Program, Northern Arizona University, Flagstaff, Arizona
*Lumbar Spine and Pelvis*

**MARCIA EPLER, PT, ATC, MEd**
Adjunct Assistant Professor, Philadelphia College of Pharmacy and Science; Orthopedic Outpatient Department, Jeanes Hospital, Philadelphia, Pennsylvania
*Gait*

**Z. ANNETTE IGLARSH, PT, PhD**
President, Orthopaedic Section, American Physical Therapy Association; Adjunct Associate Professor, University of Delaware School of Life and Health Sciences, Department of Physical Therapy, Newark, Delaware
*Temporomandibular Joint and the Cervical Spine*
*Education of Patients*

**JANNA L. JACOBS, PT, CHT**
Director of Rehabilitation Services, Meridian Healthcare Center at Brightwood, Baltimore, Maryland
*Hand and Wrist*

### BARNEY LeVEAU, PT, PhD
Professor and Chairman, Department of Physical Therapy, Georgia State University, Atlanta, Georgia
*Hip*

### DAVID L. McKINNIS, PT, MEd, OCS
Private Practice, Butler, Pennsylvania
*The Posture-Movement Dynamic*

### LYNN NOWICKI MCKINNIS, PT, OCS
Associate Professor, Adjunct Faculty, Slippery Rock University, Slippery Rock, Pennsylvania; Facility Director, Keystone Rehabilitation Systems, Indiana, Pennsylvania
*Fundamentals of Radiology for Physical Therapists*

### JAMES A. PORTERFIELD, PT, ATC
Assistant Professor of Physical Therapy, Cleveland State University, Cleveland; Adjunct Faculty, Ohio State University Division of Physical Therapy; Owner/Director, Rehabilitation and Health Center of Crystal Clinic, Cleveland, Ohio
*Lumbar Spine and Pelvis*

### JAN K. RICHARDSON, PT, PhD, OCS
Director and Professor, Graduate School of Physical Therapy, Slippery Rock University, Slippery Rock, Pennsylvania

### DANIEL L. RIDDLE, PT, MS
Assistant Professor, Department of Physical Therapy, Virginia Commonwealth University, Richmond, Virginia
*Foot and Ankle*

### PAUL ROCKAR, PT, MS, OCS
Associate Professor, Graduate School of Physical Therapy, Slippery Rock University, Slippery Rock, Pennsylvania; Adjunct Assistant Professor, Duquesne University, Pittsburgh, Pennsylvania; CORE Network, McKeesport, Pennsylvania
*Thoracic Spine*

### LYNN SNYDER-MACKLER, PT, ScD, SCS
Assistant Professor, University of Delaware, Newark, Delaware
*Temporomandibular Joint and the Cervical Spine*

## SUSAN W. STRALKA, PT, MS

Clinical Instructor, University of Tennessee School of Health Sciences; Clinical Instructor, University of Mississippi, Jackson, Mississippi; Director of Physical Therapy, Campbell Clinic, Memphis, Tennessee

*Elbow*

## KENT E. TIMM, PT, PhD, SCS, OCS, ATC

Instructor, Physical Therapy Department, University of Michigan-Flint, Flint, Michigan; Instructor, Kramert Graduate School of Physical Therapy, University of Indianapolis, Indianapolis, Indiana; Research and Development Specialist, St. Luke's Healthcare Association, Saginaw, Michigan

*Knee*

## MAE L. YAHARA, PT, MS, ATC

Assistant Professor of Physical Therapy, Florida International University, Miami, Florida

*Shoulder*

# *Preface*

In the late 1970s, the House of Delegates of the American Physical Therapy Association mandated that professional education requirements for entrance into physical therapy be elevated to a postbaccalaureate degree program. Soon after this vote, the House of Delegates once again acted to meet the rapidly growing profession by recognizing a certification process for clinical specialists.

Unfortunately, available textbooks did not parallel the expanded scope of practice in physical therapy. Traditional textbooks lacked the presentation of problem-solving and clinical decision-making skills integral to the practice of the advanced clinical specialist and required by the greater complexity of professional education. Clinicians preparing for the specialty examination were forced to use a large number of texts spanning multiple disciplines and lacking critical-thinking learning experiences and case scenarios, while educators continued to search for a comprehensive text at a reasonable cost to be used by students in the classroom.

A third, and perhaps the most clinically significant, change in physical therapy is the growing number of states permitting direct access to physical therapists as primary providers. California was the first state in which a physical therapist was permitted to evaluate a patient without a referral from a physician, and Maryland permitted physical therapists to evaluate and treat patients independently in 1979. Today more than half the states in the United States permit evaluation and/or treatment without a referral, and each year delegations of physical therapists approach their state legislatures seeking similar practice privileges. The right to evaluate and treat without referral requires that the physical therapist differentially diagnose in order to provide the highest quality of care, including making appropriate referral to others when necessary.

These three factors have altered the academic curricula for physical therapy education. The escalation of the profession was so dramatic through the 1980s that textbooks written by physical therapists for physical therapists became a publishing trend. However, these texts were intended to be reference manuals more than problem-solving diagnostic guides.

Thus, this textbook, *Clinical Orthopaedic Physical Therapy*, was created to fill this academic void. Structured in accordance with the matrix for the orthopaedic specialist examination as written in the Orthopaedic Competency Manual, each chapter in *Clinical Orthopaedic Physical Therapy* guides the reader from the basics of anatomy, biomechanics, and pathokinematics through a comprehensive, objective evaluation, differential diagnosis, and treatment plan. The case studies reinforce the clinical application of the contents of each chapter. The book is highly illustrated with line drawings and photographs to support the textural discussions and reinforce concepts. Discussion of radiology, gait, and posture complement the regional approach of other chapters. The final chapter on patient education is a practical analysis of effective teaching techniques as applied to the clinical setting, because to achieve a successful outcome, the physical therapist must teach patients life skills, methods of modifying their lives to avoid reinjury or to minimize exacerbations of a chronic illness. In addition, the therapist must also educate the patient and family about the dysfunction and treatment to ensure compliance and solicit their support and active participation. The phrase "If I treat you, I can help you today, but if I teach you, I can help you for a lifetime," expressed by Concept Care Incorporated (Pittsburgh, PA, 1982) is still apropos.

We enlisted the talents of highly regarded physical therapists who are leaders in their clinical fields to contribute their expertise to this text. Z. Annette Iglarsh and Lynn Snyder-Mackler integrate an analysis of the temporomandibular joint and the cervical spine. Richard Bowling and Paul Rockar present the thoracic spine, a region of the body often overlooked by orthopaedic texts. International experts Carl DeRosa and James Porterfield utilize their conceptual model to study the lumbar spine and pelvis. Mae Yahara approaches the shoulder from a practical and easily understood clinical perspective. Susan Stralka and Jill Brasel discuss the elbow, which is often injured in traumatic and repetitive strain injuries, and Janna Jacobs completes the discussion of the upper extremity in her chapter on the hand and wrist. Barney LeVeau eloquently presents congenital, pediatric, and adult development, pathology, and treatment of the hip. Dually certified specialist Kent Timm uses a comprehensive approach to the knee joint and its rehabilitation. Daniel Riddle simplifies the complex biomechanics and pathokinematics of the foot and ankle and relative clinical implications. Posture is reviewed from developmental and functional perspectives by David McKinnis. Normal and abnormal gait is analyzed by Marcia Epler. Lynn McKinnis presents a clinician's approach to radiology. The last chapter, Patient Education, by Z. Annette Iglarsh, is a practical discussion of effective teaching techniques for the clinical setting.

As the first competency-based, problem-oriented text, *Clinical Orthopaedic Physical Therapy* leads the physical therapist and clinical specialist through a quality orthopaedic evaluation: the development of differential diagnoses, and treatment of diverse patient populations. It is our hope that *Clinical Orthopaedic Physical Therapy* will represent the first of many texts written to meet the demands of the rapidly growing physical therapy profession and the accompanying challenges to all educational programs, as we move from baccalaureate degrees to masters degrees and ultimately doctoral degrees.

JAN K. RICHARDSON
Z. ANNETTE IGLARSH

# Contents

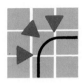

CHAPTER ■■■ *Four*

Shoulder .......................................... 159

*MAE L. YAHARA*

CHAPTER ■■■ *Five*

Elbow .............................................. 221

*SUSAN W. STRALKA, JILL G. BRASEL*

CHAPTER ■■■ *Nine*

# Foot and Ankle ........................... 483

DANIEL L. RIDDLE

CHAPTER ■■■ *Ten*

# The Posture-Movement Dynamic ........................... 563

DAVID L. McKINNIS

CHAPTER ■■■ *Eleven*

# Gait ........................... 602

MARCIA EPLER

CHAPTER ■ *Twelve*

## Fundamentals of Radiology for Physical Therapists ...................... 626

*LYNN NOWICKI McKINNIS*

CHAPTER ■ *Thirteen*

## Education of Patients ................... 688

*Z. ANNETTE IGLARSH*

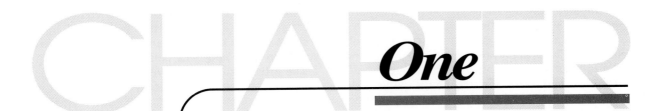

# *One*

# Temporomandibular Joint and the Cervical Spine

## Z. ANNETTE IGLARSH / LYNN SNYDER-MACKLER

## INTRODUCTION

As much as 12.1% of the population in the United States suffers annually from head and neck pain and dysfunction, yet these areas have been only minimally addressed in physical therapy professional curricula. The head and upper cervical spine should not be evaluated as separate structures because these regions are interrelated; it is the interaction of these structures that often perpetuates chronic pain and restricts the functional activities of this large population of patients.[1]

An anatomic study of the structures of the head and upper neck is the foundation of the static and dynamic biochemical analysis of these regions. Discussion of the soft tissue force on the bone structures completes the functional analysis. This basic scientific information is integral to the selection of effective evaluation procedures and the interpretation of the evaluation findings. The practitioner uses these evaluation findings initially to determine a differential diagnosis and then to design an effective treatment protocol.

Pre- and postoperative physical therapy protocols are necessary to treat a patient who has had surgical intervention. These protocols are a balance of aggressive physical therapy procedures and timing to promote effective healing of the involved tissues. Respect for the healing process is tempered by the need to encourage early movement and soft tissue relaxation.

Surgical and nonsurgical treatment protocols should include home treatment programs and education of patients and their care givers. Self-treatment and education encourage patients to modify their lifestyles to minimize parafunctional, destructive habits.

Although the terms neck dysfunction and cervical dysfunction are often used interchangeably, they are not synonymous. Neck dysfunction can be local or extending, inflammatory, and painful and can involve hypomobility or muscle weakness; and although it includes all categories of cervical dysfunction, some diagnoses may have nothing at all to do with the cervical spine. This chapter addresses problems in the posterior neck region, from the occiput to the midthorax.

Physical therapy diagnosis of neck dysfunction is even more problematic than that of low back problems. Classification schemes for low back pain are common in the literature and on the lecture circuit.[2-4] Similar characterizations of neck pain syndromes have not been as forthcoming. The pathology model fails just as much in suggesting treatment and predicting outcome of neck dysfunction as it does for low back dysfunction.[5] Many patients with radiologic diagnoses of arthritis, spondylolisthesis, disc protrusions, and bone spurs are asymptomatic. In addition, patients with neck dysfunction who have these radiologic findings present with a myriad of symptom complexes that transcend the radiologic categories.

## ANATOMY

### Temporomandibular Joint

Anatomically, the temporomandibular joint is a bilateral, moving hinge joint that is classified as a synovial joint. It is the primary moving joint and bone structure attaching the mandible to the head or skull. The sutures and cranial bones of the skull constitute the joints of the head.[6] The head also articulates with the upper cervical spine, considered to include the first and second cervical vertebrae and, in some sources, C-3.[7]

The soft tissue of the region includes the muscles of mastication and the ligaments of the temporomandibular joint, the muscles of facial expression, and the muscles and ligaments of the cervical spine, anterior and posterior aspects.

Neurologically, the region is supplied by both cranial and cervical nerves. Overlapping of branches from both types of nerves complicates the neurologic analysis of this region and may account for the extensive range of symptoms involved in head and neck pain and dysfunction.

The arterial supply and venous and lymphatic drainage can also be clinically significant in a patient with head and neck pain. These circulatory systems can be compromised by postural changes in the head and neck position, soft tissue spasm, trauma, or disease. This circulatory compromise can cause pain and functional loss.

The temporomandibular joint is suspended from the face by muscle and ligament. These soft tissue structures overcome the force of gravity as the individual maintains closed lips, produces speech, and ingests and swallows food.

This bilateral joint also articulates at the teeth. The teeth approximate in speech, chewing, and swallowing. The actual articulation of the teeth, occlusion, is determined by the interlocking teeth facets, contour of the teeth, and force of the muscles of mastication on the mandible as it travels in and beyond the temporal fossa. The extent of the influence of occlusion on temporomandibular joint dysfunction is disputed in the literature.[8] However, it is generally agreed that excessive occlusal disharmonies alter the forces on the mandible and its joints and cause soft tissue pain and occlusal dysfunction.

The temporomandibular joint is a gliding hinge joint consisting of temporal fossa, disc, and mandibular head. The biconcave disc of this joint is seated atop the convex mandibular head and modifies the mandibular head to conform to the convex articular eminence. This modification enables the mandibular head to move past the articular eminence as the mandible depresses and elevates.[9]

The disc also delineates the superior and inferior joint space, both lined with synovial membrane. The superior joint space consists of the mandibular fossa and superior surface of the disc, and the inferior joint space is delineated by the inferior disc surface and mandibular head (Fig. 1–1).

The disc's central zone, the intermediate zone, lacks vascularization and innervation and, therefore, is designed to be the weight- or force-bearing zone of the joint.[9] The anterior and posterior zones are vascularized and innervated and pain and dysfunction are produced if they are compressed by weight-bearing forces. This can occur if the disc becomes displaced, a possible cause of temporomandibular joint dysfunction. The disc is attached to the mandibular head by the medial and lateral collateral ligaments, pterygoid muscle anteriorly, and stratum and bilaminar zone pos-

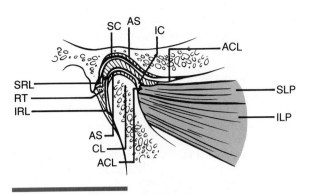

**FIGURE 1-1** ■ Temporomandibular joint with disc. SC, superior joint cavity; AS, articular surface; IC, inferior joint cavity; ACL, anterior capsular ligament; SLP, superior lateral pterygoid muscle; ILP, inferior lateral pterygoid muscle; CL, collateral ligament; IRL, inferior retrodiscal lamina; RT, retrodiscal tissues; SRL, superior retrodiscal ligament.

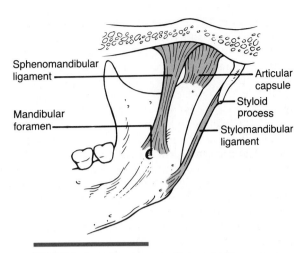

**FIGURE 1-2** ■ Temporomandibular joint ligaments.

teriorly. As the mandibular head moves anteriorly in the temporal fossa in mouth opening, the disc moves medially and posteriorly on the mandibular head until the collateral ligaments become taut. At this point the disc is seated and fixed on the mandibular head as the entire unit moves anteriorly until the anterior closed lock position is achieved with full opening. This process is reversed in closure of the mandible.

The ligaments of the temporomandibular joint complete the joint capsule. These ligaments are summarized in Table 1-1.

The ligaments and their suspensory role are shown in Figure 1-2. The ligaments of the temporomandibular joint, especially the capsular ligament, constitute the joint capsule.

The muscles of mastication act on the temporomandibular joint (Fig. 1-3, Table 1-2). The line of pull or vector force of the contractile fibers of the muscles of mastication, because of their attachments, determines the action of these muscles on the mandible (Table 1-3).

Because the temporomandibular joint is bilateral, the muscles of mastication must work in perfect synchrony; that is, the fibers must fire and relax in a regular pattern within the muscle and in a coordinated fashion with the muscles on the contralateral side. Muscles that are bruised by trauma or severed during surgery or that act parafunctionally on an unstable occlusion must be re-educated to fire once again in a synchronous fashion. The muscles can be re-educated by the use of biofeedback, functional electric stimulation, and isometric exercises.

The muscles of facial expression (Fig. 1-4, Table 1-4) enable the individual to communicate nonverbally and several of these muscles contribute to the anterior lip seal. Weakness of these

**Table 1-1.** LIGAMENTS OF THE TEMPOROMANDIBULAR JOINT

| Ligament | Attachments | Function |
|---|---|---|
| Capsular | Mandibular fossa, articular tubercle, and neck of the mandibular condyle | Stabilizes meniscus on top of the mandible |
| Temporomandibular | Zygomatic arch, articular eminence, and mandibular neck | Prevents excessive movements by the mandible as the mouth opens |
| Sphenomandibular | Spine of sphenoid and mandible near mandibular foramen | Supports mandible in wide opening |
| Stylomandibular | Styloid process of temporal bone posterior ramus of mandible malleus to medial posterior joint capsule | Limits excessive opening of mandible |
| Mandibular malleolar | Meniscus and sphenomandibular ligament | |

Data from Hiatt JL, Gartner LP: Textbook of Head and Neck Anatomy. New York: Appleton-Century-Crofts, 1982, p 221.

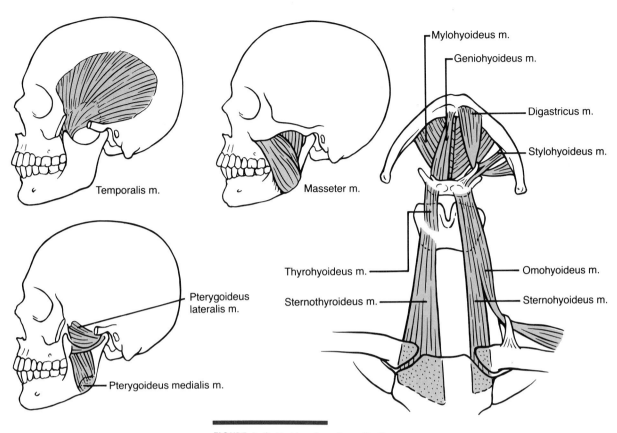

**FIGURE 1–3 ■** Muscles of mastication.

muscles is manifested by facial asymmetry, facial drooping, and altered facial expression.

As seen in the muscle charts, cranial nerves V and VII, the trigeminal and facial nerves, innervate predominantly the muscles of mastication and facial expression (Fig. 1–5). Therefore, direct trauma, demyelinating diseases, and infections of these nerves can cause facial paralysis and distorted facial expression, altered mastication, impaired word formation in speech, and disrupted anterior lip seal. A weakened anterior lip seal can permit anterior movement of the teeth, especially in individuals who protrude the tongue excessively, such as tongue thrusters.

Both rotation and translation (a combination of continued rotation, depression, and protrusion at the temporomandibular joint) occur in this joint. Rotation occurs predominantly in the inferior joint space as the mandibular head rotates anteriorly and the disc rotates posteriorly to seat itself atop the mandibular head. This portion of the joint motion can be evaluated by asking the patient to open his or her mouth as wide as possi-

ble while maintaining the tongue on the hard palate of the mouth. This range is usually the least painful for most patients and should be the functional limit of opening in the acute phase of dysfunction.

As the patient's mouth opens and the tongue loses contact with the hard palate, translation in the joint begins. Translation occurs in the superior joint space and should be avoided when the patient is in the acute phase of dysfunction. The practitioner should attempt to encourage painless translation during the early phase of treatment under controlled conditions.

## Neck Muscles

The neck muscles can be divided into three functional groups:

■ Posterior
■ Posterolateral
■ Suboccipital

**■■■■■ Table 1–2.** MUSCLES OF MASTICATION

| Muscle | Origin and Insertion | Action | Innervation |
|---|---|---|---|
| Temporalis | O. Temporal fossa and fascia<br>I. Medial and anterior coronoid | Elevates mandible and posterior fibers retract mandible | Trigeminal nerve, mandibular division, deep temporal nerve |
| Masseter | O. Superficial: lower border of zygomatic arch and maxillary process<br>I. Angle and inferior lateral surface of ramus | Elevates mandible, superficial fibers protrude mandible, slightly deep fibers retract mandible | Trigeminal nerve, mandibular division, masseteric branch |
| | O. Deeper portion: zygomatic arch<br>I. Lateral coronoid process and superior ramus | | Trigeminal nerve, mandibular division, masseteric branch |
| Lateral pterygoid | O. Superior: infratemporal crest of greater wing of sphenoid bone<br>I. Articular disc, capsule, and condyle<br>O. Inferior: lateral surface of pterygoid head plate<br>I. To anterior temporomandibular joint neck, and medial condyle | | Trigeminal nerve, mandibular branch, lateral pterygoid nerve |
| Medial pterygoid | O. Lateral pterygoid plate and pyramidal process of palative bone<br>I. Medial ramus and angle of mandible | Elevates mandible, protrudes and laterally deviates mandible | Trigeminal nerve, mandibular branch, medial pterygoid nerve |
| Digastric | O. Anterior: lower border of mandible<br>Posterior: temporal bone, area of mastoid process<br>I. Common tendon to the hyoid bone | If hyoid bone is stabilized, the muscle opens the mandible as it is pulled down and posteriorly | Trigeminal nerve, mandibular branch, mylohyoid and facial nerve |
| Stylohyoid | O. Temporal bone, styoid process<br>I. Hyoid bone | Acts in early opening of mandible; if mandible is stabilized, can retract and elevate hyoid bone | Trigeminal nerve, mandibular branch, facial nerve |
| Mylohyoid | O. Entire length of mandible<br>I. Hyoid bone (floor of mouth) | Depresses mandible if hyoid bone is fixed and conversely elevates hyoid bone if mandible is fixed | Trigeminal nerve, mandibular branch, mylohyoid nerve |
| Infrahyoid (sternohyoid, thyrohyoid, and omohyoid) | | Stabilize hyoid bone if mandible is stable; depress hyoid bone if mandible is not stable | Trigeminal nerve, mandibular branch, infrahyoid nerve |

Adapted from Hiatt JL, Gartner LP: Textbook of Head and Neck Anatomy. New York: Appleton-Century-Crofts, 1982, p 221.

**■■■■■ Table 1–3.** SUMMARY OF MUSCLE ACTIONS ON THE MANDIBLE

| Action | Muscle |
|---|---|
| Mouth closure or mandibular elevation | Masseter, temporalis with retrusion, superior head of lateral pterygoid with protrusion |
| Mouth opening or mandibular depression | Interior head of lateral pterygoid, anterior head of digastric suprahyoid muscles initiate motion if hyoid bone is fixed, masseter and medial pyterygoid muscles with protrusion |
| Retraction of mandible | Posterior temporalis with digastric and suprahyoids |
| Protrusion of mandible | Masseter, medial and lateral pterygoids |
| Lateral deviation of mandible | Lateral and medial pterygoids and contralateral temporalis, digastric, geniohyoid, and mylohyoid assist |

Data from Hertling D, Kessler RM: Management of Common Musculoskeletal Disorders, 2nd ed. Philadelphia: JB Lippincott, 1990, pp 419–421.

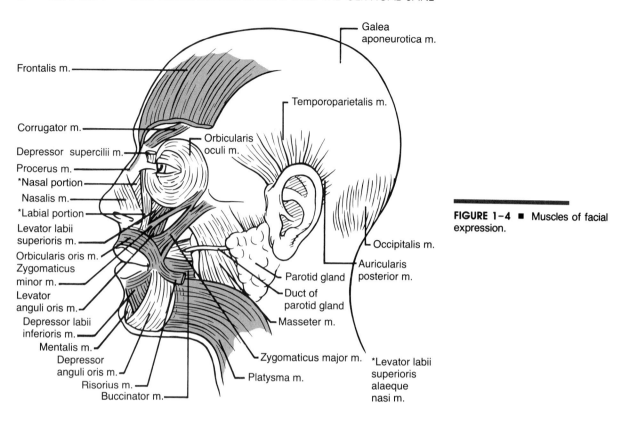

**FIGURE 1–4** ■ Muscles of facial expression.

The posterior group includes the trapezius superficially and the erector spinae groups in the deeper levels (Fig. 1–6A). The posterolateral group includes the levator scapulae, sternocleidomastoid, and scalenus (Fig. 1–6B). The suboccipital group includes all the short muscles that attach from the head to C-1 and C-2.[10,11] Although more specific descriptions of the anatomy can be undertaken, for the purposes of diagnosis and treatment of neck dysfunction this is sufficient. Table 1–5 lists the muscles of the neck region with their attachments and innervations.

## Cervical Vertebrae

There are seven cervical vertebrae. The atlas (Fig. 1–7) has no real vertebral body or spinous process. It has lateral masses with transverse processes containing the foramen transversarium, through which the vertebral artery and vein and the venous plexus travel. The superior facets are formed by the lateral masses as they articulate with the occipital condyles. The inferior facets articulate with the superior facets of C-2 (the axis). The internal surface of the anterior arch articulates with the odontoid process of the axis. The axis (Fig. 1–8) has a superior protrusion, the odontoid process (dens), and a large bifid spinous process. Superior articular facets are almost entirely in the transverse plane, and the inferior facets are typically cervical. The remaining cervical vertebrae have small vertebral bodies and transverse processes that are characterized by the presence of the vertebral foramen. Upward projections from the lateral margins of C-3 to C-6 articulate with the bodies of the vertebrae above to form the joints of Luschka (uncovertebral joints) (Fig. 1–9). The plan of the articular facets of C-2 through the transitional zone of the upper thoracic area is at approximately a 45-degree angle to the transverse plane: the superior facets face superiorly and posteriorly and the inferior facets face inferiorly and anteriorly (Fig. 1–10).[12]

Ligamentous support is much better in the cervical area than in the lumbar area (Fig. 1–11). The anterior longitudinal ligament runs from the atlas to the sacrum and is narrowest in the cervical area. It attaches to the vertebral bodies and the intervertebral discs. The anterior longitudinal ligament is taut in extension, limiting this motion. The posterior longitudinal ligament runs from the axis to the sacrum and is widest in the

■■■■ **Table 1–4.** MUSCLES OF FACIAL EXPRESSION

| Facial Muscle | Origin/Insertion | Action | Innervation |
|---|---|---|---|
| Orbicularis oris | Fibers from buccinator, levator angulioris, depressor angulioris, maxilla and mandible, and nasal septum to levator angulioris, depressor angulioris, buccinator, and oral mucosa | Compresses lips (whistle) | Facial nerve—buccal branch |
| Zygomaticus | Minor: zygomatic bone to zygomaticomaxillary suture to upper lip | Protrudes upper lip | Facial nerve—buccal branch |
| | Major: zygomatic bone to zygomaticotemporal suture to angle of mouth, levator angulioris, depressor angulioris | Raises outer margins up and outward (smile) | |
| Levator angulioris | Below infraorbital foramen to angle of mouth, lygomaticus depressor angulioris, orbicularis | Lifts angles of mouth cranially | Facial nerve—buccal branch |
| Risorius | Masseter and platysma of mouth | Raises corner of mouth laterally | Facial nerve—mandibular buccal branch |
| Buccinator | Alveolar processes of maxillar mandible (along three molars) and pterygomandibular raphe to lips | Compresses cheeks | Facial nerve—buccal branch |
| Depressor angulioris | Oblique line of mandible to angle of mouth | Lowers corners of mouth and pulls out to side | Facial nerve—mandibular and buccal branch |
| Depressor labii inferioris | Oblique line of mandible to lower orbicularis oris, depressor labii inferioris (contralateral) | Protrudes lower lip down | Facial nerve—buccal branch |
| Mentalis | Incisive fossa of mandible to chin | Pulls skin over chin cranially | Facial nerve—mandibular and buccal branch |
| Platysma | Facial pectoralis minor and deltoid muscles to muscle inferior and posterior mental symphysis, mandible below oblique line and angle of mouth | Depresses mouth and its corners downward | Facial nerve—cervical branch |

Adapted from Daniels L, Worthingham C: Muscle Testing: Technique of Manual Examination. Philadelphia: WB Saunders, 1972, pp 146, 149.

cervical area. It attaches to the vertebral margins and to the intervertebral discs. The posterior longitudinal ligament is taut in flexion, limiting extremes in this motion. The supraspinous ligament runs from spinous process to spinous process, limiting flexion, and is continuous with the ligamentum nuchae. The interspinous ligaments connect adjacent spinous processes and also limit flexion. The ligamentum flavum is actually a series of short ligaments that run from lamina to lamina and are continuous with the facet joint capsules.[12,13]

There are eight cervical nerves. Cervical nerves 1 through 7 exit above the vertebrae for which they are named. The C-8 nerve exits below the C-7 vertebral body (Fig. 1–12). Therefore, a pos-

terolateral protrusion of the C5–6 intervertebral disc affects the C-6 nerve root (Fig. 1–13). The lower cervical nerves combine with the T-1 spinal nerve to form the brachial plexus, innervating the upper back and arms.[11]

# BIOMECHANICS

## Temporomandibular Joint

The mandibular head rotates in the articular fossa and depresses and protrudes to permit full mandibular opening; thus, the temporomandibu-

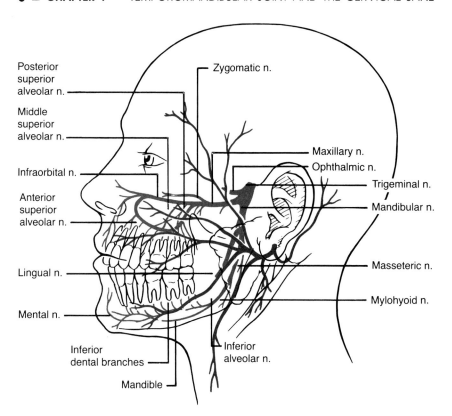

Posterior superior alveolar n.
Middle superior alveolar n.
Infraorbital n.
Anterior superior alveolar n.
Lingual n.
Mental n.
Inferior dental branches
Mandible
Zygomatic n.
Maxillary n.
Ophthalmic n.
Trigeminal n.
Mandibular n.
Masseteric n.
Mylohyoid n.
Inferior alveolar n.

**FIGURE 1–5** ■ Innervation of muscles of mastication and facial expression.

lar joint is a hinge joint with a moving axis (Fig. 1–14). The mandibular head must protrude beyond the edge of the bony articular eminence to open the mouth maximally.

The disc travels atop the mandibular head as it advances. In this position, the disc functionally flattens the point-like surface of the mandibular head and allows it to pass more easily under the eminence (Fig. 1–15). The lateral pterygoid and capsular ligaments stabilize the disc on top of the mandibular head; that is, they become taut as the mandible rotates anteriorly upon opening. This pure rotation of the disc and mandibular head occurs in the inferior joint capsule, whereas the entire movement of the disc and mandibular head beyond the fossa onto the articular eminence occurs in the superior joint capsule. This latter motion of the superior joint space is referred to as translation. If the normal position of the disc on the mandibular head is altered, this complex motion is impeded and full mandibular range of motion is limited.

Full range of motion of the temporomandibular joint is relative to the individual's stature. Researchers have identified the normal range of motion as 40 to 55 mm. Lateral deviation is one fourth of the opening range. Protrusion of the

mandible ranges from 3 to 6 mm. These ranges must be considered with respect to the patient's overbite (the extent to which the maxillary teeth overlap the mandibular teeth) and overjet (the anterior-posterior distance between the overlapping maxillary and mandibular teeth). To determine maximal opening accurately, the degree of overbite should be added to the full opening measurement and the degree of overjet should be added to the full protrusion measurement.[14]

The temporomandibular joint has two extremes of range of motion, two closed pack positions. These positions are named in relation to the end position of the mandibular head in the fossa. The soft tissue and joint capsule stop maximal opening in the anterior closed pack, and the teeth stop maximal closing in the posterior closed pack position (Fig. 1–16A and B). The region between these two extreme positions of the mandible is referred to as the "open pack" position. The soft tissue of the temporomandibular joint position is most relaxed in a specific portion of the range of open pack position known as the "freeway space." To achieve this position of relaxation, the mandible is slightly depressed and the tongue is retained on the hard palate held in

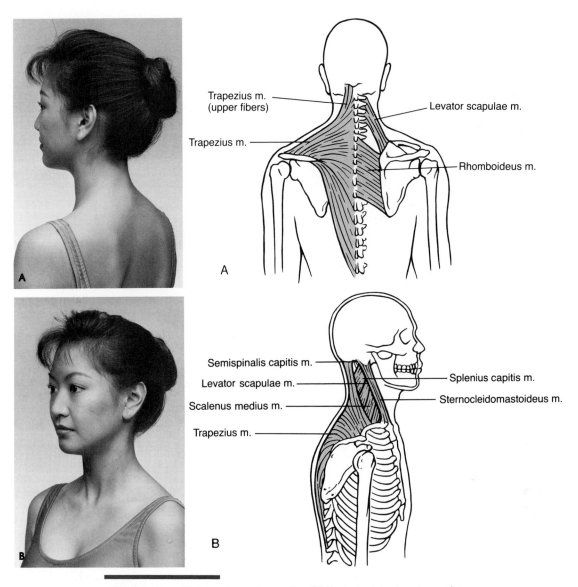

**FIGURE 1-6** ■ (A) Posterior neck muscles. (B) Posterior lateral neck muscles.

place by negative air pressure in Donder's space (Fig. 1–17). Therapists can identify this optimal position by gently placing their fourth digits with the finger pads facing anteriorly in the patient's external ear canals (Fig. 1–18). The patient is asked to close the mouth slowly until the therapist signals that the patient's mandibular heads are felt gently touching the finger pads. This should be done with great care because it is possible to push mandibular discs anteriorly with excessive force. The patient can also approach the freeway space by slowing closing the mouth so that the lips touch but the teeth do not touch.

These two ways to assume the freeway space can be closely approximated unless there is a significant malformation or a disproportionate relationship of the oral structures.

Functional mandibular range of motion differs from maximal range of motion. When the mandible is opened functionally, the muscles of mastication and ligaments are stretched to 70 to 80% of their full length. This functional range is physiologically more appropriate for the tissue because it promotes normal circulation and retains the protective mechanisms of the soft tissue. At maximal opening, the soft tissue is at

■■■■■■ **Table 1–5.** DEEP MUSCLES OF THE BACK

| Muscle | Origin | Insertion |
|---|---|---|
| Erector spinae (longitudinal group) | Series of muscles forming mass that extends from sacrum to skull. Acting unilaterally, they bend vertebral column to that side; bilaterally they extend vertebral column. They are segmentally innervated by dorsal rami of spinal nerves, as are all muscles of back listed below. | |
| Iliocostalis thoracis | Superior borders of lower seven ribs medial to angles | Angles of upper seven ribs and transverse process of seventh cervical vertebra |
| Iliocostalis cervicis | Superior borders at angles of third to seventh ribs | Transverse processes of fourth, fifth, and sixth cervical vertebra |
| Longissimus cervicis | Transverse processes of upper five or six thoracic vertebrae | Transverse processes of second through sixth cervical vertebra |
| Longissimus capitis | Transverse processes of first four cervical vertebrae and articular processes of last four cervical vertebrae | Mastoid process of temporal bone |
| Spinalis cervicis | Spines of upper two thoracic and lower two cervical vertebrae | Spines of second through fourth cervical vertebrae |

| Muscle | Origin | Insertion | Action |
|---|---|---|---|
| Semispinalis capitis | Transverse processes of upper six thoracic and seventh cervical vertebrae | Between superior and inferior nuchal lines | Extends and inclines head laterally |
| Semispinalis thoracis | Transverse processes of lower six thoracic vertebrae | Spines of upper six thoracic and lower two cervical vertebrae | Extends and inclines head laterally |
| Semispinalis cervicis | Transverse processes of upper six thoracic vertebrae | Spines of second through sixth cervical vertebrae | Extends and inclines head laterally |
| Multifidus | Sacrum and transverse processes of lumbar, thoracic, and lower cervical vertebrae | Spinous processes of lumbar, thoracic, and lower cervical vertebrae | Abducts, rotates, and extends vertebral column |
| Rotatores | Transverse processes of second cervical vertebra to sacrum | Lamina above vertebra of origin | Rotate and extend vertebral column |
| Interspinales | Superior surface of spine of each vertebra | Inferior surface of spine of vertebra above vertebra of origin | Extend and rotate vertebral column |
| Intertransversarii | Extend between transverse processes of cervical, lumbar, and lower thoracic vertebrae. Unilaterally, they bend vertebral column laterally; bilaterally they stabilize column. | | |
| Splenius cervicis | Spinous processes of third through sixth thoracic vertebrae | Transverse process of first three cervical vertebrae | Inclines and rotates head and neck |
| Splenius capitis | Ligamentum nuchae and spinous processes of upper five thoracic vertebrae | Mastoid process and superior nuchal line | Inclines and rotates head and neck |

Christensen JB, Telford IR: Synopsis of Gross Anatomy. Philadelphia: JB Lippincott, 1988.

100% of its full length and more prone to dysfunction.

## Cervical Joints

The upper cervical joints are the occipitoatloid and atlantoaxial joints. They function as a composite craniovertebral articulation, with the atlas acting essentially as a washer so that the occiput conforms better to the axis. In flexion and extension, the occiput rolls on the atlas-axis complex. There is approximately 10 to 15 degrees of both flexion and extension at this level. Occipitoatloid lateral bending is less than 10 degrees in each direction, and no rotation occurs at the occipitoatloid joint (Fig. 1–19). At the atlantoaxial joint, flexion and extension are about 10 degrees and there is no lateral bending. However, most cervical rotation occurs at the atlantoaxial joint

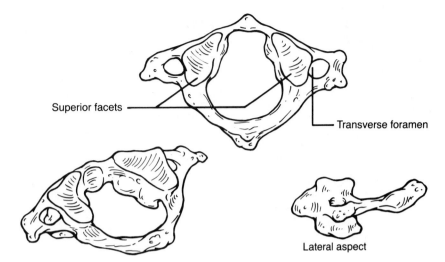

**FIGURE 1-7** ■ Atlas C-1.

with approximately 50 degrees of rotation in each direction (Fig. 1-20). This motion is checked by the alar ligament.[13,15,16]

The joints below C-2 function as concave on convex articulations. The superior facets roll and glide in a superior and anterior direction during flexion and roll and glide in an inferior and posterior direction during extension. Most cervical flexion and extension occur in the lower cervical spine (between C-4 and C-6) and the motion is about 100 degrees. Total range of motion of lateral bending is 30 degrees to each side and of rotation is 20 degrees to each side. However, cervical rotation and lateral bending are conjugate motions, always occurring together. In the cervical spine, rotation to one side is always accompanied by lateral bending to the same side.

(Note: Rotation is described with respect to the direction of movement of the vertebral body, but during examination one is most often looking at the spinous process, which moves in the opposite direction) (Fig. 1-21).[13,15,16]

## EVALUATION

When therapists can recognize the normal anatomy and kinematics of the joint structures, they can evaluate this region objectively. Evaluation of this joint, as with other regions of the body, begins subjectively and progresses to an objective evaluation consisting of observation, palpation, range of motion, muscle test, and functional analysis.

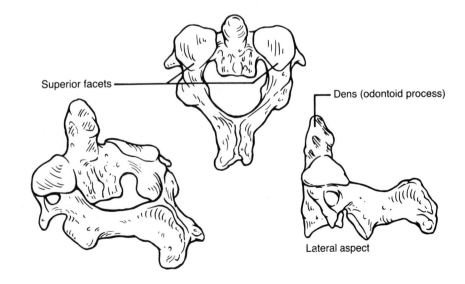

**FIGURE 1-8** ■ Axis C-2.

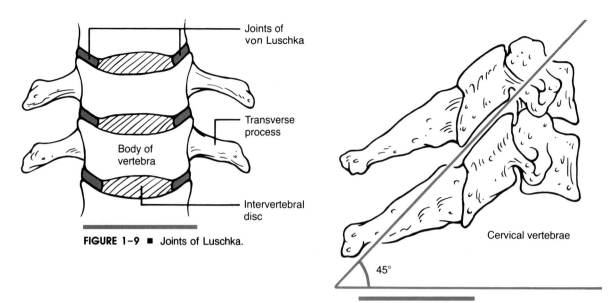

**FIGURE 1–9 ■** Joints of Luschka.

**FIGURE 1–10 ■** Plane of articular facets of C-2.

## Subjective Evaluation of the Temporomandibular Joint

In the subjective evaluation, questions are asked initially to determine the patient's predysfunctional state, onset of the pain and dysfunction, contributing factors or possible etiology, and factors that make the pain and dysfunction better or worse. What previous medical, dental, or physical therapy interventions have been effective? The patient's general stress levels, coping mechanisms, and psychosocial status should also be recorded.

The patient's attitude toward the dysfunction and expectation of the therapy protocol influence the therapist's ability to evaluate effectively, diagnose differentially, and treat appropriately. Thus, the therapist must also determine these attitudinal factors in the subjective evaluation.

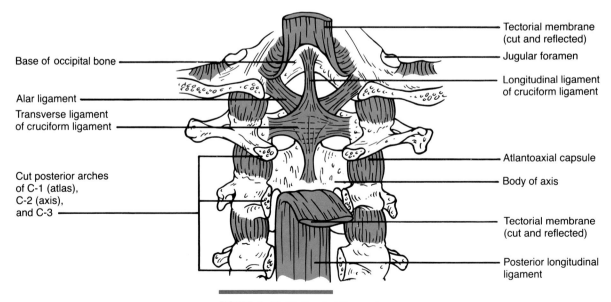

**FIGURE 1–11 ■** Cervical ligaments.

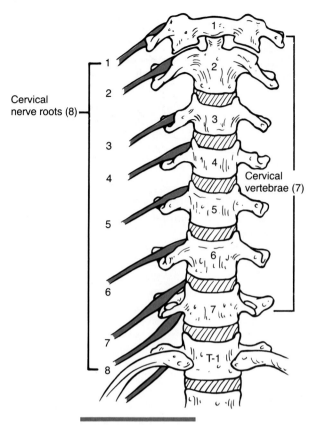

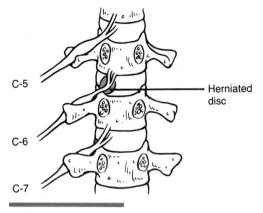

FIGURE 1-13 ■ Posterior lateral protrusion of C5-6.

FIGURE 1-12 ■ Cervical nerves.

The sample questions from the patient's questionnaire on page 17 can be used to conduct a subjective evaluation. This sample can be altered to reflect the practitioner's clinical experience or the characteristics of a population of patients.

The therapist can ask the patient, "What would your life be like if I were able to take away all of your pain tomorrow?" Patients who respond unrealistically by stating that they would be "beautiful, well-liked, rich, and happy" may not be dealing with their physical condition in an

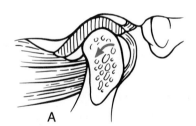

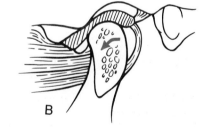

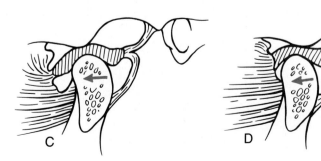

FIGURE 1-14 ■ Temporomandibular joint—a moving hinge joint.

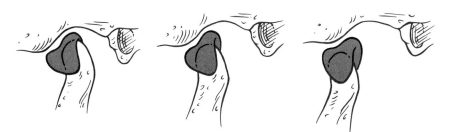

FIGURE 1–15 ■ Disc atop mandibular head.

appropriate manner. They may have "become" their pain and, despite all possible effective measures, may be consciously or unconsciously reluctant to give up their pain and dysfunction. Patients who state that, without pain, their life would be very different and admit that they would have to learn to return to full function and take their social place in the home and community, have a more appropriate reaction to their physical problem, and they should respond to therapeutic intervention more favorably.

Another component of the subjective evaluation is the Holmes and Rahe Schedule of Life Events.[17] This modified questionnaire enables patients to identify their major stressors of the past 12 months and potential stressors of the next 12 months. See Life Event Scale. In discussion, the therapist can help the patient deal with current and future sources of stress, discuss coping skills, and learn relaxation techniques. The therapist may choose to refer to a mental health practitioner those patients who have become so-

cially dysfunctional or are overwhelmed by their psychological state. Specific scales have been developed for college students, children, and other individuals.

A multidimensional approach to nominal pain scales was developed by Edeling.[18] This system is effective in determining the patient's response or lack of response to treatment procedures.

These nominal scales (periodicity, intensity, and response to analgesics), body charts, pain qualities or characteristics, precipitating and aggravating factors, and associated or concomitant systems yield a comprehensive picture of the patient's pain (see Total Pain Pattern). Although these findings cannot be analyzed statistically, they do provide an objective description of patients and nominal statistical scales that can be used to compare the same patients to themselves over time. Thus, these factors can be used to determine the patient's response or lack of response to the applied treatment protocol.

It is also important to identify the patient's

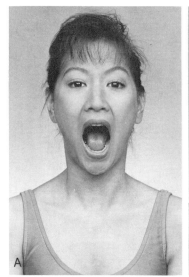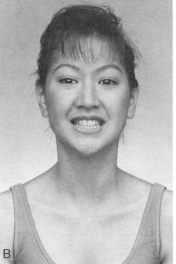

FIGURE 1–16 ■ Closed pack positions. (A) Anterior. (B) Posterior.

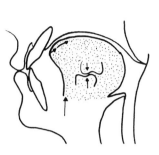

**FIGURE 1-17** ■ Donder's space. (From Rocabado M, Iglarsh ZA: Musculoskeletal Approach to Maxillofacial Pain. Philadelphia: JB Lippincott, 1992, p 58.)

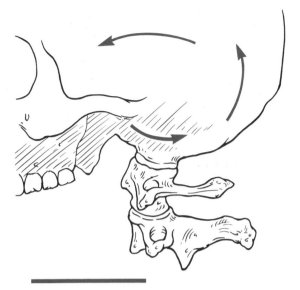

**FIGURE 1-19** ■ Motions at the occipitoatloid joint.

prior and current medical, dental, and physical therapy practitioners and, with the patient's written permission, request prior evaluation and laboratory findings. This information may help the practitioner to develop a more accurate differential diagnosis and design an effective treatment protocol with objective goals.

## Subjective Evaluation of the Cervical Structures

The history plays a critical role in the development of a hypothesis about why a patient has neck dysfunction. In addition to providing information about when the problem started and whether there was precipitating trauma, the history indicates the patient's functional limitations and the nature of symptoms. Clearly, it is important to obtain information about medical management of the patient's problem, medications, other treatment regimens, and radiographic

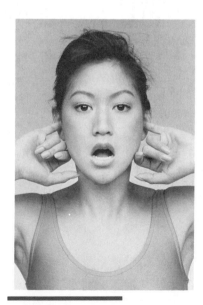

**FIGURE 1-18** ■ Freeway space palpation.

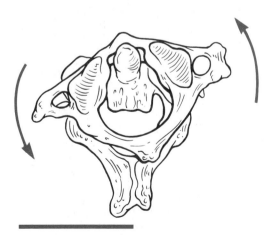

**FIGURE 1-20** ■ Motions at the atlantoaxial joint.

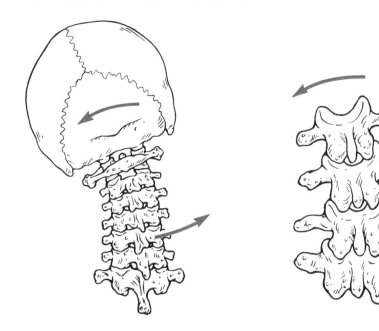

**FIGURE 1-21 ■** Vertebral body rotation.

findings. However, as stated previously, radiographic changes do not necessarily correlate with symptoms.

The therapist should ask the patient to describe the symptoms (pain, paresthesia, numbness, weakness, immobility) and their location (neck, shoulder, head, arm, forearm, hand). The symptoms may be constant, intermittent, or variable. The patient should state what improves or worsens the symptoms (position, activity, time of day). If pain is a major symptom, some attempt must be made to quantify the pain symptoms by using a pain rating scale. The most common type of rating scale is a visual analog scale (Fig. 1–22) on which the patient indicates the severity of present pain by drawing a line.

At this point, the patient's problem has been described and tentative functional goals should be agreed on by the patient and the therapist. Although the goals may be modified after the physical examination or during the course of treatment, it is important to establish them as early in the examination process as possible so that the therapist and patient are working toward the same objectives.[19]

A thorough history helps to direct the focus of the physical examination. If weakness and immobility are not symptoms, then strength testing and assessment of joint motion can take the form of screening examinations rather than being a highlight of the physical examination. The history is used to decide where to begin and to direct the progression of the physical examination.

## Objective Evaluation of the Temporomandibular Joint

### Observation

The objective evaluation begins as the practitioner observes the patient's sitting posture in the waiting room, how the patient rises up from the chair, the patient's gait pattern while walking to the treatment room, and the patient's sitting posture during the subjective interview.

**Postural Relationships.** The postural relationship of the mandible to the face, the head to the neck, and the neck to the entire axial skeleton should be analyzed.

■ The practitioner begins by analyzing the mandible's position relative to facial structures as the patient maintains the mouth in relaxed closure and relaxed full opening.
■ In both positions, how is the chin lined up vertically with the nares, the skin folds descending from the nostrils to the upper lip?
■ Did the mandible deviate as the patient opened and closed the mouth?
■ Is the head laterally shifted to one side or tilted?
■ Is the anatomic line created by the spinous processes in the posterior cervical spine in alignment?
■ Are the diagonal muscle bellies of the sternocleidomastoid muscles and the horizontal lines of the clavicles symmetric?

# SAMPLE SUBJECTIVE QUESTIONS

## Dysfunction / Pain

1. Describe your pain or dysfunction.
2. When did it begin?
3. Do you know what caused it to start?
4. How has it changed since its original occurrence?
5. What makes it better or worse?
6. Is the pain / dysfunction better in morning or at end of day?
7. How are you sleeping?
8. How do you feel upon rising in the morning?
9. Does activity make your problem better or worse?
10. Does rest make your pain better or worse?

## History

1. Does anyone in your family have similar problems?
2. Were you bottle or breast fed? How long?
3. Did you suck a pacifier or finger(s)? How long?
4. Have you had any blows to the face? When?
5. Have you had any falls onto the face? When?
6. Have you been involved in an auto accident?
7. How is your health in general?
8. Do you experience headaches? Where? How often?

## Social History

1. What is your family composition?
2. What are your major life stressors?
3. How do you cope with your stress?

## Activities of Daily Living History

1. Do you function independently?
2. Do you have difficulty chewing?
3. Do you have difficulty swallowing?
4. Do you have difficulty talking?
5. Are you employed in or out of the home?
6. What are the typical postures of your job?
7. What are the physical demands of your job?
8. What are the typical postures of your recreational activity?

## Treatment History

1. Have you been treated by other practitioners for this problem?
2. List all former and current medical and dental practitioners.
3. Which of their treatments appeared to help? Which did not?
4. Have you had extensive dental treatments?
5. Have you been hospitalized in the past 5 years?
6. Do you wear dentures? Full or partial?
7. Do you have missing teeth?
8. Have you worn braces? When?

# LIFE EVENT SCALE

NAME: _____    DATE: _____

If any of the events listed below have happened to you within the last 12 months, check in the column headed "PAST." If you anticipate that the event will happen to you in the next 12 months, check the box in the column headed "FUTURE."

| PAST | FUTURE | |
|------|--------|---|
| ____ | ____ | Death of spouse |
| ____ | ____ | Divorce |
| ____ | ____ | Marital separation |
| ____ | ____ | Jail term |
| ____ | ____ | Death of close family member |
| ____ | ____ | Personal injury or illness |
| ____ | ____ | Marriage |
| ____ | ____ | Fired from work |
| ____ | ____ | Marital reconciliation |
| ____ | ____ | Retirement |
| ____ | ____ | Change in family member's health |
| ____ | ____ | Pregnancy |
| ____ | ____ | Sex difficulties |
| ____ | ____ | Addition to family |
| ____ | ____ | Business readjustment |
| ____ | ____ | Change in financial status |
| ____ | ____ | Death of close friend |
| ____ | ____ | Change to different line of work |
| ____ | ____ | Change in number of marital arguments |
| ____ | ____ | Mortgage or loan over $10,000 |
| ____ | ____ | Foreclosure of mortgage or loan |
| ____ | ____ | Change in work responsibilities |
| ____ | ____ | Son or daughter leaving home |
| ____ | ____ | Trouble with in-laws |
| ____ | ____ | Outstanding personal achievement |
| ____ | ____ | Spouse begins or stops work |
| ____ | ____ | Starting or finishing school |
| ____ | ____ | Change in living conditions |
| ____ | ____ | Revision of personal habits |
| ____ | ____ | Trouble with boss |
| ____ | ____ | Change in work hours, conditions |
| ____ | ____ | Change in residence |
| ____ | ____ | Change in schools |
| ____ | ____ | Change in recreational habits |
| ____ | ____ | Change in church activities |
| ____ | ____ | Change in social activities |
| ____ | ____ | Mortgage or loan under $10,000 |
| ____ | ____ | Change in sleeping habits |
| ____ | ____ | Change in number of family gatherings |
| ____ | ____ | Change in eating habits |
| ____ | ____ | Vacation |
| ____ | ____ | Christmas season |
| ____ | ____ | Minor violation of the law |

# TOTAL PAIN PATTERN

## Distribution

- Patient marks a body chart.
- Patient points to pain on the patient's body.
- Therapist presses the area indicated by patient to verify painful areas and possibly reproduce pain radiation.

## Nature

- Pain quality or characteristics.
- May use pain characteristics listed in McGill Pain Questionnaire.

## Periodicity

- P1—pain on 1 day or less per month
- P2—pain on 2 or more days per month
- P3—pain on 1 or more days per week
- P4—daily but intermittent pain
- P5—continuous pain

## Intensity A

- I1—mild
- I2—more than mild but still tolerable
- I3—moderately severe
- I4—severe
- I5—intolerable, suicide inducing (worst pain patient has ever felt)

## Intensity B

- Unmarked—10-cm line that has 0 at one end and 10 at the other, the patient marks the level of pain.

## Response to Analgesics

- R1—pain decreases easily with small doses of a simple analgesic.
- R2—pain is decreased but does not disappear with a simple analgesic.
- R3—pain is completely relieved by a compound analgesic.
- R4—pain is decreased but does not disappear with a compound analgesic.
- R5—no dose of any analgesic has any effect on the pain.

## Precipitating and Aggravating Factors

- Environmental factors—temperature, air pollutants
- Emotional stress
- Diet—caffeine, chocolate, preservatives, refined sugar, and so forth
- Posture—forward head and rounded shoulders

## Associated or Concomitant Symptoms

- Ear pain, dulled hearing, or tinnitus
- Headaches
- Visual disturbances
- Dizziness or nausea

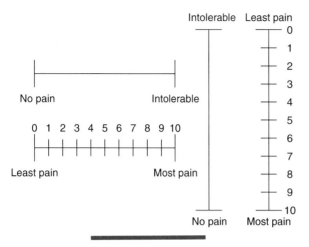

**FIGURE 1–22** ■ Pain scales.

**Structural Relationships of the Face.** Look at the structural relationships of the face (Fig. 1–23).

■ Does the right side of the face look like the left?
■ Are the eyebrows, eye pupils, ear tragus, nostrils, and corners of the mouth symmetric?
■ Does the nasal bone line up with the nares?
■ Is the upper lip frenulum aligned with the lower lip frenulum?
■ What is the relationship between the maxillary and mandibular teeth?

■ How is the chin aligned with the other midline structures?

Developmentally, the structures evolve in a proportional relationship. The top line of the frontal crease (hairline) and the nasal bone constitute the upper third of the face, the nasal bone to inferior nose constitutes the middle third, and the inferior nose to chin constitutes the lower third (Fig. 1–24). Some of these relationships are determined genetically; others are responses to the physical environment. If the tongue is not maintained on the hard palate, the palate develops with a high-domed contour and the maxilla may not expand to accommodate the full width of the tongue. If the tongue remains on the floor during development, the lower third of the face may be elongated and the mandible may become wider than the maxilla. Thus, the analysis of proportions of the face may direct the therapist to further examination of specific structures of the face.

The patient's tongue should be examined for bite marks or scalloping on the edges (Fig. 1–25). Scalloping may indicate that the patient is biting the tongue or that the tongue rests between the teeth to prevent the teeth from touching. In these cases, the tongue is too wide or is not resting on the hard palate. If the tongue is between the teeth or in the floor of the mouth, it increases the weight that must be overcome by the muscles of mastication to permit the lips to approximate. A dry or white tongue may indicate

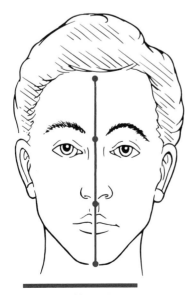

**FIGURE 1–23** ■ Facial symmetry.

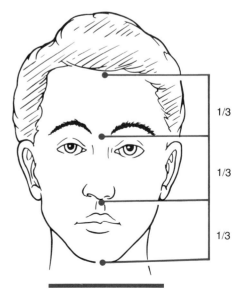

**FIGURE 1–24** ■ Facial thirds.

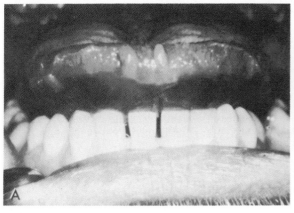 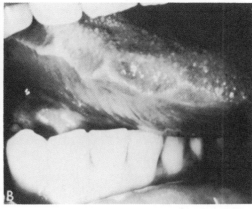

FIGURE 1-25 ■ Scalloped tongue. (From Langlais RP: Oral Diagnosis, Oral Medicine, and Treatment Planning. Philadelphia: WB Saunders, 1984, Figure 14-27.)

a medication reaction, salivary gland dysfunction, or oral yeast or bacterial infection.

Tongue thrusting should also be evaluated. Touching the lips during this phase of the examination alters swallowing. Therefore, the practitioner cannot open the lips to determine tongue thrusting. Patients are asked to bring their head onto their neck in a well-balanced head-retracted posture and attempt to swallow a glass of water. A person who tongue thrusts can do this only if the head is allowed to protrude. This is a simple method for grossly determining tongue thrust. Tongue thrusting, if present, should be documented and tongue function can be retrained in treatment.

Before completing the observation portion of the evaluation, the practitioner should summarize the observation findings. That is, which are the normal and abnormal structural or functional relationships? These determinations in combination with palpation findings guide the practitioner in the measurement phase of the evaluation.

## Palpation

If the practitioner palpates the axial skeletal structures first, the patient is less intimidated than if the practitioner begins by palpating the tender muscles of mastication. Gentle touch progressing to deep pressure helps the patient to relax during this phase of the examination.

Begin the facial palpation at the site of primary pain, because it is this pain that motivated the patient to seek care. Proceeding to anterior and then posterior structures, record tenderness to palpation on a 10-point pain scale. Muscle bulk, trigger points, tight fibrous bands, swelling, and surface contour should be recorded.

Care should be taken in palpating the muscles of mastication because they are often tender in patients with facial pain. Even light touch can produce significant irritation if the muscles of mastication are in spasm. These muscles are palpated to determine muscle bulk and the patient's response to light pressure and to compare them to the uninvolved or less involved contralateral side. Table 1-6 and accompanying figures will assist the therapist in palpating the muscles of mastication (Figures 1-26 through 1-32).

When palpating in the superior vestibule for the pterygoid muscle, the practitioner is actually palpating both the medial and lateral pterygoid muscles according to Tanaka.[20] If this area is tender, the practitioner cannot differentiate between the two groups. However, if the medial pterygoid in the angle of the mandible is not tender, one can deduce that the pain produced by superior palpation was caused by the lateral pterygoid. If the inferior palpation is also painful, the practitioner cannot implicate one muscle group (see Evaluating Medial or Lateral Pterygoid Muscles chart).

## Range of Motion

Mandibular depression, protrusion, and lateral deviation should be measured in the initial evaluation and, if dysfunctional, measured again before and after each treatment session as an objective evaluation of progress. A Boley gauge, (Fig. 1-33), triangle, or ruler (Fig. 1-34) can be

**Table 1-6.** PALPATION OF MUSCLES OF MASTICATION

| Muscle | Area of Palpation | Resisted Action to Promote Muscle Contraction |
|---|---|---|
| Temporalis (Fig. 1–26) | Temporal fossa and insertion at coronoid process as it glides out from under the zygomatic arch upon opening | Mandibular closing |
| Lateral and medial pterygoid (Fig. 1–27) | Along exterior posterior maxillary vestibule and superiorly into the inferior temporal fossa | Contralateral lateral deviation with some protrusion |

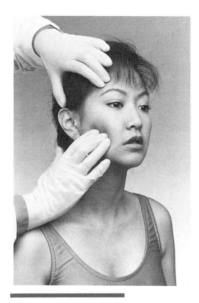

**FIGURE 1–26** ■ Palpation of temporalis muscle.

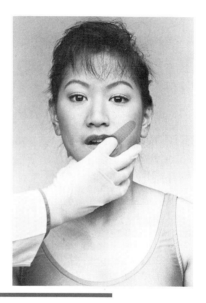

**FIGURE 1–27** ■ Palpation of medial and lateral pterygoid muscles.

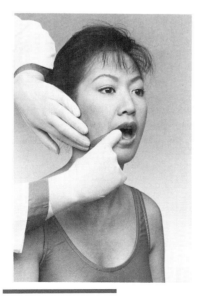

**FIGURE 1–28** ■ Palpation of medial pterygoid muscle.

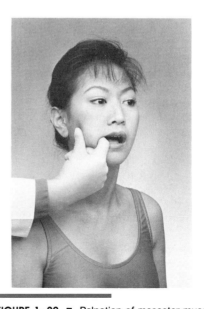

**FIGURE 1–29** ■ Palpation of masseter muscle.

**Table 1-6.** PALPATION OF MUSCLES OF MASTICATION *Continued*

| Muscle | Area of Palpation | Resisted Action to Promote Muscle Contraction |
|---|---|---|
| Medial pterygoid (Fig. 1–28) | Inside the mandible at its angle under the tongue | Contralateral lateral deviation and mandibular closing |
| Masseter (Fig. 1–29) | Posterior muscle belly of the cheek | Mandibular closing |
| Suprahyoid muscles, superior hyoid bone (Fig. 1–30) | Floor of the mouth, above the hyoid bone | Stabilize hyoid and resist mandibular depression |
| Inrahyoid muscles, inferior hyoid bone (Fig. 1–31) | Hyoid bone to the sternal notch | Elevate hyoid bone manually |

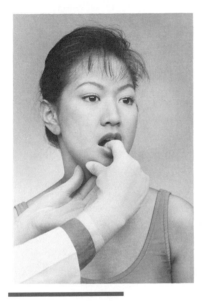

**FIGURE 1-30** ■ Palpation of suprahyoid muscle.

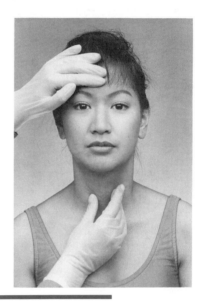

**FIGURE 1-31** ■ Palpation of infrahyoid muscles.

used to measure the range of the temporomandibular joint in millimeters.

Mandibular opening is measured between the two maxillary and mandibular incisor teeth with the device placed vertically. Lateral deviation is measured by selecting a zero point on the ruler placed between the maxillary incisors and measuring the deviation left and right of the mandible by using the center of the mandibular incisors as a guide. Lateral deviation in each direction should be approximately one fourth of opening (Fig. 1–35) Protrusion is measured as the distance through which the lower teeth can move horizontally past the maxillary teeth.

Two additional measurements may be made by referring dentists: overbite and overjet. Overbite, the degree to which the anterior maxillary teeth cover the mandibular teeth when the mouth is fully closed, is usually 2 to 3 mm. It is measured by marking the level at which the upper teeth cover the lower teeth and measuring this distance from the tip of the tooth to the line when the mouth is open (Fig. 1–36A). Overjet, normally 2 to 3 mm, is the distance that the maxillary teeth close over the mandibular and is measured as shown in Figure. 1–36B.

## Muscle Strength Testing

When testing the strength of the muscles of mastication, the practitioner attempts to determine whether the resisted motion is weak or strong and whether it produces pain. All muscles, with the exception of the orbicularis oris, can be tested and compared with the contralateral muscles.

Muscles of mastication are tested by resisting their motions and recording comparative strength

# EVALUATING MEDIAL OR LATERAL PTERYGOID MUSCLES

| PAIN UPON PALPATION | MUSCLE SPASM INDICATED |
| --- | --- |
| Superior palpation painful | Medial or lateral pterygoid |
| Superior palpation painful but not inferior palpation | Lateral pterygoid only |
| Superior and inferior palpation | Medial or lateral pterygoid |

# STRUCTURES TO BE PALPATED IN AN UPPER QUADRANT OBJECTIVE EVALUATION

## *Muscles*

- Longus colli (Fig. 1–32)
- Sternocleidomastoid
- Scaleni
- Pectoralis major and minor
- Small neck extensors

## *Joints*

- Sternoclavicular
- Acromioclavicular

## *Vertebrae*

- Cervical 1 (transverse processes)
- Cervical 2 (transverse and spinous processes)
- Cervical 3 (transverse and spinous processes)

## *Clavicles*

- Should be horizontal

FIGURE 1–32 ■ Palpation of longus colli muscle.

## *Breathing Patterns*

- Sternum protrusion and elevation during inspiration normal
- An apical breathing pattern abnormal

## *Swallowing Patterns*

- Tongue thrust
- Hyoid bone elevation/depression and slight elevation to rest at level of C-3

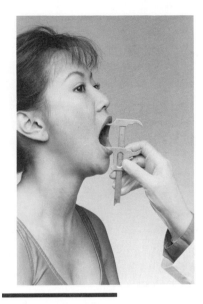

**FIGURE 1–33** ■ Boley gauge measurement.

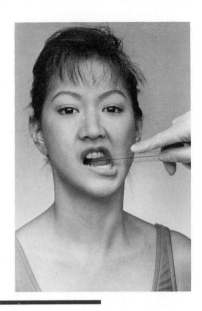

**FIGURE 1–35** ■ Measurement of lateral deviation.

and pain levels (Fig. 1–37A–E). The muscles of facial expression are tested by asking the person to attempt the specific facial expression attributed to each muscle. When testing the muscles of facial expression, with the exception of the orbicularis oris and buccinator muscles, symmetry in action may be evaluated rather than the muscle's ability to overcome applied resistance (Fig. 1–38).

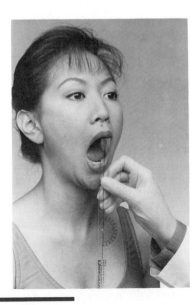

**FIGURE 1–34** ■ Ruler measurement of mandibular depression.

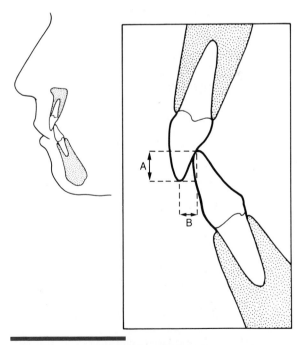

**FIGURE 1–36** ■ (A) Overbite. (B) Overjet. (From Friedman MH, Weisberg J: The temporomandibular joint. *In* Orthopedics and Sports Physical Therapy. [Gould JA III, ed], p 578. St Louis: Mosby, 1990.)

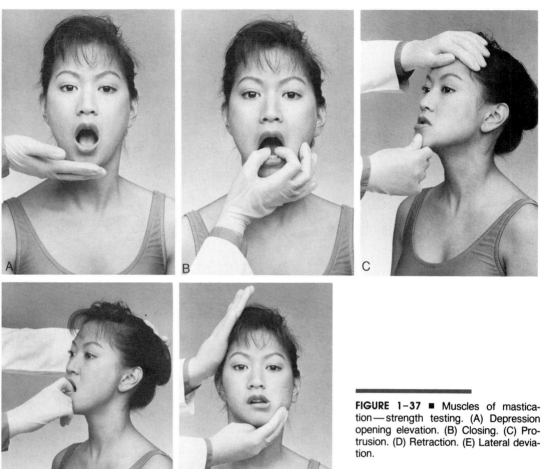

**FIGURE 1–37** ■ Muscles of mastication—strength testing. (A) Depression opening elevation. (B) Closing. (C) Protrusion. (D) Retraction. (E) Lateral deviation.

The orbicularis oris superficial fibers are tested as the patient's lips are wrapped around the practitioner's fingers. The practitioner attempts to expand the fingers laterally. The practitioner should feel the same degree of resistance bilaterally and the resisted action should not produce pain (Fig. 1–39). The deeper fibers of this muscle are tested as the patient billows air into the cheeks and the practitioner attempts to push the air out of the patient's cheeks. Whether or not the patient can keep air in the cheeks is not the focus of the test; rather, the shape of the lips resisting the escaping air is significant. If the patient can resist the loss of air by maintaining the lips in a straight line without discomfort, the deep fibers of the orbicularis oris have normal strength and function. However, a patient who resists the air loss with pursed, puckered lips has weak deep fibers and is using the superficial fibers to substitute (Fig. 1–40).

The buccinator (Fig. 1–41) is tested as the practitioner places a finger in the vestibule between the cheek and the maxilla. After the patient contracts the buccinator to hold the practitioner's finger along the patient's maxillary teeth, the practitioner attempts to pull the finger laterally. The practitioner should not be able to move the finger from the patient's maxillary teeth. This action should not be painful.

All test actions, resisted motions, and attempted facial expressions are also used as exercises to rehabilitate muscles with identified

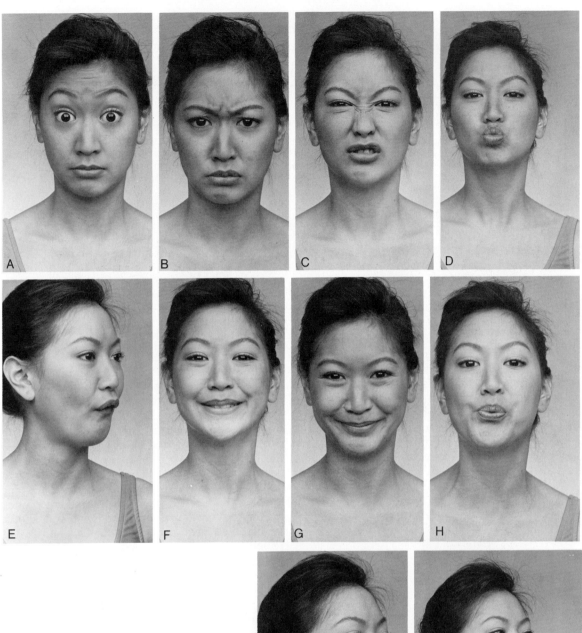

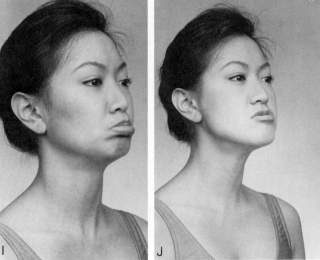

**FIGURE 1-38** ■ Muscles of facial expression. (A) Frontalis. (B) Corrugator supercilii. (C) Procerus. (D) Orbicularis oris. (E) Zygomaticus minor. (F) Zygomaticus major. (G) Risorius. (H) Buccinator. (I) Depressor labii inferioris. (J) Platysma.

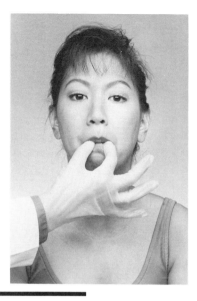

**FIGURE 1-39** ■ Testing orbicularis oris internal fibers.

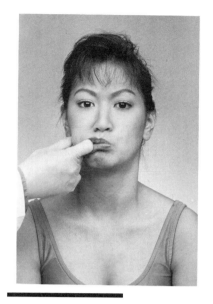

**FIGURE 1-41** ■ Testing buccinator muscle.

weakness. Patients are instructed to repeat the test procedures at home to strengthen weakened muscles. Thus, they can easily see how the action identified the weakness and the familiar action can be repeated to promote strengthening.

It is important that the internal (tongue) and external (lips) forces of the face must be kept in balance to avoid excessive forces on the teeth. If the upper lip is shortened, the lower lip must

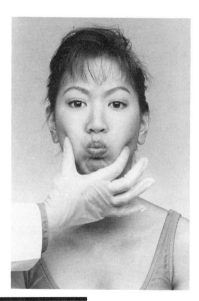

**FIGURE 1-40** ■ Testing orbicularis oris external fibers.

elevate forcibly to close the lips. This excessive closure increases the external forces on the teeth. The length of the upper lip can be evaluated by observing the extent to which it covers the maxillary teeth. The lip should cover two thirds of the upper teeth at rest. If it does not, it is considered short. However, if the patient can draw the lip actively over the upper teeth so that the dark line around the lip or vermilion border is not visible, the lip is considered functional and does not require treatment. If the patient cannot, the lip is considered nonfunctional and should be stretched as shown in Fig. 1-42A and B. The patient should be evaluated after orthodontic or orthgnathic procedures have been completed because these procedures affect lip length.

The strength of the muscles acting on the tongue can also be tested. The practitioner resists the tongue in lateral deviation, protrusion, retraction, and elevation. As with the muscles of mastication, these test positions are used as exercise activities for muscles of determined weakness (Figs. 1-43 to 1-46).

Upper extremity muscle strength should also be evaluated because temporomandibular joint dysfunction is often an upper quadrant problem. Cervical spine, range of motion, and head or neck posture should be evaluated using objective parameters.

Attempts should be made to identify symptoms in the soft tissue of the head and neck and then attempt to differentiate the symptoms and

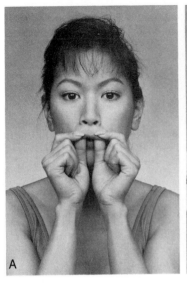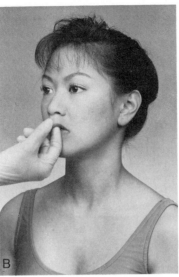

FIGURE 1–42 ■ (A) Self-lip stretch. (B) Passive lip stretch.

develop a differential diagnosis. An effective treatment plan for each of the differentiated diagnoses can then be formulated. The comprehensive evaluation forms outline a subsequent objective approach to evaluating the patient with temporomandibular joint pain (see samples provided on pages 36 through 38.

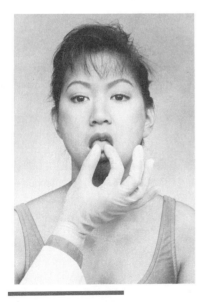

FIGURE 1–43 ■ Testing tongue protrusion.

## Objective Evaluation of the Cervical Spine

### Observation

The first step in any physical examination is to observe the patient. Head position during standing, walking, and sitting; stiffness or awkward postures; and painful facial responses should be observed early in the patient-therapist interaction. More formally, observation should include inspection of the patient's sitting and standing postures (Fig. 1–47A and B). The entire spine should be examined, even if complaints are regional. (A forward head can often be totally corrected by correcting a lumbar kyphosis) (Fig. 1–48A and B). The anterior-posterior spinal curves, pelvic position, and lateral curves should be identified. Any obvious deformity or scar should be noted.[21,22]

### Palpation

Areas to be palpated are also determined from the patient's history. Common bone landmarks that are palpated during physical examination of the neck include the following:

The mastoid processes (temporal bone)
Superior nuchal lines (occipital bone)
Occipital protuberance
The C-1 transverse processes

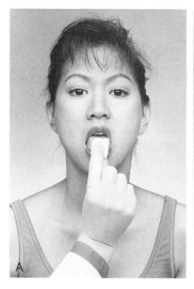
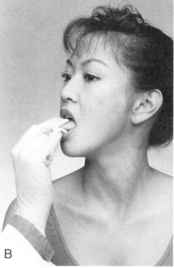

FIGURE 1–44 ■ Testing tongue retraction.

The C-2 spinous process
The transverse and spinous processes of C-3 to C-6 and the C-7 and T-1 spinous processes (Fig. 1–49)

Soft tissue palpation may include the following (Fig. 1–50A and B):

Sternocleidomastoid muscle
Neck extensors
Trapezius muscle
Rhomboid muscle
Levator muscle of scapulae and scalene muscle

These areas are palpated to evoke systems and/or to serve as landmarks for measurements.[22,23]

### Range of Motion

It is often helpful to begin the examination of joint motion by having the patient perform motions actively, holding the neck in neutral or slight axial extension. This allows the therapist to observe the patient's willingness and ability to move the neck. If motion is limited and/or symptoms are evoked by an active motion, the motion is tested passively and end feel is as-

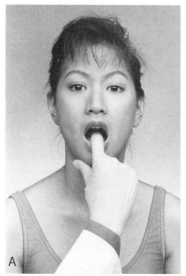
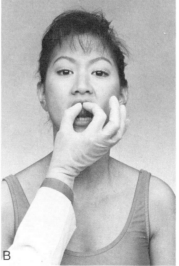

FIGURE 1–45 ■ Testing tongue elevation.

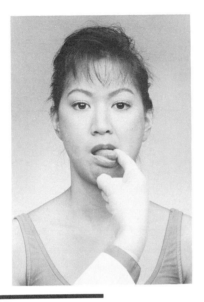

FIGURE 1–46 ■ Testing tongue lateral deviation.

sessed using overpressure. (The therapist applies a force to the patient's end range at the point where the patient's active range of motion stops). The occipitoatloid joint is assessed actively by having the patient nod the head and passively by moving the neck into forward and backward bending (Fig. 1–51). The atlantoaxial joint is assessed actively by having the patient rotate the neck and passively by superimposing rotation to one side on full contralateral lateral bending (Fig. 1–52). Mid- to lower cervical and upper thoracic

motion is assessed actively by having the patient sequentially nod, laterally bend, and rotate the neck and passively using the same motions. Limited motion should be measured using a goniometer or inclinometer (Fig. 1–53). Abnormal end feels should be noted.[23]

When motion is limited and end feel can be assessed, accessory motion (joint play) testing should follow joint motion measurements. Tests of the entire cervical spine include distraction (Fig. 1–54), compression (Fig. 1–55) and side glide (Fig. 1–56). Motion at individual spinal segments can be assessed using passive intervertebral motion techniques. The patient's neck is flexed passively and motion is palpated as it occurs at C-3 through T-3. The spinous processes should move sequentially and symmetrically upward as the neck is flexed. Anterior glides of one vertebra on another and rotation of one vertebra on another are also assessed (Fig. 1–57A). Accessory motions are graded as hypermobile, normal, and hypomobile. Usually, the presence of pain with accessory motion testing is also noted and may indicate an acute injury or inflammation (Fig. 1–57B and C).

When symptoms are evoked with joint motion or when they radiate, certain movement tests can be used to help determine which remedial exercises and neck positions might be helpful in managing them. The patient's responses are categorized in one of five ways: the symptoms are worsened or improved; there is a transient increase or decrease in symptoms; the movement

*Text continued on page 38*

FIGURE 1–47 ■ (A) Sitting posture. (B) Standing posture.

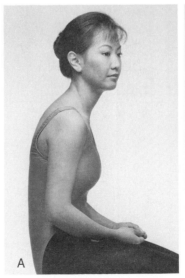
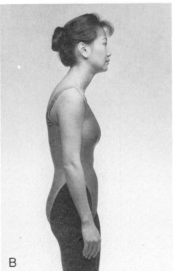

# INFORMATION FORM FOR PATIENTS WITH UPPER QUARTER DYSFUNCTION

Name _____ Today's Date _____

Birth Date _____ Age _____

Sex _____ Height _____ Weight _____

General Health Prior to the Onset of Your Current Medical Problem

_____

_____

_____

General Dental History Prior to Onset of Your Current Pain

_____

_____

_____

Do You Have Dentures? _____ Full or Partial? _____

Chief Complaint (reason for seeking medical care)

_____

_____

Pain Distribution (please shade in areas of pain and place an "X" over a(n) area(s) of specific pain)

When you experience your chief/major pain, are you aware of any other symptoms which occur with or after the beginning of your major pain? _____
_____
_____

When did your major pain begin? _____

Was there a specific reason or action that caused your pain to start? _____
_____

Do other members of your family suffer from a similar problem? _____
_____

Have you ever received previous medical care, dental treatment, or physical therapy care for this problem? _____

If so, where?
Practitioner's Name _____   Practitioner's Name _____
Address _____   Address _____
Treatment Received _____   Treatment _____
_____

Practitioner's Name _____   Practitioner's Name _____
Address _____   Address _____
Treatment Received _____   Treatment _____
_____

Are you aware of any factors that start your pain or make your pain worse? _____
_____

Are you aware of any factors that make your pain better or stop your pain? _____
_____

How does rest affect your pain? _____

How does activity affect your pain? _____

Is your pain better in the morning or at night? _____

Is your pain different when sitting or standing? _____

Have you had this pain before? _____   If so, what did you do for it? _____
_____

Do you have trouble sleeping? _____

How do you feel upon rising in the morning? _____

Do you suffer from any of the following symptoms?

Change in vision ———

Change in hearing ———

Change in balance (do you feel dizzy) ———

Headaches ———

Does your pain change when you:    yawn    ———

cough    ———

sneeze    ———

swallow    ———

What treatments do you apply at home which may relieve your symptoms? ———
———————————————————————————————

Have you been diagnosed as having any of the following:

Hypertension ———          Rheumatoid arthritis ———

Diabetes ———              Osteoarthritis ———

Sinusitis ———

Over the past five years, have you experienced any of the following: Surgeries (date and description) ————————————————————————
———————————————————————————————

Hospitalizations (date and description) ——————————————————
———————————————————————————————

Auto Accidents (date and description) ————————————————————
———————————————————————————————

Falls or Blows to the face (date and description) ———————————————

Extensive Dental Work (date and description) ————————————————
———————————————————————————————

Quality or Nature of Pain (please circle all that apply)

Severe      Mild        Moderate

Burning     Throbbing   Tingling

Sharp       Dull        Stabbing

Other ———————————————————

Pain Occurrence: (circle one)

P1—pain on one day or less per month

P2—pain on two or more days per month

P3—pain on one or more days per week

P4—pain is daily but intermittent

P5—continuous pain

Pain Intensity: (please circle one)

    I1—absent or mild

    I2—more than mild but tolerable

    I3—moderately severe

    I4—severe

    I5—intolerable or worst pain you have ever experienced

Please mark the line at an appropriate level for your pain:

0 (no pain) – – – – – – – – – – – – – – – – – – – – – – – – – – –10 (excruciating pain)

Response to analgesics (pain killers): (please circle one)

    R1—pain decreased easily with a small dose of a single analgesic, i.e. aspirin or Tylenol

    R2—pain is decreased but does not disappear with a single analgesic

    R3—pain is completely relieved by a compound analgesic

    R4—pain is decreased but does not disappear with a compound analgesic

    R5—no dose of any analgesic has any effect at all on the pain

Occupation _____

    Lifting requirements at workplace:

| _____ | _____ | _____ |
|---|---|---|
| light | moderate | heavy |

    Standing requirements at workplace:

| _____ | _____ | _____ |
|---|---|---|
| infrequently | about half of my day at work | most of the time |

    Environment at the Workplace:

Air Quality

| _____ | _____ |
|---|---|
| normal | may have impurities or irritants |

Sound Levels

| _____ | _____ |
|---|---|
| normal | loud and irritating |

Are there any other factors in your medical or social history which may be helpful in determining the source of your problem and designing an effective treatment plan?

_____

_____

_____

(From Rocabado M, Iglarsh ZA: Musculoskeletal Approach to Maxillofacial Pain. Philadelphia: JB Lippincott, 1992, p 228–229.)

# EVALUATION OF UPPER QUARTER MUSCULOSKELETAL DYSFUNCTION

Date of Evaluation _____

Patient's Name: _____

Therapist Conducting Evaluation _____

I. Subjective Evaluation          Completion Date _____
II. Objective Evaluation
   A. Posture
      <u>Frontal</u> <u>view</u>

Head position on neck _____

Shoulder height _____

Hip ASIS levels _____

Patella position _____

Foot placement _____

      <u>Side</u> <u>view</u>        Left        Right

Head position on neck _____

Shoulder position _____

Degree of cervical lordosis _____

Degree of thoracic kyphosis _____

Degree of lumbar lordosis _____

      <u>Posterior</u> <u>view</u>

Head position on neck _____

Shoulder height _____

PSIS _____

Popliteal crease height _____

Knee genu valgum or varum _____

Achilles tendon alignment _____

   B. Face observation
      1. Segment proportions        upper third _____

                                middle third _____

                                lower third _____

      2. Symmetry               eye level _____

                                nasal bone _____

                                nostrils _____

                                mandibular posturing _____

      3. Areas of swelling or soft tissue atrophy: _____

_____

_____

C. Pain
  x — Trigger point
  xx — Muscle spasm
  xxx — Referral site/zone

  Pain line   0 – – – – – – – – – – – – – – – – – – – – – – – – – – – – – –10

  Does/does not patient appear to understand use of pain line?
D. Cervical spine alignment

  C-1 _____

  C2-7 _____

  T1-8 _____

  Clavicular alignment _____
E. Range of motion

| Cervical spine | Active/passive | Active/passive |
|---|---|---|
| Rotation | (L) | (R) |
| Side flexion | (L) | (R) |
| Flexion | (L) | (R) |
| Extension | (L) | (R) |

| Shoulder | Left active/passive | Right active/passive |
|---|---|---|
| Forward flexion | | |
| Extension | | |
| Abduction | | |
| Internal rotation | | |
| External rotation | | |

  TMJ

  Opening _____ mm       Left/right deviation

  Lateral deviation    Left _____ mm    Right _____ mm

  Protrusion _____ mm
F. Manual muscle test
  Shoulder

| | | |
|---|---|---|
| Forward flexion | Left | Right |
| Extension | Left | Right |
| Abduction | Left | Right |

| Muscles of mastication | Normal | Weak | Painful | Painless |
|---|---|---|---|---|
| Elevators | | | | |
| Depressors | | | | |
| Lateral deviators | | | | |

  Lips
    Internal orbicularis
    External orbicularis

  Other _____
       _____
       _____

  Grasp    Left _____    Right _____    Dominant _____

G. Lip function    normal _____
                   short functional _____
                   short nonfunctional _____

H. Tenderness to Palpation                    Left              Right
    Temporalis
    Temporalis tendon
    Posterior occiput
    TMJ: Anterior/lateral capsule
    Posterior capsule
    Zygomatic arch
    Masseter
    Medial/lateral pterygoid
    Longus colli
    Anterior neck swelling

I. Sensory
   1. Cranial nerves    I _____    VI _____    XI _____
                        II _____    VII _____    XII _____
                        III _____    VIII _____
                        IV _____    IX _____
                        V _____    X _____

   2. Cervical nerves
      a. C-5 (shoulder posterior/lateral to wrist) _____
      b. C-6 (thumb and index) _____
      c. C-7 (middle 3 digits) _____
      d. C-8 (last 3 digits) _____
      e. T-1 (ulnar wrist area) _____
      f. T-2 (inner elbow to shoulder) _____

J. Thoracic outlet:    Left _____    Right _____

K. Pectoralis syndrome:    Left _____    Right _____

III. Treatment Goals
IV. Planned Treatment Regimen
 V. Treatment Schedule
VI. Physical Therapy Diagnosis _____
_____

_____   ____
Physical Therapist    lic. #

has no effect on the symptoms. The patient's responses may be mixed. For example, the patient may have a transient increase in some symptoms during a test movement but an overall improvement of symptoms after the test movements are completed. All movements begin with the neck in neutral or axial extension. Single, repeated (10 times), and sustained forward bending and backward bending are performed with the patient sitting (Fig. 1–58). If symptoms worsen with a single movement to the point that the examination must be terminated, repetitive and sustained motions may not be tested.[4]

### Neurologic Testing

Neurologic testing is indicated if the patient reports diminished or altered sensation or muscle

# RECORD OF TREATMENT SESSION

Patient's Name: _____

Date: _____

Patient Subjective Statement: _____

_____

_____

Pain Distribution:

Pain Line:   0 – – – – – – – – – – – – – – – – – – – – – – – – – – – – –10

Pain Quality:   Severe _____   Mild _____   Moderate _____

Burning _____   Throbbing _____   Tingling _____

Sharp _____   Dull _____   Stabbing _____

Other _____

Pain Frequency:   (circle one)
P1—pain on one day or less per month
P2—pain on two or more days per month
P3—pain on one or more days per week
P4—pain is daily but intermittent
P5—continuous pain

Pain Intensity:   (circle one)
I1—absent or mild
I2—more than mild but tolerable
I3—moderately severe
I4—severe
I5—intolerable or even suicide producing

Response to Analgesics:   (circle one)

        R1 — pain decreased easily with a small dose of a single analgesic, i.e., aspirin or Tylenol

        R2 — pain is decreased but does not disappear with a single analgesic

        R3 — pain is completely relieved by a compound analgesic

        R4 — pain is decreased but does not disappear with a compound analgesic

        R5 — no dose of analgesic has any effect at all on the pain

Changes in:   Social Environment
              Physical Environment
              Stress
              General Health

Treatment Regimen:

Patient Response to Treatment (Related to Goals)

                  Pretreatment           Posttreatment

ROM

MMT

TTP

Assessment:

Plan:

Treatment Modifications for Next Treatment:

Schedule:

                                 Physical Therapist      lic. #

weakness in the upper back, head, shoulders, or upper extremities. Multimodal sensory testing, including light touch, pain, temperature, and vibration sense of peripheral nerve, cord, trunk, and dermatomal distributions, is critical to the determination of the pattern of neurologic involvement. Triceps (C-7), biceps (C-5), and brachialis (C-6) deep tendon reflexes may also be tested (Fig. 1–59). Because spinal cord compression may result from cervical spine pathology, the therapist should attempt to elicit the Babinski (Fig. 1–60) and Hoffmann (Fig. 1–61) reflexes and wrist clonus.[24]

## Muscle Strength Testing

Resisted isometric muscle testing is used to distinguish the presence of gross muscle weakness and to identify muscle actions that evoke pain. Muscles are graded as weak or strong and painful or painless. A strong and painless response indicates that contractile structures (muscle, tendon, nerve) are functioning normally. Strong and painful and weak and painful responses usually indicate a problem with the muscle or tendon structures. A weak and painless response suggests a peripheral nerve prob-

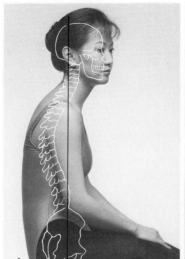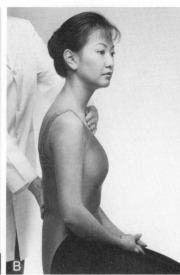

**FIGURE 1–48** ■ Spinal curves.

lem. Resisted isometric testing is performed with the neck in neutral and includes flexion, extension, lateral bending, rotation (C-1), and shoulder shrugging (C2-4). Resisted isometric testing of the upper extremities may also be used to help clarify the site of pathology. If muscle weakness is detected, more precise and quantitative muscle testing techniques can be used to determine how weak it is and for documentation purposes.[26] Usually, manual muscle testing, electromechanical dynamometry, or hand-held dynamometry is used. If a painful response is noted with resisted isometric testing, techniques that isolate the action of specific muscles (e.g., placing the joint in a particular position) can be used to locate the muscle or tendon that is most problematic.[25]

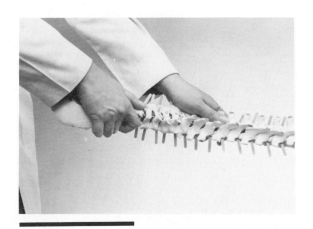

**FIGURE 1–49** ■ Bone landmarks of the cervical spine.

## Cervical Special Tests

Some special clinical tests are commonly performed during an examination of a patient with neck dysfunction. Cervical spine compression is usually performed in weight bearing (with the patient seated) (Fig. 1–62) but may be performed without weight bearing (with the patient in a supine position). Although cervical distraction can be performed with the patient sitting, it is most often done with the patient supine (Fig. 1–63). As a rule, patients who have worsening of symptoms with compression usually notice improvement of symptoms with distraction and vice versa. Worsening of symptoms with distraction implicates the capsule of ligaments, whereas worsening of symptoms with compression implicates the articular structures. Although there are notable exceptions to this rule (impingement), compression-distraction testing is helpful in determining treatment regimens for these patients.

The vertebral artery can be compromised during neck rotation in patients with cervical arthritis or instability. Before initiating any joint mobilization treatment, a test should be performed to determine whether vertebral arterial circulation is compromised during cervical rotation. The patient is supine and the neck is extended slightly and passively fully rotated to one side (Fig. 1–64). The therapist looks into the patient's eyes. Positive signs include nystagmus, tinnitus, dizziness, nausea, and syncope. This test can be performed with the patient sitting (Fig. 1–65). The alar ligament test is used to detect rupture of the

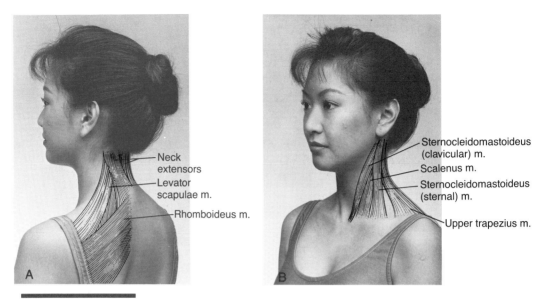

FIGURE 1-50 ■ Soft tissue of the posterior cervical spine. (A) Posterior lateral view. (B) Anterior lateral view.

alar ligament and/or fracture of the odontoid process. This is a rare but dangerous situation. The patient is supine and the therapist's index finger is placed next to the C-2 spinous process. The therapist then tilts the patient's head laterally to the opposite side (Fig. 1–66). The C-2 spinous process should immediately rotate into the therapist's finger. Any delay in rotation or failure of the spinous process to rotate is indicative of alar ligament involvement and should be treated as an emergency. If this test is negative, it should be repeated with the patient sitting.[22,27]

## DIFFERENTIAL DIAGNOSIS

### Temporomandibular Joint

In general terms, abnormal function of the temporomandibular joint can be categorized as hypomobile and hypermobile. These are actually

FIGURE 1-51 ■ Passive neck forward and back bending.

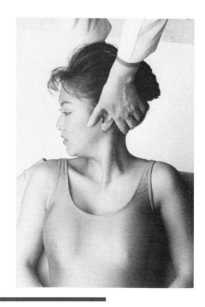

FIGURE 1-52 ■ Atlantoaxial joint assessment.

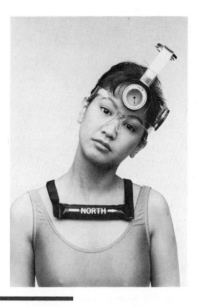

FIGURE 1–53 ■ Measurement of cervical range of motion.

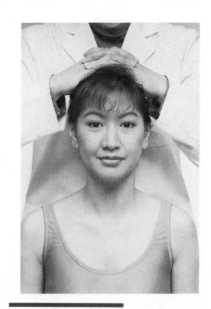

FIGURE 1–55 ■ Cervical compression test.

physical therapy diagnoses. Hypomobility is classified as a mandibular opening of less than 25 or 33 mm and hypermobility as an opening of more than 50 mm. Several conditions can contribute to loss of motion or excessive motion in the joint.[14]

Hypomobility can be caused by joint degeneration, disc displacement, spasm in the muscles of mastication, soft tissue contractures or adhesions, capsular tightness, joint dislocation, bone spurs, loose bodies in the joint, or an abnormal mass growth in the joint. Obviously, some of these processes are progressive or require surgical intervention. In the majority of these cases, the therapist can identify the specific muscles in spasm or tight soft tissue to relax or stretch. Weakened muscles can be strengthened and asynchronous joint action re-educated.

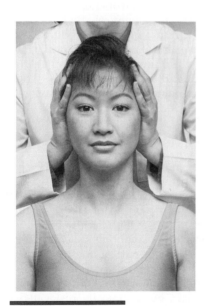

FIGURE 1–54 ■ Cervical distraction test.

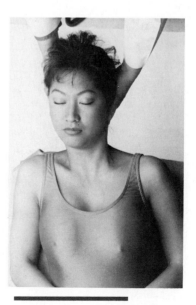

FIGURE 1–56 ■ Cervical glide test.

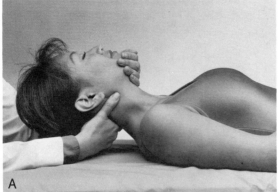

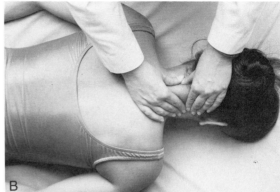

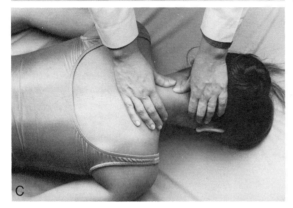

**FIGURE 1-57** ■ (A) Anterior glide assessment. (B) Accessory motion testing using transverse vertebral pressure. (C) Accessory motion testing using transverse vertebral pressure.

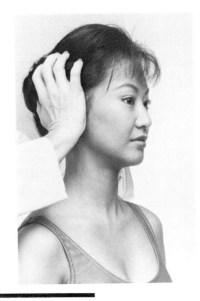

**FIGURE 1-58** ■ Cervical forward and back bending.

Structures that are overstretched in hypermobile joints can be identified and stabilized. As in hypomobility, asynchronous muscle function can be re-educated. Parafunctional habits that contribute to hypermobility of the temporomandibular joint include prolonged bottle feeding and pacifier use and finger sucking in children, excessive nail biting and gum chewing, mouth breathing, and nocturnal bruxers. These habits must be eliminated through behavior modification.

### Disc Displacement[9]

The disc normally rests in the 12 o'clock to 1 o'clock position on the mandibular head. Predisposing conditions, degenerative processes, systemic disease, malocclusions, oral dysfunction, or trauma can cause the disc to be pulled into a more anterior position on the mandibular head. The force-bearing part of the disc shifts from its noninnervated central portion to the posterior pole, which is innervated and can produce pain. The disc can be chronically dislocated or reseat itself or "reduce" to return to its place atop the mandibular head, often producing the audible or

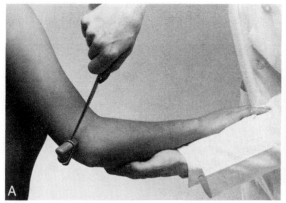

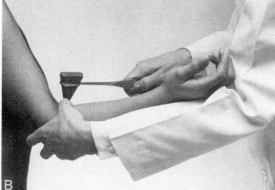

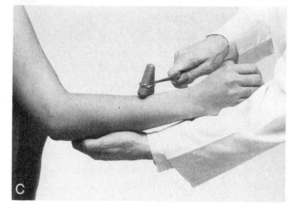

**FIGURE 1-59** ■ Deep tendon reflexes. (A) Triceps reflex. (B) Biceps reflex. (C) Brachioradialis reflex.

palpable click characteristic of many temporomandibular joint patients.

The degree of disc displacement can be graded into stages:

**Stage 1 of derangement**—The disc may be positioned slightly anteriorly and medially on the mandibular head. The click is inconsist-

ent, if present at all, and occurs early in the opening cycle. Pain is mild or absent.

**Stage 2 of derangement**—The disc has slipped more medially and anteriorly on the mandibular head. The reciprocal click is present more consistently and occurs in the early phase of opening and late in the phase of closing, and the disc reseats itself on the

**FIGURE 1-60** ■ Babinski reflex test. (A) Negative. (B) Positive.

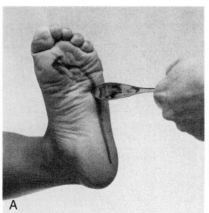

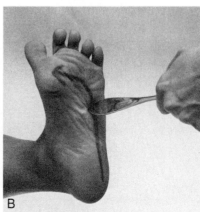

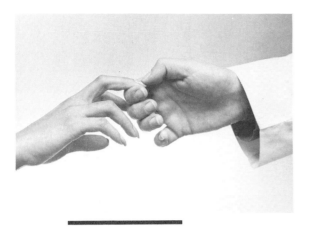

FIGURE 1–61 ■ Hoffmann reflex test.

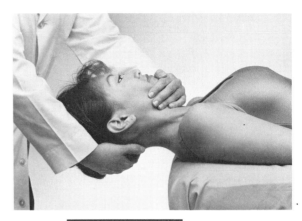
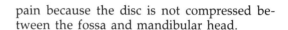

FIGURE 1–63 ■ Cervical distraction.

mandibular head. Pain becomes more severe and consistent as innervated portions of the disc are compressed between bone surfaces.

**Stage 3 of derangement**—The click is more consistent and occurs later in the cycle of opening and earlier in the phase of closing. The mandibular head must rotate considerably in the fossa before the disc clicks into place and rotates in reverse only a slight degree before dislocation upon closing. This is often the most painful phase.

**Stage 4 of derangement**—A click is rare in this late stage because the disc is usually so far out of place that it can no longer relocate atop the mandibular head. There may be no

pain because the disc is not compressed between the fossa and mandibular head.

## Adhesive Capsulitis or Capsular Tightness and Contractures

The capsule of the temporomandibular joint and its associated ligaments can become contracted or scarred. The shortening or loss of flexibility in the joint's connective tissue restricts joint motion and can dislocate the disc from its normal, painless relationship with the mandibular head. Trauma can cause capsular tightness as joint fibers are torn and bleeding infiltrates the fibers and causes scarring and connective tissue fiber disorganization.

Bilateral joint tightness limits motion of the mandible, especially translation, whereas unilateral joint tightness causes relative degrees of

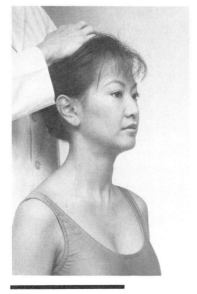

FIGURE 1–62 ■ Cervical compression.

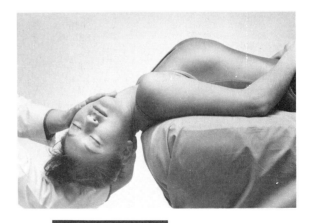

FIGURE 1–64 ■ Supine vertebral artery test.

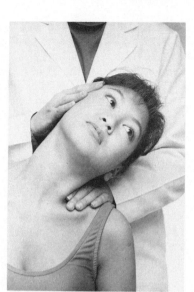

**FIGURE 1-65** ▪ Sitting vertebral artery test.

asymmetric mandibular depression and elevation. This latter type of dysfunction causes the mandible to deviate toward the side of capsular tightness. Pain may occur as the innervated portion of the disc is compressed between the mandibular head and articular eminence.

Local inflammation caused by mechanical irritation of the joint surfaces or bacterial or viral infection can also cause tissue scarring and motion limitations. Practitioners should attempt to

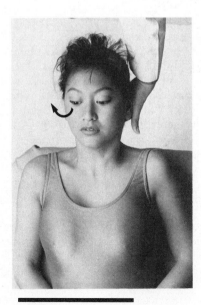

**FIGURE 1-66** ▪ Alar ligament test.

increase circulation and minimize mechanical irritation while treating the patient pharmacologically to eliminate the viral or bacterial infection.

### Spasm in Muscles of Mastication

Spasms in the muscles of mastication cause pain in the muscles themselves, alter the mandibular head and disc relationship, and restrict normal temporomandibular joint function in chewing and speaking. Detailed subjective and objective techniques can be used to determine the specific muscle in spasm.

Temporalis muscle spasm can cause headaches in the temporal region. Palpation can elicit pain at trigger points in the body of the muscle or at its insertion on the coronoid of the mandible. A patient who has a significant number of muscle fibers inserting on the inferior orbit of the eye may experience visual changes. Although vision is not impaired, the patient experiences difficulty in seeing or coordinating the eye muscles. The patient may feel pressure behind the eye, have increased eye fatigue, and have difficulty seeing in poor light or at dusk.

Spasm in the lateral and medial pterygoid muscles causes pain deep in the cheek area, pain upon chewing, and pain in the ear. The ear symptoms occur as the muscle spasm draws the mandibular head into the middle ear, causing pain, tinnitus, muffled or dampened hearing, a "swimmer's ear" sensation, and even dizziness.

The longus colli spasm is felt as a "sore throat" by the patient, but no throat irritation is visualized via bronchoscopy. Failure to substantiate the symptoms often leads patients to feel as if they are imagining them. These symptoms can be validated if palpation of the longus colli behind the larynx in the anterior neck, anterior to the spinal column and medial to the external belly of the sternomastoid muscle, produces pain. The "wet feather–like" nonspasmed muscle feels like a "worm" when in spasm and produces pain upon palpation. Clinically, these patients experience pain upon swallowing and feel a lump in their throat. Some of these patients also develop yeast infections in the mouth with changes in tongue texture and taste.

Muscles in the anterior neck can also go into spasm. The sternocleidomastoid muscle in spasm can restrict head on neck motion and cause spasmatic torticollis. It can also cause pain upon breathing. A spasm in the scaleni muscles can cause a "soft" thoracic outlet syndrome with radiating neurologic and vascular symptoms. This spasm can raise the lateral portion of the clavicle and cause anterior chest pain.

Suprahyoid muscle spasm causes pain in the floor of the mouth and, by maintaining the hyoid bone in an elevated position, alters swallowing and increases the caudal forces on the mandible. The suprahyoid muscle counterparts, the infrahyoid muscles, normally maintain the hyoid bone in a depressed position after swallowing; therefore, in the hyoid's abnormal elevated position, these muscles indirectly add caudal forces to the suprahyoid muscles and mandible. Spasm in the anterior neck muscles also contributes to a forward head and anterior shoulder posture.

### Osteoarthritis

Degenerative joint disease, often a unilateral or uneven bilateral process, alters the force-bearing surfaces of the temporomandibular joint, creating cracks in the articular surfaces, osteophytes or bone spurs, and abnormal joint surface modeling. The cracks in the joint surface contribute to joint erosion and irregular joint motion. The osteophytes impede motion and joint surface remodeling, permanently altering the relationship of the joint components. These sharp edges of bone can also perforate the disc.

In these cases, pain is at its lowest level when the patient rises in the morning and becomes worse as the day progresses and the patient moves the joints. Excessive chewing and talking increase joint pain because they mechanically irritate the joint surfaces and reduce the synovial fluid bathing the joint surfaces. Gentle distraction and lateral glides increase the synovial fluid covering the joint surfaces and can slow the progression of osteoarthritis.

### Rheumatoid Arthritis

Rheumatoid arthritis, a systemic disease, can involve the temporomandibular joint. In cases of juvenile rheumatoid arthritis, it is often the first joint involved. Patients with rheumatoid arthritis experience greater pain and stiffness upon arising in the morning. Appropriate levels of non–weight-bearing or non–force-bearing motion in the joint relieve some of this morning pain. The patient goes through the day with a significant level of chronic pain, balancing therapeutic levels of active motion and avoiding excessive motion that irritates the synovial lining.

In the early phases of the disease, bone changes may not be visible on x-ray examination but can be detected in laboratory tests of hematocrit levels. As the disease progresses, the panus formation invades the articular surfaces, causes cystic lesions, and softens the bone. These bone changes are often bilateral. As the disease progresses, the patient with rheumatoid arthritis can experience fever, multiple joint pain, and anorexia.

### Lyme Disease

Lyme disease, a tick-borne disease, is increasing in prevalence in deer-populated regions of the United States and Canada. The spirochete can cause neurologic symptoms, general malaise, and rheumatoid-like joint symptoms. Often confused with migraine or cluster headaches, Epstein-Barr, chronic fatigue syndrome, systemic lupus erythematosus, and rheumatoid arthritis, Lyme disease may involve the temporomandibular joint. In this case a symptom-based physical therapy treatment plan gives the patient only short-term palliative relief. Healthy joint function is maintained at the highest possible level while the patient is treated pharmacologically to attack the disease-causing spirochete.

### Referred Pain

Pain in the face can be referred segmentally from cervical nerve roots or trigger points. The cervical nerves refer pain in specific dermatomal patterns, which may be complicated by overlying cranial nerve influence. That is, the trigeminal nerve can refer to the palate, throat, forehead, temple, or ear, and the glossopharyngeal nerve refers to the ear, tonsil, larynx, or tongue.

Trigger points in skeletal muscle are tender when palpated, contain a tight fibrous band, produce a local twitch response, and cause muscle weakness without atrophy. The trigger points can be treated to reduce pain at the referral site. It is often effective to treat the referral zone as well. Prolonged trigger point irritation of a referral zone may cause local physiologic reaction requiring treatment of the zone as well (Fig. 1–67).

Patients may seek repeated help for treatment of pain referred to the teeth or temporomandibular joint. If the source of referred pain is not described, the patient may agree to surgery or tooth extraction. Unfortunately, treatment of only the referral zone does not affect the trigger point or the pain.

When the trigger point is mechanically, chemically, or electrically irritated, the patient feels the

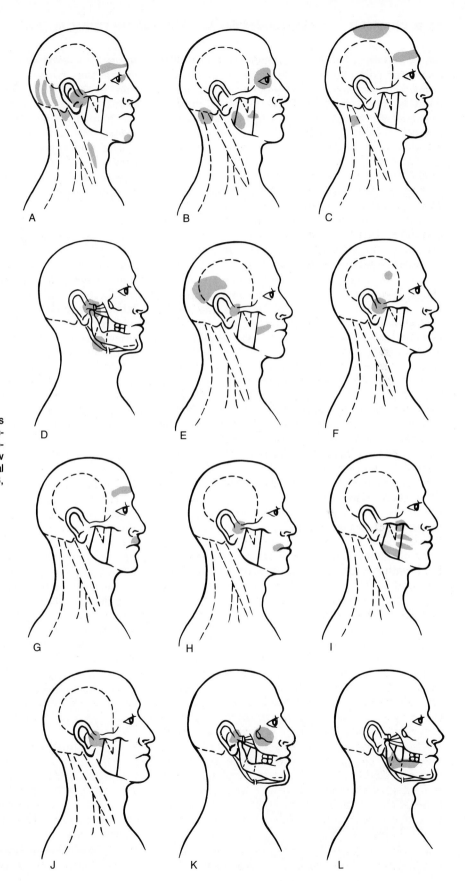

**FIGURE 1-67** ■ Referral zones of the face. (Redrawn from Fricton J, Kroening R, Haley D: Myofascial pain syndrome. A review of 168 patients. Oral Surg Oral Med Oral Pathol 60:615–623, 1982.)

referred pain. If the practitioner cannot reproduce the pain when injecting or irritating the point, the treatment is not effective. The treatment is more effective if the involved joint is stretched passively after the trigger point is irritated.[28]

### Cranial Nerve Neuralgias

**Trigeminal Neuralgia.** The etiology varies with the patient, including focal nerve demyelination, viral infection, vascular abnormalities, and extensive dental procedures. The mandibular or maxillary branches of the trigeminal nerve are most commonly involved.

The pain is usually described as like an electric shock. It begins as the individual touches nose or lips, talks, chews, shaves, or brushes the teeth. The symptoms may remit but do not end. Despite the pain, sensory loss is rarely experienced by the patient.

**Glossopharyngeal Neuralgia.** The unilateral pain is abrupt and lasts only a minute. The pain often awakens the patient and can last for weeks to months. The symptoms may remit for months to years. Swallowing, chewing, coughing, and yawning can trigger the pain. The pain may be caused by peripheral nerve lesions, Eagle's syndrome (ossified styloid ligament), or ninth and tenth nerve compression.[29]

### Reflex Sympathetic Dystrophy

The etiology may be maxillofacial surgery, penetrating trauma (i.e., bullet or knife), head injury, or extensive dental procedures. These events may cause increased central nervous system excitability, self-exciting neuronal loop in dorsal horn, or dysfunction of a "cerebral biasing mechanism in the brain or abnormal tissue neuromas."[30]

The patient complains of burning pain, allodynia, hyperpathia, trophic changes, localized edema, and surface temperature changes. These symptoms may have been categorized previously as atypical facial pain.

### Etiologic Models

Etiologic analyses of temporomandibular disorders may be as simple as the three-part pie model of Gelb[31] (Fig. 1–68) or as complex as laboratory mazes for mice. The "dynamic model" is flexible and functional in helping the practitioner to delineate contributing factors and develop an effective treatment regimen.[32]

The masticatory system is a balance between orthofunction (normal to adaptive supernormal) and pathofunction (abnormal). The individual can adapt toward orthofunction (hyperfunction) or toward pathofunction (Fig. 1–69), biomechanically overloading the joint and promoting degeneration and disc perforation and deformation.

Adaptation results from the individual's attempt to achieve homeostasis in the masticatory system. The system can adapt physiologically, functionally, or behaviorally. Several factors influence adaptability: trauma, health, nutrition, structure, and coping mechanisms. Gender may be an additional factor because females may have condyles that are retropositioned compared to those in males, predisposing females to anterior disc dislocation.

Conversely, several factors would make a person more prone to hyperfunction: forward head

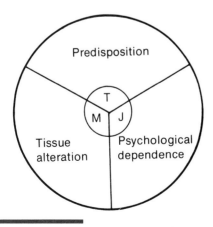

FIGURE 1–68 ■ Gelb's model. (From Gelb H, ed: Clinical Management of Head, Neck, and TMJ Pain and Dysfunction, p. 95, Figure 11–1. Philadelphia: WB Saunders, 1985.)

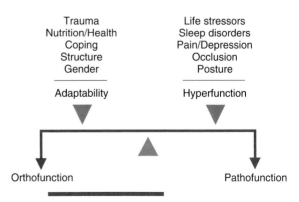

FIGURE 1–69 ■ Dynamic etiologic model.

and shoulder posture, occlusion (especially asymmetric), pain and depression, sleep disorders, and life stressors. The latter three factors also affect the pain threshold, another characteristic leading toward hyperfunction.

## Neck Dysfunction Syndromes

Physical therapists treat movement dysfunction. In most cases, patients have either inflammatory, muscle performance, or mobility problems. It is helpful to use categories like these to guide diagnosis and treatment of neck dysfunction. Treatment is largely symptom driven. That is, exercise, mobilization, and other treatments that increase the patient's symptoms are avoided and those that improve the symptoms are encouraged. Most neck dysfunction syndromes can be classified into one of the following categories: impingement, hypomobility, inflammation, muscle weakness, muscle spasm, extension dysfunction, and flexion dysfunction. These are not necessarily mutually exclusive categories, although one problem may have to be resolved before another can be uncovered.

### Impingement

Impingement syndrome is characterized by a sudden onset (often without any memorable trauma) of sharp unilateral neck pain with restricted movement. The most restricted and painful motions are those that close or compress the facet joint on the painful side: extension and rotation toward the side of pain (Fig. 1–70). Lateral bending toward the side of pain may be painful but is usually much less evocative of symptoms than extension and rotation. Compression in weight-bearing and non–weight-bearing positions is also painful. Distraction often helps to localize the pain to a specific vertebral level. Patients use words like "sharp" and "excruciating" to describe the symptoms. They complain of a "stiff neck." Passive intervertebral motion often cannot be assessed because of significant muscle spasm and guarding.

**Treatment.** The symptoms can usually be relieved with manual distraction and a rotation mobilization to the side away from that of pain (Fig. 1–71). Occasionally, a rotation mobilization toward the painful side may be necessary to restore full, pain-free motion.[25] Unfortunately, several treatments may be needed to relax the patient enough so that the mobilization can be

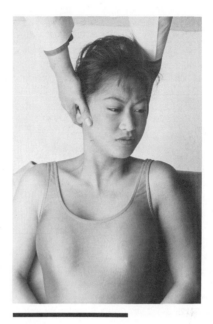

FIGURE 1–70 ■ Impingement syndrome.

performed. The use of electrical or thermal agents is helpful in the early stages of impingement syndrome to relax the patient. Thermal agents (most often vapor coolant sprays or ice massage) can be helpful in relieving any soreness that occurs after mobilization.[33,34]

Patients usually feel immediate relief of pain and return of full motion after the mobilization. Some practitioners recommend that the patients

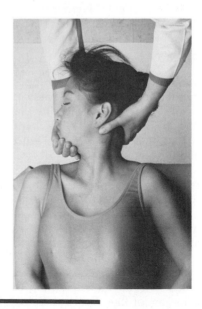

FIGURE 1–71 ■ Manual distraction and rotation.

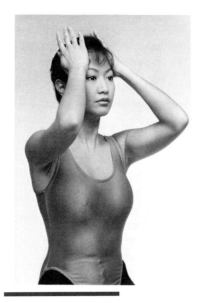

**FIGURE 1–72** ■ Cervical flexion exercises.

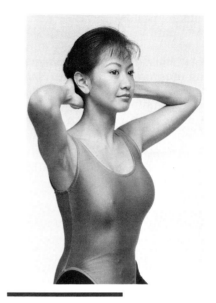

**FIGURE 1–73** ■ Cervical retraction exercises.

return as often as five times per week for "adjustments," ostensibly to prevent future occurrences. Repetitive manipulation can lead to joint hypermobility. Hypermobility may actually precipitate impingement because it results in more joint motion and a larger joint space where the synovium and other neural structures may become pinched. Rather than repetitive manipulation, neck positioning (cervical pillow for sleeping, seating modifications) and remedial exercise are stressed. Exercises include isometric neck flexion, extension, side bending, and rotation (Figs. 1–72 and 1–73).[35]

### Hypomobility

Hypomobility syndromes can be diagnosed when there is a true loss of passive range of neck motion. The loss of mobility may be accompanied by acute signs of inflammation or muscle spasm that must be addressed before the hypomobility can be assessed or treated adequately.

The articular pattern of loss of range of motion in the cervical spine consists of equal loss of rotation and lateral bending to the side opposite that of restriction and loss of extension. (By contrast, with impingement, rotation toward the side of pain is restricted.) Unilateral, single joint restriction may not be diagnosed without careful passive intervertebral motion testing (see Objective Evaluation of the Cervical Spine) because hypermobility of an adjacent segment may make

gross motion measurements appear normal. In these cases, the patient may actually present with an impingement of the hypermobile joint and the hypomobility may be masked until the impingement is resolved. Bilateral involvement is characterized by restriction of rotation and lateral bending to both sides and loss of extension. Multilevel involvement is usually bilateral and loss of motion is more profound because the compensation afforded by unrestricted adjacent levels is absent. In all cases of articular restriction, distraction causes a stretching discomfort that is not long-lasting.

**Treatment.** Traction is often used to treat these patients. Mechanical traction (Fig. 1–74)

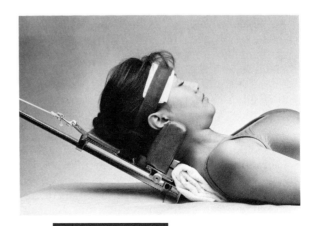

**FIGURE 1–74** ■ Mechanical cervical traction.

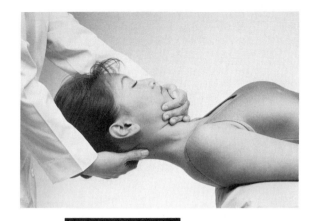

**FIGURE 1-75** ■ Manual cervical traction.

can be used for a prolonged stretch, and manual traction (Fig. 1-75) can be used to direct the stretch to particular vertebral levels. Specific joint mobilization (usually grade III and grade IV oscillations) into the restricted range of motion is used to treat segmental restrictions.[36] Indirect mobilization (muscle-energy techniques) can also be used to move the joints, using reverse action of the muscles that attach to the bone as the mobilization force. Multisegmental problems are more likely to reflect age-related bone changes that may not be amenable to mobilization. It is important to include remedial exercise stressing range of motion because when motion is increased by joint mobilization, the patient must learn to incorporate the newly acquired motion into activities of daily living. In all cases, educating the patient regarding neck positioning and environmental modifications (e.g., seating, desk top alterations) is an integral part of the treatment plan.

Loss of range of motion in a nonarticular pattern may reflect an injury to one part of the joint capsule or may result from prolonged immobilization in a position other than neutral.

## Inflammation

When signs of acute inflammation (redness, swelling, heat, and pain) are apparent, classification of the neck dysfunction into any of the other categories is nearly impossible.

**Treatment.** Treatment is directed at reducing the inflammation and controlling pain. Rest and the use of aspirin or some other nonsteroidal, anti-inflammatory medication are usually the first course of action. Physical agents such as ice and sensory-level electrical stimulation may also be used.[33,34] Exercise is limited to gentle range-of-motion exercises in the patient's pain-free range. When the inflammation has been reduced and physical examination is possible, the patient may be reclassified into one of the other categories and treated appropriately.

## Muscle Spasm

Muscle spasm often accompanies the early stages of neck dysfunction. Like acute inflammatory signs, muscle spasm may prevent an accurate diagnosis and usually must be treated before a physical examination can be completed. Accurate assessment of passive range of joint motion and joint play is compromised in the presence of muscle spasm. Muscle spasm can be treated using many physical agents (see the later section on physical agents), contract-relax exercise techniques, and soft tissue mobilization (e.g., by massage). Treatment may also include the use of antispasmodic medications prescribed by a physician. As in the case of the inflammation, when the muscle spasm has been reduced the physical examination can be completed and the problem can be reclassified.

## Muscle Weakness

Although muscle weakness may develop after prolonged disuse, it is rarely a significant feature of neck dysfunction in the absence of neurologic involvement. When muscle weakness is identified during a physical examination, the degree of weakness should be quantified during manual muscle testing, electromechanical dynamometry, or hand-held dynamometry. Other muscles innervated by the same peripheral nerve, brachial plexus trunk and cord, and cervical nerve root should also be tested. Many upper extremity compression neuropathies and brachial plexopathies can cause muscle weakness (Fig. 1-76). Careful examination of sensation should accompany motor testing. If frank weakness is identified, with or without sensory changes, the patient should be referred to a neurologist.

## Disc-like Syndromes: Extension and Flexion Dysfunction

Many patients with neck dysfunction have intermittent or variable symptoms that can be re-

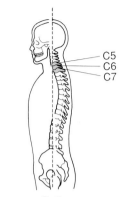

## C5 Neurologic level

A     Dermatome

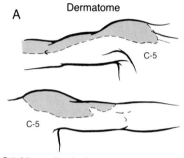

Muscle test of muscles innervated by C-5

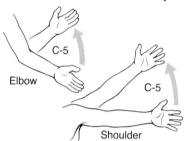

Reflex

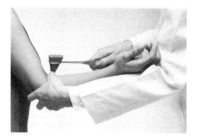

## C6 Neurologic level

B     Dermatome

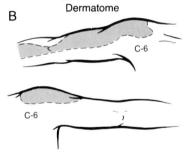

Muscle test of muscles innervated by C-6

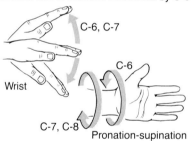

Reflex

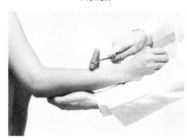

## C7 Neurologic level

C     Dermatome

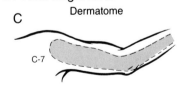

Muscle test of muscles innervated by C-7
See
C-6 neurologic level

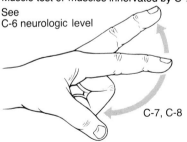

Reflex

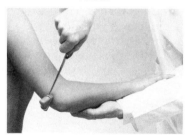

**FIGURE 1–76** ■ Upper extremity compression neuropathies.

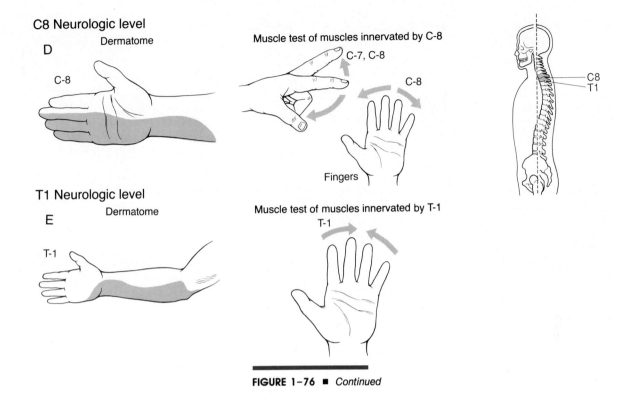

**FIGURE 1–76** ■ *Continued*

produced reliably with certain positions or movements. These patients can be treated by using the movements or positions that alleviate the symptoms to treat the dysfunction. The patients generally fall into two categories: those for whom neck flexion improves symptoms and those for whom neck extension improves symptoms. Improvement in both cases is defined as a decrease in the extent or intensity of the peripheral symptoms. Patients in both categories usually report that traction alleviates their peripheral symptoms. For patients in the flexion category, mechanical traction is administered with the neck in slight flexion. For patients in the extension category, traction is administered with the neck in neutral or slight axial extension. Remedial exercise is the most important component of the treatment regimen. Exercise is performed with the neck in slight axial extension. Extension syndrome patients begin with retraction and extension exercises, and flexion syndrome patients begin with flexion exercises. The ultimate goal is to restore full, pain-free motion in all directions, so rotation, lateral bending, flexion, and extension exercises are used when the symptoms are under control (Fig. 1–77). Education of the patient is critical to successful management of these types of problems. Patients must be aware of the positions, situations, and motions that worsen the symptoms and of strategies for controlling the symptoms.

## TREATMENT OF TEMPOROMANDIBULAR JOINT PAIN

The most effective treatment approach is based on objective evaluation findings. These enable the practitioner to establish baseline descriptions of joint, muscle, and soft tissue function; treat each symptom or group of symptoms specifically; determine objectively the effectiveness or lack of effectiveness of the treatment regimen; and modify the treatment as appropriate.

It is beneficial to have an orientation to treatment that the patient understands:[9]

■ Treat the pain—this is usually the symptom that brings the patient to your office for treatment.

■ Identify any structures that are not in their normal location (bone or soft tissue).

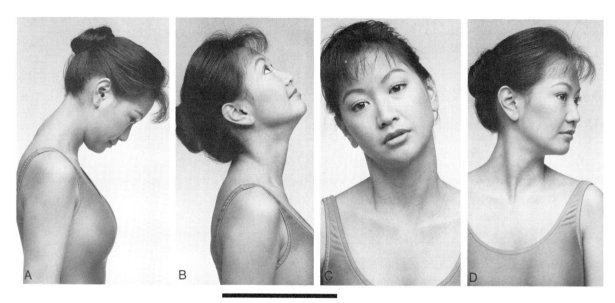

**FIGURE 1–77** ■ Cervical exercises.

■ Relax the soft tissue around these structures (to assist mobilization).

■ Relocate these structures into their normal position (using direct or indirect, passive or active forces).

■ Teach the patient this new position and any new structural relationships (visual feedback and repetitive motion). The patient must know the new positions to effect a life skill or permanent behavioral change.

■ Strengthen the soft tissue around these relocated structures to maintain the new positions (if the surrounding tissue is not strengthened, the structures will not remain in their new positions).

## Treatment by Symptoms

The patient with temporomandibular joint pain or dysfunction often presents a complicated clinical picture, challenging even experienced therapists. The practitioner who attempts to treat a diagnosis rather than a collection of symptoms will be perplexed by the patient's unpredictable or inconsistent response to treatment.

Consequently, the therapist who performs effective objective measurements and designs a treatment plan specific to the evaluation findings is more successful in treating patients with temporomandibular joint dysfunction. The practitioner must resist routinely applying "cookbook"

treatment protocols. Despite the similarity of symptoms among patients, each must be treated uniquely. Therapists must trust their cognitive skills in problem solving and treatment planning and their manual skills in palpating, massaging, and mobilizing patients.

The following presentation of treatment protocols describes effective modalities and procedures, but the therapist must modify each of these in accordance with patient-specific treatment protocols.

Procedures used in treating the temporomandibular joint should not be painful, with the exception of friction massage and trigger point irritation. Painful procedures may cause microtrauma, local inflammatory reactions, and protective muscle spasm. These conditions can slow and even prevent a patient's progress.

Modalities are applied to reduce pain and swelling and to prepare the soft tissue for mobilization, massage, exercise, or stretching procedures. In some cases modalities can be applied after mobilization, massage, exercise, or stretching to reduce pain, swelling, and local inflammatory reactions resulting from these treatments (see Modality Application to the Face).

These protocols can be combined in a comprehensive regimen to treat any patient with complex temporomandibular joint dysfunction. The components of the regimen are selected on the basis of the objective evaluation findings. When the regimen is initiated, the objective findings should be re-evaluated to determine the patient's response to treatment and treatment modifications should be made as needed. The protocols presented are not rigid but rather guidelines upon which to create an individualized, flexible treatment regimen.

### Physical Agents for Treating Neck Dysfunction

Physical agents have a role to play in the management of neck dysfunction. However, they should be used on the basis of sound hypotheses about how each agent effects therapeutic change rather than as a generic treatment for neck dysfunction. A specific diagnosis warrants a specific treatment. The use of ice, heat in some cases, and electrical stimulation may be warranted for pain and other inflammatory symptoms.

Muscle spasm can be treated with a host of modalities (e.g., motor-level electrical stimulation, vapor coolant sprays, ice massage, ultrasound, sensory-level electrical stimulation). Often the soreness that follows mobilization or stretching

*Text continued on page 65*

# MODALITY APPLICATION TO THE FACE

## Suggested Modifications

| MODALITY | MODIFICATION |
|---|---|
| Hot pack | Use conventional packs or face masks |
| Cold pack | Use conventional packs or face masks |
| Ultrasound (Fig. 1–78) | Use 0.75 to 1.0 W/cm² at 50 to 100% cycle, use 3-MHz instead of 1-MHz sound heads |
| High-voltage stimulation (Fig. 1–79) | Use positive electrode as treatment electrode; set at high rate. Use TENS-type pads, hand-held or internal probe; avoid muscle contraction; patient should perceive the impulse only minimally |
| Transcutaneous electrical nerve stimulator (TENS) | Use at minimal perceivable levels with low rate and wide width (slow rise to peak or gradual ramp) |
| Pain suppressor | Designed for head application and pain treatment |
| Microcurrent | Use probes or current applied through hands |

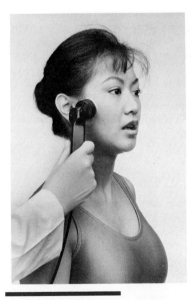

**FIGURE 1–78** ■ Application of ultrasound.

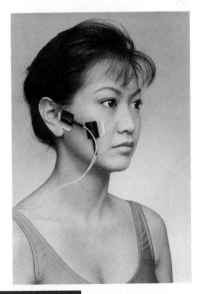

**FIGURE 1–79** ■ Application of high-voltage stimulation.

| MODALITY | MODIFICATION |
|---|---|
| Electric point stimulation (Fig. 1–80) | Treat face and neck points bilaterally; use moldable, tightly adhering delivery pads |

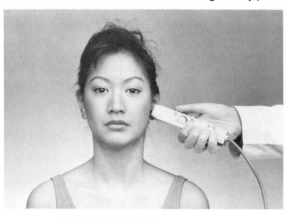

**FIGURE 1–80** ■ Application of Neuroprobe.

| MODALITY | MODIFICATION |
|---|---|
| Vapocoolant spray | Spray from trigger point to trigger zones while joint is passively stretched; cover eyes for protection and do not let the patient become chilled |
| Re-educate position of head on neck (Fig. 1–81A and B) | Restore head on neck to decrease excessive stretch on muscles of anterior neck and mandible |
| | Reduce biomechanical forces on small neck extensors |
| | Decrease compressive forces between posterior occiput and spinous process of cervical vertebra 2 |
| Active exercises of mandible (Fig. 1–82) | Repetitious midline mandible exercise to restore synchrony to muscles of mastication |
| Ice massage | Local anesthetic response |

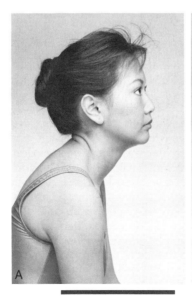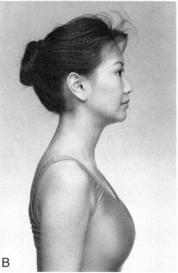

A          B

**FIGURE 1–81** ■ Re-education of head on neck posture.

## Suggested Applications by Symptom

### Swelling

| MODALITY | RATIONALE FOR APPLICATION |
| --- | --- |
| Cold packs | Reduce swelling |
| High-voltage stimulation | Reduces swelling and can be applied intraorally with Teflon probe |
| TENS | Application of electric stimulation at home over extended periods of time |
| | Minimal muscle contraction will promote swelling reduction |
| Iontophoresis | Application of local inflammatory medications can reduce swelling in the deep tissue |

| PROCEDURE | RATIONALE FOR APPLICATION |
| --- | --- |
| Intraoral massage (Fig. 1–83) | Gentle release technique reduces swelling in the oral mucosa |
| Active range-of-motion exercises of temporomandibular joint | Active contraction of the muscles of mastication reduces swelling if the patient does not force opening into painful range |
| Ice massage | Swelling locally reduced by massage with an ice cube or cold probe |

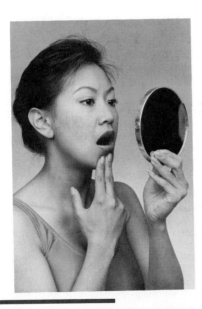

**FIGURE 1–82** ■ Active exercise of mandible.

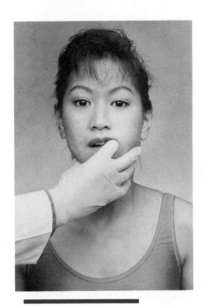

**FIGURE 1–83** ■ Intraoral massage.

### Muscles of Mastication Spasm

| MODALITY | RATIONALE FOR APPLICATION |
| --- | --- |
| Moist heat | Relax soft tissue, increase circulation |
| High-voltage stimulation | Decrease nerve conduction velocity |
| TENS | Provide prolonged use of electric stimulation at home |

| MODALITY | RATIONALE FOR APPLICATION |
|---|---|
| Ultrasound | Relax soft tissue, increase circulation |
| Iontophoresis | Introduce an anti-inflammatory agent into the muscles in spasm |
| Vapocoolant spray | Apply spray and stretch the soft tissue and to reduce the referred pain |
| Trigger point stimulation | Electric stimulation to reduce trigger points |
| Biofeedback (Fig. 1–84) | Teach the patient active relaxation of muscles in spasm |

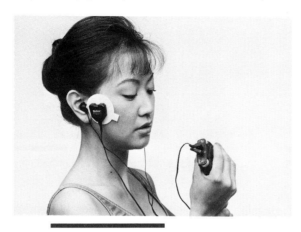

**FIGURE 1–84** ■ Application of biofeedback.

## Pain

| MODALITY | RATIONALE FOR APPLICATION |
|---|---|
| Cold packs | Reduce swelling |
| | Anesthetic procedure |
| Heat packs | Relax soft tissue |
| | Increase circulation |
| High-voltage stimulation | Reduce swelling |
| | Decrease pain |
| | Slow nerve conduction velocity |
| TENS | Continue benefits of electric stimulation at home |
| | Apply a local treatment for a local problem |
| | Give the patient an active form of self-treatment |
| Ultrasound | Relax soft tissue |
| | Increase circulation |
| | Apply hydrocortisone to reduce a local inflammatory effect (phonophoresis) |
| Iontophoresis | Apply lidocaine anesthetic to reduce pain |
| | Apply dexamethosone, an anti-inflammatory medication, to deep tissues and in greater concentration than phonophoresis |
| Vapocoolant | Stretch soft tissue |
| | Reduce a trigger point and eliminate referred pain |

| PROCEDURE | RATIONALE FOR APPLICATION |
|---|---|
| Intraoral massage | Reduce spasm of muscles of mastication |
| | Reduce swelling |
| | Reduce trigger points |
| Long axis distraction of mandible (Fig. 1–85) | Reduces force of head of mandible pressing against ear, thus reducing ear pain |
| | Relaxes muscles in spasm by applying a prolonged stretch to muscles of mastication |
| Contract-relax exercises of mandible | Fatigues the muscle and relaxes the spasm |
| Long axis distraction of mandibular head | Provides prolonged stretch on the soft tissue, which relaxes the spasm |
| Head and neck posture re-education exercises | Reduce stretch on fatigued muscles of mastication in spasm |
| Ice massage | Reduces myotonic stretch response |

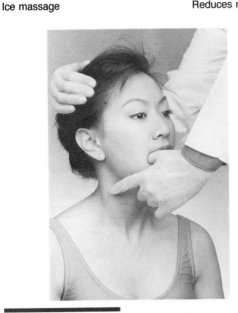

**FIGURE 1–85** ■ Long axis distraction of mandibular head.

## Forward Head Posture

| MODALITY | RATIONALE FOR APPLICATION |
|---|---|
| Moist heat | Relaxes soft tissue to upper quarter muscle |
| High-voltage stimulation | Relaxes soft tissue of neck and upper quarter |
| Ultrasound | Relaxes soft tissue of posterior cervical spine, anterior spine, and anterior shoulders |

| PROCEDURE | RATIONALE FOR APPLICATION |
|---|---|
| Massage | Relaxes soft tissue of posterior cervical spine, anterior spine, and anterior shoulders |
| Mobilization | Retracts head, anterior-posterior derotate and descend lateral clavicles, sternum, and anterior rib attachments |

| PROCEDURE | RATIONALE FOR APPLICATION |
|---|---|
| Exercises | Head nod (Fig. 1–86)<br>Head retraction on neck (Fig. 1–87)<br>Prone head extension (Fig. 1–88)<br>Arms overhead (Fig. 1–89)<br>Open door stretch (Fig. 1–90A and B) |

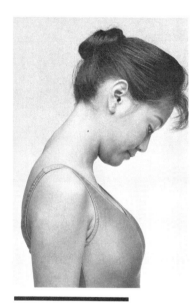

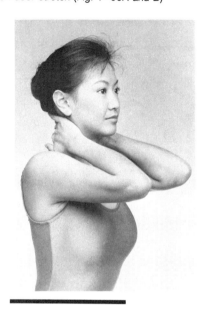

**FIGURE 1–86** ■ Head nod exercises.

**FIGURE 1–87** ■ Head traction exercises.

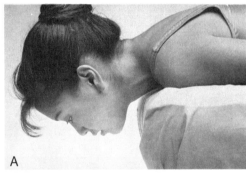

A

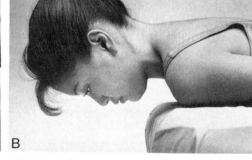

B

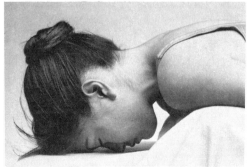

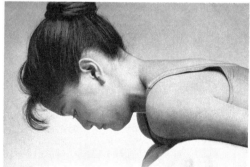

**FIGURE 1–88** ■ Prone head extension exercises.

| PROCEDURE | RATIONAL FOR APPLICATION |
|---|---|
| Breathing exercises | Body of sternum protrudes anteriorly and elevates diaphragmatic breathing |

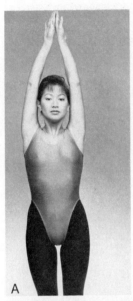
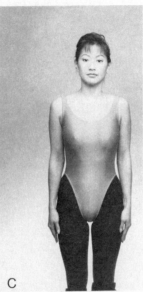
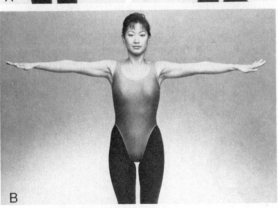

**FIGURE 1–89** ■ Arms overhead exercises.

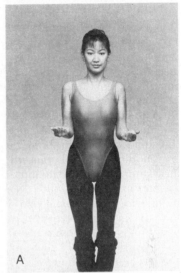
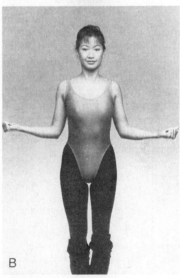

**FIGURE 1–90** ■ Open door stretch exercises.

## Hypomobile Temporomandibular Joint

| MODALITY | RATIONALE FOR APPLICATION |
|---|---|
| Moist heat | Relaxes the soft tissue, increases circulation |
| High-voltage stimulation | Reduces pain, relaxes the soft tissue, decreases swelling |
| TENS | Continue effects of electric stimulation at home |
| Ultrasound | Relaxes the soft tissue, increases circulation |
|  | Apply an anti-inflammatory medication |
| Iontophoresis | Apply an anti-inflammatory medication to deep tissue |
| Vapocoolant spray | Stretches soft tissue, decreases referred pain |

| PROCEDURE | RATIONALE FOR APPLICATION |
|---|---|
| Intraoral massage | Relaxes soft tissue |
| Mobilization to the mandible | Stretches soft tissue of the joint capsule and muscles of mastication |
|   Distraction | |
|   Protrusion | |
|   Lateral tilt | |
| Self-mobilization | Application of Therabite (Fig. 1–91) or tongue blades (Fig. 1–92) |
| | Bidigital mandibular (Fig. 1–93) stretching of soft tissue |
| Contract-relax exercises | Stretching of soft tissue |
| Isometric exercises | Prolonged stretch of muscles of mastication |

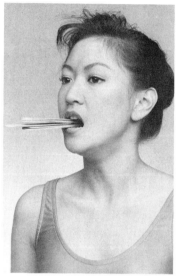

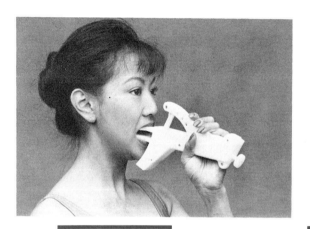

**FIGURE 1–91** ■ Application of Therabite.

**FIGURE 1–92** ■ Application of tongue blades.

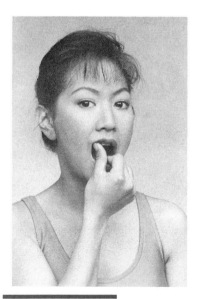

**FIGURE 1–93** ■ Bidigital self-mobilization.

## *Hypermobile Temporomandibular Joint*

| MODALITY | RATIONALE FOR APPLICATION |
|---|---|
| Not appropriate for this symptom. Apply modalities for concomitant symptoms. | |

| PROCEDURE | RATIONALE FOR APPLICATION |
|---|---|
| Limited range of motion | Limit opening to rotation (allow patient to open only as wide as possible while leaving the tip of the tongue on the hard palate). |
| Isometric exercises | Re-educate the muscles of mastication to synchronous function and reduced opening (Fig. 1–94) |
| Mandibular midline exercises | Restore synchronous function to muscles of mastication |
| Head and neck posture re-education exercises | Stretch contracted small neck extensors and relax taut muscles of anterior neck and shoulder triangles. |

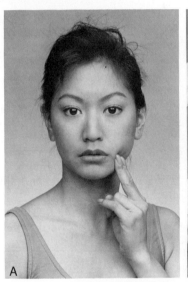
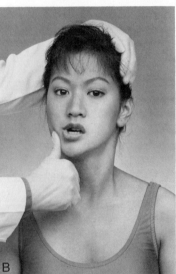

**FIGURE 1–94** ■ Isometric mandibular exercises.

can be ameliorated with the use of cold thermal agents after the treatment.

If a therapist diagnoses hypomobility of the left C5-6 facet joint, treatment should be directed at that problem; the therapist has no justification for treating the patient with hot packs and sensory-level electrical stimulation. This is not to be construed as an indictment of modalities; each physical agent has physical effects that should be used to evoke physiologic responses. As long as the therapist has a hypothesis about the patient's problem which indicates that certain modalities might be helpful, they should be included in the treatment plan.

## PHYSICAL THERAPY FOR THE ORAL SURGERY PATIENT

Pre- and postoperative physical therapies are essential components of a comprehensive program for treating temporomandibular joint dysfunction. The first phase, preoperative care, consists of teaching the patient about temporomandibular joint dysfunction and about posture; the latter phase, postoperative care, is discussed in the next section.

## Preoperative Physical Therapy

1. Initiate the patient-therapist relationship.
2. Conduct postural, functional, and objective musculoskeletal evaluation of the face, neck, and upper quadrant.
3. Discuss mandibular and postural re-education exercises.
4. Perform soft tissue stretching of the structure of the face, neck, and upper quadrant, if needed.
5. If the patient can attend more than one preoperative session, treat the soft tissue. Pain, swelling, and muscle spasm should be reduced and exercises should be performed to improve temporomandibular joint synchronous function and head and neck posture.

## Postoperative Physical Therapy

Postoperative rehabilitation can take up to 6 months or a year. Initially, during the acute inflammatory phase from 0 to 72 hours, the therapist can overtreat and irritate the patient's condition as easily as treat it effectively. Therefore, the practitioner must develop good rapport and communication with the patient to ensure effective feedback regarding treatment and healing. The patient is truly the expert regarding symptoms; this information is essential for modification of the treatment protocol. Involvement of the patient ensures compliance because the patient acts as a copractitioner, an active not passive participant.

1. Establish postoperative joint integrity status and rehabilitation goals with the oral surgeon.
2. Conduct a postoperative evaluation of mandibular and head and neck postural relationships.
3. Apply modalities and procedures to reduce pain, swelling, or muscle spasm of scarred or contracted tissue.
4. Limit mandibular opening to that which allows the patient to leave the tongue on the hard palate. This limits the patient to rotation only in the joint, a noncompressive force.
5. Limit lateral deviation to 5 mm on the side opposite the surgery (Fig. 1–95).
6. Limit the patient to a soft diet for up to 3 months, depending on the extent of surgery and possible scar tissue growth.

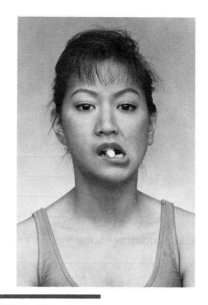

FIGURE 1–95 ■ Lateral deviation of the mandible.

7. Educate the patient in restoration of retracted head on neck posture, midline mandibular function, and limiting activities of daily living that promote forward head posture.
8. Encourage the patient to maintain the tongue on the hard palate and the teeth separated in the freeway space.
9. Instruct the patient in decreasing tongue thrust, if present, and teach the patient swallowing exercises.
10. Encourage the patient to apply home palliative techniques to decrease any postoperative pain:

Application of cold, progressing to heat
Posture modification
Self-mobilization
Stimulation of face acupuncture points
Application of transcutaneous electrical nerve stimulator (TENS), if appropriate

## Follow-up Office Visits

Frequency of office visits depends on treatment goals and extent of rapport with the patient. If the patient is compliant with prescribed home exercises and modification of activities of daily living, the frequency of visits can be based on treatment goals. If the patient is not consistently compliant, treatment sessions may have to be scheduled more frequently to guide healing of

# EXAMPLE OF POSTARTHROSCOPIC TREATMENT REGIMEN

## Preoperative

Evaluation

       Posture
       Muscular status of face and upper quarter
         Strength
         Spasm
         Tenderness to palpation
       Temporomandibular joint
         Range of motion
         Function
         Parafunctional habits

Posture re-education
Introduction to exercise protocol
  Midline mandible

## Postoperative

Inflammatory phase (0 to 72 hours)

       Ice/cryotherapy to reduce edema
       Electric stimulation (TENS, microcurrent) to reduce pain
       Soft tissue massage to relax tissue
       Iontophoresis or phonophoresis to reduce local inflammatory reactions
       Limit range of motion to rotation, avoid translation
       Postural activities
       Neuromuscular techniques

Repair phase (72 hours to 6 weeks)

       Add lateral excursion to limit adhesion formation
         To side opposite surgery to 5 mm
         To side of surgery beyond 5 mm (to 8 to 10 mm)
       Add long axis distraction
         Manual—in pain-free range
         Self-distraction—home program
         1. Bidigital
         2. Tongue blades
       Neuromuscular techniques
         Add contract-relax to increase range of motion
         Add isometrics to re-educate soft tissue environment, restore muscular synchrony
       Modify modalities as needed
       Limit parafunctional habits

Restore function (beyond 6 weeks)

Periodic physical therapy to:

Re-evaluate temporomandibular joint muscular status
Note and reduce muscle spasm
Modalities to decrease pain as appropriate
Isometric exercise to decrease any edema
Maintain range of motion
    Exercises—contract-relax
    Mobilization
    Progress 2 to 3 mm/week to maximum of 40 mm (if cannot open beyond 30 mm, add protrusion)
Modify diet from soft nonchewy to soft chewy to firmer chewing
Monitor neuromuscular re-education
Possible addition of functional distraction appliance (FDA)—worn at night, 2 to 3 hours in day
    Spring force at rear molars to apply slight mandibular head distraction.
May need occlusal splint to maintain relationship between mandible and maxilla

(Data from Rocabado M, Iglarsh ZA: Musculoskeletal Approach to Maxillofacial Pain. Philadelphia: JB Lippincott, 1992, p 47.)

tissue post surgery. Visits can be scheduled three times a week to allow the patient's tissue to heal between sessions, unless the soft tissue is so painful that the patient needs daily treatment to reduce severe pain and spasm. Range-of-motion activities may also have to be performed in the clinic daily if progress is slow or if the patient is not effective in self-mobilization.

As progress levels off and the patient appears to be doing the exercises consistently at home, the frequency of visits can be decreased; the patient can be weaned to once a week or even once a month. These sessions over longer intervals can be scheduled to re-evaluate the patient and revise the home exercises accordingly. The practitioner should document these less frequent visits objectively to substantiate the necessity of care. An example of a postarthroscopic treatment regimen follows.

It is essential that the practitioner communicate with the referring dentist to coordinate treatment plans. If the patient was not referred to you by a dentist, ask the patient's permission to contact his or her family dentist. This practitioner can give the therapist the patient's dental history and serve as a referral for splint fabrication or a more detailed dental evaluation. Treatment plans in dentistry and physical therapy should be coordinated to sequence interventions more effectively.

The patient should be treated by the therapist to reduce pain and soft tissue tightness before a dental procedure that requires increased mandibular depression, and pain and swelling reduction modalities and procedures should be applied by the therapist after a painful dental session. Another example of coordinated scheduling is that bite guards need repeated modification as the therapist reduces the patient's forward head posture and indirectly alters the patient's occlusion.

## SUMMARY

The physical therapist should seek further knowledge about dental and medical visualization procedures, oral and cervical surgery, and splint therapy to complement the information in this chapter. This information should include in great detail the specific structural changes associated with specific types of temporomandibular joint and cervical dysfunction, soft tissue and bone tissue operative changes, and the impact of splint therapy on occlusion and soft tissue. The therapist should acquire dental terminology to enable the therapist, dentists, and physicians to communicate more effectively with patients about the team approach to their care.

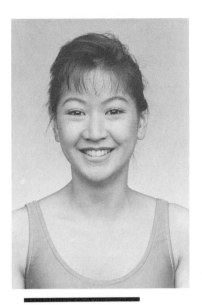

**FIGURE 1–96** ■ Goals achieved.

Temporomandibular joint and cervical patients do require a team approach to their complex problem. The dentist is often the case manager, primary referrer, and splint fabricator. The oral surgeon or orthopaedist may be the case manager or simply a consultant providing a second opinion on the conservative, soft tissue approach to treatment. The ear, nose, and throat specialist rules out or treats sinus and ear problems and the ophthalmologist rules out vision changes. The neurologist evaluates and treats headaches or radiating pain. The psychologist or psychiatrist helps the patient identify and cope with stressors and may reduce stress and muscle spasm with biofeedback. The final member of the team, the physical therapist, treats the musculoskeletal and postural components of the patient with temporomandibular joint and cervical spine pain and dysfunction. These components are often the most debilitating and affect most significantly the patient's ability to function in the activities of daily living.

Physical therapists can treat patients with temporomandibular joint and cervical spine dysfunction effectively if they can interpret the displayed pathokinematics, identify the objective characteristics of the symptoms, formulate a precise differential diagnosis, plan a symptom-specific treatment regimen based on objective goals, implement the regimen in response to the patient's reaction to treatment, and reassess the patient in terms of the objective goals, modifying the regimen accordingly. The primary treatment goal is

to increase the patient's function. If pain or discomfort is lowered to a level that the patient can control or handle with home treatment techniques, function increases; thus treatment goals are achieved (Fig. 1–96.).

## CASE STUDY 1

▼ Mrs. B. is a 43-year-old woman who does child care in her home. She was referred for physical therapy 10 days after an artificial disc was inserted into the left temporomandibular joint and an open joint lavage and condylar remodeling was performed on the right temporomandibular joint.

Approximately 5 years before, Mrs. B. fell on a cement pavement during an ice storm. She fractured her mandible along both rami and was fixated for several weeks. Upon removal of the wires she noted severe bilateral ear pain and temporal headaches. Her pain increased with chewing and prolonged talking and decreased, but did not disappear, with heat and rest.

She has been treated intermittently with pain medication, muscle relaxants, and mouth splints. Because these conservative approaches have not been effective in the long term, she agreed to undergo surgery.

Her immediate postoperative course was normal with no excessive swelling or pain noted. In the 10 days since the surgery she states that her pain has decreased from 10 of 10 to 6 of 10 on a pain scale. She is receiving a liquid diet. Mrs. B. sleeps fairly well with the assistance of her pain medication.

She presents with headaches, temporomandibular joint pain, and decreased motion in the temporomandibular joint as her chief complaints. Her posture evaluation reveals a decreased lordotic curve and moderately forward head. She is extremely thin, which she attributes to her long-standing pain upon chewing.

Her cervical range of motion is normal but some painful tightness is noted with overpressure at the end of the range. Temporomandibular joint range-of-motion values are 20 mm of opening and 3 mm right and 4 mm left lateral deviation. Upon opening, the mandible deviates to the left. There is no weakness of the muscles of mastication and muscles of facial expression. She has a functional upper lip of normal length. There are no audible joint sounds.

Palpation reveals significant swelling in the oral mucosa bilaterally. Trigger points are palpable in the masseter muscles, medial pterygoid muscle, and superior mucosa over the buccinator muscles, all bilaterally. The lateral and medial pterygoid muscles, temporalis insertion, transverse process of the first cervical vertebra, and preauricular soft tissue are all tender to palpation bilaterally.

The treatment goals for this case were as follows:

1. Eliminate internal mucosal swelling and trigger points.
2. Decrease pain to 0 to 2 of 10 in all activities of daily living and chewing of semisolid foods.

3. Increase temporomandibular joint range of motion to 38 to 42 mm in opening and 9 to 10 mm bilaterally in lateral deviation.

4. Institute synchronous function of muscles of mastication to permit opening and closing in midline.

The treatment protocol in this case was as follows:

1. Moist heat and electric stimulation of the facial muscles with bilateral electrode placement over the inferior zygomatic arch trigger points and anterior to the tragus of the ear. These modalities decrease pain, relax the patient, and possibly reduce swelling.

2. Ultrasound at 0.75 w/cm$^2$ with a 10% hydrocortisone coupling agent to the preauricular soft tissue for 5 min to 8 min to each point. This modality warms the soft tissue and relaxes the muscle spasm. The hydrocortisone decreases a local inflammatory reaction. This modality will be discontinued if patient experiences rebound pain.

3. Oral massage to the internal oral mucosa, using gentle circular strokes to decrease swelling and trigger points.

4. Self-stretching performed by the patient. The patient could use the bidigital technique and/or tongue blade or Therabite device. The stretching should be performed into the stretching range and not significantly into the painful range of motion. The patient can use moist heat after stretching. Bidigital stretching can be done every 2 to 3 hours (5 to 10 repetitions) if it is not painful, and tongue blade or Therabite stretching can be done two or three times per day for 15 minutes to each side. For the first 2 to 3 weeks the patient may be limited to the degree of opening that keeps the tongue in contact with the hard palate.

5. Lateral deviation should be emphasized, using a surgical tube or dental cotton roll as a pivot. The patient should seek to attain 5 mm to each side because surgery involved both joints. Lateral deviation may promote improved synovial fluid motion, promote healing, and reduce fibrous adhesion formation.

6. Active exercise should be performed in front of a mirror to encourage visual feedback for re-education of the muscles of mastication. Gentle placement of fingers on the mandible may give proprioceptive feedback.

7. Contract-relax exercises of the muscles of mastication can also be part of the home program. These exercises reduce muscle spasm and increase range of motion.

8. The patient should be instructed in postural exercises including head retraction and strengthening of the neck extensors.

9. Cervical range-of-motion exercises may relieve tightness and pain at the end of the range of motion.

Treatment continued until goals were met. The patient was seen three times a week for 3 weeks, twice a week for 3 weeks, and once a week for 2 weeks. The patient was then seen only as needed for the next 2 to 3 months. The patient progressed and appeared pleased with the results. Unfortunately, the patient returned for a re-evaluation after 8 months complaining of returning headaches, ear pain, and facial pain. Joint motions were more painful and angular and produced joint sounds bilaterally. Magnetic resonance imaging revealed osteophyte formation on the right and a torn artificial disc on the left. A second surgery was planned for osteophyte and artificial disc removal.

## CASE STUDY 2

▼Mr. A. was injured in an auto accident 30 days ago. This 50-year-old salesman complains of headaches that begin at the base of his head and of limited neck motion. The headaches radiate to the temporal region bilaterally.

Mr. A. rates his pain as 7 to 8 of 10 today but 10 of 10 at its worst. The pain is severe upon rising, decreases after a hot shower, and then increases by the end of the day. He has increased pain after driving, reading, and using his computer. He has found that rest, moist heat, and medication reduce his pain to 4 of 10. Mr. A. also reports that he had similar problems after an auto accident 3 years ago. These symptoms resolved completely with a 6-week course of physical therapy.

Upon examination, Mr. A. presents with a forward head and shoulder posture. Cervical spine motion is limited in rotation (left) and side tilt (right). Both forward flexion and extension are within normal limits but extension is painful. Both active and resistive motions of the head and neck are painful. Upper extremity motion is full and pain free.

C-1 is rotated to the right and testing of C-3 reveals a positive spring test with a hard end feel. The patient reports that the pain radiates from the posterior occiput to both temporalis muscles and to the right upper trapezius but sensation is intact (patient reports no neurologic symptoms radiating to extremities.)

Temporomandibular joint evaluation reveals no joint sounds upon opening and closing, but there is a slight deviation of the mandible to the left. The muscles of mastication are mildly tender on the left but range of motion is 42 mm of opening, 10 mm of lateral deviation to the right, and 12 mm to the left.

Trigger points are not palpable in the muscles of mastication but are found in the muscle belly and insertion of the left temporalis muscle. Trigger points and muscle spasms are palpable in the posterior occiput. The rhomboid muscles on the right are in moderate spasm and are tender to palpation.

The treatment goals for this case were as follows:

1. Decrease pain to 0 to 2 of 10 in all activities of daily living.

2. Eliminate muscle spasms in the left temporalis, right upper trapezius, and right rhomboid muscles.

3. Restore posture to head on neck and shoulders retracted.

4. Derotate C-2 and restore C-3 to its normal position with normal soft tissue tests and end feel.

5. Restore cervical spine motion in rotation on left and side tilt on right to be equal to those on the contralateral side with a 0 to 2 of 10 level of pain.

6. Restore synchronous function of the temporomandibular joint.

The treatment protocol in this case was as follows:

1. Moist heat and electric stimulation to posterior occiput and right upper trapezius. These modalities decrease pain and relax the patient.

2. Ultrasound to be added with 10% hydrocortisone if other modalities do not decrease pain in two or three sessions.

3. Instruction of the patient in posture exercises and strengthening of posterior musculature of cervical spine and scapular abductors (when rhomboid pain and spasm are reduced).

4. Massage of posterior occiput and right upper quadrant to relax the soft tissue.

5. Use of indirect mobilization techniques to restore C-1 and C-3 to their normal positions.

6. If trigger points persist, use of spray and stretching and/or iontophoresis with dexamethasone and lidocaine.

7. Instruction of patient in self-care for the temporomandibular joint (midline mandible exercises and application of heat or cold).

8. Instruction of the patient in active range-of-motion exercises of cervical spine with towel used to stabilize the first rib.

9. Discussion and modification of the patient's driving and sleeping posture.

10. Institution of an upper quadrant conditioning program using hydrofitness, upper body ergometry, upper extremity progressive resistive exercises, and modified cervical resistance if tolerated.

11. Instruction of patient in a general conditioning exercise program that does not promote forward head motion.

The patient was seen three times a week for 2 weeks, twice a week for 2 weeks, and once a week for 2 weeks. The patient responded to treatment well as modalities were gradually reduced after the first 2 weeks and emphasis was placed on postural and conditioning exercises. By the end of the sixth week all treatment goals were met with only slight pain (2 of 10) noted at the end of the range of cervical motion in rotation left and side tilt right. Despite excellent recovery, the patient was asked to continue his exercises and to contact the therapist to modify the exercise program as needed or if his musculoskeletal status regressed.

## REFERENCES

1. Von Korff M, Dworkin SF, LeResche L, et al: An epidemiologic comparison of pain complaints. Pain 32:173–183, 1988.
2. Erhard RE, Bowling RW: Management of Low Back and Sciatic Pain. New York: Churchill-Livingstone (in press).
3. Maitland GD: Vertebral Manipulation 5th ed. Boston: Butterworth, 1986.
4. McKenzie RA: The Lumbar Spine. Lower Hutt, NZ: Spinal Publications, 1981.
5. Haldeman S: Failure of the pathology model to predict low back pain. Spine 15:718–724, 1990.
6. Hiatt JL, Gartner LP: Textbook of Head and Neck Anatomy. New York: Appleton-Century-Crofts, 1982, p 73.
7. Hertling D, Kessler RM: Management of Common Musculoskeletal Disorders, 2nd ed. JB Lippincott, Philadelphia: JB Lippincott, 1990, p 496.
8. Weinberg LA, Chastin JK: New TMJ clinical data and the implication on diagnosis and treatment. J Am Dent Assoc 120:305–311, 1990.
9. Rocabado M, Iglarsh ZA: The Musculoskeletal Approach to Maxillofacial Pain. Philadelphia: JB Lippincott, 1991, p 47.
10. Kendall F, McCreary E: Muscle Testing and Function, 3rd ed. Baltimore: Williams & Wilkins, 1983.
11. Williams PL, Warwick R, eds: Gray's Anatomy, 36th British ed. Edinburgh: Churchill-Livingstone, 1980.
12. White AA, Panjabi MM: Clinical Biomechanics of the Spine. Philadelphia: JB Lippincott, 1975.
13. White AA: Biomechanical analysis of clinical stability in the cervical spine. Clin Orthop 109:85–96, 1975.
14. Dworkin et al: Epidemiology of signs and symptoms in temporomandibular disorders: clinical signs in cases and controls. J Am Dent Assoc 120:273–281, 1990.
15. Kapandj IA: The physiology of the joints. In The Trunk and the Vertebral Columns, Vol. 3. New York: Churchill-Livingstone, 1974.
16. White AA, Panjabi MM: Clinical Biomechanics of the Spine Philadelphia: JB Lippincott, 1975.
17. Holmes TH: The social readjustment rating scale. J Psychosom Res 11:213–218, 1967.
18. Edeling J: Manual Therapy for Chronic Headaches. London: Butterworth, 1988.
19. Echternach JL, Rothstein JM: Hypothesis-oriented algorithms. Phys Ther 69:559–561, 1989.
20. Tanaka T: Recognition of the pain formula for head, neck, and TMJ disorders: the general physical examination. Calif Dent Assoc J May 4:3–9, 1984.
21. Kendall FO, Kendall FP, Boynton DA: Posture and Pain Baltimore: Williams & Wilkins, 1952.
22. Hoppenfeld S: Physical Examination of the Spine and Extremities. New York: Appleton-Century-Crofts, 1976.
23. Clarkson HM, Gilewich GB: Musculoskeletal Assessment: Joint Range of Motion and Manual Muscle Strength. Baltimore: Williams & Wilkins 1989.
24. Kimura J: Electrodiagnosis in Diseases of Nerve and Muscle. Philadelphia: FA Davis, 1983.
25. Cyriax J: Textbook of Orthopaedic Medicine, Vol. 1, 8th ed. London, Bailliere Tindall, 1982.
26. Sapega AA: Muscle performance evaluation in orthopaedic practice. J Bone Joint Surg [Am] 72:1562–1572, 1990.
27. Magee D: Orthopedic Physical Assessment, 2nd ed. Philadelphia: WB Saunders, 1987.
28. Travell J: Myofascial Pain and Dysfunction: The Trigger Point Manual. Baltimore: Williams & Wilkins, 1983, Part 1, p 165.
29. Zarmen A, Bigelow WC, McCoy JM, et al: "Eagle's syndrome: a comparison of intraoral versus extraoral surgical approaches. Oral Surg Oral Med Oral Pathol 62:625–629, 1986.
30. Jaeger B, Singer E, Kroening R: Reflex sympathetic dystrophy of the face. Arch Neurol 43:693–695, 1986.

31. Gelb H: Clinical Management of Head, Neck, and TMJ Pain and Dysfunction. Philadelphia: WB Saunders, 1977.

32. Parker MW: A Dynamic Model of Etiology in Temporomandibular Disorders. J Am Dent Assoc 120:283–290, 1990.

33. Michlovtz S: Thermal Agents in Rehabilitation, 2nd ed. Philadelphia: FA Davis, 1990.

34. Snyder-Mackler L, Robinson AJ: Electrophysiology: Electrotherapy and Testing Procedures, Baltimore: Williams & Wilkins, 1989.

35. Kisner C, Kolby LA: Therapeutic Exercise: Foundations and Techniques, 2nd ed. Philadelphia: FA Davis, 1990.

36. Maitland GD: Vertebral Manipulation, 5th ed. Boston: Butterworth, 1986.

37. Rocabado M: Facial and oral pain. J Craniomandib Dis 3:75–82, 1989.

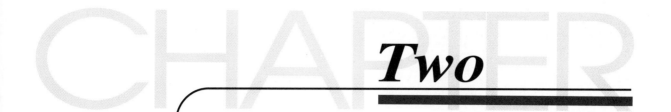

# Two

# Thoracic Spine

## RICHARD W. BOWLING / PAUL ROCKAR

## INTRODUCTION

The realm of physical therapy for the thoracic spine, as for other regions, encompasses recognizing and managing movement dysfunction. Pathologies of the musculoskeletal and other systems give rise to symptoms in the thoracic region. Many of these are not amenable to physical therapy management, however, and the practitioner must be adept at identifying the need for referral to other disciplines. In order to accomplish this, the physical therapist must have knowledge and skills in differential diagnosis. Practitioners must be able to distinguish between movement disorders that can be managed and those that cannot be managed with physical therapy intervention. In addition, they must be able to identify symptoms arising from other systems that mimic pathologies of musculoskeletal dysfunction.

Information pertaining to pathology and dif-ferential diagnosis of medical conditions is available from other sources.[1,2] This chapter provides only a brief overview with selected references to these topics. The focus of this chapter is on identifying and managing movement disorders of the thoracic spine.

## ANATOMY AND MECHANICS

### Osteology

There are 12 thoracic vertebrae (Figs. 2–1 and 2–2). The mass of the bodies of the thoracic vertebrae increases from T-1 through T-12. In addition to changes in size, the bodies change in shape, with the upper thoracic vertebrae resembling cervical vertebrae and the lower thoracic vertebrae appearing more similar to lumbar vertebrae. Similarly, the contour of the spinal canal

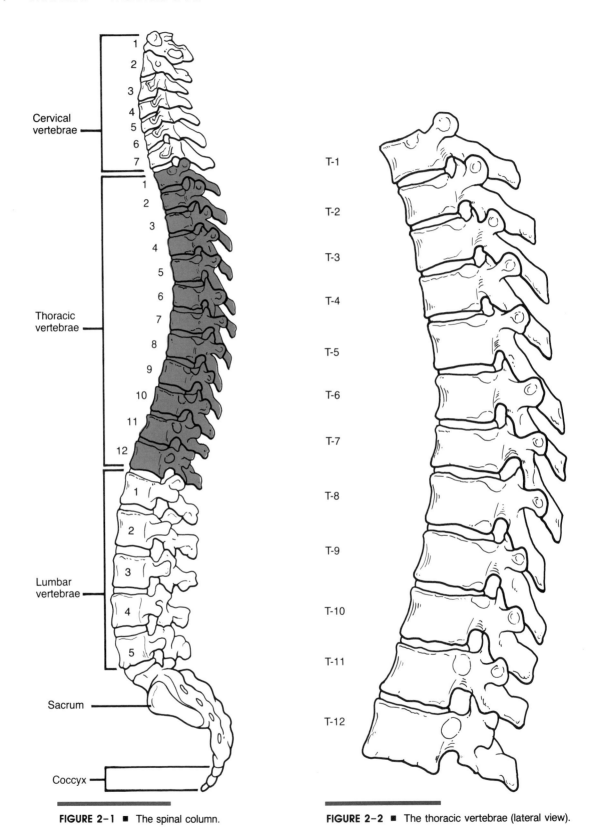

**FIGURE 2-1** ■ The spinal column.

**FIGURE 2-2** ■ The thoracic vertebrae (lateral view).

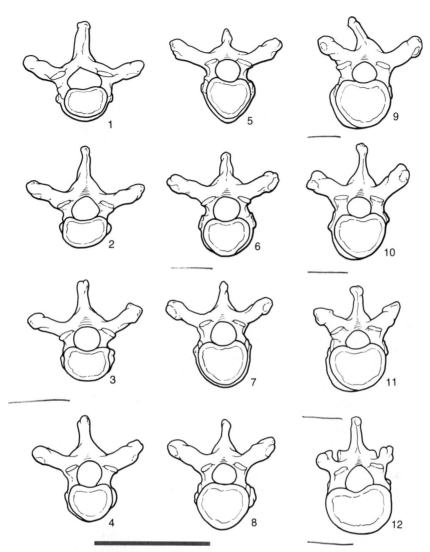

**FIGURE 2-3** ■ The thoracic spine (superior view).

changes from an oval orientation in the upper extent to trefoil in the lower thoracic region (Figs. 2–3 and 2–4).

Transitional changes are also evident in the transverse, spinous, and articular processes. The transverse processes can be seen to diminish in spread from T-1 through T-12, where the processes are short and blunt and resemble those of an upper lumbar vertebra. The orientation of the thoracic spinous processes varies from one region to another.[3] In the upper fourth of the thoracic spinal column (T1–3), the tip of the spinous process lies in the same transverse plane as the corresponding body and transverse processes. In the next region of the thoracic spinal column (T4–6) the tip of the spinous process lies in a transverse plane that passes between the corresponding body and transverse processes and those of the vertebrae below. The third region contains T-7 through T-9. Here the tip of the spinous process lies in the same transverse plane as the body and tips of the transverse processes of the lower vertebrae. The lowest region (T10–12) vertebrae with characteristics of all of the foregoing groups. The spinous process of T-10 is one level below the body, that of T-11 is half the distance of the vertebrae below, and the spinous process of T-12 is located at the same level (see Figs. 2–3 and 2–4).

The orientation of the articular processes in the

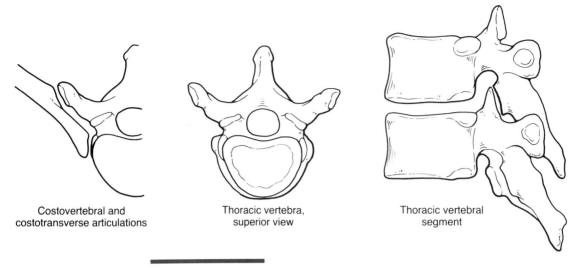

Costovertebral and
costotransverse articulations

Thoracic vertebra,
superior view

Thoracic vertebral
segment

**FIGURE 2-4** ■ Distinguishing features of the thoracic spine.

upper thoracic region resembles that of a lower cervical vertebra in that the superior articular surfaces are directed posteriorly and superiorly. The remaining articular surfaces face posteriorly and laterally, with the exception of those located on the inferior articular processes of T-12. These are directed in a lateral direction (see Figs. 2–3 and 2–4).

There are 12 pairs of ribs that articulate posteriorly with the thoracic vertebrae. The upper 10 pairs are also connected anteriorly with the sternum via the costal cartilages. The lower two pairs have no anterior attachment. (Fig. 2–5)

## BIOMECHANICS

Motion of the spine represents a summation of the movements that occur in all of the functional units. In order to develop an understanding of motion of the spinal column as a whole, the physical therapist must first comprehend motion of the basic unit or segment.

## Vertebral Motion Segment — Arthrokinematics

The term **joint motion** or **arthrokinematics** refers to the movement of one joint surface in relation to another. The arthrokinematics of a joint are governed by the shape of the articular surfaces and by the soft tissues that limit or restrain motion.

The functional spinal unit consists of two vertebrae and the intervening soft tissues. Each vertebral segment is a three-joint complex: (1) a fibrous joint between the vertebral bodies formed by the intervertebral disc and (2 and 3) the paired, synovial, facet or apophyseal joints.

The fibrous intervertebral joint is a symphysis and, if capable of moving independently of the other joints in the segment, would be multiaxial. However, the symphysis is coupled functionally to the facet joints. At each region of the spine, the facet joints by orientation control the motion permitted in the region. Thus, the symphysis permits segmental motion while the facets control or direct movements.

A typical spinal joint has three degrees of freedom. The motions of flexion and extension occur in the sagittal plane, lateral flexion or lateral bend is permitted in the frontal plane, and rotation occurs in the transverse plane. During flexion, the disc is compressed anteriorly and both facet joints glide in a cranial direction. The converse occurs with extension, allowing the posterior aspect of the disc to be compressed as the superior facets glide caudally.

The motion of lateral flexion is permitted in the frontal plane. During this motion, the disc is compressed on the side of the concavity created by the movement. The facet joint on the side of the concavity glides in an inferior or caudal direction while the contralateral joint glides in a superior or cranial direction.

Rotation occurs in the transverse plane about an axis that lies in the frontal and sagittal planes.

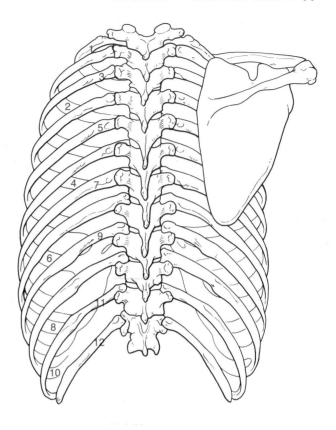

**FIGURE 2-5** ■ The thorax.

The disc undergoes torsion while both facet joints glide in the direction opposite the rotation of the vertebral body.

Kapandji states that flexion and extension are "pure movements" that can occur independently of the other motions.[4] There appears to be minimal agreement regarding the nature of rotation and side bending. It has been said that these movements are "coupled." That is, neither can occur in the absence of the other. This confusion appears to have arisen from inconsistent usage of the terms arthrokinematic (referring to movement of joints) and osteokinematic (referring to movement of bones).

It has been observed that single-plane joint motion may produce a displacement of vertebra in two cardinal body planes. If this were the only consideration, the analysis of lumbar and thoracic motion would not be difficult. However, these joints are components of an articular system. The position of an individual joint axis in space is influenced by the position of the joints that are situated inferiorly. That is, as the joints distal to a given segment move, the axis of the joint in question is repositioned in space. The resulting motion produced when that segment moves is different than that produced when the distal joints are in the resting or neutral position.

For example, the position of the axis of side bending of L-1 is altered by concomitant side bending of all of the lumbar joints situated inferior to it. The motion in space of the L-1 vertebra is changed because of this phenomenon. The vertebral motion is altered because of the change of the position of the joint axis in space and not because of a change in arthrokinematics. The joint motion occurs at a right angle to the axis of motion regardless to the position of the axis.

The vertebrae in the motion segment are connected by ligaments and by muscles (Figs. 2–6 to 2–11). These soft tissue structures are instrumental to normal motion of the spinal unit. The ligament functions to restrain motion of the joint, and there is an optimal ligament length for this purpose. If the ligament becomes too short, motion is abnormally restrained and the clinical condition of hypomobility results. If the ligament is too long, motion of the joint is excessive or the joint is hypermobile.

The function of the muscles at the segmental level is twofold. First, when the muscle functions in a concentric manner, motion is produced. Sec-

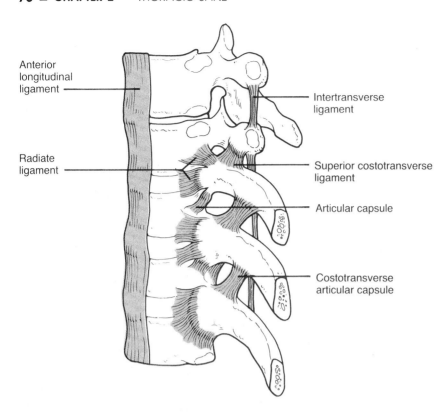

Anterior longitudinal ligament

Radiate ligament

Intertransverse ligament

Superior costotransverse ligament

Articular capsule

Costotransverse articular capsule

**FIGURE 2-6 ■** Costovertebral articulation and its ligamentous attachments.

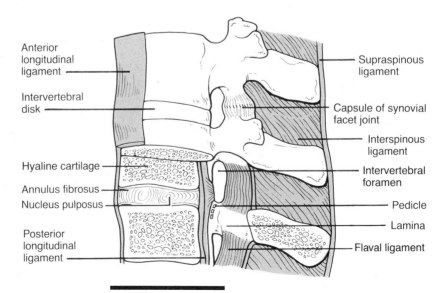

Anterior longitudinal ligament

Intervertebral disk

Hyaline cartilage

Annulus fibrosus

Nucleus pulposus

Posterior longitudinal ligament

Supraspinous ligament

Capsule of synovial facet joint

Interspinous ligament

Intervertebral foramen

Pedicle

Lamina

Flaval ligament

**FIGURE 2-7 ■** Ligaments of the spinal column.

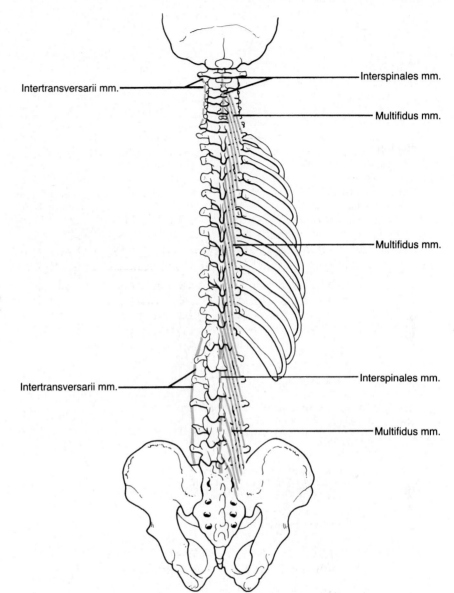

Intertransversarii mm.

Interspinales mm.

Multifidus mm.

Multifidus mm.

Interspinales mm.

Intertransversarii mm.

Multifidus mm.

**FIGURE 2–8** ■ Muscles of the spinal column, the multifidi, interspinales, and intertransversarii.

ond, eccentric contraction of the muscle retards or decelerates motion of the segment; for example, as the segment is undergoing flexion the movement is decelerated by the contraction of the extensor muscles of the segment. Insufficient deceleration function could result in increased stress on the posterior ligaments of the segment. This may lead to lengthening of these ligaments and ultimately instability. Alternatively, if the muscle is unable to lengthen sufficiently, motion of the segment is impeded, resulting in loss of range of motion. In summary, it is clear that a harmonious interaction between the ligaments

and muscles is essential for normal motion to occur at each segment.

## EVALUATION

Examination of the thoracic spine is rarely undertaken as an isolated procedure. More often than not, thoracic pain is a complication of a cervical and/or lumbar syndrome. Furthermore, the upper thoracic spine and upper ribs are functionally connected to the cervical spine, whereas the lower thoracic spine is best exam-

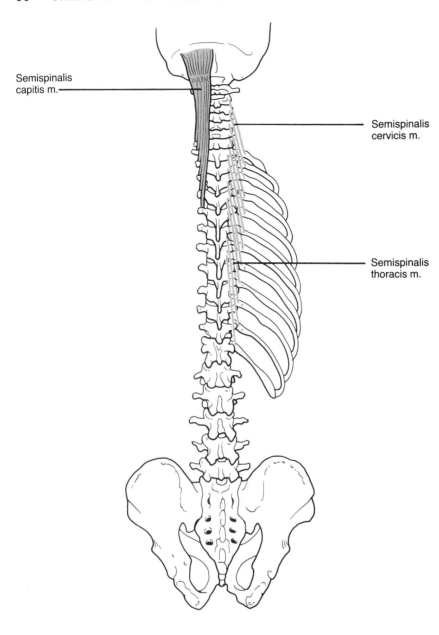

Semispinalis capitis m.

Semispinalis cervicis m.

Semispinalis thoracis m.

**FIGURE 2-9** ■ Muscle of the spinal column, the semispinalis.

ined with the lumbar region. Therefore, for clinical purposes, the thoracic region consists of vertebral levels T-3 to T-10 and the rib articulations.

## Subjective Evaluation

A thorough history of a patient with spinal pain is necessary to arrive at a tentative diagnosis. The information obtained from a carefully performed subjective examination is essential in formulating an objective examination scheme.

## Initial Observation

If feasible, the patient should be called from the reception area by the examiner. This provides the examiner with an opportunity to observe the skills of a few basic activities of daily living (sitting, standing, and walking) before the patient is placed in a formal examination setting. At times the patient's behavior is not consistent with that found upon performance of the objective examination. The examiner notes what resting position the patient has chosen in the waiting area. For example, if the patient is found standing in an uncrowded waiting area or has difficulty in rising

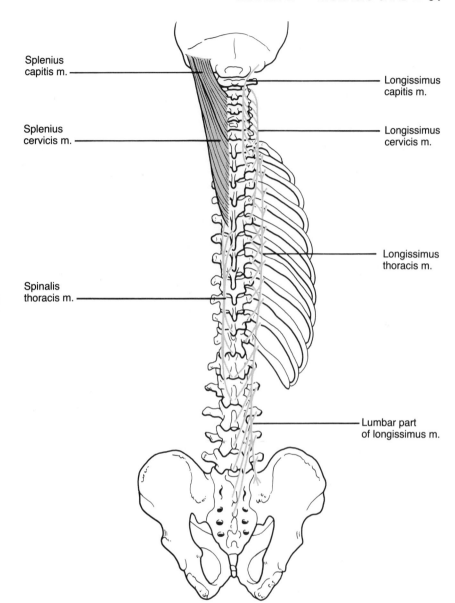

Splenius capitis m.

Splenius cervicis m.

Spinalis thoracis m.

Longissimus capitis m.

Longissimus cervicis m.

Longissimus thoracis m.

Lumbar part of longissimus m.

**FIGURE 2–10** ■ Muscles of the spinal column, the spinalis, splenius, and longissimus.

from the seated position, the patient's willingness or ability to sit is already determined. This information is correlated with the patient's account of what activities worsen or ease that status of the condition.

The patient's gait can also be observed while walking into the examination area. Pertinent to examination of the thoracic area is any evidence of a spastic or guarded gait pattern. This should lead the examiner to questions dealing with function of the central nervous system, such as the presence of bilateral paresthesias versus an abnormal gait pattern resulting from splinting secondary to muscular spasm.

Once in the examination area, the patient is again allowed to select the posture of choice for continuing the subjective examination. This simple procedure allows the examiner to formulate an initial impression of the nature and severity of the patient's problem.

## History

The goals of taking a history are to determine whether

■ The client is suitable for mechanical diagnosis
■ The individual has a mechanical problem, a nonmechanical problem, or both
■ The condition is acute or subacute
■ The physical examination can be performed vigorously or the examiner should proceed with caution

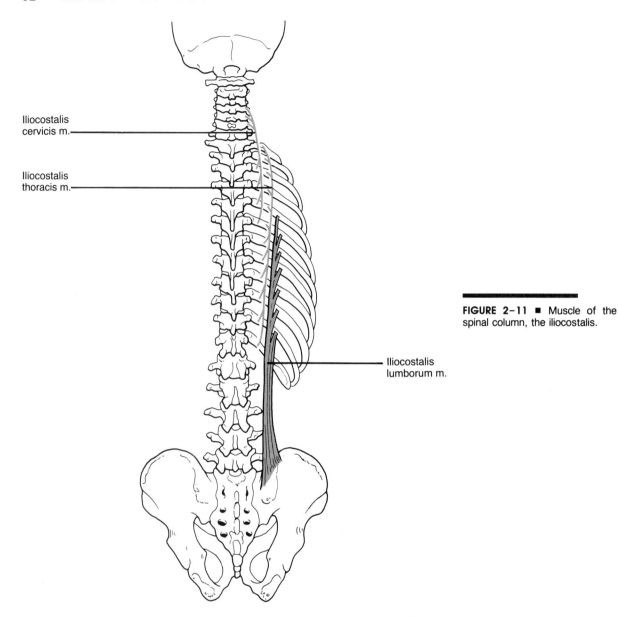

Iliocostalis
cervicis m.

Iliocostalis
thoracis m.

Iliocostalis
lumborum m.

**FIGURE 2–11** ■ Muscle of the spinal column, the iliocostalis.

## Current History

The examiner first determines the nature and location of the patient's present symptoms. The locations of pain, paresthesias, and anesthesia are recorded on a body diagram (Fig. 2–12)

The next query is directed at the patient's impressions of the cause of the problem. The response to this line of questioning falls into one of two categories:

■ The problem began for no apparent reason
■ The patient describes a specific activity during which the problem began

Subsequently, the examiner determines what ac-

tivity the patient was engaged in before the occurrence of symptoms. This may be difficult to determine when the patient is uncertain about the cause of the problem or when the onset was gradual. This line of questioning is pursued to ascertain whether the patient was involved with any activity or sustained posture before the precipitating event that may have predisposed to the onset of thoracic spinal pain. It is sometimes necessary for the examiner to direct the questioning to specific activities when the patient reports "not doing anything" before the onset of pain. Extensive sitting is often not perceived by the patient as an activity. One is most often searching for sustained flexed positions of the

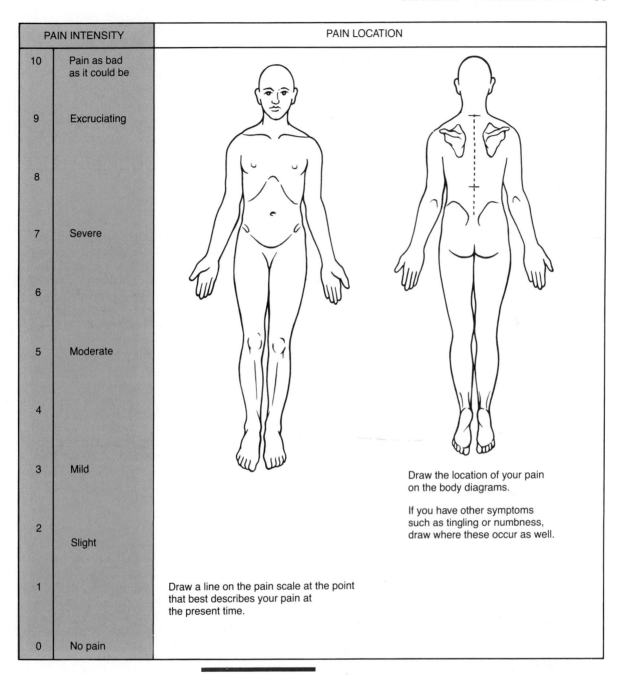

| PAIN INTENSITY | | PAIN LOCATION |
|---|---|---|
| 10 | Pain as bad as it could be | |
| 9 | Excruciating | |
| 8 | | |
| 7 | Severe | |
| 6 | | |
| 5 | Moderate | |
| 4 | | |
| 3 | Mild | |
| 2 | | |
| | Slight | |
| 1 | | |
| 0 | No pain | |

Draw the location of your pain on the body diagrams.

If you have other symptoms such as tingling or numbness, draw where these occur as well.

Draw a line on the pain scale at the point that best describes your pain at the present time.

**FIGURE 2-12** ■ Body diagram with pain scale.

thoracic spine such as may occur while working at a desk. For instance, a patient may ascribe the onset of symptoms to a trivial lifting incident while he or she was in a prolonged malaligned sitting posture just before the occurrence of "injury."

It is important to establish the type and location of symptoms at onset and to correlate these with symptoms at the time of subjective examination to determine whether the condition is static, improving, or worsening. The mode of onset of the symptoms must be investigated to determine whether there is a history of trauma and, if so, whether the symptoms occurred immediately or gradually after the incident. Likewise, if the onset had no apparent cause, the examiner must determine whether the symptoms developed rapidly or slowly.

The patient should also be questioned regarding previous treatment received for the current episode. This should include medications, bed rest, changes in work and activity status, previous mechanical interventions, and use of orthoses and assistive devices. Equally important is the assessment of the results of such treatment. When considering the outcome of a treatment, the examiner must endeavor to determine the patient's compliance with the treatment. The patient may proclaim that a medication prescribed by a physician was of no benefit in alleviating symptoms, but when the patient is asked if the medication was taken as prescribed, the answer is frequently negative.

### Determination of Suitability for Mechanical Diagnosis

The aim of this line of questioning is to resolve whether the patient has a mechanical pain syndrome that is appropriate for mechanical diagnosis and treatment. Of special interest is knowing whether the patient's symptoms are constant or intermittent. Mechanical pain is more often than not cyclic, whereas chemical pain or nonmechanical pain is consistent. Often a patient describes pain as constant when in fact it is not. Most of these individuals are not symptom magnifiers but are merely attempting to emphasize the intensity of symptoms or the severity of their situation to the examiner. Further questioning often discloses periods of time during which the individual is pain free. If the physical therapist determines that the pain is truly constant, it is important to know whether the intensity varies. Fluctuation of intensity may be related to activity, may reflect temporal variations, or both. If the intensity of symptoms varies with activity, a combination of mechanical and nonmechanical pain is possible.

The patient is next questioned regarding ability to sleep without disturbance. It has long been thought that sleep disturbances are indicators of serious pathology. This may or may not be the case and is related to the manner in which sleep is disturbed.

Sleep disturbance may be manifested in the following ways:

- ■ The individual may be unable to fall asleep because of the intensity of pain.
- ■ The individual may be awakened by pain that

has increased in intensity, often at a particular time.
- ■ The patient may report falling asleep, being awakened by pain during a movement such as turning, and then falling back to sleep.

The most troubling problem is that of the individual who is awakened by pain not related to posture or position. If the patient describes a sleep disturbance of this nature, serious pathology must be suspected.

### Special Questions

The examiner must determine the effects of deep respiration and of coughing or sneezing. Movement dysfunction of the rib articulations may be worsened with these activities. However, any acute condition may be aggravated by jarring associated with coughing or sneezing, and therefore this is not of any specific diagnostic import.

The patient is also questioned regarding any alteration in the function of the bladder or bowel with particular reference to incontinence or loss of sphincter control. In addition, questions should be directed to whether there are bilateral paresthesias in the lower extremities. If either of these symptoms is present, the patient's physician must be notified immediately. These may be indicators of a central disc protrusion with compression of the spinal cord.

The patient is questioned regarding any change in body weight. One must determine the extent and direction of the change, the reason for the change, and the time period over which the change has occurred. Unexplained (non-diet-related) weight losses in individuals who have probably been more sedentary than usual because of pain are of significance. Such weight loss must be recognized as a possible warning signal of medical pathology such as a carcinoma or diabetes.

### Radiologic Examination

If the patient has had a traumatic onset of pain or the pain is severe, an adequate radiologic examination should be performed. If this has been done, the examiner should at least obtain the report of these studies if the radiographs cannot be viewed. If x-ray studies have not been performed, the physician should be consulted to determine whether radiologic examination is appropriate.

## Previous Episodes

The patient is next questioned regarding previous episodes of back pain or related symptoms. Often, it is necessary to clarify what is meant by related symptoms. If the patient reports previous episodes of back pain or related symptoms, the location, pattern, and other characteristics of past symptoms should be identified. It is benefical to determine the location of symptoms in a chronologic manner from first episode to the current episode in an attempt to determine progression of the disorder. The patient is questioned about the number of past occurrences and whether the occurrences are becoming more or less frequent. Treatment and results of treatment should be recorded and analyzed.

## Aggravating and Easing Factors

Next, the examiner determines the general effects of activity on the patient's status. The patient is asked to rate whether activity makes the status better, worse, or unchanged. If the condition is unchanged by activity, nonmechanical causes may be suspected. When patients report that their condition is improved by activity, other possibilities should come to mind. Activity customarily aggravates mechanical pain and may frequently relieve pain of nonmechanical genesis. Conversely, rest usually relieves mechanical pain and aggravates nonmechanical pain. For example, thoracic pain of a mechanical nature is often relieved by rest in a reclining position. If a patient reports feeling worse after rest in bed and the posture for rest is not faulty, the physical therapist may suspect that a nonmechanical disorder such as ankylosing spondylitis is present. This inference would be supported if pain was relieved by movement.

It is also important to determine what activities the patient is engaged in on a day-to-day basis. This includes vocational and avocational pursuits. The examiner must determine whether the patient is required to lift and, if so, how much weight is lifted and how frequently. It may also be of benefit to identify the various positions utilized for lifting. The percentage of time spent lifting is compared to that spent sitting, walking, and standing.

## Provisional Diagnosis

If the goals of subjective examination have been met, the practitioner has determined whether additional examination of the patient is appropriate or a referral or consultation is required.

At this juncture in the examination process, the evaluator must formulate a hypothesis about the patient's condition based on responses to questions. The examiner now knows the following:

- What stage of the inflammatory process the patient is in at the moment
- Whether the problem is mechanical, nonmechanical, or a combination of both
- Whether a movement examination can be performed at this time
- If a movement test can be performed, whether caution is required to avoid exacerbation or the patient must be stressed to elicit the symptoms
- Whether a referral or consultation is required

## Objective Evaluation

### Lower Quarter Screening Examination

After the initial observation and history, a lower quarter screening examination is performed on patients who are suitable for mechanical evaluation. The screening examination allows the examiner to identify the area, or body region, of the problem so that the specific examination can be directed to the proper structure(s). It has been arranged to collect as much data as feasible in a short time with minimal stress to the client. The screening examination is ordered to allow a progression of test items from standing to sitting to supine to lying prone.

OBJECTIVES

- To identify the clients who are appropriate for movement testing
- To identify clients with a medical and/or surgical problem that may preclude further mechanical evaluation or treatment
- To identify patients who display nonorganic pain behavior
- To determine the stage of inflammation of the patient's condition
- To determine which areas or regions of the body require further examination and which can be ruled out or deferred for evaluation at a later time

The evaluation form used for this is illustrated in Figure 2–13.

LOWER QUARTER SCREENING EXAMINATION        Name:_____

| OBSERVATION OF STANDING POSTURE |
|---|

**Lordosis**
Increased ☐
Normal ☐
Reduced ☐

**Scoliosis**
Convex Rt ☐
Convex Lt ☐
Normal ☐

**Lateral Shift**
Right ☐
Left ☐
Normal ☐

**Lower Extrem.**
Feet ☐
  Pron Rt ☐
  Pron Lt ☐
Normal ☐

**Knees**
Lt Varus ☐
Valgus ☐
Normal ☐
Rt Varus ☐
Valgus ☐
Normal ☐

Flex ☐
Recurv ☐

Flex ☐
Recurv ☐

**Hips**
Lt Int Rot ☐
Ext Rot ☐
Normal ☐
Rt Int Rot ☐
Ext Rot ☐
Normal ☐

| HEEL/TOE WALKING |
|---|

**Heel Walk**    + Rt ☐
                 + Lt ☐
**Toe Walk**     + Rt ☐
                 + Lt ☐
**WNL**          ☐

| PELVIC LANDMARKS: Standing |
|---|

**Iliac Crest High**  Rt ☐      **Iliac Crest High**  Rt ☐
  (Posterior)  Lt ☐        (Anterior)  Lt ☐
             WNL ☐                   WNL ☐
**PSIS High**   Rt ☐      **ASIS High**   Rt ☐
                Lt ☐                      Lt ☐
              WNL ☐                     WNL ☐

| AXIAL LOADING | + ☐    − ☐ |
|---|---|

| TRUNK RANGE OF MOTION |
|---|

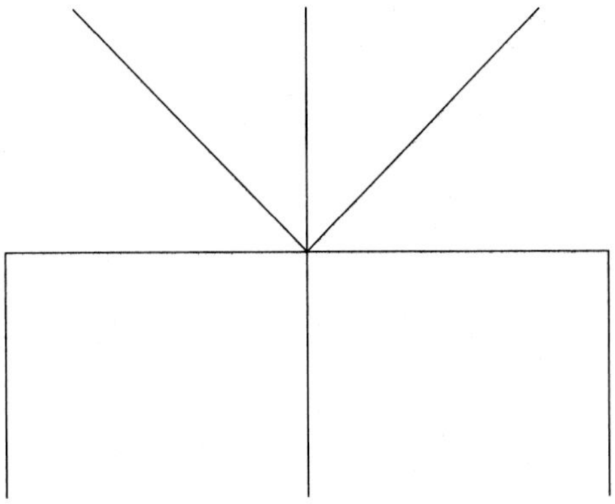

|      | INC | WOR | DEC | IMP | ISQ |
|------|-----|-----|-----|-----|-----|
| FB   |     |     |     |     |     |
| BB   |     |     |     |     |     |
| RSB  |     |     |     |     |     |
| LSB  |     |     |     |     |     |
| RPT  |     |     |     |     |     |
| LPT  |     |     |     |     |     |
| ERPT |     |     |     |     |     |
| ELPT |     |     |     |     |     |

| OBSERVATION OF GAIT |
|---|

_____

_____

_____

**FIGURE 2-13** ■ Lower quarter screening examination.

LOWER QUARTER SCREENING EXAMINATION        Name:_____

| LUMBAR PELVIC RHYTHM | STANDING FLEXION | ROTATION |
|---|---|---|

**LUMBAR PELVIC RHYTHM**

FLEXION     LUMBAR > = < PELVIC
EXTENSION   LUMBAR > = < PELVIC

**STANDING FLEXION**

RT  +     −
LT  +     −

**ROTATION**

POS  ☐
NEG  ☐

POSTERIOR SHEAR     POS ☐   NEG ☐     LEVEL:_____

## SITTING EXAMINATION

### OBSERVATION OF POSTURE

**Lordosis**
Increased  ☐
Normal     ☐
Reduced    ☐

### PELVIC LANDMARKS: Sitting

**Iliac Crest High**   Rt ☐       **Iliac Crest High**   Rt ☐
(Posterior)   Lt ☐          (Anterior)   Lt ☐
              WNL ☐                        WNL ☐
**PSIS High**   Rt ☐          **ASIS High**   Rt ☐
                Lt ☐                          Lt ☐
                WNL ☐                         WNL ☐

### SEATED FLEXION TEST

RT  +     −
LT  +     −

### MOTOR EXAMINATION

Seated ☐        MOTOR EXAMINATION        Supine ☐

| | | 5 | 4 | 3 | 2 | 1 | 0 | +/− |
|---|---|---|---|---|---|---|---|---|
| HIP FLEX | RT | | | | | | | |
| | LT | | | | | | | |
| KN EXT | RT | | | | | | | |
| | LT | | | | | | | |
| ANK DFL | RT | | | | | | | |
| | LT | | | | | | | |
| HAL EXT | RT | | | | | | | |
| | LT | | | | | | | |

### REFLEXES

| | ABS | CAPS | WNL |
|---|---|---|---|
| KJ  RT | | | |
| KJ  LT | | | |
| AJ  RT | | | |
| AJ  LT | | | |
| SEATED SLR    +    − | | | |
| REGION WEAK    +    − | | | |

MEDIAL HIP ROT          LT  > = <  RT

## SUPINE EXAMINATION

### STRAIGHT LEG RAISE

| | DEG | LBP | LEG | IPS | CON |
|---|---|---|---|---|---|
| RT | | | | | |
| LT | | | | | |

### DOUBLE SLR

DEGREES _____

MEDIAL HIP ROT

RT  > = <  LT

### HIP RANGE OF MOTION

| | FABR +/− | CAPS | NON CAPS | WNL | IMBAL |
|---|---|---|---|---|---|
| RT | | | | | |
| LT | | | | | |

**FIGURE 2-13** ■ *Continued*

*Illustration continued on following page*

LOWER QUARTER SCREENING EXAMINATION          Name:_____

### SENSORY EXAMINATION

|        | ABS | DIM | WNL |
|--------|-----|-----|-----|
| L-3    |     |     |     |
| L-4    |     |     |     |
| L-5    |     |     |     |
| S-1    |     |     |     |
| S-2    |     |     |     |
| S-4    |     |     |     |
| NONANATOMIC | + | − | |

### BABINSKI

| RT | + | − |
|----|---|---|
| LT | + | − |

### CLONUS

| RT | + | − |
|----|---|---|
| LT | + | − |

### PERIPHERAL PULSES

|              |    | PRES | ABS |
|--------------|----|------|-----|
| POST TIBIAL  | RT |      |     |
|              | LT |      |     |
| DORSAL PED   | RT |      |     |
|              | LT |      |     |
| ABDOM AORTA  |    | +    | −   |

| LONG SITTING TEST | + | − |
|-------------------|---|---|

### PRONE EXAMINATION

#### HIP ROTATION

|             | DEGREES |
|-------------|---------|
| MED  ROT  RT |        |
| MED  ROT  LT |        |
| LAT  ROT  RT |        |
| LAT  ROT  LT |        |

#### HAND-KNEE ROCK

| FLEXION   | LUMBAR  >  =  <  PELVIC |
|-----------|-------------------------|
| EXTENSION | LUMBAR  >  =  <  PELVIC |

#### FEMORAL NERVE

| RT | + | − |
|----|---|---|
| LT | + | − |

PALPATION_____

_____

_____

### SPRING TESTING

|       | HYPO | HYPR | WNL | SX LOC | SX DIST |
|-------|------|------|-----|--------|---------|
| SAC   |      |      |     |        |         |
| L-5   |      |      |     |        |         |
| L-4   |      |      |     |        |         |
| L-3   |      |      |     |        |         |
| L-2   |      |      |     |        |         |
| L-1   |      |      |     |        |         |
| SUPER-FICIAL | | OVER-REACTION | | NON-ANATOM | |
| + | − | + | − | + | − |

### SUMMARY

**STAGE I**                                    ☐
  MOVEMENT TESTING LUMBAR                       ☐
  PAIN MODULATION                               ☐

**STAGE II**                                   ☐
  POSTURAL EXAM                                 ☐
  FITNESS EXAM                                  ☐
  BACK SCHOOL                                   ☐

**STAGE III**                                  ☐
  PHYSICAL CAPACITY EXAM                        ☐
  WORK CAPACITY EXAM                            ☐

**NONORGANIC PAIN BEHAVIOR**                   ☐

REFERRAL _____

**FIGURE 2-13** ■ *Continued*

Standing Examination

**Observation of Posture.** The individual's posture is observed from the posterior, lateral, and anterior aspects of the body. Observation is initially performed from a distance of 5 to 7 feet. The alignment of the spine is noted in the sagittal and frontal planes.

The lumbar curve is assessed and classified as normal, decreased, or increased. A normal lumbar curve may vary from one body type to another but is characterized by a gentle concavity or lordosis facing posteriorly.

The thoracic curve is assessed and judged as normal, decreased, or increased. It is somewhat difficult to describe a "normal" curve because the normal kyphotic curve can vary considerably from one body type to another. At this juncture in the examination the examiner should be most concerned with extreme variations from the customary curve. It is relatively easy to identify these individuals (Figs. 2–14 to 2–16).

The frontal plane deformities of rotoscoliosis and lateral shift should be noted. The difference between these two deformities can be subtle, but it is important to distinguish them. **Rotoscoliosis** is a lateral malalignment of the thoracolumbar region and includes a rotational component in the transverse plane.[3] This condition is often found in conjunction with leg discrepancies. In the presence of rotoscoliosis, the pelvis lies beneath the shoulder girdle in the frontal plane. A scoliotic curve is classified as a C curve, which presents as a primary curve, or an S curve, which presents as a primary curve with a secondary lesser curve to the opposite direction. In addition, curves are defined as either right or left depending on the side on which the apex of convexity occurs. A lateral shift is characterized by a shifting of the shoulder gridle in the frontal plane in relation to the pelvic girdle so that the shoulders lie to the right or left of the midline of the body (Fig. 2–17).

The major joints of the lower extremity are observed for postural deviations, and an assessment is made of the statis position of the feet. It is important to assess the height of the medial longitudinal arches and the inclination of the calcaneus in the frontal plane.

Three patterns are observed in static postural analysis of the feet:

■ The high arched foot associated with a calcaneal varus
■ The low arched foot associated with a vertical or valgus position of the calcaneus
■ Asymmetric feet

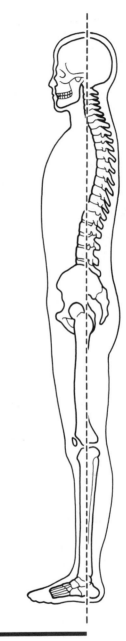

**FIGURE 2–14  ■** Ideal postural alignment.

The foot on the side of a long lower extremity often has a lower arch than the opposite foot. This represents an attempt to compensate for the leg length differential because pronation of the subtalar joint can produce functional shortening of the limb. If unilateral pronation of the foot is present as a compensatory mechanism for another osseous or soft tissue deformity, it may create a functional leg length imbalance. For these reasons, it is important to determine the levels of the iliac crests in the standing position with both subtalar joints in neutral positions. Otherwise, false impressions of leg lengths may be obtained.

The posture of the knees is observed. The knees may assume a flexed or hyperextended attitude in relaxed stance. Varus or valgus deformities may also be observed at the knee joints. It is important to note any asymmetry in the position of the knee joints because this may also be associated with leg length discrepancies. The position of the hip joint can be evaluated in relationship to foot placement. The degree of in-toeing and out-toeing is noted.

**Observation of Gait.** The individual's gait is then observed. The examiner should note the symmetry of pelvic list and lumbar side bending during ambulation. This is observed as the patient walks away from and then toward the examiner. The function of the lower kinetic chain is also observed with particular attention to transverse plane motion of the knee and the degree and timing of pronation and supination of the foot. The examiner must also note any lack of symmetry of swing of the upper extremity and thoracic rotation. Diminished amplitude of arm swing on the opposite side of lateral shift deformities is often observed. This may be related to the handedness patterns and is seen frequently in individuals who habitually carry objects such as a briefcase in the same hand, or it may be due to inability to clear the arm during swing because of the position of the pelvis. When this phenomenon is noted during gait observation, the patient can be encouraged to exaggerate swing of the upper extremities. If this gait pattern is influencing the patient's back pain, symptoms may be increased by increasing the amplitude of swing of the involved upper extremity.

**Heel and Toe Walking.** Heel walking and toe walking are performed at this time to assess the strength of the ankle dorsiflexors and plantarflexors, respectively. Any pain reported during these tests is also noted. Heel walking is often painful for the patient with low back pain. However, the patient who complains of pain on toe walking is the exception. The same individual who reports pain on this test is generally scored positively on three or more of the signs of Waddell et al.[5] Heel walking and toe walking are performed to provide a quick assessment of the motor function of the L4-5 and S1-2 myotomes.

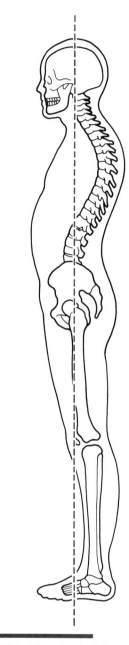

**FIGURE 2–15** ■ Kyphotic-lordotic posture.

**Axial Loading.** Axial loading of the spine is performed by pressing downward on the top of the patient's head.[5] The patient is instructed to report any pain. If the patient states that pain is produced in the lower back with this maneuver, the test is reported as positive. This examination

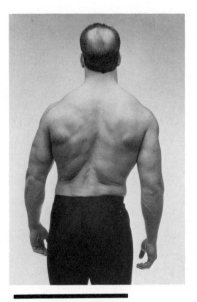

**FIGURE 2–17** ■ Right lateral shift.

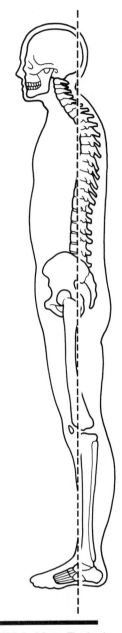

**FIGURE 2–16** ■ Flat back posture.

technique has been designed as a simulation and is typically negative in patients with organic back pain. The patient may state that pain is produced in the cervical region. If this is the case, the test is negative. Interpretation of this test procedure must be reserved until completion of the entire lower quarter screening examination. A positive response to this test associated with positive re-

sponses to other test procedures has been reported by Waddell et al. to be indicative of non-organic pain behavior.

**Pelvic Landmarks.** The examiner must next assess the symmetry of the pelvic landmarks including the posterior superior iliac spines (PSISs), anterior superior iliac spines (ASISs), and iliac crests. These are observed to determine whether any asymmetry of the pelvic girdle is present.

The iliac crests can be evaluated from the posterior aspect of the patient using a pelvic level (Fig. 2–18). The bars of the pelvic level are placed over the most superior aspect of the patient's iliac crests. The examiner observes the bubble of the level to determine whether one iliac crest is situated more superiorly than the other crest. This finding may indicate either a leg length discrepancy, an iliac rotation, or both. Asymmetry of the iliac crests must be correlated with the positional findings for the PSISs and ASISs to determine underlying dysfunction.

The PSIS levels are determined by placing the tips of the index fingers directly beneath the inferior shelves of the PSIS on each side and visually comparing the levels in a superior to inferior relationship. The same procedure is used to compare the levels of the ASISs. If the PSIS and the ASIS of one side are superior in relation to those of the opposite side, and that side demonstrated a high iliac crest, then the extremity of that side is most likely long. If the ASIS is high on the side of the high iliac crest and the PSIS is low on

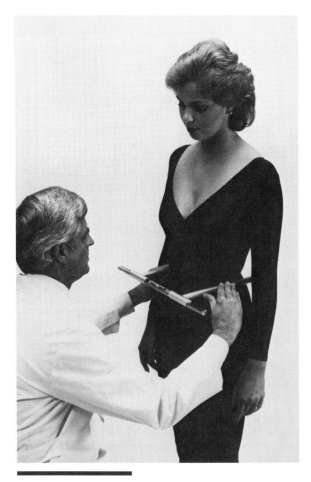

FIGURE 2–18 ■ Use of the pelvic med-level. (Courtesy of Ballert International, Inc., Northbrook, IL.)

**Active Range of Motion.** Active range of motion of the thoracolumbar spine is examined. The purpose of these procedures is to determine the following:

■ The range of motion present in each direction
■ The behavior of the patient's symptoms during and immediately after the movement in question

The following movements are examined:

■ Right side bending
■ Left side bending
■ Backward bending
■ Forward bending
■ Right pelvic translocation
■ Left pelvic translocation
■ Backward bending in right pelvic translocation
■ Backward bending in left pelvic translocation

For ease of recording the range of motion present and the location of symptoms, a movement diagram and a shorthand system to denote where symptoms are produced are used (Fig. 2–19). In addition to recording the range of motion and production and location of symptoms, it is important to note whether the patient's status has changed as a result of performing the movement. The appropriate box is checked to indicate whether the patient's status worsened or improved because of the movement, whether the patient's symptoms increased or decreased during the movement, or whether the individual's condition was unchanged during and after the movement test.

the same side, an iliac rotation may be present. This may be a posteriorly rotated innominate on the side of the high ASIS or an anteriorly rotated innominate on the side of the low ASIS.

The possibility of concomitant iliac rotations and anatomic leg length discrepancies is high. In fact, a posteriorly rotated innominate appears to be a common compensation for a long lower extremity. In cases of long leg compensation through posterior rotation of the innominate bone, the iliac crest and the ASIS are high on the side in question and the PSIS may be equal to that on the opposite side. If the compensation is incomplete, the PSIS is also high on the same side but not as high as the ASIS or crests in relation to the counterparts. For the purposes of the screening examination, it is important only to identify leg length asymmetries and iliac rotations. These findings indicate whether it is necessary to perform the lower kinetic chain evaluation to clarify the clinical picture.

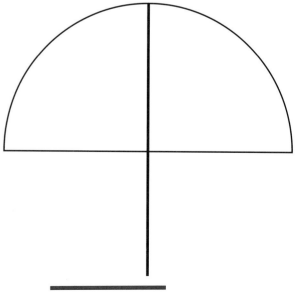

FIGURE 2–19 ■ The movement diagram.

**Lumbar Pelvic Rhythm.** Forward bending and backward bending are complex movements that involve motion of the thoracic and lumbar intervertebral segments and sagittal plane movement of the pelvic girdle at the hip joints. It is important to determine the ratio of lumbar movement to pelvic movement in forward and backward bending. Abnormal pelvic motion may be a risk factor for the development of spinal pain syndromes.

Different types of patterns of lumbopelvic rhythm can be observed. On forward bending two abnormal patterns are observed. In one group of patients the range of motion of the pelvis is markedly restricted while the range of lumbar flexion is excessive. Other patients can easily touch the floor without reversal of their lumbar lordosis into convexity. In the latter case, the range of pelvic motion is excessive and the range of lumbar flexion is clearly limited.

In the first example the hip extensors—hamstrings and gluteus maximus—are excessively tight. This limits the range of hip flexion and places excessive strain on the thoracic and lumbar spine. Over time, the demand for compensatory flexion in these regions produces excessive movement or hypermobility. In the second example the range of hip flexion is excessive and there is no need for compensatory movement of the spinal joints.

During backward bending similar abnormal patterns are observed. It is common to see individuals with limited pelvic extension associated with excessive lumbar extension.

Another type of patient demonstrates excessive extension of the pelvis with little or no extension of the lumbar spine.

**Standing Flexion Test.** The tips of the examiner's index fingers are placed directly beneath the inferior shelves of the posterior superior iliac spines.[3] The fingers are directed against the inferior margin of the PSISs with maintenance of a cephalic or upward pressure. The examiner's dominant eye is positioned directly between the tips of the index fingers at the same level. The patient is instructed to bend forward as far as possible while the examiner observes for symmetry of cranial movement of these bone landmarks. As the pelvis rotates into flexion, the examiner must rise to a standing position so that the movement of the PSISs can be monitored. Normally, the superior movements of the PSISs should be equal. If a pelvic joint dysfunction is present, the excursion or observable eruption of one PSIS may be greater than that of the other. Mitchell states that if one PSIS moves more cra-

nially in the standing flexion test, an iliosacral restriction is present and the side of greater PSIS movement is the side of the restriction.[3]

**Posterior Shear.** The standing posterior shear test is performed by instructing the patient to assume a comfortable standing position with hands crossed over the lower abdomen. The examiner stands at the patient's side and places one arm around the patient's abdomen over the hands, while the heel of the opposite hand stabilizes the pelvis and the index or middle finger palpates the L-5–S-1 interspinous space. The examiner produces a posterior shearing force through the patient's abdomen and an anteriorly directed stabilizing force with the opposite hand. The index or middle finger palpates to determine the extent and nature of the movement thus produced at L-5–S-1. The test is repeated at the other lumbar intervertebral segments. Normally, when this test is performed the examiner should feel an approximation of the spinous processes as during extension of a segment. Posterior translocation of the superior spinous process in the segment in relation to the inferior segment is suggestive of hypermobility.

**Rotation.** Thoracolumbar rotation assessment is best performed with the patient seated. Rotation in standing as a simulated test can be performed as described by Waddell et al.[5] In this test maneuver the patient is instructed to place the hands over the lateral aspect of the proximal thighs. The examiner's hands are placed over the patient's hands and produce a rotation of the pelvis. Care is taken to ensure that the lumbar spine is *not* rotated but is merely carried with the pelvic rotation. This test is generally not painful for individuals with organic pain unless there is involvement of the hip joint(s). If the hip joints are involved, this is determined at a later point in the examination.

### Sitting Examination

**Observation of Posture.** At this point the patient is instructed to assume a seated position at the edge of the examination table. It is important that the examiner not begin immediate observation of the patient's spine. Many patients become immediately aware of their posture upon observation and therefore assume an erect position. It is best that the examiner take a few moments to review the data already collected while the patient sits naturally in a normal resting posture. As was the case with observation of standing posture, the thoracic kyphosis is recorded as increased, reduced, or normal. The presence of rounded shoulders, concave or convex anterior chest, and forward or hyperextended head is noted. Any deviation in the frontal plane is noted as well.

**Observation of Pelvic Landmarks.** The levels of the iliac crests are observed from the anterior and posterior aspects. The PSIS levels are evaluated from the posterior aspect. Interpretation of the position of these landmarks is correlated with that found with the patient in the standing position. Any abnormality of the landmarks in either position is an indication for a specific pelvic examination.

**Seated Flexion Test.** The seated flexion test is performed in the same way as the standing flexion test. Mitchell et al. interpret a positive seated flexion test as an indication of a disturbance of sacral motion within the innominates.[3] A positive test result indicates the need to perform a pelvic examination

**Reflexes.** The examiner evaluates the patient's knee jerks and ankle jerks bilaterally. These are reported as increased, normal, or decreased and correlated with other objective signs of neurologic involvement.

**Resisted Tests.** Key muscles to each lumbar and sacral myotome are evaluated.[2] These key muscles include the hip flexors (L1-2), knee extensors (L3-4), ankle dorsiflexors (L4-5), and great toe extensors (L-5). The ankle plantarflexors have been evaluated during toe walking (S1-2). Two typical patterns emerge when weakness is present. The weakness may be isolated to a specific anatomic distribution of a nerve root or a peripheral nerve or may be nonanatomic. The latter is indicative of nonorganic pain behavior.[5] The former warrants a more detailed neurologic examination including electromyography and nerve conduction velocity studies.

**Seated Straight Leg Raise.** The seated straight leg raise (SLR) maneuver is not an isolated test but a subtest of the evaluation of motor function. As resisted knee extension is performed in the seated position, the patient is required to assume a position involving 90 degrees of hip flexion with full knee extension. The same is true if the examiner tests ankle dorsiflexion or great toe extension with the knee extended. In any case, lack of pain with this test position is correlated with the straight leg test in the supine position. If a seated SLR is possible but a supine SLR produces pain, nonorganic pain behavior is suspected.[5]

Supine Examination

**Straight Leg Raise.** The test is performed by standing at the patient's side to be examined. A goniometer is placed along the lateral aspect of the patient's lower leg at the greater trochanter. The opposite hand is placed around the medial aspect of the patient's knee to facilitate palpation of the hamstring tendons. The extremity is raised with neutral rotation to the point where hamstring spasm or insufficiency limits the movement, and the degrees of movement are noted on the goniometer. The examiner should not abort the test when the patient reports pain. A painful arc may be present.[2] If the extremity is moved carefully into the pain, it may be discovered that the pain abates and movement proceeds without pain to the available limit. The opposite leg is examined in the same way. The noninvolved lower extremity is usually examined first. After each test, the examiner records the range of motion permissible and whether pain was reported by the patient to be present in the back, the ipsilateral leg, or the contralateral leg. Patients with neurologic involvement typically demonstrate limitation of one SLR to less than 40 degrees. The opposite side is usually also limited and pain is often produced in the contralateral (involved) limb.

Other low back pain syndromes may produce limitation of SLR or pain during SLR but at a greater range of motion. Occasionally, neurologically limited SLR may occur at a slightly higher degree in females, particularly those who present with hypermobility.

After the single SLR tests, the examiner proceeds to examine double SLR. This is tested in the same manner as single SLR except that both legs are raised simultaneously. Double SLR through a greater range of motion than the most limited single SLR represents evidence of pelvic joint involvement, because double SLR produces less torque on the pelvic joints than single SLR.

**Range of Motion of the Hip Joints.** The examiner performs the Patrick test (also called fabere sign, for flexion, abduction, external rotation, extension) of both hips. This is done by placing the heel of the lower extremity to be tested over the knee of the opposite leg. The patient is then instructed to relax and allow the knee of the leg being examined to fall laterally toward the examination table. The range of motion is observed and the patient is questioned concerning the production and location of pain.

If an arthrosis of the hip joint is present, the involved extremity does not move through as great a range of motion as its counterpart. Pain caused by stressing the hip joint in this manner is generally reported in the anteromedial thigh (groin). Occasionally, the sacroiliac joint is stressed by this maneuver and may produce pain in the same area. The joint may also cause discomfort in the PSIS or gluteal area during this test procedure. It is not common for this movement to be limited secondary to involvement of the sacroiliac joint.

The ranges of motion of hip flexion, extension, abduction, internal rotation, and external rotation are assessed. If motion is restricted, it is recorded as either a capsular or noncapsular pattern. The capsular pattern of the hip as defined by Cyriax is a gross limitation of flexion, abduction, and internal rotation with slight limitation of extension and minimal or no limitation of external rotation.[2] In either case, a specific evaluation of the hip joint is indicated.

Restriction of SLR concurrently with limited hip flexion and a noncapsular pattern of restriction of range of motion of the hip joint constitutes what Cyriax terms the "sign of the buttock."[2] As a rule, this aggregation of signs signifies serious pathology in the pelvic or gluteal region. Possible causes include osteomyelitis of the femur, chronic septic sacroiliac arthritis, ischiorectal abscess, septic bursitis, neoplasm of the upper femur, or fractured sacrum. This syndrome was observed in a patient who was referred for strengthening exercises of the quadriceps with a diagnosis of chondromalacia patellae. The patient suffered pain only at the medial aspect of the knee joint and was unable to perform an active SLR. The lower quarter screening examination showed that the patient had good plus quadriceps and fair minus hip flexor strength in the seated position. Straight leg raising was limited, as was hip flexion. A noncapsular pattern of hip restriction was present. The patient was referred to the attending physician for further evaluation of the hip joint and a malignancy of the proximal femur was identified upon radiologic examination.

**Peripheral Pulses.** The posterior tibial and dorsalis pedis pulses are evaluated to rule out the possibility of vascular insufficiency. Lack of or diminished pulses are grounds for referral or consultation, particularly when the history is characteristic of peripheral vascular disease.

**Resisted Tests.** The resisted tests of hip flexion, knee extension, ankle inversion, and ankle eversion may be done with the patient supine if they were not done with the patient seated. Frequently, the patient cannot stay in a seated position long enough to permit evaluation of motor status of the lower extremities. This evaluation is performed in the same manner as that described for sitting. The examiner notes the presence of regional versus anatomic weakness as described in relation to the seated examination.

**Sensory.** Sensory examination includes light touch and pinprick. Areas of abnormal sensation are recorded on a body chart. A sensory examination is generally not necessary if the patient denies any symptoms in the lower extremities, if SLR was normal, and if the results of motor assessment were within normal limits.

**Babinski Reflexes.** The Babinski reflexes are tested bilaterally to rule out the presence of long tract signs. If pathologic reflexes are present, a complete neurologic examination is required.

**Long Sitting Test.** The long sitting test is performed to determine whether there is any limitation of motion of the joints of the pelvic girdle. The patient is in the supine position and the examiner stands at the foot of the examination table. The therapist's thumbs are placed inferior to the patient's medial malleoli, and the relative leg length is estimated visually by comparing the levels of the malleoli. The patient is then instructed to assume a seated position with the hips flexed as much as possible and the knees fully extended. At the completion of the movement, the examiner again observes the relative leg lengths to determine whether there has been an apparent change in the levels of the malleoli. If a change occurred, the test is recorded as positive. The direction of change is not important at this point in the examination. A positive test result means that an evaluation of the pelvic joints must be performed.

**Girth Measurements.** The circumferences of the thighs and calves are measured with a tape measure. Care is taken to measure the girths at the same location on both lower limbs. It is important to measure the girths at specified distances above and below the medial joint line of the knee because this landmark is reproducible.

### Prone Examination

**Hand-Knee Posture.** The patient is instructed to assume a position on the hands and knees. The examiner offers no assistance in the assumption of this position and should observe the ease or difficulty with which the patient rolls over from supine to prone and then assumes the hand-knee position.

The patient's hand-knee posture is observed with particular reference to the position of the thoracic-lumbar-pelvic-hip complex.[6] Considerable information can be gathered from this procedure. Three posture types may be observed. In one posture type the femurs are inclined posteriorly away from the body, a marked kyphosis exists in the thoracic spine, and the lumbar spine is also kyphotic or flat. Another type is characterized by inclination of the femurs under the trunk, hips flexed more than 90 degrees, a lordotic position of the lumbar column, and a relatively normal thoracic curve. If neither of these extremes is present, the posture is classified as normal.

The posture of the hips and lower legs is also observed from the posterior aspect of the patient. The presence of hip abduction or rotation is noted, as is the presence of tibial rotation.

**Hand-Knee Rock.** The patient is now instructed to assume a posture with the arms and thighs vertical.[6] The knees are placed together with the medial malleoli approximated and the feet in a plantarflexed position. The examiner instructs the patient to keep the hands in position on the table while attempting to approximate the buttocks to the heels by allowing the body to move in a posterior downward direction. This involves flexion of both hips and knees, and the test may not be possible if pathology is present in any joint that would preclude the performance of this movement. The thoracolumbar spine is also flexed during this movement. The examiner notes the relative proportion of pelvic-femoral movement in relation to lumbar movement. Two abnormal patterns that might be noted with this movement are actually accentuations of the posture observed in the preceding test position. The patient who exhibits hip extension with flattening or kyphosis of the lumbar spine moves into posterior rock. Because the hip joints are unable to flex to normal range, the patient's trunk moves posteriorly and the pelvic girdle assumes a more vertical orientation in space. The degree of kyphosis of the lumbar spine increases.

The patient who exhibits a flexed postural attitude of the femurs in the kneeling position rocks in a posterior direction with minimal change in the position of the pelvis or the lumbar spine, because ample movement is available at the hip joint to accomplish this movement without lumbar movement.

The former example is reported as lumbar movement greater than pelvic and the latter as pelvic movement greater than lumbar. The patient then returns to the neutral position and is instructed to rock forward to bring the pelvis to the table while maintaining extension of the elbows. Again, two typical abnormal patterns might be observed. One type includes the patient who allows the pelvis to approximate the table surface almost entirely through hip extension. This individual exhibits minimal to no lumbar extension. The second type includes the patient who demonstrates an inordinate amount of lumbar extension with restriction of hip extension. This excessive lumbar extension typically occurs in a limited portion of the lumbar spine at one or two segments.

**Internal Hip Rotation.** Internal rotation of the hips is measured with the hips at 90 and 0 degrees of flexion. The range of motion is assessed visually in both positions to determine whether there is a consistent limitation of internal rotation on one side or fluctuation of the sides of restriction as the patient is assessed at 0 and 90 degrees of hip flexion. If a difference is observed in the range of motion of internal rotation of the hips and the side of the limitation is consistent at 0 and 90 degrees of hip flexion, then either a restriction is present at the joint (capsular) or a femoral anteversion is present. However, if the side of restriction changes as the patient's position of hip flexion is changed, then the restriction is most likely due to muscular imbalance. In either case, a detailed examination of the lower kinetic chain is warranted.

**Gluteal Tone.** The gluteal muscle mass is observed for symmetry. Frequently, one side is seen to have diminished bulk compared to the contralateral side. The examiner places the fingertips over the gluteus maximus and presses them in a ventral direction in an attempt to assess the tone of the muscle. Muscle that appears to be wasted often feels soft or lacking in tone. This can occur in the presence of hip joint or sacroiliac joint dysfunction and indicates the need to perform a lower kinetic chain examination. Less frequently, diminished mass and tone of the gluteus maximus is observed in lumbar spine syndromes.

**Femoral Nerve Stretch.**[2] The femoral nerve stretch consists of two subtests:

■ Prone knee flexion
■ Reverse bent leg raising

In prone knee flexion, the examiner passively

flexes the patient's knee in the prone position. In reverse bent leg raising, the knee is flexed to 90 degrees and the hip is extended passively. These tests are designed to place tension on the femoral nerve in much the same way as the SLR test places tension on the sciatic nerve. When these tests produce positive results, irritation of the third lumbar root is usually present.

A positive test result is recorded by noting the production and location of pain on both tests. Test interpretations could include several variations. Both tests may cause pain in either the lumbar spine or anterior thigh. Reverse bent leg raising causes extension of the lumbar segments, and if pain is localized in the low back it may be mechanical pain. Anterior thigh pain on reverse bent leg raising is probably caused by irritation of the third lumbar nerve root. Prone knee flexion causes the quadriceps to be placed under tension and may cause discomfort in this region in normal subjects. If the rectus femoris is tight, flexing the knee produces extension in the lumbar spine because of anterior tilting of the pelvis. This may produce lower back pain of mechanical rather than neurologic origin. If both tests produce pain in the anterior thigh, irritation of the third lumbar nerve root may be indicated, especially if the range of motion is markedly limited. Both tests producing pain in the lower back may be interpreted as a positive test result, but not as consistently as the former example. If prone knee flexion causes anterior thigh pain and reverse bent leg raising causes lower back pain, the result is interpreted as negative.

**Spring Test.** Spring testing is performed over the sacrum and over the spinous processes of the vertebrae from L-5 through T-6.

The sacral spring test is a provocation test. That is, if a painful dysfunction is present at the sacroiliac joints, pain may be produced by delivering a sharp thrust over the dorsal aspect of the sacrum. The pain experienced by the patient during this test may be local and confined to one or both sacroiliac joints, or distal, peripheral to the lesion. The examiner stands at the patient's side and places the hand closest to the patient's head over the sacrum with the palmar surface of the hand conforming to the sacrum as closely as possible. The elbow and wrist are maintained in full extension, and the opposite hand is placed over the dorsal aspect of the hand. A sharp, anterior thrust is delivered perpendicular to the sacrum. If pain is produced by this test, a detailed examination of the sacroiliac joint is indicated.

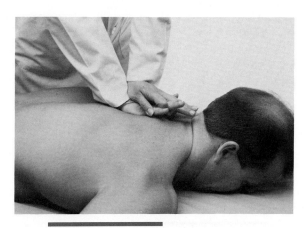

**FIGURE 2–20** ■ Spring test for thoracic spine.

The vertebral spring tests are both provocations and tests of mobility of the thoracic and lumbar segments. These are also performed with the examiner at the patient's side. The tests are performed first at L-5 and progress in a cranial direction until all vertebrae from L-5 to the midthoracic region have been tested. When testing at or distal to the apex of the lumbar lordosis, the examiner uses the hand nearest the patient's head. Proximal to the apex of the lordosis, the opposite hand is used to facilitate application of a perpendicular thrust to the vertebra. The examiner places the hypothenar eminence over the spinous process of the vertebra to be tested. The contact point of the hand is just distal to the pisiform. When the examiner's hand is positioned appropriately, the wrist and elbow are extended, and a gentle but firm anteriorly directed pressure is applied to the spinous process. The force is applied by allowing the body weight to be extended through the arms (Fig. 2–20). The patient is instructed to report any change in symptoms during the test. The examiner should also note the ease with which the vertebrae are translated anteriorly and record the results as normal, hypomobile, or hypermobile at these levels. Spring testing is also performed over the rib angles (Fig. 2–21).

**Palpation.** Palpation of the thoracic, lumbar spine, and gluteal regions proceeds from superficial to deep structures. The skin and subcutaneous tissues are palpated first to assess the patient's general reaction. The examiner places the tips of the middle and ring fingers on either side of the lumbar spinous processes and gently pushes the skin in a cranial direction, allowing a

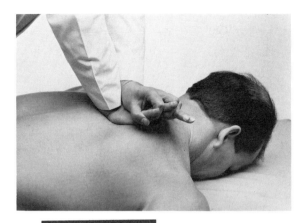

**FIGURE 2-21** ■ Spring test over the rib angles.

small roll of skin to gather in front of the fingertips. The fingertips are then moved upward slowly while the skin roll is moved in a cranial direction, much like the movement of a wave. It is not uncommon for the patient to report discomfort as the examiner's fingers move through a narrow area of the back. The discomfort may be present unilaterally or bilaterally and is often accompanied by an "orange peel" appearance of the skin in this zone. The examiner also notes increased resistance to movement of the skin in a cranial direction in this area. One must be suspicious when the patient reports widespread superficial tenderness of the lumbar region because this may represent nonorganic pain behavior.[5]

Next, the muscles are palpated for abnormal tone and tenderness. The superficial layers of the erector spinae are assessed by moving the fingertips transversely across the fibers of the muscle, beginning on one side. The examiner attempts to move the muscle fibers in a transverse direction in relation to the underlying tissues. The deep spinal extensors are palpated with the fingertips or thumb tips placed on either side of the spinous processes. The fingers are moved in a diagonal direction, laterally and superiorly, while deep pressure is applied over the belly of the muscles. The examiner then moves the hands to the gluteal region and begins palpation by identifying the iliac crest. Deep pressure is applied with the fingertips to assess for tenderness of the proximal attachment of the gluteus medius, gluteus minimus, and tensor fascia lata as the fingertips are moved from the posterior to the anterior aspect just beneath the flare of the posterior pelvic crests.

The piriformis muscle is palpated by locating the midpoint of the body of the sacrum and the greater trochanter of the femur. Deep pressure is exerted between these bone landmarks to search for spasm or tenderness of the piriformis muscle. The greater trochanter of the femur is palpated with the thumb tip. The examiner locates the trochanter with the palm of the hand and then places the tip of the thumb at the posterior, distal extent of the bone landmark. Deep pressure is applied first at this location. The thumb is moved proximally to palpate the superior aspect of the trochanter. Tenderness at any point along the posterosuperior aspect of the greater trochanter is indicative of trochanteric bursitis. The ischial tuberosity is palpated similarly. The landmark is first identified with the palm of the hand, and then the thumb tip is used to probe the area for tenderness. This may be indicative of ischial bursitis or tendinitis of the proximal hamstring attachment.

The iliotibial tract is palpated along the lateral aspect of the thigh toward the attachment on the lateral aspect of knee.

In the thoracolumbar region, the tips of the spinous processes are palpated for tenderness over the interspinous ligaments. Normal ligaments are not tender to palpation, and point tenderness at an interspinous space may confirm suspicion of hypermobility. All interspinous spaces are assessed from the L-5–S-1 junction through the thoracic area. The ribs must also be assessed for tenderness.

SUMMARY OF LOWER QUARTER SCREENING EXAMINATION

At the completion of the lower quarter screening examination, the examiner makes a decision to continue with further evaluation or conclude. If further evaluation is indicated, a thoracolumbar examination, an examination of the lower kinetic chain, or both are involved.

If the examiner decides to conclude, it is generally because signs have been found that indicate the need for referral to another practitioner for additional evaluation. These signs might indicate the presence of a nonmusculoskeletal problem or a serious problem that requires medical intervention. There may also be signs of nonorganic pain behavior. In the latter case, further examination may or may not be indicated. Several tests for nonorganic pain behavior throughout the lower quarter screening examination have been described. These have been grouped by Waddell et al. into the following categories:[5]

■ Tenderness that is superficial or nonanatomic
■ Simulations
■ Distractions

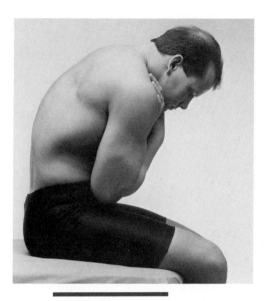

**FIGURE 2-22** ■ Thoracic flexion.

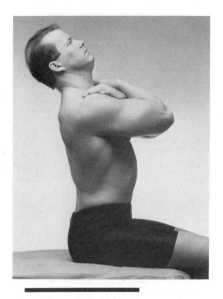

**FIGURE 2-23** ■ Thoracic extension.

■ Regional disturbances
■ Overreaction

If the patient has a positive test result in three or more of these categories, the examiner should suspect nonorganic pain behavior. Further examination of these individuals is usually difficult because the examiner depends on the individual's subjective reports of alteration in symptoms. This may pose a problem, and referral for psychologic evaluation may be indicated.

## Active Range of Motion (Physiologic Movements)

The physiologic motions of thoracic flexion, extension, rotation, side bending, and cervical flexion are assessed. The excursion of inspiration and expiration is observed to assess rib movement (Figs. 2-22 to 2-28) Active range-of-motion testing determines the willingness of the patient to move, the ability of the patient to move, the available active range, and the irritability of the condition. It is not diagnostic in and of itself.

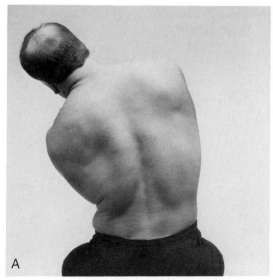
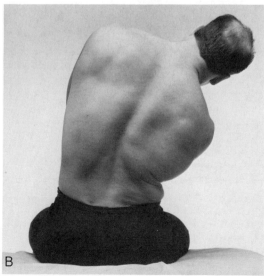

**FIGURE 2-24** ■ Thoracic side bending to left (A) and right (B).

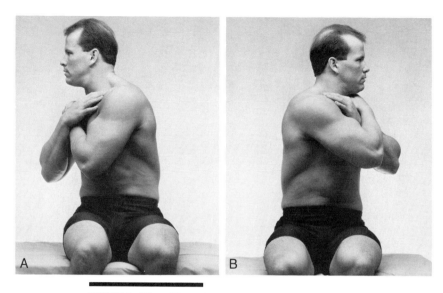

**FIGURE 2-25** ■ Thoracic rotation to right (A) and left (B).

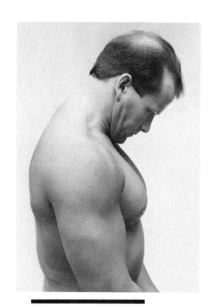

**FIGURE 2-26** ■ Cervical flexion.

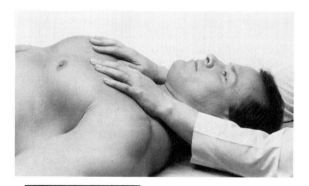

**FIGURE 2-27** ■ Observation of rib elevation (inspiration).

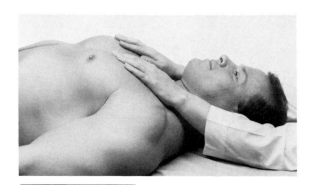

**FIGURE 2-28** ■ Observation of rib depression (expiration).

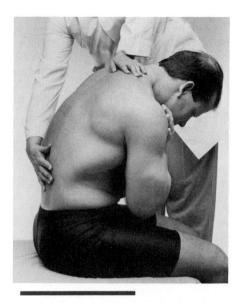

**FIGURE 2–29** ■ Thoracic flexion (passive).

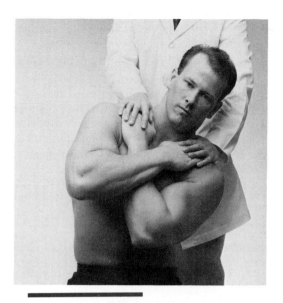

**FIGURE 2–31** ■ Thoracic side bending (passive).

## Passive Range of Motion (Physiologic Movements)

Passive range of motion is assessed to determine the amount of true movement available. This is performed for thoracic flexion, extension, rotation, side bending, and cervical flexion (Figs.

2–29 to 2–32). Often it is difficult for the patient to relax, so the examiner may need to use overpressure at the end of the active range to determine the degree of passive movement available. The examiner should note the quality of the movement and the motion barrier encountered.

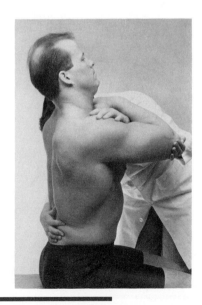

**FIGURE 2–30** ■ Thoracic extension (passive).

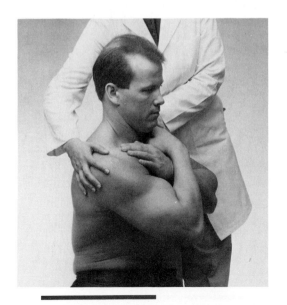

**FIGURE 2–32** ■ Thoracic rotation (passive).

## *Mobility Testing (Scandinavian Approach)*

The movement available at a specific segment is determined by mobility testing. It is necessary to conduct this test so that treatment can be directed at the specific restriction. The movement is classified as normal, hypomobile, or hypermobile. The following are the Scandinavian techniques for the thoracic spine and rib cage.

## Thoracic Spine[7,8]

### FLEXION (Fig. 2–33)

### Patient's Position

The patient is sitting on a chair or near the edge of the table. The arms are crossed in front of the chest.

### Physical Therapist's Position

The examiner stands or sits at the patient's side facing the lateral aspect of the patient's trunk.

### Hand Placement

One of the examiner's hands is used to palpate the interspinous space.

The other arm is placed beneath the patient's arms.

### Procedure

The hand supporting the patient's arms allows the trunk to fall forward into flexion as the other hand palpates the gapping of the interspinous space. If the patient has a difficult time relaxing, the operator may have to grasp the patient's shoulder and place his or her own shoulder in the patient's axilla to bring the trunk into flexion.

### EXTENSION (Fig. 2–34)

### Patient's Position

The patient is sitting in a chair or near the edge of the table. The arms are clasped behind the head with the arms brought forward in front of the face.

### Physical Therapist's Position

The examiner stands or sits at the patient's side facing the lateral aspect of the patient's trunk.

### Hand Placement

One hand is used to palpate the interspinous spaces.

The other arm is placed beneath the patient's arms.

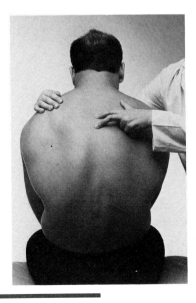

**FIGURE 2–33 ■** Mobility testing (thoracic flexion).

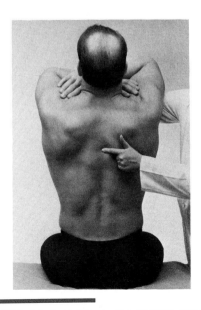

**FIGURE 2–34 ■** Mobility testing (thoracic extension).

## Procedure

The arm placed beneath the patient's arms is used to bring the patient's trunk into extension. The other hand palpates the approximation of the spinous processes and provides a counterforce to the extension.

### SIDE BENDING (Fig. 2–35)

#### Patient's Position

The patient is sitting in a chair or near the edge of the table. The arms are crossed in front of the chest.

#### Physical Therapist's Position

The examiner stands or sits at the patient's side facing the lateral aspect of the patient's trunk.

#### Hand Placement

One hand is used to palpate the interspinous space.

The other arm is brought around the anterior aspect of the patient. The hand is placed on the patient's shoulder. The shoulder of this arm may be placed in the patient's axilla nearest the therapist.

#### Procedure

The patient's trunk is side bent by means of the therapist's hand, while the opposite hand palpates the gapping or approximation of the spinous processes.

### ROTATION (Fig. 2–36)

#### Patient's Position

The patient is sitting in a chair or near the edge of the table.

The arms are crossed in front of the chest.

#### Physical Therapist's Position

The examiner stands or sits at the patient's side facing the lateral aspect of the trunk.

#### Hand Placement

One hand is used to palpate the interspinous space.

The other hand is brought around the anterior aspect of the patient and grasps the shoulder away from the therapist. The shoulder of this arm may be placed in the patient's axilla nearest the therapist.

#### Procedure

The patient's trunk is rotated while the palpating hand evaluates the movement of the upper spinous process with respect to the lower spinous process.

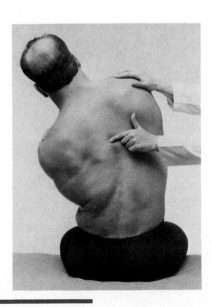

FIGURE 2-35 ■ Mobility testing (thoracic side bending).

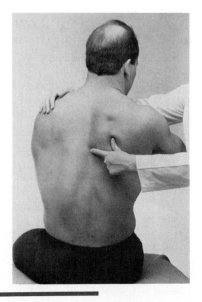

FIGURE 2-36 ■ Mobility testing (thoracic rotation).

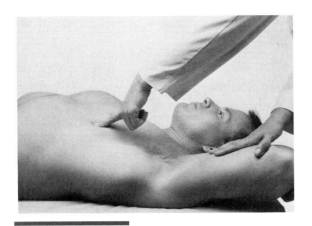

FIGURE 2–37 ■ Mobility testing (rib elevation and depression of upper ribs).

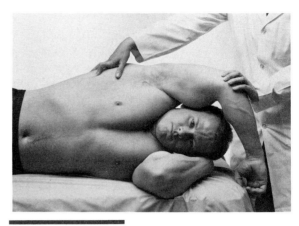

FIGURE 2–38 ■ Mobility testing (rib elevation and depression of the lower ribs).

## Rib Cage[7,8]

### RIB ELEVATION AND DEPRESSION (UPPER RIBS) (Fig. 2–37)

#### Patient's Position

The patient is supine with the arm overhead.

#### Physical Therapist's Position

The examiner is standing at the side of the patient's elevated arm.

#### Hand Placement

One hand palpates the intercostal spaces over the anterior chest wall.

The other hand holds the patient's humerus.

#### Procedure

For elevation (inspiration) the humerus is pulled superiorly while the rib separation is assessed with the palpating hand.

For depression (expiration) the humerus is released while the rib approximation is assessed with the palpating hand.

### RIB ELEVATION AND DEPRESSION (LOWER RIBS) (Fig. 2–38)

#### Patient's Position

The patient is lying on one side with the upper arm elevated overhead.

#### Physical Therapist's Position

The examiner stands at the side of the patient's elevated arm.

#### Hand Placement

One hand palpates the intercostal space over the lateral chest wall.

The other hand holds the patient's humerus.

#### Procedure

For elevation (inspiration) the humerus is pulled superiorly while the palpating hand assesses the separation of the ribs.

For depression (expiration) the humerus is released while the palpating hand assesses the approximation of the ribs.

### Provocation Testing (Australian Approach)

In provocation testing, a posterior-to-anterior force is produced centrally and unilaterally over the thoracic vertebrae and the rib angle. The examiner assesses the quantity and quality of motion available and whether the movement caused the pain to begin, to increase, or to decrease. This information is utilized with the other examination data to determine which movement is appropriate for the treatment of pain or mobility changes.[9]

The technique of providing a posterior-to-anterior force was discussed in the section on spring testing during the screening process.

### Positional Testing (Osteopathic Approach)

The osteopathic approach to examination involves assessment of the position of the vertebra in relation to the level above and to the level below. This information can be utilized to determine which specific mobilization techniques are required to increase the movement of the segment. The following techniques are utilized for the thoracic spine.

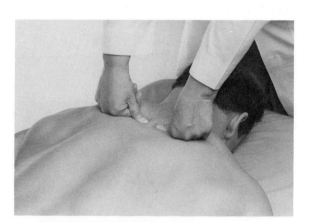

**FIGURE 2-39** ■ Positional examination (neutral).

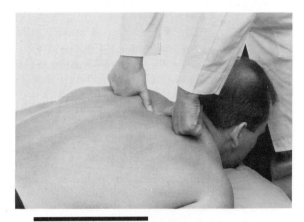

**FIGURE 2-40** ■ Positional examination (extension).

## POSITIONAL EXAMINATION[3]
### Neutral Position

The patient lies prone. The examiner stands with the dominant eye positioned over the midline of the patient to facilitate observation of symmetry of the transverse processes in relation to the frontal plane. (Fig. 2–39)

### Extended Position

The patient lies prone. An extension moment is produced by pressing anteriorly on the transverse processes with the thumbs. The examiner observes the symmetry of the transverse processes at the end range of extension (Fig. 2–40).

### Flexed Position

The patient sits on a stool or stands and flexes the neck and upper back. The examiner stands behind the patient to compare the symmetry of the transverse processes in relation to the frontal plane (Fig. 2–41).

## INTERPRETATION[3]
### Neutral Position

If a group of vertebrae exhibit transverse processes that are more posterior on one side, a type I lesion is present. This is termed an NSR (neutral, side bent, rotated) lesion. Subscripts on R and S are used to denote the direction of the rotation and side bending. In neutral lesions the side bending and rotation occur to opposite sides.

### Extended Position

If a vertebra has one transverse process more posterior than the counterpart, a type II lesion is present. This is termed an FRS (flexed, rotated, side bent) lesion. Subscripts on R and S are used to denote the direction of the side bending and rotation. In type II lesions the rotation and side bending occur to the same side.

### Flexed Position

If a vertebra has one transverse process more posterior than the counterpart, a type II lesion is present. This is termed an ERS (extended, rotated, side bent) lesion. Subscripts on S and R are used to denote the direction of the side bending and rotation.

## Thoracic Outlet Syndrome Testing

Thoracic outlet syndrome is due to compression of the neurovascular bundle in the superior aperture of the thorax. It is a complex pathologic process that is characterized by pressure on one or all of the following structures: the brachial plexus, the subclavian artery, and the subclavian

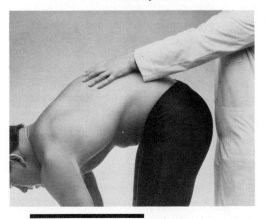

**FIGURE 2-41** ■ Positional examination (flexion).

## ADSON OR SCALENE MANEUVER (Fig. 2–42)

The patient is instructed to 1) take and hold a deep breath; 2) extend the neck fully; and 3) turn the chin toward the side being examined. The examiner holds the upper extremity in slight abduction and external rotation. The examiner monitors the radial pulse and notes any change or reproduction of the symptoms.[1,13]

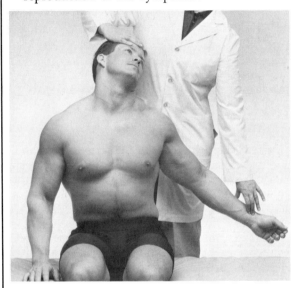

**FIGURE 2–42**

## COSTO-CLAVICULAR MANEUVER (Fig. 2–43)

The patient's shoulders are placed in an exaggerated military position. The examiner monitors the radial pulse and notes any change or reproduction of the symptoms.[13]

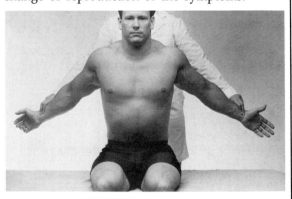

**FIGURE 2–43**

## HYPERABDUCTION MANEUVER (Fig. 2–44)

The patient's arm is placed overhead. The examiner monitors the radial pulse and notes any change or reproduction of the symptoms.[13]

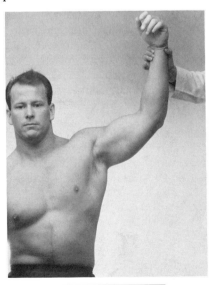

**FIGURE 2–44**

## HYPEREXTENSION MANEUVER (Fig. 2–45)

The patient's arm is placed in extension. The examiner monitors the radial pulse and notes any change or reproduction of the symptoms.[15]

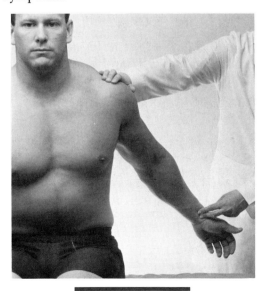

**FIGURE 2–45**

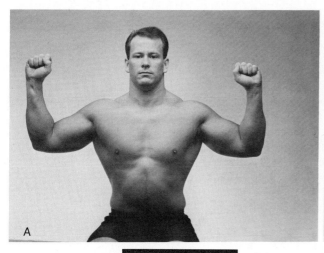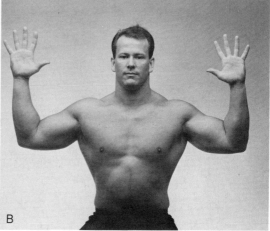

FIGURE 2–46 ■ Elevated arm stress test. (A) Hands closed; (B) hands open.

vein. The signs and symptoms can be neurologic and or vascular. Nerve compression causes distress in approximately 90% of the cases encountered.[10-13]

Thoracic outlet syndrome includes many syndromes that have been designated according to a presumed cause-and-effect relationship. These include cervical rib syndrome, scalenus anticus syndrome, hyperabduction syndrome, and costoclavicular syndrome. Symptoms alone do not allow an accurate diagnosis. Differential diagnosis by objective testing is mandatory. The examination must include a thorough neurologic evaluation in addition to muscle length and strength tests. Common associated pathologies include cervical disc disease and carpal tunnel syndrome.[10-13]

Various diagnostic manuevers have been designed to inculpate the different areas of involvement. Although useful in the examination process, these are not exclusively diagnostic. During these tests the examiner monitors the onset of the patient's symptoms. It has been recommended that the radial pulse also be monitored in positional tests to determine if obliterations or decreases occur. However, this may occur in normal individuals and because 90% of the cases are neurologic this does not appear to be the most important aspect of the test. In addition, other signs indicate vascular compromise, including tropic changes, pallor, and cyanosis.[1,12-14]

The most commonly performed positional tests are as follows:

1. Adson or scalene maneuver[1,13]
2. Costoclavicular maneuver[13]

3. Hyperabduction maneuver[13]
4. Hyperextension maneuver[15]

In addition, an active maneuver is often assessed. This test is termed the elevated arm stress test (EAST).[14] The patient is sitting. Both extremities are abducted, rotated externally at the shoulder, and flexed to 90 degrees at the elbow. While in this position, patients are asked to open and close their hands for 1 to 2 minutes. The examiner monitors the onset of symptoms (Fig. 2–46).

## DIFFERENTIAL DIAGNOSIS

The problems associated with clinical diagnosis and management of spinal pain are numerous. Pain that is experienced in the thoracic spine can be caused by a variety of pathologic conditions. Some of these pathologies are mechanical in nature and arise from the musculoskeletal system whereas others are nonmechanical (See Chart—Unsuitable Patients, p. 108). Conditions with a mechanical component typically involve fluctuation of symptom intensity, with symptoms aggravated by some activities or postures and improved by others. Conditions with no mechanical element do not involve symptom alteration related to posture or movement. Symptoms of patients with nonmechanical pain syndromes are often constant and unremitting and demonstrate temporally related variations in intensity. The magnitude of symptoms often increases at night and awakens the patient from sleep. No position or movement can be found that influences the

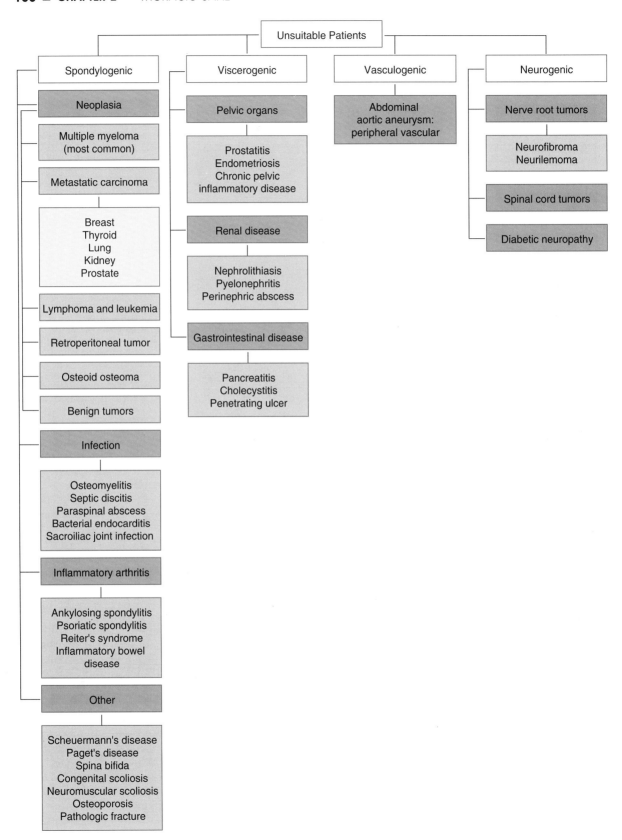

patient's symptoms. To attempt treatment of nonmechanical pain by mechanical means is fruitless.

Furthermore, naming of a pathology or disease process often provides little guidance for management of the patient's problems with physical therapy. For example, a patient with degenerative arthritis of a spinal joint may present with vastly dissimilar problems. One problem might be asymptomatic while another problem involves a movement dysfunction characterized by severe pain on all active or passive movements.

It follows that the single most important aspect of differential diagnosis as it pertains to physical therapy is segregation of patients with problems that can be resolved by interventions. It is important that attention is focused on describing syndromes that can be improved by intervention rather than on merely naming pathologic or disease processes.

## Classification of Patients

Physical therapy management of thoracic spinal pain involves the use of

- Active movement, sustained posture, immobilization or rest from function, and physical agents to modulate symptoms of patients with acute pain syndromes
- Exercise to enhance elements of muscle performance (strength, endurance, coordination, and flexibility)
- Training and educational protocols to enhance the performance of the cardiovascular system and facilitate appropriate motor behavior for functional activities

A person who is suitable for treatment must have a problem that is likely to respond favorably to one of the foregoing interventions. Problems that meet this criterion include

- Pain that is related to movement
- Movement dysfunction of the trunk (hypomobility or hypermobility of spinal or costovertebral joint)
- Muscular performance deficits
- Aerobic deficits
- Inappropriate motor behavior for functional activity including vocational and avocational

A narrow therapeutic approach to spinal pain often leads to failure or increased probability of recurrences. It is inappropriate simply to discharge a patient from management when the acute episode is controlled. Most patients require

therapeutic strategies directed toward factors that may predispose them to a relapse or recurrence. This therapeutic sequence of managing the acute problem followed by managing putative risk factors is outlined in the following as phases of treatment.

The first level of differential diagnosis or classification of the patient involves determining whether an individual should be

1. Managed independently by a physical therapist,
2. Referred to a medical practitioner, or
3. Managed by a physical therapist in consultation with another practitioner.

Clearly, patients with mechanical spinal pain are most often managed independently by the physical therapist. The patient with nonmechanical pain or no identifiable problem that would respond to physical therapy must be referred to another practitioner. A consultation is most often required for the patient with a mechanical syndrome who also has a significant inflammatory (chemical) component. Such patients require physical therapy but may respond more rapidly if given anti-inflammatory medications.

## Stage of Spinal Pain Syndromes

If the decision is made to intervene in a patient's spinal pain problem(s), the physical therapist must next assign the patient to a functional stage and treatment category. It has proved convenient to classify movement disorders into stages. These divisions are arbitrary, but one can develop a comprehensive management approach by viewing the individual as moving from one stage to another. Staging criteria are related to severity of disability and not to chronicity of the condition.

The operational definition and criteria for inclusion in each stage or category are described.

### Stages of Mechanical Spinal Pain

**Stage I.** A patient is classified in stage I if pain interferes with the ability to sit, stand, or walk. These activities are best thought of as foundations for other purposeful activities. If individuals cannot perform these foundation activities, it is illogical to expect them to perform a more complex activity in any of these positions. The symptoms of a person who is classified in stage I must be modulated before progression to stage II or stage III is possible.

An individual is classified in stage I if unable

to stand for 15 minutes, sit for 30 minutes, or walk one quarter of a mile. The Oswestry score in stage I typically ranges from 30 to 75%, although there are some exceptions.[16]

**Stage II.** A diagnosis of stage II can be made if disability does not interfere with sitting, standing, or walking. However, the condition precludes the performance of purposeful activities such as vacuuming or lawn mowing. Modified Oswestry disability scores are usually in the range of 10 to 30%.[16]

**Stage III.** Disability in stage III is less than that in stage II. Individuals in stage III are generally asymptomatic but have become deconditioned because of a lengthy period of inactivity. These individuals typically rate their disability at 10% or less on the Oswestry scale.[16]

**Syndromes.** Each of the preceding stages can be further subdivided into syndromes. Categorization into a syndrome dictates the treatment protocol. The syndromes are as follows:

*Stage I Syndrome*
Active movement improves:
    Flexion
    Extension
Passive movement improves:
    Capsular pattern
    Noncapsular pattern
        Opening dysfunction
        Closing dysfunction
    Rib dysfunction
        Inhalation
        Exhalation
Movement worsens:
    Bed rest
    Rest from function
    Immobilization (corset, orthosis)

*Stage II Syndrome*
Strength deficits
Flexibility deficits
Endurance deficits (muscular)
Coordination deficits

*Stage III Syndrome*
Aerobic deficits (cardiovascular)
Inappropriate motor behavior (body mechanics)

## TREATMENT

As discussed in section on differential diagnosis, patients are classified in the categories of suitable for treatment and nonsuitable for treatment. This section is an overview of various treatment approaches for patients who are deemed suitable for treatment by physical therapists. The goal is to familiarize the reader with the various techniques that are used in the treatment for each stage.

It is, however, difficult to encompass every possible clinical scenario. Therefore the treatment approaches are delineated according to the goal established for the specific stage. These can be summarized as follows:

■ To reduce pain
■ To increase mobility
■ To reduce mobility
■ To prevent recurrence[17]

## Pain Management

Pain can be controlled in a variety of ways in the patient with spinal problems. These fall in the following categories:

**Modalities.** A specific discussion of this area is not feasible here. Physical agents that are most commonly utilized include moist heat, cold, electricity, traction, and ultrasound. The reader is referred to texts on this subject.[18–20]

**Immobilization.** If the condition causes significant pain at rest, is irritable, and is unresponsive to movement therapy, the patient may require immobilization until these aspects of chemical pain decrease in intensity. This can be accomplished by general immobilization (bed rest) or by specific immobilization (bracing, corsets).

**Procedures.** As with physical agents, therapeutic procedures are adjuncts available to the physical therapist. These procedures include mobilization, manual traction, manipulation, proprioceptive neuromuscular facilitation, and massage.

**Mobilization.** The lower grades of the mobilization techniques—"piccolo" and "slack" in the Scandinavian system and grades I and II in the Australian system—are based on activation of the joint receptors and may help in pain control. It is important to recognize that the symptoms do not always call for a hands-off approach by the physical therapist.[9,17]

## Hypomobility

Decreased movement may be observed in the soft tissues surrounding the joint and in the joint complex. The treatment goal is to increase mo-

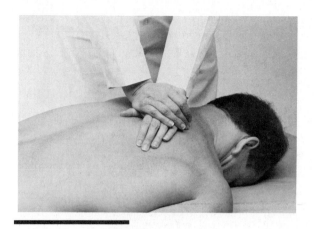

**FIGURE 2-47** ■ Transverse friction massage to superficial muscles.

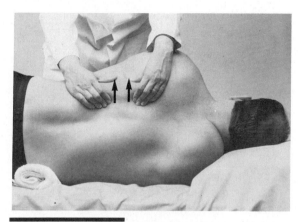

**FIGURE 2-49** ■ Transverse friction massage to back extensor muscles.

bility in these structures to return the patient to pain-free function. Various treatment approaches are available. The techniques discussed correlate with the discussion presented on examination and are an excellent starting reference for the entry-level clinician.

### Soft Tissue Mobilization[7]

**Transverse Friction Massage to the Superficial Muscles** (Fig. 2–47). The patient is prone. The thumb and thenar eminence are placed parallel to the fibers of the superficial muscles and apply a stretching force to the muscle tissue.

**Transverse Friction Massage to the Deep Muscles** (Fig. 2–48). The patient is prone. The physical therapist places one thumb on the deep muscles on one side directed caudally. The other thumb is placed on the opposite side directed cranially. The thumbs provide a stretching force

by working in unison, pressing caudally on one side and cranially on the other. This is repeated in a gentle rhythmic pattern.

**Transverse Friction Massage to the Back Extensor Muscles** (Fig. 2–49). The patient lies on one side with the knees flexed and the head supported. The physical therapist faces the anterior aspect of the patient. The fingers of each hand are placed on the most medial aspect of the paravertebral muscle mass. The forearms may rest on the patient's shoulder girdle and lower trunk. A side-bending force is provided to the muscle mass by means of simultaneous superior and lateral movements of the hands.

**Scapulothoracic Mobilizations** (Fig. 2–50). The interscapular muscles can be mobilized by using scapulothoracic mobilizations. Refer to the chapter on the shoulder complex for a review of these techniques.

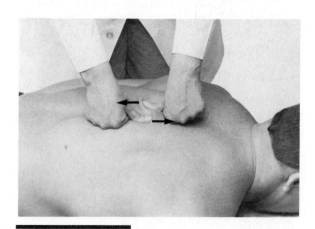

**FIGURE 2-48** ■ Transverse friction massage to deep muscles.

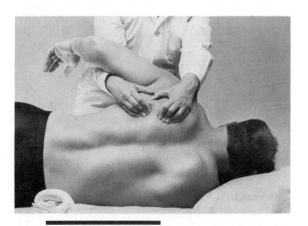

**FIGURE 2-50** ■ Scapulothoracic mobilization.

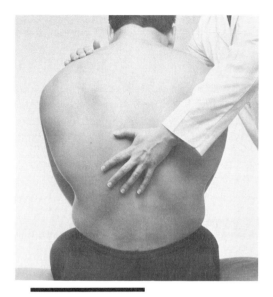

FIGURE 2-51 ■ Mobilization (thoracic flexion).

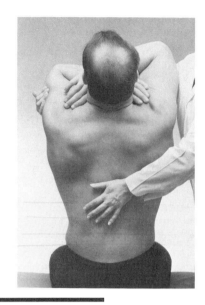

FIGURE 2-52 ■ Mobilization (thoracic extension).

## *Mobilization of the Joint Complex*

SCANDINAVIAN APPROACH[7]

Thoracic Spine

The mobilizations for the thoracic spine are extensions of the mobility tests with the addition of proper stabilization and maintenance of force. The stabilization includes the following:

## Mobilizations for Thoracic Spine

**FLEXION** (Fig. 2-51)

The palpating hand is converted to a stabilizing hand. It provides stabilization by providing a caudal and anterior force to the spinous process of the lower vertebra.

**EXTENSION** (Fig. 2-52)

The palpating hand is converted to a stabilizing hand. It provides stabilization by providing a posterior-to-anterior force to the spinous process of the lower vertebra.

**SIDE BENDING** (Fig. 2-53) **AND ROTATION** (Fig. 2-54)

The palpating hand is converted to a stabilizing hand. It provides stabilization by grasping the spinous process of the lower vertebra by means of a key grip.

## Manual Traction to Mobilize the Thoracic Spine

### Patient's Position

The patient is sitting on the treatment table.

For traction to the more cranial portion of the thoracic spine the patient's hands are clasped behind the head with the arms brought forward in front of the face (Fig. 2-55).

For traction to the more caudal portion of the thoracic spine the patient's arms are crossed (Fig. 2-56).

### Physical Therapist's Position

The physical therapist stands behind the patient with the knees slightly flexed.

### Hand Placement

For the cranial portion of the thoracic spine both hands are inserted between the patient's upper arms and forearms.

For the caudal portion of the thoracic spine the hands grasp the crossed arms of the patient.

### Procedure

The physical therapist straightens the knees and leans backward to provide a traction force. The patient is then slowly returned to the starting position. This is repeated 8 to 10 times.

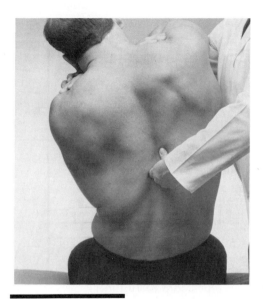

**FIGURE 2-53** ■ Mobilization (thoracic side bending).

Rib Cage

Mobilizations in the rib cage are similar to the mobility testing procedures. The operator must provide stabilization and mobilization force.

## Mobilizations in the Rib Cage

### ELEVATION (INSPIRATION) RESTRICTIONS
(Fig. 2-57)

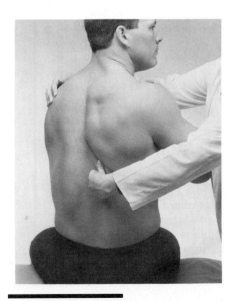

**FIGURE 2-54** ■ Mobilization (thoracic rotation).

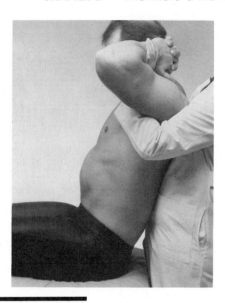

**FIGURE 2-55** ■ Manual traction of the upper segments of the thoracic spine.

### Patient's Position

If there is an upper rib lesion, the patient is supine.

If there is a lower rib lesion, the patient is lying on the side.

The arm on the involved side is elevated overhead.

### Physical Therapist's Position

The physical therapist stands at the side of the elevated arm.

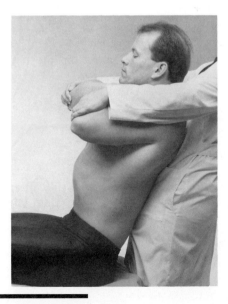

**FIGURE 2-56** ■ Manual traction of the lower segments of the thoracic spine.

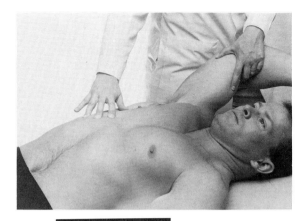

FIGURE 2–57 ■ Mobilization (rib elevation).

### Hand Placement

The web space of the stabilizing hand is on the inferior rib of the lesioned segment. The mobilizing hand grasps the elevated humerus.

### Procedure

The patient takes a deep breath. The inferior rib is stabilized while an elevation is provided through the humerus. This is held for 8 to 10 seconds. The patient relaxes and the downward force on the inferior rib is maintained. This is repeated 8 to 10 times.

### DEPRESSION (EXPIRATION) RESTRICTIONS (Fig. 2–58)
### Patient's Position

If there is an upper rib lesion, the patient is supine.

If there is a lower rib lesion, the patient is lying on the side.

The arm on the involved side is elevated overhead.

### Physical Therapist's Position

The physical therapist is standing on the side of the elevated arm.

### Hand Placement

The stabilizing hand is on the superior rib of the lesioned segment. The mobilizing hand grasps the elevated arm.

### Procedure

The patient takes a deep breath. While the patient exhales forcibly, the therapist provides a downward force with the stabilizing hand and an elevation force to the humerus with the mobilizing hand. This is held for 8 to 10 seconds and then repeated 8 to 10 times.

AUSTRALIAN APPROACH[9]

The mobilizations of the Australian approach are oscillatory. They include anteroposterior central vertebral pressure, anteroposterior unilateral vertebral pressure, and transverse vertebral pressure.

### ANTEROPOSTERIOR CENTRAL VERTEBRAL PRESSURE (Fig. 2–59)
### Patient's Position

The patient lies prone.

### Physical Therapist's Position

The physical therapist stands at the patient's side or head.

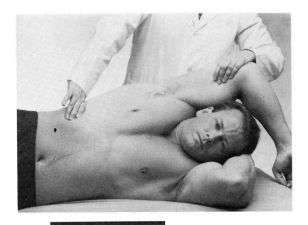

FIGURE 2–58 ■ Mobilization (rib depression).

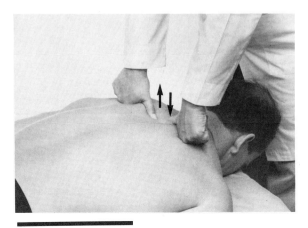

FIGURE 2–59 ■ Anteroposterior central vertebral pressure.

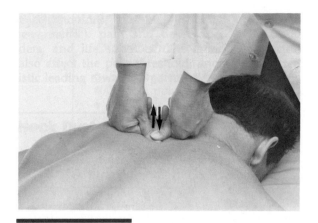

**FIGURE 2–60** ■ Anteroposterior unilateral vertebral pressure.

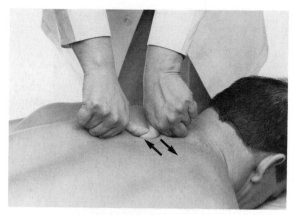

**FIGURE 2–61** ■ Transverse vertebral pressure.

## Hand Placement

The pads of the thumbs are placed on the spinous process pointing transversely across the vertebral column.

## Procedure

An anteroposterior oscillatory pressure is produced by the body and transmitted to the thumbs by the arms.

## ANTEROPOSTERIOR UNILATERAL VERTEBRAL PRESSURE (Fig. 2–60)

### Patient's Position

The patient lies prone.

### Physical Therapist's Position

The physical therapist stands at the patient's side or head.

### Hand Placement

The thumbs are placed on the transverse process of the involved segment pointing toward each other.

### Procedure

An anteroposterior oscillatory pressure is produced by the body and transmitted to the thumbs by the arms.

## TRANSVERSE VERTEBRAL PRESSURE (Fig. 2–61)

### Patient's Position

The patient lies prone.

### Physical Therapist's Position

The physical therapist stands at the side of the patient at the level that is to be treated.

## Hand Placement

The pads of the thumbs are placed on the side of the spinous process of the vertebra to be treated.

## Procedure

A transverse oscillatory pressure is provided to the spinous process by the thumbs through the arms.

---

OSTEOPATHIC APPROACH[3]

The lesions identified by positional testing are of type I (NSR) and type II (FRS, ERS). The following are examples of treatment techniques used to correct these dysfunctions. These techniques can be adapted for the specific lesion found upon examination.

---

## NS(R)R(L) (NEUTRAL SIDE BENT (RIGHT) ROTATED (LEFT)) (Fig. 2–62)

### Patient's Position

Sitting on a stool or treatment table with hands clasped behind the neck.

### Physical Therapist's Position

Standing at the side of the patient opposite to the side of the side bending restriction. The physical therapist reaches under the patient's nearest arm to place the right hand on the top of the patient's left shoulder. The right hand is used to monitor the interspinous space below the vertebra to be treated.

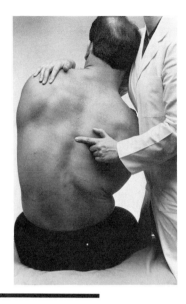

**FIGURE 2-62** ■ Mobilization—NS(R)R(L) lesion.

## Procedure

1. The patient is side bent to the left at the level of involvement.

2. The patient is rotated in the appropriate direction: toward the physical therapist if level is at apex of curve or below, away from physical therapist if the level is above the apex.

3. The patient is instructed to side bend to the right with 10 to 15 pounds of force against the physical therapist's unyielding resistance; the force is maintained for 5 to 8 seconds and the patient is instructed to relax.

4. The side bending and rotation are relocalized.

5. Steps 3 and 4 are repeated three times and then the patient is re-examined.

## ERS(L) (Fig. 2-63)
### Patient's Position

Supine on the treatment table with hands clasped behind the neck.

### Physical Therapist's Position

Standing at the side of the patient.

### Procedure

1. The patient's elbows are used to rotate the patient toward the physical therapist.

2. The right hand is placed behind the patient and the pisiform makes contact with the right transverse process of the lower vertebrae in the segment. The flexed fingers contact the left transverse process of the superior vertebrae in the segment.

3. This contact is maintained and the patient is rolled back to the supine position.

4. With the left hand, the physical therapist uses the patient's elbows to flex the patient to the level being treated. The patient's elbows are cradled by gripping over the superior aspects of the forearms with the right hand.

5. The physical therapist takes up the slack in the soft tissues and maintains a downward and cranial force along the shafts of the humeri for 8 to 10 seconds.

6. This is repeated three times and the patient is reassessed.

## FRS(L) (Fig. 2-64)
### Patient's Position

Prone on the treatment table.

### Physical Therapist's Position

Standing at the patient's left side (side of the most posterior transverse process).

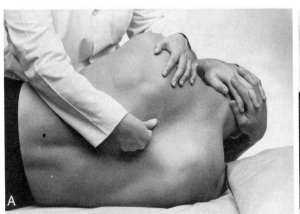
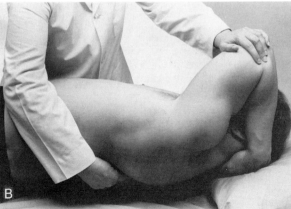

**FIGURE 2-63** ■ Mobilization—ERS(L) lesion.

## Procedure

1. The physical therapist's right hand is placed on the left transverse process (posterior process) with the fingers pointing cranially.

2. The left hand makes contact with the right transverse process of the same level with the fingers directed caudally. Use skin locking to improve the effectiveness of the technique.

3. The patient is instructed to take a deep breath. As the patient exhales a force is applied with the right hand directed upward and cranially and the left hand directed downward and caudally.

4. Repeat this 8 to 10 times and reassess.

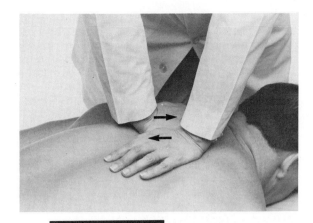

FIGURE 2–64 ■ Mobilization—FRS(L) lesion.

## Hypermobility

Hypermobility is detected by mobility testing. It is best treated by use of bracing, corsets, and exercise programs designed to stabilize the structures of the trunk. Clinically, the use of braces or corsets for the thoracic spine is usually limited to a Cash orthosis (Ballert International) or a Jewett hyperextension brace in the management of compression fractures. Because of the nature of the three points of pressure and the lack of cosmetic appeal of these devices, compliance may be a factor.

Numerous clinicians have written extensively on exercise programs for postural correction. The principles put forth by Kendall and co-workers[21,22] and Sahrmann[6] are most beneficial. Refer to these resources.

## Prevention of Recurrence

To prevent recurrence of a problem, education of the patient must be an ongoing process from the initiation of treatment to its conclusion. The most significant aspects of the program for the thoracic spine are knowledge of a postural exercise program[6,21,22] and the possible need for environmental adjustment.

Over the past decade, more individuals have become involved in occupations in which a significant amount of time is spent sitting. The computer operator sitting at the visual display terminal for an extended period of time is a classic example. The physical therapist must be aware of possible adaptations to the work environment that may prevent habitual poor postures that ultimately lead to musculoskeletal imbalance and pain. A job analysis may be the most important part of the treatment process. The occu-

pational health literature can assist the reader in learning the specifics of various workplace environments and provide recommendations for modifications.[23,24]

## CONCLUSION

The thoracic spine and rib cage require a thorough examination to determine whether a patient is suitable or not suitable for treatment by the physical therapist. After this examination, goals and treatment protocols can be established based on the identified signs and symptoms. This protocol must be individualized to the patient and cannot be based strictly on pathology.

## CASE STUDY 1

▼This outpatient was a 15-year-old female referred to the physical therapist by a vascular surgeon for a postural exercise program. Radiographs revealed the presence bilaterally of cervical ribs. The patient complained of right arm numbness and tingling that began in the middle of the school day. These symptoms worsened as the day progressed. She stated that these symptoms were present for approximately 6 months. She also had occasional back and neck pain.

Objective evaluation revealed a slouched posture with rounded shoulders and a forward head. Range of motion of the cervical spine was within normal limits but produced some discomfort in the neck musculature. Range of motion of the upper extremities was within normal limits. Neurologic evaluation of the upper extremities was within normal limits for all myotomes and dermatomes. The patient's symptoms were reproduced with the Adson maneuver, the costoclavicular maneuver, the hyperabduction maneuver, and the elevated arm stress test.

The goals of treatment were to improve the postural malalignment and decrease the symptoms of thoracic outlet syndrome. The patient was instructed in a posture correction program including chin retraction, middle and lower trapezius strengthening, and scapular stabilization. She was also educated regarding the nature of thoracic outlet syndrome and the effects of posture on its progression. The patient became independent in the exercise program and performed a home program on a regular basis with compliance. After six sessions the patient was able to control her symptoms throughout the day and was discharged. The importance of continuing the exercise program was stressed to the patient.

## CASE STUDY 2

▼The patient was a 78-year-old female who suffered the onset of back pain after a fall at home. She was admitted to the hospital through the emergency room. She was evaluated by the orthopedic department and a thoracic compression fracture was suspected. A compression fracture of T-11 was confirmed by radiologic examination. She was referred to the physical therapist for ambulation and increased activity. The patient was placed in a Cash orthosis (Ballert International) to maintain the spine in a neutral position and prevent flexion. The patient was instructed in ambulation with a walker for balance and safety and in application and removal of the brace. The patient became independent in ambulation and was discharged from the hospital with home care services.

## References

1. Cailliet R: Neck and Arm Pain. Philadelphia: FA Davis, 1964.
2. Cyriax J: Textbook of Orthopaedic Medicine, Vol 1, 8th ed. London: Bailliere Tindall, 1982.
3. Mitchell FL, Moran PS, Pruzzo NA: An Evaluation and Treatment Manual of Osteopathic Muscle Energy Procedures. Valley Park, MO: Mitchell, Moran, and Pruzzo, 1979.
4. Kapandji IA: The Physiology of the Joints, Vol 3, The Trunk and Vertebral Column. New York: Churchill Livingstone, 1974.
5. Waddell G, McCulloch J, Kummel E, et al: Non-organic physical signs in low back pain. Spine 5(2):117–125, 1980.
6. Sahrmann S: A program for correction of muscular imbalance and mechanical imbalance. Clin Manag 3(4):23–28, 1983.
7. Kaltenborn FM: Mobilisation of the Spinal Column. Wellington, NZ: New Zealand University Press, 1970.
8. Stoddard A: Manual of Osteopathic Technique. London: Hutchinson, 1980.
9. Maitland GD: Vertebral Manipulation, 5th ed. Boston: Butterworths, 1986.
10. Dale WA, Lewis MR: Thoracic outlet syndrome. *In* Vascular Surgery (Edwards WH, ed). Baltimore: University Park Press, 1976, pp. 211–229.

11. Judy KL, Heymann RL: Vascular complications of thoracic outlet syndrome. Am J Surg 123:521–531, 1972.
12. Urschel HC, Paulson DL, McNamara JJ: Thoracic outlet syndrome. Ann Thorac Surg 6(1):1–9, 1968.
13. Lord JW, Rosati LM: Thoracic outlet syndromes. Clin Symp 23(2):1–32, 1974.
14. Roos DB: Congenital anomalies associated with thoracic outlet syndrome. Am J Surg 132:771–778, 1976.
15. Smith KF: The thoracic outlet syndrome: a protocol of treatment. J Orthop Sports Phys Ther 1(2):89–99, 1979.
16. Fairbank JCT, Couper J, Davies JB, et al: The Oswestry low back pain disability questionnaire. Physiotherapy 66:271–273, 1980.
17. Kaltenborn FM: Manual Mobilization of the Extremity Joints, 4th ed. Oslo: Olaf Norlis Bokhandel, 1989.
18. Mannheimer JS, Lampe GN: Clinical Transcutaneous Electrical Nerve Stimulation. Philadelphia: FA Davis, 1984.
19. Michlovitz SL: Thermal Agents in Rehabilitation, 2nd ed. Philadelphia: FA Davis, 1990.
20. Scully RM, Barnes MR, eds: Physical Therapy. Philadelphia: JB Lippincott, 1989.
21. Kendall HO, Kendall FP, Boynton DA: Posture and Pain. Malabar, FL: Robert E. Krieger, 1952.
22. Kendall FP, McCreary EK: Muscles—Testing and Function, 3rd ed. Baltimore: Williams & Wilkins, 1983.
23. Arndt R: Working posture and musculoskeletal problems of VDT operations—review and reappraisal. Am Ind Hyg Assoc J 44:437–446, 1983.
24. VDT's Preliminary Guidelines for Selection, Installation, and Use. New York: AT&T Bell Laboratories, 1983.

## Bibliography

Basmajian J, Nyberg R (eds): Rational Manual Therapies. Baltimore: Williams & Wilkins, 1993.
Boissonnault WG (ed): Examination in Physical Therapy Practice. Screening for Medical Disease. New York: Churchill Livingstone, 1991.
Ferguson D, Duncan J: Keyboard design and operating posture. Ergonomics 17:731, 1974.
Goodman CC, Snyder TE: Differential Diagnosis in Physical Therapy. Philadelphia: WB Saunders, 1990.
Goss CM (ed): Gray's Anatomy of the Human Body, 29th American ed. Philadelphia: Lea & Febiger, 1973.
Grandjean E, Hunting W, Piderman M: VDT workstation design: preferred settings and their effects. Hum Factors 13:117, 1971.
Grant JC: Grant's Atlas of Anatomy. Baltimore: Williams & Wilkins, 1962.
Grant R (ed): Physical Therapy of the Cervical and Thoracic Spine, Vol 17, Clinics in Physical Therapy. New York: Churchill Livingstone, 1988.
Grieve GP (ed): Modern Manual Therapy of the Vertebral Column. New York: Churchill Livingstone, 1986.
Magee DJ: Orthopedic Physical Assessment, 2nd ed. Philadelphia: WB Saunders, 1992.
O'Rahilly R: Anatomy. A Regional Study of Human Structure, 5th ed. Philadelphia: WB Saunders, 1986.
Williams PL, Warwick R, Dyson M, et al: Gray's Anatomy, 37th British ed. New York: Churchill Livingstone, 1989.

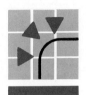

# CHAPTER

# *Three*

# Lumbar Spine and Pelvis

## CARL DeROSA / JAMES A. PORTERFIELD

## INTRODUCTION

Low back pain is among the most common ailments in industrialized societies. Although spinal disorders have a very low mortality rate, the cost to society in terms of health care, disability, and lost productivity is quite high (Fig. 3–1). It has been noted that the costs for treatment and compensation for low back pain in industry are greater than the total amount spent on all other industrial injuries combined.[1,2] In the United States the number of individuals disabled because of low back pain grew at a rate 14 times that of population growth during the decade from 1971 to 1981.[3] Mooney[4] notes that there has been a greater growth of low back disability than of any other medical disability. Of even greater concern is that the dramatic increase in low back disability occurred at the same time as a dramatic increase in knowledge of ergonomics and biomechanics and that diagnosis was aided by the development of increasingly sophisticated equipment.

The problem is obviously complex and presents many dilemmas for the clinician. One of the most confounding aspects is the prevalence of low back pain. It is generally accepted that nearly 80% of the general population experience low back pain at some time in their life and, even more impressive, that 20 to 30% are experiencing it at any given time.[5–7] Another aspect of concern is that despite considerable research efforts toward identifying the etiology of low back pain, only syndromes that are associated with neurologic compression of the nerve roots have reasonably well understood clinical presentations.[8] Experts agree that the precise diagnosis is unknown in 80 to 90% of patients with low back pain. Nachemson[9] notes that we do not have the pathologic understanding to delineate the anatomic source of pain in most patients with low back pain.

We obviously still have much to learn and perhaps need to reconsider our past approach to dealing with low back pain. It is well recognized that there can be many sources of low back pain and that naming the exact tissue involved during the evaluation process is most unlikely. This chapter is designed to provide a general background on the functional anatomy of the lumbar spine and pelvis. The primary focus of this chapter is on activity-related mechanical low back disorders, because these patients are the group most indicated for physical therapy. Differential diagnostic considerations are addressed but only to alert the examining physical therapist of the many disorders that have the potential to result in low back pain. Lastly, treatment considerations, with particular emphasis on the objectives of treatment, are discussed.

## ANATOMY AND MECHANICS

The lumbopelvic complex consists of the five lumbar vertebrae, sacrum, paired innominate bones, and articulating femurs, with intervening soft tissues including the intervertebral discs, ligaments, and muscles.

## Osteology

### Lumbar Vertebrae

The lumbar spine is composed of five individually segmented vertebrae. Occasionally the caudal region varies in segmentation. This variation results in either the first sacral vertebra failing to fuse with the rest of the sacrum (lumbarization of the first sacral vertebra) or fusion of the fifth lumbar vertebra to the sacrum (sacralization of the fifth lumbar vertebra).

The components of the lumbar vertebrae are shown in Figure 3–2. The vertebral body consists of spongy bone covered by a thin shell of cortical bone. The size of the vertebral bodies increases from the first lumbar vertebra to the fifth. The posterior aspect of the vertebral body, which helps form the anterior limitation of the spinal canal, is generally concave in the upper lumbar segments and slightly convex in the lower.

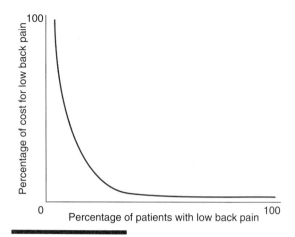

**FIGURE 3–1** ■ Cost of the low back pain problem. Fewer than 20% of patients with low back pain are responsible for over 80% of the costs.

The pedicles are two short, stout bony projections from the posterolateral aspects of the vertebral body. Because most of the musculature of the lumbar spine attaches to the various posterior processes of the vertebrae, the force of muscle contraction is ultimately transmitted to the vertebral body through the pedicles.

The paired laminae originate from the posterior aspect of the pedicles. The pars interarticularis is the part of the lamina that lies just superior to the articular surface of the inferior articulating process. This bony structure assists in counterbalancing the anterior shear force of the antigravity posture. Its clinical importance lies in the fact that it is often the region of fracture in spondylolisthesis.

Above and below the pedicles of the vertebrae are the superior and inferior notches. When two lumbar vertebrae are placed together, the superior and inferior notches of the articulating vertebrae come together to form the intervertebral foramen, through which the spinal nerve exits and begins to divide into the anterior and posterior rami.

Each lumbar vertebra has two superior facets, which face superiorly and medially, and two inferior facets, which face anteriorly and laterally (Fig. 3–3). It is important to note that the inferior articulating process lies medial to the superior articulating process. Understanding this anatomic relationship helps the clinician to visualize the forces generated into and through this joint as movement analysis is carried out during the assessment process. The facet is the portion of the articular process that meets the facet of its

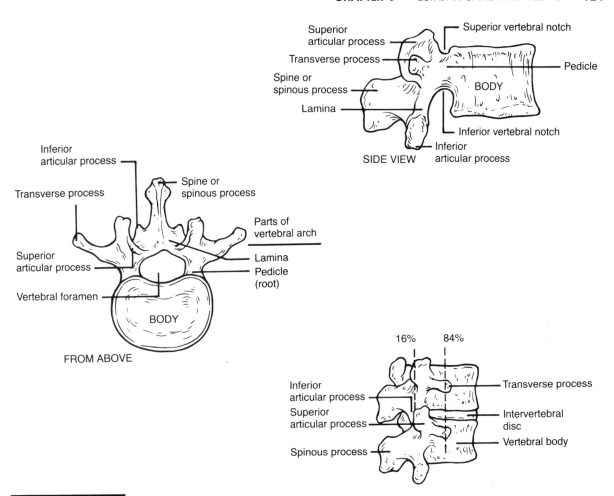

**FIGURE 3-2** ■ Components of the lumbar vertebrae: body, pedicle, transverse process, superior facets, inferior facets, transverse process, mammillary process, accessory process, lamina, and spinal canal.

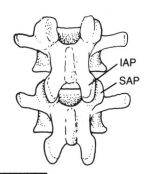

**FIGURE 3-3** ■ Posterior view of two lumbar vertebrae showing medial relationship of the inferior articulating process (IAP) to the superior articulating process (SAP). (From Porterfield JA, DeRosa CP: Mechanical Low Back Pain: Perspectives in Functional Anatomy. Philadelphia: WB Saunders, 1990.)

joint partner. The correct anatomic term for the synovial joint formed is zygapophyseal joint, although the term facet or apophyseal joint is used quite often. On the posterior surface of the superior articulating process is the mammillary process, which serves as an attachment for the multifidus muscle.

Just anterior to the facets are the laterally projecting transverse processes, which serve as attachments for muscles. The accessory process is on the posterior surface of the transverse process and serves as a point of attachment for the multifidus and intertransverse muscles.

The spinous processes of the lumbar vertebrae project directly posteriorly. Generally, the spinous processes of the third and fourth lumbar vertebrae are larger than those of the fifth. The spi-

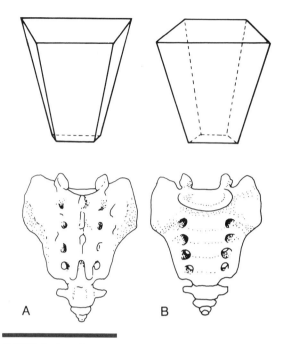

**FIGURE 3–4** ■ The sacrum is wider superiorly than inferiorly and wider anteriorly than posteriorly. (From Porterfield JA, DeRosa CP: Mechanical Low Back Pain: Perspectives in Functional Anatomy. Philadelphia: WB Saunders, 1990.)

nous processes serve as attachments for the multifidus muscles and posterior layer of thoracolumbar fascia.

### Sacrum

The sacrum consists of five fused vertebrae. The sacrum is wider superiorly and anteriorly than it is inferiorly and posteriorly (Fig. 3–4). It resembles a truncated pyramid. From a superior to inferior perspective, the anterior aspect of the sacrum is concave and the posterior aspect is convex. The lamina of the fifth sacral vertebra does not usually fuse during development and the sacral hiatus is formed. This hiatus is continuous with the epidural space and can serve as a portal of entry for epidural injections.

The sacrum articulates with the fifth lumbar vertebra via the articulations between the superior facets of the sacrum and the inferior facets of the fifth lumbar vertebra, forming the lumbosacral junction. The intervertebral disc also serves as an articulating link between the body of the fifth lumbar vertebra and the cranial aspect of the sacral surface. The sacrum also articulates with the ilium, forming the sacroiliac joint.

### Innominate Bone

The innominate bone is formed by the fusion of the ilium, ischium, and pubis. It contributes to the formation of the sacroiliac joint, pubic symphysis, and hip joints. The ring formed by the articulation of the paired innominates with the sacrum is termed the pelvis. The pelvis serves as an attachment for many trunk and lower extremity muscles. With the foot fixed to the ground in the upright standing posture, contraction of these muscles can alter the relationship of the pelvis to the lumbar spine and hence the weight-bearing characteristics of the lumbar spine. This is discussed later. The reader is referred to Chapter 7 for the detailed anatomy of the hip and pelvis.

## Connective Tissues

### Intervertebral Disc

Two vertebral bodies are linked by the intervertebral disc. Typically the intervertebral disc is described as consisting of an outer annulus fibrosus and inner nucleus pulposus. However, from a histologic perspective, the cartilaginous end plate can also be considered part of the intervertebral disc because of the intimate relationship between the collagen framework of the vertebral end plate and the annulus fibrosus (Fig. 3–5).

The shape of the lumbar intervertebral discs is roughly elliptic. Generally the anterior height of the last two lumbar discs is nearly twice their posterior height. This 2:1 relationship re-

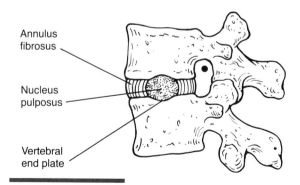

Annulus fibrosus

Nucleus pulposus

Vertebral end plate

**FIGURE 3–5** ■ Structure of the intervertebral disc demonstrating the components of the disc and the concentric rings of the annulus fibrosus. (From Porterfield JA, DeRosa CP: Mechanical Low Back Pain: Perspectives in Functional Anatomy. Philadelphia: WB Saunders, 1990.)

sulting in a wedge shape for the disc is nearly always present in the L-5–S-1 disc. Although the anterior inclination of the sacrum is a contributing factor, the wedge shape of the disc contributes greatly to the development of the lumbar lordosis.

Approximately 12 to 15 concentric rings of fibrocartilage form the annulus fibrosus (see Fig. 3–5). Each layer of fibers is obliquely offset from the next layer, with the fibers forming an approximately 30-degree angle with the horizontal.[10] In the anterior annulus, the lamellae are quite thick and are fairly distinguishable. In contrast, the posterior annulus is thinner and the lamellae tend to be compressed and merged together. The proportion of collagen increases from the inner to outer annulus, and there is also a variation of the type of collagen within the intervertebral disc. Type I collagen, the type that is structured to counter tensile forces, is found mainly in the annulus. Type II collagen, which counters compressive forces, is in the nucleus.

The nucleus pulposus is primarily a hydrated gel of proteoglycans consisting of sulfated glycosaminoglycans bound to a protein core, with a small number of cells of collagen present. Water typically accounts for more than 80% of the weight of the nucleus. Because of the presence of negatively charged sulfate groups, water is attracted to the proteoglycan macromolecule, hence the term hydrophilic. One of the most striking age-related changes of the nucleus pulposus is loss of water. This loss is generally attributed to changes in the glycosaminoglycan content of the nucleus pulposus.

The major components of the intervertebral disc are collagen fibers, proteoglycans, and water. The histochemistry changes from the periphery to the center. A more densely arranged collagen framework is evident in the peripheral annulus, whereas a greater concentration of proteoglycans and less collagen are found in the central nucleus pulposus. Because the water content depends on the water-binding properties of the proteoglycans, there is a greater amount of water in the nucleus pulposus. It is beyond the scope of this text to discuss in detail the types and behavioral characteristics of the specific types of collagen and proteoglycans, and the reader is encouraged to review sources providing this information.[11-15] As the intervertebral disc ages, it is difficult to distinguish the nucleus pulposus from the annulus fibrosus.

The cartilaginous end plates consist of hyaline cartilage over the subchondral bone plates of the vertebral body. The cartilage is approximately 0.6 mm thick and is generally thicker peripherally and thinner toward the center. The vertebral end plates are connected directly to the lamellae that form the inner one third of the annulus fibrosus. The cartilage resembles the intervertebral disc in that it has a higher concentration of proteoglycans and water than collagen toward the center and more collagen than proteoglycans peripherally. Multiple perforations in the cartilage end plate permit contact with the vascular buds from the marrow of the cancellous bone of the vertebral body. This vascular communication plays an important role in the nutrition of the intervertebral disc. Because of these vascular contacts and the thinness of the cartilage, diffusion of nutrients such as oxygen and glucose is facilitated. The intervertebral discs are essentially avascular. Two sources of nutrition for the disc are the vertebral blood vessels ramifying close to the nucleus and annulus in the cartilaginous end plates and the blood vessels that enter the periphery of the annulus fibrosus.

Because collagen fibers reinforce a tissue if the applied stress is in the axial direction of the fiber, it should be apparent that the orientation of the collagen fibers of the annulus fibrosus allows restraint of nearly all motions of the spine. For example, twisting (torsion), anterior shear forces that accompany weight bearing, or forward bending of the spine results in tension being applied to specific regions of the annulus fibrosus (Fig. 3–6). Any motion of the lumbar spine can be seen to place specific annular regions under tension.

Both the annulus fibrosus and the nucleus pulposus also function to resist compression. The proteoglycan-water component of the nucleus provides a hydrostatic mechanism to help distribute compressive forces tangentially toward the annulus, which increases the tension of the annular rings, further stabilizing the intervertebral disc (Fig. 3–7). Compression of the disc raises the pressure in the nucleus, which stretches the collagen fibers of the inner annular lamellae. Attraction and binding of water by the proteoglycans result in a swelling pressure that ultimately allows the intervertebral discs to support compressive loads. Note also that contraction of the muscles of the spine causes compression between the vertebrae as a result of the muscle fiber direction (see later). In fact, intervertebral compressive forces that ultimately increase intradiscal pressure are dependent on, in probable decreasing order of influence, muscle

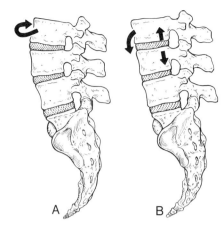

FIGURE 3-6 ■ Oblique orientation of the annulus fibrosus helps limit any motion of the lumbar spine. This example shows tension being applied to annular fibers during torsion (A) and forward bending (B).

contraction, preload by the ligaments, and super-incumbent weight. The combined function of the annulus and nucleus stabilizes the disc complex to direct forces properly and restrict movement, maintains the size and shape of the neurofora-men, and ensures that the apophyseal joint maintains a midrange position during weight bearing.

### Zygapophyseal Joints

The facets of the zygapophyseal joints have both a sagittal and a frontal plane orientation (Fig. 3–8A and B). The superior lateral facet is slightly concave, and the inferior medial articulation has a slightly convex orientation. The joints are thus oriented to limit both anterior shear and torsional stresses. Because of the lumbar lordosis, a continuous anterior shear stress results from the force of gravity, especially at the lumbosacral junction and the L4-5 articulation. Because of the two-plane arrangement of the joint structure, the cartilaginous surface of the facet oriented in the frontal plane is the first region of the joint to show early signs of degeneration.[16,17]

The zygapophyseal joints are the only true diarthrodial joints in the lumbar spine. Therefore they contain a fibrous joint capsule with a synovial lining. Motions allowed between the lumbar facets are largely flexion and extension motions. Minimal lateral bending or rotation occurs at the lumbar joints. The average range of flexion and extension at each segment is 15 degrees, and the average segmental rotation is 2.5 degrees.[18]

Since the facet articular cartilage is aneural, pain does not arise directly from that structure. Possible sources of pain from degeneration of the joints include the following:[19-21]

- Overloading of the subchondral bone trabeculae
- Microfractures of bone trabeculae
- Mechanical deformation or chemical irritation of joint capsule nociceptors
- Internal derangements from joint loose bodies
- Meniscoid synovial folds
- Vascular disturbances in the bone or soft tissues
- Joint inflammation

Overloading of the articular cartilage is recognized as potentially accelerating the degenerative process. Underloading of articular cartilage also results in degenerative changes because of de-

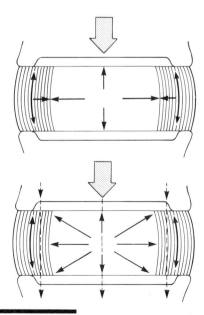

FIGURE 3-7 ■ Compressive forces applied to the intervertebral disc are distributed peripherally toward the annular rings. (From Bogduk N, Twomey LT: Clinical Anatomy of the Lumbar Spine. New York: Churchill-Livingstone, 1987).

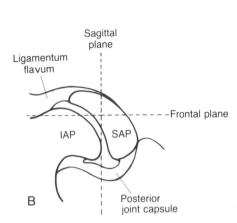

**FIGURE 3–8** ■ Frontal plane (A) and sagittal plane (B) orientation of the zygapophyseal joints of the lumbar spine. (From Porterfield JA, DeRosa CP: Mechanical Low Back Pain: Perspectives in Functional Anatomy. Philadelphia: WB Saunders, 1990.)

creased proteoglycan synthesis of the chondrocyte and cartilage softening.[22] It should be recognized that the apophyseal joint is under a constant variety of loads because of its position in the weight-bearing chain and muscular contraction. Adams and Hutton[23] have noted that in the upright posture, compressive force on the lumbar vertebrae is distributed in such a way that 86% of the force is borne by the bone-disc complex and 14% by zygapophyseal joints. The degree of lumbar flexion or extension alters the magnitude of this compressive force. When the lumbar spine is in more flexion, the zygapophyseal joints have less compressive force while there is more compression intervertebrally. Extension of the lumbar spine increases the compressive force between the articulating facets and compresses the posterior aspect of the disc, creating an anterior shear of the vertebrae above on the vertebrae below.

The joint capsules of the zygapophyseal joints deserve special mention. These fibrous structures are thick posteriorly, and anteriorly they are formed by the lateral extension of the ligamentum flavum (Fig. 3–9). The joint capsules are innervated from branches of the posterior rami of the spinal nerves, especially the medial and intermediate divisions.

### Sacroiliac Joint

The sacroiliac joint is formed by the articulation between the sacrum and the ilium.[24] The iliac surface is composed of thin fibrocartilage, and the articular surface of the sacrum is formed by hyaline cartilage that is 1.7 to 5 times thicker than the iliac cartilage.[25,26]

From the lateral aspect, the sacral articular surface can be divided into a cranial and a caudal surface (Fig. 3–10). As an individual ages, the topography of the joint surface changes from being relatively smooth to having numerous elevations and depressions. The fit of the various curvatures into corresponding depressions contributes to the inherent stability of the joint.

Because the sacrum is wider anteriorly than posteriorly, the joint plane is oblique, which means that it is aligned between a sagittal and a frontal plane orientation. In general, only the first three sacral vertebrae contribute to the formation of the sacroiliac joint. Horizontal sections of the joint indicate that the plane of the joint may vary at each level (Fig. 3–11).

Much controversy has surrounded the types, amounts, and relevance of sacroiliac joint movements. The axis of motion has been described as occurring at the junction of the cranial and caudal aspects of the sacral surface,[27] as well as just posterior to the pubic symphysis.[28] Most likely, these two fixed-axis theories represent points on a continuum of instantaneous axes of motion at the sacroiliac joint.[29]

With the axis of motion located at the sacrum, the iliac motion at the sacrum is typically described as anterior or posterior torsion, whereas sacral motion on the ilium is described as nuta-

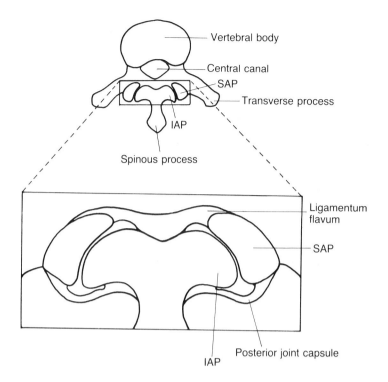

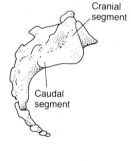

**FIGURE 3-9** ■ Horizontal view of the zygapophyseal joints showing how the ligamentum flavum helps form the anterior limitation of the joint capsule. (From Porterfield JA, DeRosa CP: Mechanical Low Back Pain: Perspectives in Functional Anatomy. Philadelphia: WB Saunders, 1990.)

**FIGURE 3-10** ■ Lateral view of sacral surface showing the cranial and caudal aspects. (From Porterfield JA, DeRosa CP: Mechanical Low Back Pain: Perspectives in Functional Anatomy. Philadelphia: WB Saunders, 1990.)

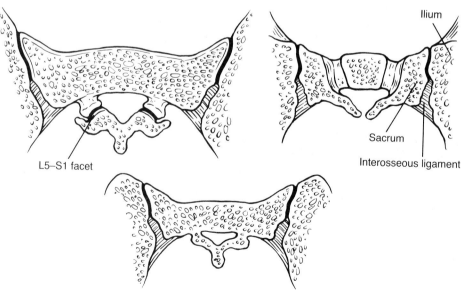

**FIGURE 3-11** ■ Horizontal section of the sacroiliac joint at three different levels. Note the variability of the joint plane at the different levels and the relationship of the interosseous ligament to the sacroiliac joint.

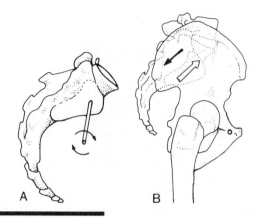

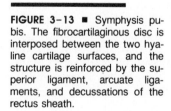

**FIGURE 3-12** ■ Two different theoretical axes of the sacroiliac joint. The axis through the sacrum (A) allows torsional movements of the ilium or nutation-counternutation of the sacrum. The axis behind the pubic symphysis (B) allows translational motion at the sacroiliac joint. Both stresses occur simultaneously. (From Porterfield JA, DeRosa CP: Mechanical Low Back Pain: Perspectives in Functional Anatomy. Philadelphia, WB Saunders, 1990.)

tion (flexion) or counternutation (extension). With the axis of motion posterior to the pubic symphysis, motion at the sacroiliac joint would consist of translations (Fig. 3-12). In reality, this articulation is under constant load and the joint structure permits deformation of the two cartilaginous surfaces, allowing a combination of rotary and shear stresses to be attenuated simultaneously.

The amount of motion is minimal because of the joint topography and reinforcing ligaments. Weisel[30] reported 5.6 mm, Sashin[31] reported 4 degrees, and Sturesson and co-workers[32] found 1

to 2 degrees of movement at the sacroiliac joint. On average, there are approximately 3 degrees of flexion, 0.8 degrees of lateral bending, and 1.5 degrees of axial rotation.[33] There has been no controlled, randomized study demonstrating that sacroiliac joint motion can be palpated to determine evidence of hypermobility or hypomobility.

## Pubic Symphysis

The articulation between the medial aspects of the pubic bones forms a cartilaginous joint. The complete articular surface of each bone is covered by hyaline cartilage. Between the two articulating surfaces is a fibrocartilaginous interpubic disc that is generally thicker in females than males. The superior pubic ligament, arcuate pubic ligament, and decussations of the rectus sheath help reinforce the joint (Fig. 3-13).

The joint does not normally allow movement.[34,35] However, during pregnancy the ligaments associated with the joint soften and allow some degree of separation between the joint surfaces.[36,37] This separation is approximately 2 mm.

## Ligaments

**Anterior Longitudinal Ligament.** The anterior longitudinal ligament is a very strong structure in the lumbar spine. It runs the entire length of the spine and typically is fixed firmly to the annulus fibrosus and more loosely blended with the periosteum of the vertebral bodies.

**Posterior Longitudinal Ligament.** The posterior longitudinal ligament runs the entire length

**FIGURE 3-13** ■ Symphysis pubis. The fibrocartilaginous disc is interposed between the two hyaline cartilage surfaces, and the structure is reinforced by the superior ligament, arcuate ligaments, and decussations of the rectus sheath.

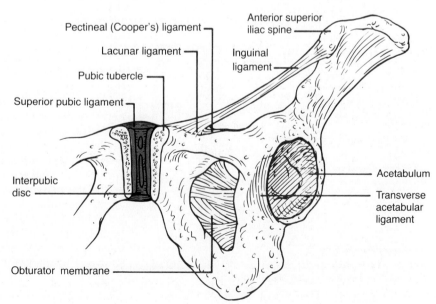

Pectineal (Cooper's) ligament
Lacunar ligament
Pubic tubercle
Superior pubic ligament
Interpubic disc
Obturator membrane
Anterior superior iliac spine
Inguinal ligament
Acetabulum
Transverse acetabular ligament

of the spine. It has an hourglass arrangement because of the location of the pedicles on the posterior aspect of the vertebral body. It fans out over the posterior aspect of the intervertebral disc to which it is connected (Fig. 3–14). All of the spinal ligaments contain free nerve endings and complex unencapsulated endings; however, the posterior longitudinal ligament appears to have the greatest density of nerve endings.[38]

**Ligamentum Flavum.** The paired ligamenta flava run from one lamina to the adjacent one. Each is attached to the front of the lower border of the lamina above and passes downward and backward to the back of the upper border of the lamina below. Because the ligament has a high elastin fiber content, it is more yellow than other spinal ligaments. The different histochemistry allows greater elastic properties. As mentioned earlier, the lateral extent of the ligament forms the anterior limitation of the zygapophyseal joint capsule.

**Interspinous Ligaments.** The interspinous ligaments are present in the complete spine but are most completely developed in the lumbar region. These ligaments run in an oblique fashion superiorly and posteriorly from one spinous process to the next (Fig. 3–15). The ligaments occupy the space between the supraspinous ligament and the ligamentum flavum.

**Supraspinous Ligaments.** The supraspinous ligaments attach to the tips of the spinous processes, terminate at approximately the third lumbar segment, and are reinforced in the lower lumbar region by the decussation of the posterior layer of thoracolumbar fascia. In general, the su-

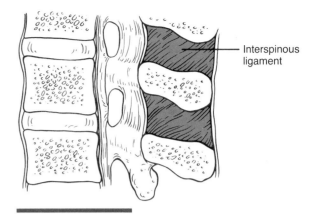

FIGURE 3–15 ■ Course of the interspinous ligament between adjacent spinous processes.

praspinous ligament is continuous with the posterior edge of the interspinous ligaments.

**Iliolumbar Ligaments.** The iliolumbar ligaments connect the fifth and occasionally the fourth lumbar transverse processes with the ilium. The ligament is broad and stout and typically continues to reinforce the anterosuperior aspect of the sacroiliac joint.[39] The ligament is a major stabilizer of the L-5 vertebrae on the sacrum.

The iliolumbar ligament is present only in adults. In children it is represented by muscle tissue. Luk and colleagues[40] suggest that the iliolumbar ligament is an example of metaplasia because age-related changes of the quadratus lumborum result in a replacement of the lower muscle fibers of the quadratus lumborum with thick connective tissue of the iliolumbar ligament, perhaps as a result of the gravitational forces on the lumbar lordosis in the upright posture.

**Sacroiliac and Interosseus Ligaments.** The posterior sacroiliac ligaments lie just anterior to the multifidus muscle and course in two directions to counter the inferior and anterior components of the inferiorly directed trunk force. The posterior sacroiliac ligaments are separated from the next layer, the interosseus ligament, by the dorsal rami of the sacral spinal nerves and blood vessels that course between the two ligaments.

The interosseus ligament is the major stabilizer of the sacroiliac joint and forms the chief bond between the two bones (see Fig. 3–11). Any potential movement between the sacrum and ilium must deform this ligament, which is one of the strongest ligaments in the human body.

The anterior sacroiliac ligaments travel later-

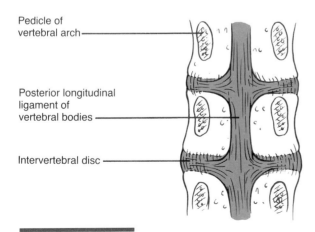

Pedicle of vertebral arch

Posterior longitudinal ligament of vertebral bodies

Intervertebral disc

FIGURE 3–14 ■ Relationship of the posterior longitudinal ligament to the intervertebral disc and pedicles.

ally, inferiorly, and laterally from the ilium to the sacrum. These ligaments blend with the inferior aspect to the iliolumbar ligament to strengthen the anterior aspect of the sacroiliac joint.

**Sacrotuberous and Sacrospinous Ligaments.** The sacrotuberous and sacrospinous ligaments are attached to the sacrum and the ischial tuberosity and ischial spine, respectively. Their attachments allow extrinsic stability of the sacrum as it is wedged between the ilia, especially in the upright standing posture. With the theoretical axis of motion through the junction of the cranial and caudal aspects of the sacrum, both ligaments are positioned to help check excessive nutation of the sacrum and posterior torsion of the ilium (see Fig. 3–12A). The sacrotuberous ligament tends to be broader than the sacrospinous ligament. Part of the posterior sacroiliac ligament blends with the sacrotuberous ligament.

### Muscles and Fascia

**Thoracolumbar Fascia.** Most of the muscles of the low back are covered and encased by the thoracolumbar fascia, which is thick and extremely well developed in the low back.[41] The posterior layer of the fascia attaches to the spinous processes. From this attachment it courses laterally and then anteriorly to surround the erector spinae and multifidus muscles of the lumbar spine. Anteriorly it attaches to the lumbar

transverse processes (Fig. 3–16). Occasionally another anterior layer, quite thin, is described covering the anterior aspect of the quadratus lumborum.

The juncture of the posterior layer of thoracolumbar fascia with the relative anterior layer attached to the transverse processes occurs at the lateral aspect of the erector spinae. This juncture is referred to as the lateral raphe. The lateral raphe is attached inferiorly to the iliac crest and laterally blends in with the aponeuroses of the latissimus dorsi, transversus abdominis, and occasionally the obliquus internus abdominis.

Considerable attention has been given to the theoretical biomechanics of the thoracolumbar fascia. Noting that its attachment to the spinous processes affords it the longest lever arm at the lumbar spine, it has been suggested that it contributes greatly to the stability of the lumbar spine from the flexed posture.[42] The attachments of the obliquus internus abdominis and transversus abdominis potentially exert a pull on the fascia, increasing its tension and providing stability of the lumbar spine.[43] Noting that the erector spinae and multifidus muscles are encased within the thoracolumbar fascia, it has been suggested that the broadening of the muscles during a contraction helps fill the fascial envelope and provides an increase in spinal stability.[42,44] The potential of the latissimus dorsi muscle to exert a tensile force on the fascia and thus contribute to

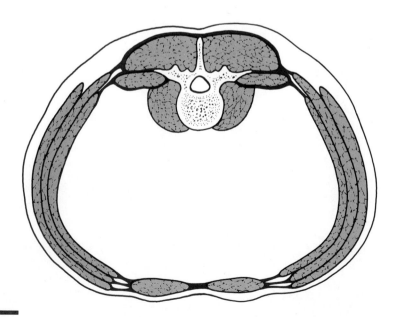

**FIGURE 3–16** ■ Cross-sectional view of the abdomen and lumbar spine. The attachments of the thoracolumbar fascia to the spinous and transverse processes and the relationships of the muscles to the fascia should be noted.

stability of the lumbar spine has also been proposed.[45]

Regardless of which mechanism is most accurate, it is readily apparent that the thoracolumbar fascia has the potential to contribute to both passive and active stabilization of the lumbar spine by virtue of its bone and muscle attachments. The fascia is a strong tissue with a well-developed latticework of collagen fibers, whose function may be described broadly as that of a type of extensor muscle retinaculum.[41]

**Erector Spinae.** Studies of the erector spinae have clearly demonstrated that these muscles can be divided into two separate anatomic and functional components in the low back, the superficial (thoracic) and deep (lumbar) components.[46]

The superficial erector spinae attaches to the pelvis and sacrum via the erector spinae aponeurosis and courses superiorly to attach to the ribs. The superficial erector spinae can be further subdivided into a lateral iliocostalis lumborum and a medial longissimus thoracis. These two divisions of the superficial erector spinae act over the thoracic vertebrae and ribs, which results in indirect action over the lumbar spine. The lever arm afforded by these two divisions allows it to increase the lumbar lordosis actively. With the trunk nearly completely bent forward, the superficial erector spinae becomes electromyographically silent as stabilization of the trunk occurs via connective tissue structures such as the fascia and joint capsules.[47,48]

The deep erector spinae can also be subdivided into the lumbar iliocostalis and the lumbar longissimus.[46] These names are chosen because these divisions, which originate on the ilium and lateral aspect of the sacrum, attach directly to the transverse processes of the lumbar vertebrae. Thus, these muscles travel superiorly from the pelvis and course anteriorly and medially (Fig. 3–17). Because the muscles are attached to the transverse processes, the lever arm for extension is not as great as that of the superficial erector spinae or multifidus muscles. The posterior-to-anterior inclination of the deep erector spinae allows it to exert a posterior shear force on the lumbar vertebrae, providing dynamic stabilization in the form of countering anterior shear in the sagittal plane. Muscular stabilization via an anterior-posterior guy wire effect is suggested by analysis of the vectors of the psoas major and deep erector spinae.[49] Both divisions of the erector spinae are innervated by branches of the posterior rami.

**Multifidus Muscles.** The multifidus muscles course the complete length of the spine but are most completely developed in the lumbar spine. These muscles arise from the dorsal surface of the sacrum and, in fact, are the largest soft tissue structures between the skin and the sacrum. The muscles also attach to the mammillary processes and joint capsules of the lumbar vertebrae. From these origins, the muscles insert two to four levels above into the spinous processes. The at-

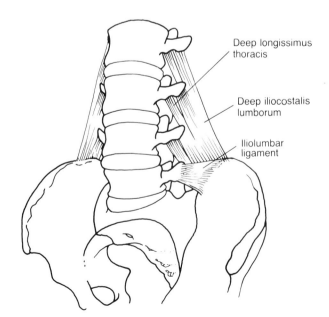

Deep longissimus
thoracis

Deep iliocostalis
lumborum

Iliolumbar
ligament

**FIGURE 3–17** ■ Vector analysis of the deep erector spinae muscle as suggested by its attachments. Note the potential to impart a posterior shear force to the lumbar vertebrae. (From Porterfield JA, DeRosa CP: Mechanical Low Back Pain: Perspectives in Functional Anatomy. Philadelphia: WB Saunders, 1990.)

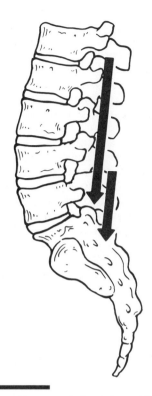

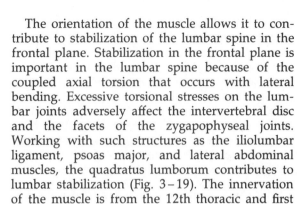

The orientation of the muscle allows it to contribute to stabilization of the lumbar spine in the frontal plane. Stabilization in the frontal plane is important in the lumbar spine because of the coupled axial torsion that occurs with lateral bending. Excessive torsional stresses on the lumbar joints adversely affect the intervertebral disc and the facets of the zygapophyseal joints. Working with such structures as the iliolumbar ligament, psoas major, and lateral abdominal muscles, the quadratus lumborum contributes to lumbar stabilization (Fig. 3–19). The innervation of the muscle is from the 12th thoracic and first lumbar nerves.

**Psoas Major.** The psoas major muscles are attached to the anteromedial aspect of the transverse processes, the anterolateral aspect of the bodies of the lumbar vertebrae, and the intervertebral disc. From this attachment the muscle courses inferiorly and descends to join the ten-

**FIGURE 3–18** ■ Vector analysis of the multifidus muscle as suggested by its attachments. The attachment to the spinous processes provides an excellent lever arm for lumbar extension.

tachments to the spinous processes give the muscle an excellent lever arm for lumbar extension (Fig. 3–18).

Although typically described in textbooks of anatomy as a rotator of the spine, the multifidus does not have an appreciable lever arm or fiber orientation to be effective in this action. It has also been speculated that the capsular attachment of the muscle allows active retraction of the joint capsule to avoid impingement between the facet surfaces.[39] All of the fascicles of the multifidus muscle are innervated by the medial branch of the dorsal ramus.

**Quadratus Lumborum.** Although typically studied with muscles of the posterior abdominal wall, the quadratus lumborum is an important muscle of the low back. From its attachment to the pelvis the muscle courses superiorly, anteriorly, and medially to gain attachments to the 12th rib (iliocostal division) and lumbar transverse processes (iliotransverse division). Occasionally, a third division courses from the 12th rib to the lumbar transverse processes (costotransverse division).

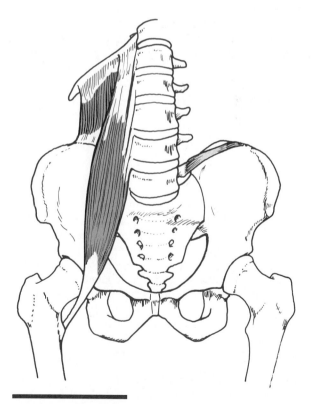

**FIGURE 3–19** ■ Frontal plane stabilization of the lumbar spine by the quadratus lumborum muscle, iliolumbar ligament, and psoas major muscle.

don of the iliac muscle, and together they travel inferiorly and laterally over the pelvic brim to attach to the lesser trochanter. In close relation and covering portions of the psoas major are the abdominal aorta, inferior vena cava, and most of the large intestine and colon. All of these structures are in turn covered by the greater omentum and muscles and fascia of the abdominal wall. The psoas major is obviously a very deeply placed muscle with numerous visceral structures completely covering its anterior and lateral surfaces.

In addition to being a strong flexor and external rotator of the hip joint, the psoas major appears to have the potential to exert many different forces on the lumbar spine, and indirectly on the pelvis, when a vector analysis is performed. If the fixed end of the muscle is considered to be the lesser trochanter, psoas major contraction exerts on the lumbar vertebrae an anterior translational stress that is most likely countered by the posteriorly directed vector of the deep erector spinae, causing a sagittal plane check and balance. The muscle can also cause a resultant anterior torsional moment of the innominate bone at the sacroiliac joint because it descends over the pelvic brim and dives posteriorly to attach to the lesser trochanter. Furthermore, contraction of the psoas major muscle from a supine position exerts a pull on the lumbar spine, and through indirect action the pelvis can be flexed at the hip joints toward the sitting position. It has already been noted that the psoas major can also contribute to sagittal and frontal plane stability of the lumbar spine. In noting that the psoas major is electromyographically active in nearly all postures and movements of the lumbar spine, Nachemson[50] suggests that it plays an important role in lumbar spine stabilization. The psoas major is innervated by directed branches from the lumbar plexus.

**Abdominal Muscles.** The abdominal muscles are typically grouped in four separate divisions: rectus abdominis, obliquus externus, obliquus internus, and transversus. A complete description of their attachments and role in posture is available elsewhere.[49] Only a brief summary is provided here.

The paired rectus abdominis muscles are individually encased within a fascial envelope and course vertically from the pubic crest to the xiphoid of the sternum and fifth through seventh ribs. Concentric contraction of the muscle approximates the thorax and pelvis. When the muscle contracts and the pelvis rotates upward, a flexion moment is imparted to the lumbosacral junction.

The external oblique muscle is prominent both posterolaterally and anterolaterally. It courses from the lower eight ribs and inserts into the iliac crest, and its aponeurosis blends in with the fascia of the thigh. The internal oblique muscle fibers are oriented at approximately 90 degrees to the fibers of the external oblique muscle. It is attached to the inguinal ligament and iliac crest and has extensive attachments to the pubis, linea alba, and lower ribs. The transversus abdominis arises from the inner surfaces of the lower ribs and the inner aspect of the iliac crest and attaches to the linea alba and pubis. The abdominal muscles are innervated by branches of the 8th to 12th intercostal, iliohypogastric, and ilioinguinal nerves.

Most functional anatomy textbooks describe the abdominal muscles as flexors and rotators of the trunk, with the exception of the rectus abdominis, which flexes only the trunk. It is intuitively obvious that in the standing position these muscles do not contribute significantly to this action, because it is the eccentric muscle activity of the spinal and hip extensors that controls the descent of the trunk by decelerating it as gravitational forces cause it to flex forward.

The abdominal muscles are extremely important in controlling the manner in which forces traverse the lumbar spine. Because the abdominal muscles also control the abdominal contents and regulate pelvic position, they directly influence the amount of flexion or extension in the spine. It was noted earlier that compression forces are shared by the vertebral body–disc complex (86%) and the posterior joints (14%). When the line of gravity of the trunk falls too far anterior to the transverse axis of motion of the spine, the resultant forward bending moment must be countered by increasing the amount of lumbar extension (Fig. 3–20). As a postural habit, this has the potential to load the posterior joints excessively. The abdominal muscles offer a means of controlling the position of the line of gravity of the trunk as well as the sagittal plane position of the lumbar spine, thus helping to reduce vulnerability of the lumbar spine.

## FUNCTIONAL NEUROSCIENCES

An understanding of back pain requires knowledge of the relevant neuroanatomy and neurophysiologic mechanisms. Pain occurs when the peripheral nerve endings known as nociceptors are stimulated by mechanical, chemical, or thermal stimuli. Activation of nociceptors related

cartilage of the zygapophyseal joints. By definition, then, any structure in the low back can serve as a source of the painful experience.

Of particular importance when considering the innervation of the low back are the posterior primary rami and the sinu-vertebral nerves (Fig. 3–21). Most of the posterior spinal structures, including the joints, are supplied by the medial and lateral branches of the posterior primary rami. The sinu-vertebral nerves innervate structures related to the spinal canal.

The sinu-vertebral nerve usually branches from the initial part of the spinal nerve and courses back through the intervertebral foramen to supply tissues within the spinal canal. Each nerve typically supplies at least two intervertebral discs, both the disc at the point of entry and the disc at the next superior level.[39] The nerve also innervates the posterior longitudinal ligament and dura mater.

Parke and Watanabe[51] have noted that the ventral dura mater in the lumbar spine is often fixed to the ventral canal surface by numerous connective tissue strands. These connective tissue attachment points are distinct from the ligaments of Hoffman, which anchor the dura mater to the spinal canal. Fixation of the ventral dura is most noticeable at the L4-5 level, which corresponds to the apex of curvature of the lumbar lordosis. The clinical implication is that elevation of this ventral dura by a herniated nucleus pulposus has the potential to produce pain.

The nerve roots in the lumbosacral spine are anatomically and physiologically unique compared to nerve roots in the other areas of the spine. Because the spinal cord ends at the upper lumbar levels, the nerve roots must traverse in a downward and lateral direction to reach their respective intervertebral foramen of exit (Fig. 3–22).

Nutrition appears to be derived from two distinct sources: a fine vasculature of the root and diffusion from the cerebrospinal fluid.[52,53] The nerve roots receive fine blood vessels from medullary (spinal cord) branches and peripherally from radicular arteries whose origins are the lumbar arteries. These proximal and distal vessels anastomose within the nerve root. This intrinsic circulation can be impeded at either the arterial or venous end of the vascular network of the nerve root. If neural ischemia results, an inflammatory state with possible spontaneous depolarization of the axon cylinders exists. Note that an inflammatory state, with its consequent fibrosis, can result in physical disruption of the diffusion of nutrients via the cerebrospinal fluid mecha-

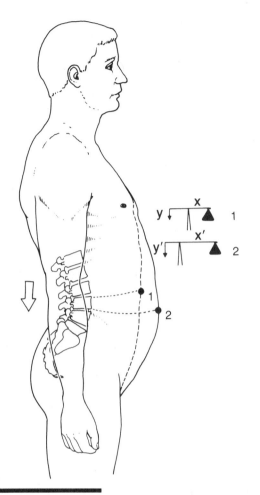

**FIGURE 3–20** ■ Lever arm and resultant extension moment on the lumbar spine. The abdominal muscles help control the position of the line of gravity of the trunk. x is the lever arm length, y is the amount of counterbalance force needed to balance the system, x' is the lever arm length with increased abdominal wall length, and y' is the amount of force needed to counterbalance x'. The greater the counterbalance force, the greater the compressive and shear forces at the lumbosacral junction. (Adapted from White AA, Panjabi MM: Clinical Biomechanics of the Spine. Philadelphia: JB Lippincott, 1978.)

to low back pain is typically due to mechanical or chemical stimuli, so the remainder of the discussion focuses on these two causative mechanisms. Upon stimulation of the nociceptive nerve endings, an afferent discharge of signals is sent toward the central nervous system, where reflex connections at both the segmental and suprasegmental levels ultimately determine the response to the painful stimuli.

All of the structures in the low back are supplied by nociceptive nerve endings with the exception of the innermost aspect of the annulus fibrosus, the nucleus pulposus, and the hyaline

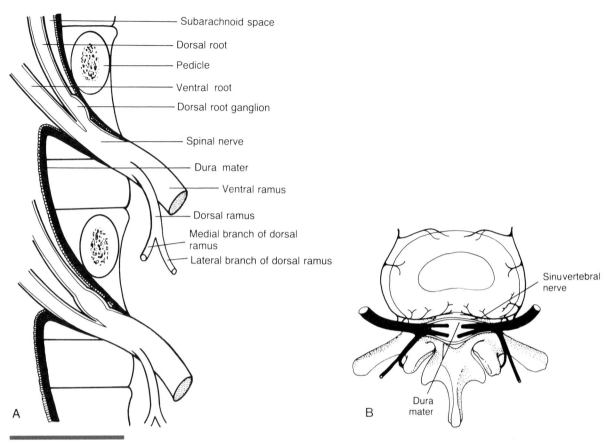

A

B

Subarachnoid space
Dorsal root
Pedicle
Ventral root
Dorsal root ganglion
Spinal nerve
Dura mater
Ventral ramus
Dorsal ramus
Medial branch of dorsal ramus
Lateral branch of dorsal ramus

Sinuvertebral nerve

Dura mater

**FIGURE 3–21** ■ (A) Formation of the spinal nerve with the anterior and posterior primary rami. (B) The sinu-vertebral nerve can also be noted as it travels back through the spinal canal to innervate spinal canal structures. (From Porterfield JA, DeRosa CP: Mechanical Low Back Pain: Perspectives in Functional Anatomy. Philadelphia: WB Saunders, 1990.)

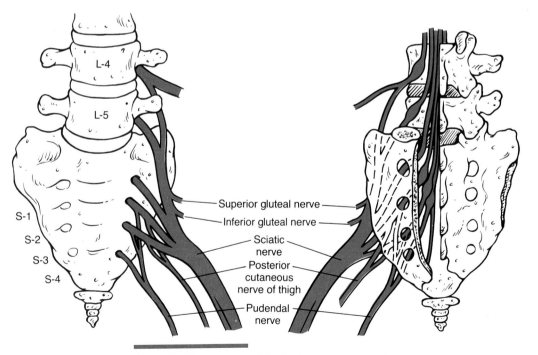

L-4
L-5
S-1
S-2
S-3
S-4

Superior gluteal nerve
Inferior gluteal nerve
Sciatic nerve
Posterior cutaneous nerve of thigh
Pudendal nerve

**FIGURE 3–22** ■ Course of the lumbosacral nerve roots.

nism. The result is an inflamed nerve root. The inflamed, irritated nerve root is one that can generate pain when mechanically distorted. In contrast, compression of normal nerve roots does not generate pain.[54]

Besides nerve root ischemia and vascular edema, another potential cause of nerve root inflammation is nuclear material that has leaked through breaches in the annulus fibrosus.[55] A chemically induced radiculitis, or inflammation caused by a possible autoimmune response to the proteoglycans of the nucleus, can render the nerve root vulnerable to producing pain when mechanically stressed (see later).

The dorsal root ganglion must also be recognized as a potential source of neurogenic low back pain. It is located in the subpedicular recess, just in front of the superior facets. The dorsal root ganglion consists of cell bodies whose peripheral axon processes supply the numerous receptors in the body and whose central axon processes terminate in the central nervous system.[49] Neurogenic inflammatory mediators such as substance P and other peptides are also manufactured and housed in the cell bodies of the ganglia neurons, and these neuropeptides are distributed via axoplasmic transport to both the central and peripheral axon processes. As a result, these peptides are transported to the spinal cord as well as the peripheral innervated tissues.

The clinical implication is that the neuropeptides released can influence the inflammatory process substantially by acting on the blood vessels and stimulate the release of leukotrienes and other chemotactic agents that attract and stimulate polymorphonuclear leukocytes besides acting at the substantia gelatinosa of the spinal cord.[56] The major difference between nerve root injury and dorsal root ganglion injury is that the former involves axons and the latter involves the all-important cell body. The ganglion is mechanically sensitive and the uninjured nerve root is not.

## BIOMECHANICS

The lumbopelvic region can be considered a hub of weight bearing, a crossroads of trunk and ground forces (Fig. 3–23). Injury can be most simply defined as acute injury or loss of cells or matrix. From a biomechanical perspective, this means inability of the tissue to accept, endure, or attenuate the stresses placed on it. The previous description of the functional anatomy makes it evident that the tissues of the low back are continually subjected to stresses such as compression, tension, and shear. When these or other stresses exceed the physiologic capacity of the tissues, injury results. All tissues of the human body have a common denominator; that is, they respond to consistent stresses placed on them. Each tissue in turn has an optimal loading zone. If the tissue is loaded within this physiologic zone, it remains healthy and uninjured (Fig. 3–

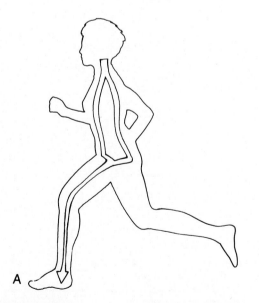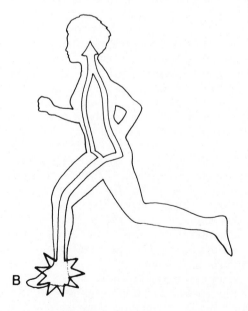

**FIGURE 3–23** ■ Trunk (A) and ground (B) forces converge into the lumbopelvic region. (From Porterfield JA, DeRosa CP: Mechanical Low Back Pain: Perspectives in Functional Anatomy. Philadelphia, WB Saunders, 1990.)

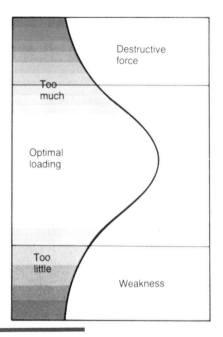

**FIGURE 3–24** ■ Optimal loading zone of tissues. To maintain health of the tissue, it must be loaded within its optimal loading zone. Injury or accelerated degeneration results if the tissue is loaded too much or too little, respectively.

24). If the tissue is loaded excessively or too little, it begins to break down.

Several factors alter the optimal loading zone of tissue. One is age. Because of the age-related changes of connective tissue structures, the limit of the optimal loading zone for tissues is less than when we were young. The strength and resilience of connective tissue decrease as we age because of changes in the biochemistry of macromolecules of connective tissue. Injury also alters the optimal loading zone. The physiologic capacity of the tissue to accept and attenuate the various forces imparted to it are much less after injury than when healthy. Simply put, a tissue that has been injured no longer has the same properties as before. This concept is important because the primary goal of rehabilitation of patients with mechanical low back pain is to teach them how to remain within the optimal loading zone of their injured tissue. By analyzing the stresses that reproduce the patient's familiar pain in the evaluation, the goal of treatment becomes one of teaching the patient movement patterns to help minimize the stresses.

Two examples may illustrate this. Consider how the hips, pelvis, and lumbar spine work as a functional unit in attenuating various forces. If an individual has a limitation of hip range of motion so that it is not possible to move the hip joint into hyperextension, the upright standing posture results in an increased anterior torsional stress of ilium on sacrum and an increased hyperextension moment on the lumbosacral zygapophyseal joints (Fig. 3–25). The facets of the lumbosacral joints now have increased weight-bearing demands and are loaded in the upper end of the optimal loading zone. The lamina and articular processes of the posterior arch are more prone to thickening in response to meeting the demands of these increased stresses, with stenosis being a possible result.

As a second example, note the biomechanics of a frontal plane asymmetry resulting from a short leg. On the ipsilateral side of the short lower extremity, there are increased abduction of the femur, increased compression at the sacroiliac joint, and increased tensile stress on tissues originating from the right iliac crest that travel superiorly toward the lumbar spine. On the contralateral side of the short lower extremity, there are increased adduction at the femur, increased shear force at the sacroiliac joint, narrowing of the intervertebral foramen, and compression of the zygapophyseal joints because of their placement in the close-packed position (Fig. 3–26).

These two examples illustrate the synergistic relationships between many tissues of the complete lumbopelvic region. In this region, which is a hub of weight bearing and must attenuate ground and trunk forces, many tissues work to-

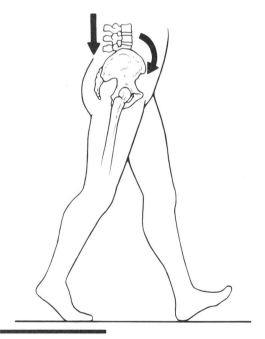

**FIGURE 3–25** ■ Forces on the pelvis and lumbar spine resulting from tightness in the hips. Note the anterior torsional moment on the ilium and the increased extension moment at the lumbosacral joint as terminal right stance.

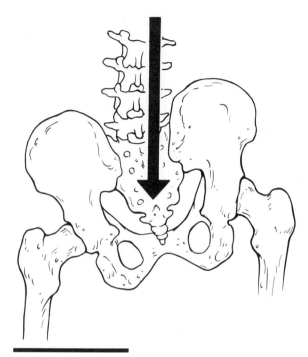

**FIGURE 3–26** ■ Forces on the pelvis and lumbar spine resulting from left frontal plane asymmetry. Note the adduction of the right hip, greater shear force at the right sacroiliac joint, and close-packed position of the right zygapophyseal joints on the contralateral side of the shorter lower extremity.

gether via control of the central nervous system. It should also be apparent that mechanical stresses, both normal and abnormal, affect multiple tissues. Therefore it is important to recognize that it is not the tissue that is injured that is of major concern in activity-related low back disorders but rather the excessive forces converging into a region that mechanically or chemically stimulates the nociceptive system and results in the experience of pain.

## EVALUATION

### History

The history should provide the examiner with an understanding of the past medical history of the patient, the main complaint of the patient, the site of the symptoms, and the behavior and irritability of the symptoms. Questions related to these characteristics allow the examiner to begin to discern pain caused by mechanical activity-related disorders from pain with nonmechanical sources. Detailed question schemes are described in other sources.[49,59]

Taking a history from a patient with complaints of low back pain should be done in a consistent manner. This allows the clinician to compare responses from patient to patient. Consistency is also extremely important for the objective examination. Throughout the history, the clinician should be ascertaining the nature of the pain:

■ Does the patient have an acute injury?
■ Is the pain exacerbated by a previous injury?
■ Is the patient suffering from chronic pain syndrome?

This is important because the objectives of treatment are dissimilar for the three types of patients.

The low back history should focus on the chief complaint that the individual has. The majority of individuals seek help because of pain, but occasionally deformity or loss of function is the reason for pursuing professional help. Determining how and when this episode or similar episodes occurred is essential for beginning to reconstruct the mechanics of injury. Asking the individual what exacerbates the pain, or increases familiar symptoms, is extremely important. It not only helps to determine the nociceptive biomechanics but also begins to provide information about whether this is a mechanical activity-related disorder or one that is nonmechanical in nature (see section on differential diagnosis). This differentiation is especially important when the physical therapist is the first clinician the patient sees. There should be some evidence in the history of mechanical factors, such as movements, positions, or loads, that increase familiar symptoms, especially from the upright standing position, in which maximal loading of low back tissues occurs. Changes in the site and intensity of a patient's symptoms should be related to variations in activities, movements and positions, and periods of rest when the musculoskeletal system is unloaded, and it is important to gain this type of information in the history and subjective questioning. Further referral is indicated if symptoms cannot be provoked mechanically.

Nonmechanical disorders include pelvic and abdominal disorders and disease processes of the musculoskeletal system. The general health of the patient and any relevant weight loss, as well as medications for other disorders, should be gleaned from the history. These are important considerations for all patients but especially those for whom the physical therapist is the initial entry into the health care system.

An occupational history is important. Again, this enables the examiner to visualize the biomechanical demands on the low back, which will influence the direction of treatment. Previous surgeries, treatments, and past medical history should be noted.

Questions should be asked so that the examiner clearly understands the location of the complaints. A clear description of the area, outlined and drawn if possible, with a description of the depth and quality of pain, is helpful. Because pain is a subjective experience and has a different meaning for different individuals, this is often difficult; individuals cannot see their low back and hence cannot visualize it in the same way they can peripheral joints. Words such as "pulsating" or "throbbing" or complaints of temperature disturbances should alert the examiner that the pain may not be mechanical in nature but, in fact, may be vascular in origin. Severe or intractable night pain, fevers, and malaise are not typical manifestations of mechanical musculoskeletal disorders and suggest further referral for diagnostic tests. Likewise, bladder retention or saddle anesthesia is suggestive of cauda equina compression and must be evaluated medically.

Nearly all structures in the low back have been shown to refer pain distally when noxiously stimulated, so care must be taken to ascertain whether it is the peripheralization of pain into the lower extremity or the low back area itself that is the chief complaint. In general, pain that is worse in the lower extremity than in the low back should be considered as due to nerve root irritation or injury of the lower extremity tissues until proved otherwise. Radicular pain of this sort usually involves leg pain worse than back pain. Hearing this, the examiner should be prepared to scrutinize motor, sensory, and reflux mechanisms during the objective portion of the examination. Low back complaints that are worse than the lower extremity complaints can be referred from any injured tissue in the spine. It is important to note that irritated tissues can refer pain below the knee and even into the foot.[57,58] Therefore, caution should be used in interpreting this symptom as purely radicular in nature.

## Objective Evaluation

Tests for evaluating the low back are legion. Many are based on various physiopathologic hypotheses that are yet to be validated or shown to be reliable between different examiners. The examiner should realize that the precise diagnosis is unknown in 80 to 90% of all cases of low back pain. Therefore, performing a physical examination in order to determine the anatomic source of pain leads to great frustration for the clinician and ultimately for the patient. Establishing a universally acceptable classification scheme for idiopathic low back pain is a top priority for clinical researchers.[60,61]

Tests used to examine the low back should have nearly the same meaning for all clinicians if we are to make progress in curtailing the low back problem. It is tempting to judge the result of a test on the basis of a physiopathologic hypothesis, but the clinician should recognize that such a diagnosis is nominal at best. Clinical experience demonstrates quite dramatically that many patients with low back problems have been given several different "diagnoses" over the course of their back pain experience. The danger of making even a nominal diagnosis based on a perceived physiopathologic hypothesis is that simple low back pain is given a diagnosis that is being considered by the patient and clinician to be substantive, when in fact it is not.[62] The possible end result is to convert simple low back pain into low back disability.[62]

The intent of the low back evaluation should be to introduce a series of stresses into the low back region in order to reproduce familiar symptoms. When these various stresses provoke symptoms, they should be substantiated or reproduced with the patient in the supine, prone, and side lying positions. The standing evaluation is the most important aspect of the mechanical low back pain examination. From this weight-bearing position, the spine must counter gravitational forces. Most activity-related low back pain complaints arise when the patient is in the weight-bearing, upright position, and symptomatic relief usually occurs when the patient is recumbent. Stiffness after prolonged periods of rest is also common. Therefore, the examiner usually comes closest to assessing the nociceptive biomechanics that are the primary complaint of the patient when analyzing movements and the response to the application of various stresses with the patient in the upright antigravity position. McCombe et al.[63] note that there is justification on the grounds of reproducibility for recording pain on movement in all planes of spinal motion.

### Standing Evaluation

*Posture Analysis.* Note at least two postural planes:

**Sagittal Plane.** Envision the weight line (postural line) traversing the lumbosacral tissues.

Consider that in the standing, upright posture, weight is borne 85% by the bone-disc-bone interface and 15% by the apophyseal joints. Note how the degree of lumbar flexion or extension alters this.

**Frontal Plane.** Envision the weight line traversing lumbosacral tissues. With frontal plane assymetry note the closed pack position on one side (compression) and tensile stress on the opposite side. Note the compression and shear at the sacroiliac joint. Note the relative abduction or adduction at the hip joints. Is there a list? Does correction of the list peripheralize pain?

Palpation points for visualizing pelvic base:
- Waist angle
- Anterior superior iliac spine
- Iliac crest
- Posterior superior iliac spine
- Greater trochanter

Complete skeletal examination with view of foot and ankle, knee, and upper quarter with the goal of determining if these might be a factor in the mechanical disorder.

### Gross Movement Testing—Standing

Forward bending
Backward bending
Quadrant testing—various combinations of three planes of movement.
Application of overpressure. Stabilize the pelvis and sacral base to apply tensile forces in forward-bending combinations, and direct the line of force to load tissues posteriorly in backward-bending combinations.
Standing neurologic screen
  Walk on toes
  Walk on heels
Seated neurologic screen
  Gastrocnemius soleus reflex
  Quadriceps reflex
  Posterior tibialis reflex
  Extensor hallucis longus manual muscle testing
  Anterior tibialis manual muscle testing
  Peroneus manual muscle testing
  Sensory check

After the structural and gross movement testing portion of the examination, the supine, prone, and side lying portions are done. Watch for "matches," that is, tests in these gravity-eliminated, unloaded postures that substantiate the pain pattern found in the upright posture.

### Supine Lying Examination

Hip range of motion. When does the movement cease to be iliofemoral and become iliosacral accommodation and then lumbar flexion?

Figure 4 (fabere sign) test. When is the motion hip range of motion, then iliosacral stress, then rotation of pelvis on lumbar spine? Note any limitation of hip motion and correlate with standing examination.

Straight leg raising. Add femoral adduction and internal rotation to further increase stretch to sciatic nerve and associated nerve roots.

Continue neurologic screen. Repeat extensor hallucis longus, anterior tibialis, peroneus manual muscle testing.

Stresses to the sacroiliac joint:
  Use the long axis of the femur to shear the ilium on sacrum.
  Test "gapping" force of posterior aspect of sacroiliac joint by placing femur in slight adduction, pushing down through long axis of femur, and, while maintaining this slight compression, adducting femur slightly.

### Prone Lying Examination

Passive knee flexion. Does the pelvis tilt anteriorly because of rectus femoris tightness?

Passive femoral extension. First stabilize ilium; then when the limits of hip hyperextension are reached, allow the test to impart an anterior torsional stress of ilium on sacrum and then a subsequent extension stress of the pelvis on lumbar spine.

Recheck hip range of motion especially for symmetry in rotation.

Sacroiliac stresses. Posterior-to-anterior stress centrally over sacrum and over the sacral sulcus. If a problem with sacroiliac tissues is suspected, you can stabilize sacrum and pull ilium upward on sacrum (shear of ilium on sacrum).

Posterior-to-anterior stress over lumbar spine. Does this correlate with standing examination (extension and compression)? Patient can also prop up in extension (support on elbows) and posterior-anterior pressures can again be applied to substantiate effect of extension and compression.

Rotational stresses by posterior-to-anterior stress over region of lumbar transverse processes.

Completion of neurologic screen
  Quadriceps manual muscle testing
  Hams manual muscle testing

### Palpation

Tissues above the iliac crest up to the last rib.
Tissues below the iliac crest.

### Side Lying Examination

Lumbar stresses. This can be done to assess response to flexion-extension, rotation, or side bending.

Sacroiliac stresses. Although many sacroiliac stresses have already been tested, torsional stresses as well as gapping stresses can be applied from this position.

It is clear that there is little reliability in assessing quantity in small intersegmental movements such as lumbar rotation, lumbar side bending, and sacroiliac motion. However, the response of the patient to these stresses—that is, whether familiar pain is reproduced—can provide useful information.

The degree of asymmetry of the zygapophyseal joints in the lumbar spine has been estimated to be at least 23%.[44] Therefore, it should not be assumed that asymmetries seen with movement assessment are truely contributing factors to the problem. Just as age-related degenerative changes seen in x-ray studies correlate poorly with low back symptoms and must be interpreted cautiously, so too must asymmetries of spinal motion. In addition, the neuromuscular control of any movement pattern, especially in the presence of pain, is probably the single biggest influence on the quality and quantity of motion. For the examining clinician, it is much more important to assess whether the motion pattern reproduces familiar pain in standing and whether application of the same type of stress in the supine, prone, or side-lying position can substantiate the findings of the standing examination. Figure 3–27A–F shows several tests that are part of the lumbosacral spine objective examination.

Upon completion of the examination, the examiner should have a clearer picture of the nociceptive biomechanics that may contribute to the symptoms. Because the ultimate goal of all low back pain rehabilitation is restoration of function, this information is important because it allows the clinician to develop an active approach to rehabilitation. With the type of biomechanical understanding gained from the evaluation, it is possible to avoid specific activities that increase loads or stresses on the spine so that functional healing can take place. Several studies have demonstrated that patients suffering from low back pain or sciatica can do selected activities without increasing their pain.[62,64]

## DIFFERENTIAL DIAGNOSIS

One of the most important decisions the physical therapist makes is whether the history and physical examination present symptoms and signs consistent with activity-related injuries to the low back. This involves differentiating between activity-related mechanical disorders, which respond to physical therapy interventions, and nonmechanical ones, which require referral for further medical evaluation.

As an expert in pathokinesiology, the physical therapist diagnoses differentially the movement disorders that occur as a result of low back pain. Posture, adaptive changes that result in altered spinal mechanics, and patterns of muscle weakness that lead to placement of abnormal loads on the spine are all diagnostic considerations and provide indications for physical therapy.

Differential diagnosis means distinguishing by a specific difference, characteristic, or symptom.[65] It is important for the physical therapist to recognize the wide array of characteristics and symptoms of other diseases that can be manifested as low back pain. This knowledge, coupled with an understanding that the primary focus of the low back musculoskeletal examination is to determine nociceptive biomechanics, makes the physical therapist a valuable member of the health care team. The therapist serves as both a primary care provider and a referral practitioner to ensure that the patient receives prompt and total assessment when signs and symptoms are clearly seen to differ from those of activity-related mechanical disorders of the musculoskeletal system. This section describes other low back pathologies in order to familiarize the physical therapist with signs and symptoms of other sources of low back pain.

## Bone Lesions of the Low Back

### Infections

Infections of the spine resulting in osteomyelitis of the vertebrae or septic arthritis of the joints are typically a result of hematogenous spread from other sources. The most common cause of pyogenic osteomyelitis is *Staphylococcus aureus*, although many other organisms can be infectious agents. Nonpyogenic organisms include the tuberculosis bacillus, *Brucella*, and fungus.

The origin of the infectious agent is extremely variable and includes

■ Infections from other bones
■ Skin lesions
■ Respiratory tract infections
■ Genitourinary tract infections

When an adult or child with a history of urinary tract infections suffers from acute-onset low back

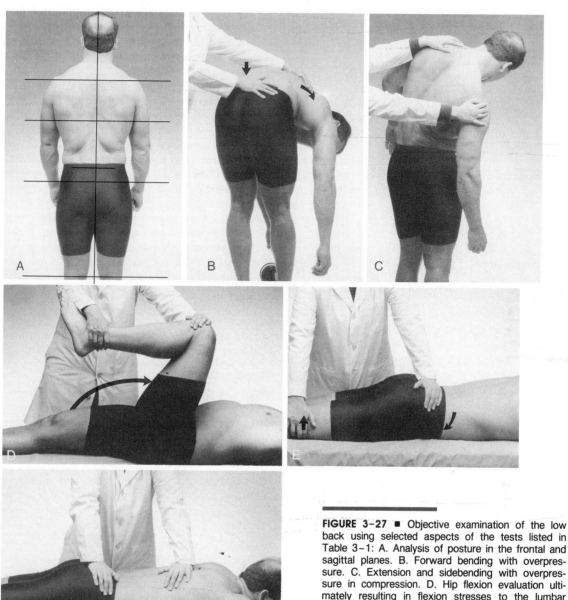

**FIGURE 3-27** ■ Objective examination of the low back using selected aspects of the tests listed in Table 3-1: A. Analysis of posture in the frontal and sagittal planes. B. Forward bending with overpressure. C. Extension and sidebending with overpressure in compression. D. Hip flexion evaluation ultimately resulting in flexion stresses to the lumbar spine. E. Shear force of the ilium on the sacrum using the long axis of the femur. F. Posterior-anterior pressure over the sacrum from the prone position.

pain, vertebral infection should be suspected unless proved otherwise. Any open wound or surgical procedure has the potential to cause infection of the vertebrae or joints.

The vertebral bodies are typically affected most often by vertebral osteomyelitis because of their rich vasculature, especially the large venous plexuses. The close proximity of the spinal canal, with its associated meninges and nervous system structures, to the vertebral body requires that prompt medical attention be given. Infections of the vertebral body may also spread and result in disc space infections.

The typical pain pattern is deep centralized back pain with a diffuse spread. The onset is usually rapid but may be insidious, depending on the infectious agent. Many of the signs of an infectious process may be present, including elevated temperature, fever, and malaise. Pronounced muscle spasm is evident in the spinal extensors and proximal thigh muscles and the muscles are tense and stiff to palpation. Pain may be aggravated by motion or percussion of the spine, and having the patient assume weight-bearing positions may intensify the pain dramatically.

Because mechanical low back pain resulting from musculoskeletal lesions is very uncommon in children, there should be a high index of suspicion for infections, especially if the child has had a recent respiratory tract infection. Laboratory evaluation, including erythrocyte sedimentation rate, white blood cell count, and blood culture, is essential. Failure to recognize and treat infection promptly can result in lysis of the bone, potentially leading to complete destruction of the vertebrae with spread to adjacent soft tissue structures.

## Fractures

A complete discussion of the diagnostic features of spine fractures and dislocations is beyond the scope of this chapter, and the reader is encouraged to review textbooks devoted to this topic.[66-68] Some of the important aspects of fracture related to disorders of the low back are discussed here.

Fractures of the lumbar spine are of many different types. Compression fracture usually results in collapse of the anterior aspect of the vertebral body and is classically associated with a flexion-compression force. On x-ray films, the anterior or anterolateral aspect of the vertebral body shows loss of vertical height. Vertical compression force resulting in fracture can also occur when a fall on the buttocks produces a force of high magnitude that is absorbed by the lumbar vertebrae. Collapse of the anterior aspect of the vertebrae results in a tensile force at the posterior arch, and tension failure may also occur posteriorly.[69] Compression forces may also result in burst fractures of the lumbar spine.

Motor vehicle accidents occasionally cause the seat belt or Chance fracture.[70,71] This injury occurs when acute flexion of the lumbar spine around the axis of the anterior abdominal wall results in tension failure of the posterior aspect of the vertebrae and compression failure anteriorly. In addition to effects on the lumbar vertebrae, abdominal injuries usually occur.

Fracture-dislocation of the lumbar vertebrae is due to combinations of compression, rotation, tension, and shear stresses. Isolated fractures of the articular processes of the lumbar spine can occur with excessive torsional stresses because of the sagittal plane orientation of the facet.[68] With a torsional stress, the inferior articular facet is compressed into the superior articulating facet of the subjacent vertebrae, and if the force is excessive facet fracture can occur.

Fractures can also be sequelae of osteoporosis. Osteoporosis is a generalized bone disorder that results in a reduction in the total volume of mineralized and unmineralized bone. Although the causes of osteoporosis are multiple, including malabsorption syndromes, endocrine disorders, and excessive steroid use, the elderly population is most often affected by idiopathic osteoporosis. Females typically have a higher incidence of idiopathic osteoporosis than males. Fractures of osteoporotic lumbar vertebrae can result from trivial trauma and multiple levels of the spine may be affected. Therefore, low back pain in an elderly population or a population with a high risk of osteoporosis should be evaluated medically.

Pain with fractures is localized, and often the history makes one suspect this as an etiology of the patient's back pain. Any history of trauma or a clinical suspicion of trauma should be evaluated radiographically or with various imaging techniques. Goals of further evaluation are to determine whether the fracture is stable or unstable, whether the patient is at risk of neurologic compromise, and whether hemorrhage from associated soft tissue injuries is present.

## Spondylolisthesis

Fractures of the pars interarticularis can result in spondylolisthesis (Fig. 3–28). Spondylolysis is the term used to designate a defect in the pars interarticularis; the actual slipping forward of a superior vertebra on an inferior vertebra is referred to as spondylolisthesis (Fig. 3–29). Although a fracture of the pars interarticularis can result in spondylolisthesis, slippage of the vertebrae can be due to other etiologies, such as elongation of the pedicles or a congenitally defective, dissolved, or stretched pars interarticularis.

Children and adolescents are most typically affected by spondylolisthesis and usually complain of pain after activities requiring running, jumping, bending, and twisting, such as gymnastics. Adults can also be affected, especially after

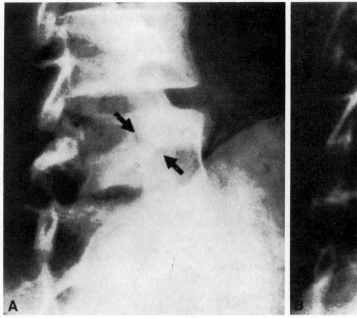
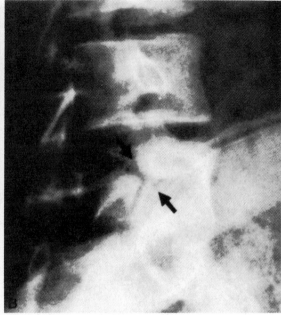

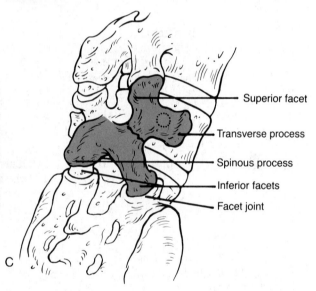

**FIGURE 3-28** ■ This 13-year-old boy felt a "snap" in the low back during a swimming racing turn. (A) X-ray demonstrates spondylolysis of the pars interarticularis (arrows). The narrow, irregular appearance suggests recent injury. (B) Despite cast immobilization the fracture did not heal. X-ray 6 months later demonstrates blunting of the bone ends and widening of the gap (arrows). The patient was asymptomatic. (From Taveras: Ferruccis Radiology: Diagnosis—Imaging—Intervention. Philadelphia: JB Lippincott.) (C) Representation of spondylolysis "scotty dog with collar" from the posterior oblique view. (Redrawn from Magee D: Orthopedic Physical Assessment, 2nd ed. Philadelphia: WB Saunders, 1992.)

Superior facet

Transverse process

Spinous process

Inferior facets

Facet joint

working with the arms overhead for long periods of time or after prolonged periods of standing if the patient lacks the abdominal muscle strength and endurance to minimize extension stress at the lumbosacral junction by postural correction.

Usually the nerve roots are not compromised, but any lower extremity tightness noted by the examiner should be evaluated carefully because it might represent not adaptive changes of the muscle tissue but rather muscle spasm caused by nerve root irritation. In more severe cases, a palpable step between the L-4 and L-5 spinous

processes occurs when the L-5 vertebra slips forward on the sacrum. Because the defect is in the pars, the posterior arch, which includes the spinous process of L-5, remains in place while the anterior elements slide forward. As a result of L-5 slipping forward on the sacrum, the L-4 spinous process is felt to be more anterior than L-5.

Spondylolisthesis is usually graded according to the amount of slippage from 1 to 4 based on x-ray study or tomography. Forward slippage of L-5 of less than 25% of the anterior-posterior diameter of the sacrum is given grade 1, and

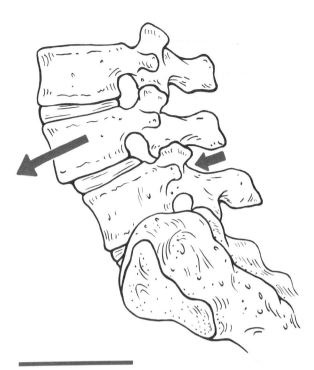

**FIGURE 3-29 ■** Translation of the L-4 vertebra on L-5 during flexion of the spine, representing spinal instability.

slippage of 25 to 50% is given grade 2. In general, extension stresses, posterior-to-anterior shear forces, and compression through the shoulders from the standing position that accentuates the lumbar lordosis aggravate low back pain resulting from spondylolisthesis.

### Paget's Disease

Paget's disease is a metabolic bone disease involving bone breakdown (osteolysis) followed by stages of immature bone proliferation and abnormal new bone growth (osteosclerosis). The onset is usually in the middle to late adult years. Because the spine is one of the most common sites of Paget's disease, it should be considered as a possible source of low back pain in adults over the age of 40.

Paget's disease of the spine has several sequelae. Enlargement of the vertebral body in the osteosclerosis stage can cause stenosis of the neural canal in the lumbar spine. The stenotic compromise in the canal can result in claudication or neural compression. The neurologic claudication phenomenon is related primarily to the vascular dysfunction that occurs as a result of narrowing of the spinal canal.

During the phases of osteolysis and immature bone proliferation, fracture of the vertebrae is possible. The clinician should also be aware that osteogenic sarcoma is 30 times more common in patients with Paget's disease than in the rest of the population.[72]

### Stenosis

Stenosis affecting the lumbar spine can occur in various locations of the spinal canal, such as the central region, the lateral recesses, the intervertebral foramen, or a combination of regions. The syndrome is most common in elderly patients who demonstrate age-related degenerative spinal changes.

Narrowing of the spinal canal may be due to bone changes in the spinal canal itself or the presence of space-occupying lesions. Causes include bone hypertrophy of the lamina, ligamentum flavum buckling or hypertrophy, and enlargement of the inferior facets as a result of the degenerative process. Disc bulging or osteophytes over the posterior margins of the vertebral body can further narrow the lumbar spinal canal.

Symptoms and signs occur because of vascular compromise, notably of the venous plexus related to the cauda equina, or pressure on the nerve root complex. The symptoms and signs of spinal stenosis suggest that vascular embarrassment is the important aspect of the pathogenesis. Pain and sensory changes can be present in one or both legs. When both legs are affected, the symptoms in the legs are often different in location and severity. The patient reports having to rest because of leg pain after walking some specified distance. Forward bending at the waist with the hands resting on the anterior thighs to support the flexed trunk helps provide temporary relief. Instead of sensory or motor disturbances that follow a single nerve root distribution, the changes tend to be broader and more diffuse. Typically more than one nerve root supplying a lower extremity is affected, and the other lower extremity may be affected with different nerve root patterns. In some instances the patient may complain of numbness in the complete lower extremity. Extension of the lumbar spine, which further narrows the spinal canal, makes symptoms and signs worse, and flexion relieves them. Imaging techniques are used to confirm the diagnosis, and decompression is often needed to relieve spinal canal pressure.

### Segmental Instability

Segmental instability has been defined as "a condition where there is a loss of spinal stiffness, such that normally tolerated external loads will result in pain, deformity, or place neurologic structures at risk."[73] Kirkaldy-Willis[74] proposed three stages of the degenerative process: dysfunction, an unstable phase, and stabilization. The causative mechanism of the unstable phase, which correlates with the instability problem, is successive episodes of trauma in which healing of structures such as the annulus fibrosus and joint capsule is less complete because the strength of the repair collagen is less than that of normal collagen.

Radiographic signs considered to be important for diagnosing segmental instability include abnormal translations in one or more planes of one vertebra on another as the patient flexes and extends the spine from the standing position. However, just as there is little relationship between clinical symptoms and radiologic changes of degeneration, there is a question regarding the relationship between translation of the vertebrae during flexion and extension and clinical symptoms. Normal males can demonstrate as much as 8 mm translation at the L4-5 segment with an average of 3 mm.[75] Paris[76] has suggested that the abnormal translations of some spinal instability problems can be palpated and, coupled with observation of hypertrophied bands of muscle and perhaps "catching" of the spine during bending, can provide some physical evidence of segmental instability. At this time, objective evidence for the role of segmental instability in low back pain is indeterminate.

## Sacroiliac Joint Pathology

The role of the sacroiliac joint in low back pain remains controversial with the exception of the spondyloarthropathies. For example, any young adult male with diffuse low back pain of insidious onset in the sacroiliac region who presents with stiffness and difficulty in spinal movements should be evaluated medically to rule out ankylosing spondylitis (see later). Sprain, strain, and subluxation hypotheses involving the sacroiliac joint and related structures continue to provide lively debate among clinicians.

The joint is considered to be a potential source of pain because it is innervated and has characteristics of other synovial joints. Inflammatory processes related to tissue injury can therefore cause low back pain. Those who do not agree that the sacroiliac joint is a source of pain point out its extremely stable nature, with a joint surface topography that allows negligible movement. In addition, fibrosus and bony ankylosis of

the joint are evident between the fourth and fifth decades. Although there is a lack of controlled scientific studies confirming the sacroiliac joint as a source of low back pain, minor dysfunctions in the form of sprain or strain appear reasonable, especially in multiparous females. Subluxation of the joint has been suggested, but it is more reasonable to assume that asymmetries of the pelvis seen with low back pain episodes are the result of abnormal states of muscle contraction and pain. In fact, much of the pain directly over the region of the joint may be due to the sustained contraction by muscles that overlie the joint.[74] Special tests that purport to detect hypermobility or hypomobility of the sacroiliac joint are most likely evaluations of the rate and amounts of lumbopelvic muscle contraction rather than measures of joint movement.

## Arthritides of the Low Back

Degenerative joint disease (osteoarthritis) is the most common of the arthritis patterns affecting the low back. It is a disease of articular cartilage that ultimately affects the subchondral bone. All of the stages of the degenerative process, including cartilage fibrillation, denudation of the articular surface, and osteophyte formation, occur with age-related changes of the low back.

Whether these changes are the source of low back problems remains controversial. It has been noted that low back pain appears to cause the greatest problems in the middle adult years with the peak age of 40.[62] If degenerative changes were responsible for low back pain and disability, we would expect the peak to be during later life when degeneration is much more evident.

When degenerative joint disease is responsible for low back pain, other joints can be affected, most often the hip and knee. Interphalangeal joints as well as the carpal-metacarpal joints of the thumb are also target areas for degenerative joint disease.

Although pain is the chief complaint, stiffness and difficulty with movement upon arising in the morning are common. Osteophytes of the articular processes or vertebral body can result in spinal stenosis.

Other sources of arthritis symptoms are the spondyloarthropathies. These are a group of disorders that share many common features. The best defined of the spondyloarthropathies is ankylosing spondylitis.

The disease process begins in the low back, specifically the sacroiliac and lower lumbar zygapophyseal joints. The involved joints are marked by enthesopathy, an inflammation at the site of ligamentous attachment to the bone; periodic episodes of joint pain that progresses to fibrous ankylosis; and ultimately bony ankylosis. Typically, the ankylosing process begins in the low back and continues toward the upper thoracic spine, resulting in the radiologic appearance of a "bamboo" spine. Involvement of the thoracic spine can restrict chest wall expansion. As a result of this ankylosing process, complaints of stiffness accompany those of pain. The onset is insidious, and because the disease process is inflammatory it can be accompanied by fatigue, malaise, and fever. There is a tendency for involvement of other joints, the eye, or the aorta, so it is important that the patient be managed medically by a rheumatologist or specialist in inflammatory disorders. The HLA-B27 antigen is present in the majority of patients with ankylosing spondylitis. Although the presence of HLA-B27 is not diagnostic of the disease, when combined with the clinical picture just described it is strongly suggestive of ankylosing spondylitis.

Related seronegative spondyloarthropathies include psoriatic arthritis, Reiter's syndrome, and arthritis associated with inflammatory bowel disease. Although the symptoms of spondylitis occur in each disease, the characteristic ossification process of ankylosing spondylitis is absent except in rare cases.

Another disease process characterized by ossification of the vertebral column is diffuse idiopathic skeletal hyperostosis. Although complaints such as back pain and stiffness may be similar to those in ankylosing spondylitis, the disease is typically limited to the middle to lower thoracic spine and to involvement of the vertebral bodies. The zygapophyseal joints are not usually affected.

## Visceral Sources of Low Back Pain

It is important to recognize that diseases of the abdominal or pelvic organs can refer pain to the low back. Kidney disorders, urinary tract infections, nephrolithiasis, prostatitis, pancreatitis, diseases of the small or large intestine, aneurysm of the abdominal aorta, and gynecologic disorders including endometriosis, pelvic infections, and ovarian cysts are a few of the sources of viscerogenic low back pain. Textbooks are available that provide complete descriptions of viscerogenic causes of low back pain as well as evaluation procedures for differential diagnosis.[77-79] Diagnosis must be confirmed by medical evaluation and laboratory studies.

Viscerogenic sources of low back pain can present a confusing clinical picture, even when complaints of low back pain are minimal and diffuse pelvis or abdominal pain is the patient's primary complaint. Tests of full range of motion at the spine and hips that fail to reproduce familiar back pain, inability to find any position of rest to relieve the pain, and inability to position or load the spine and increase pain should alert the examiner that there might be a nonmusculoskeletal source of pain. Many abdominal or pelvic disorders involve spasm of the trunk and hip muscles, especially the abdominals, so limitations of motion should be interpreted carefully as they might be due to increased efferent output to the muscle rather than adaptive changes in the connective tissue.

## Tumors Related to the Spine

The classification of bone tumors that has been developed by the World Health Organization is based on the cell types or products of tumor cells. Therefore, tumors are typically classified as bone forming, cartilage forming, and so forth. Tumors that affect spinal structures are listed in Table 3–1.

### Osteoid Osteoma  —bone

Osteoid osteoma is usually a small lesion approximately 1 cm in diameter. Although it is more common in long bones, it is occasionally found in the spine. The age group most affected is younger than 30, and extremely severe, deep pain that is worse at night is a distinctive clinical feature of this solitary lesion.

### Ewing's Sarcoma — marrow

Ewing's sarcoma is a highly malignant tumor. The histogenesis of the tumor is largely unknown. The age group most affected is under 30,

**■■■■■ Table 3–1.** SELECTED TUMORS RELATED TO THE SPINE

| Bone | Cartilage | Marrow |
|------|-----------|--------|
| Osteoma | Osteochondroma | Ewing's sarcoma |
| Osteoid osteoma | Chondroma | Plasma cell myeloma |
| Osteosarcoma | Chondrosarcoma | Eosinophilic granuloma |
|  |  | Lymphoma |

and the tumor is seen in childhood. It often affects the long bones of the lower extremity but is also seen in the spine, particularly in the vertebral body. The pain and swelling are similar to those of infectious processes, being extremely severe and unrelenting. The tumor typically occupies the medullary cavity as small, densely packed cells that can grow through the bony cortex, lifting the periosteum and expanding into the surrounding soft tissues.

### Plasma Cell Myeloma — bone

Plasma cell myeloma, also known as multiple myeloma, is a malignant tumor of bone. The age group most affected is late adult, with the average age of approximately 60.[72] The disease is characterized by proliferation of precursors of plasma cells known as myeloma cells. The bones most affected are those containing red marrow. For this reason, the vertebrae and ribs are the two areas most commonly affected. The tumor begins in the bone marrow and becomes osteolytic as it systematically attacks the surrounding bone. Spontaneous fracture of the vertebral body is common and is responsible for much of the severe spinal pain of the disease; neurologic involvement resulting from vertebral collapse is a distinct possibility. Pain is typically described as deep, severe, and constant.

### Chordomas — spinal cord

Chordomas are seen most commonly in the sacrococcygeal region. They are uncommon tumors of notochord origin. Chordomas are slow-growing, osteolytic tumors with a gelatinous consistency. They can metastasize, and the consistency of the tumor makes it difficult to remove completely by surgery.

### Other Malignant Tumors — from other places

Malignant tumors elsewhere in the body have the potential to metastasize to bone. The prevalence of metastatic lesions is demonstrated by the fact that metastatic carcinoma is the most common tumor found in bone, frequently present as multiple deposits. The tumors result from hematogenous spread of the carcinoma, most often from breast, prostate, lung, kidney, stomach, or thyroid. Most metastatic tumors are osteolytic and can result in pathologic fracture of the bone. Any age group can be affected, but there is a greater incidence in those over 50 years.[65] Low back pain that is not activity related in patients in this age group who have a medical history that includes a previous diagnosis or surgical removal of tumors should be evaluated medically to rule out metastatic bone tumor.

## Lesions of the Intervertebral Disc

The intervertebral disc is the largest avascular structure in the human body. Its health is maintained by a sophisticated diffusion process and the mechanical pumping action resulting from movement and weight-bearing activities. Unfortunately, because of this the intervertebral disc has a limited capacity for repair compared to other connective tissue structures.

The intervertebral disc exhibits several age-related changes, such as cleft formation in the nucleus, thinning and fissuring of the annulus, tears of the annulus at its junction with the bone, progressive loss of water, and cleft formation in the cartilaginous end plate. There is a paucity of controlled studies that would enable us to determine whether the age-related changes in the intervertebral disc are the primary source of low back pain or have the potential to cause low back pain.

In addition to age-related changes, intervertebral discs are subject to injury. Tears, fissures, and delamination of the annular rings are well described in the literature. These are thought to be due to excessive mechanical stresses that exceed the physiologic capacity of the annular collagen. In normal intervertebral discs, the annulus and cartilaginous end plates are strong enough to prevent displacements of the nucleus. When weakened, the annulus can no longer apply an equal and opposite force to counter the pressure of the hydrophilic nucleus pulposus. The nucleus pulposus then pushes against annular rings that have lost their inherent stiffness. Bulging of the disc, leakage of the nuclear pulp through defects in the annulus to enter the spinal canal, or a combination of nuclear and annular material occupying the spinal canal results. It is important to recognize that desiccation of the nucleus must precede any "movement" of nuclear material through the annular rings; that is, the nucleus must be degenerated or partially broken down. Yasuma et al.[80] note that herniation of the intervertebral disc can be thought of histologically as either protrusion of the nucleus pulposus, protrusion of the annulus fibrosus, or a mixed type in which both factors act together to cause the herniation. Events leading to disc pathology are summarized in Table 3–2.

**Table 3-2.** EVENTS LEADING TO INTERVERTEBRAL DISC PATHOLOGY

| Nucleus Events | Annulus Events |
| --- | --- |
| Fracture, defect in cartilaginous end plate | Viscoelasticity of annulus exceeded |
| Circulation in direct contact with nucleus through cartilage defect | Stiffness of annular rings lost |
| Exposure of nuclear matrix to circulating antibodies | Annulus yields easily to nucleus pressure |
| Fragmentation of nuclear matrix from inflammatory reaction | Buckling or tearing of annulus–posterior longitudinal ligament |

Since Mixter and Barr's[81] classic report, herniation of the lumbar disc has been considered a common cause of low back pain and associated radiculopathy. Surgical relief has been successful for carefully selected patients with nerve compression syndromes that fail to resolve naturally.[82] However, a nonoperative, aggressive physical rehabilitation program for herniated nucleus pulposus with radiculopathy can also be a successful method of treatment.[83] Weber[84] reported that the results of disc surgery for patients with radiculopathy were significantly better than the results of conservative treatment after 1 year of observation, but after 4 years there was no significant difference in results between operated and nonoperated patients. Furthermore, it has been shown that in at least 30% of spinal canals with significant disc protrusions onto the neural elements, there are no symptoms.[85,86] Disc lesions, therefore, present a compound problem—understanding the etiologic factors leading to disruption of the disc and determining whether the disruption is significant.

A number of hypotheses have been put forth to explain how lesions of the intervertebral disc contribute to low back pain. One hypothesis is that pain is caused by mechanical compression of innervated tissues in the spinal canal. Because the posterior longitudinal ligament is richly innervated, pressure on the annulus leading to distortion of this ligament is a potential source of pain.

Another possible mechanism involves the peripheral annulus itself. The outer aspect of the intervertebral disc is known to be innervated and contains a blood supply, and pressure on the weakened annular rings by the nucleus may cause mechanical distortion and chemical irritation of the nociceptive endings. Pain directly from the disc caused by mechanical or chemical

irritation of the nociceptive nerve endings is thus a possibility. This is the etiologic basis of pain in diskography.

Still another mechanism of pain associated with pathology of the intervertebral disc involves the nerve roots. As previously mentioned, normal, uninjured nerve roots are not typically sensitive to mechanical stimulation.[54] However, if the nerve root is inflamed it becomes sensitive to any mechanical distortion and can cause radicular pain. Various lesions of the intervertebral disc appear to have the potential to alter the chemical environment of the nerve root and render it mechanosensitive. A chemical radiculitis caused by nuclear material in the spinal canal,[87] an autoimmune response to leaking nuclear material,[55] and mechanical compression of the perivascular network of the nerve root via disc protrusion which leads to fluid stasis, ischemia, hypoxia, and a decrease in axoplasmic transport[88,89] have all been proposed as etiologic factors that alter the chemical environment surrounding the root. It is clear that mechanical compression of the nerve root by the intervertebral disc is not sufficient to induce radicular pain. Mechanical factors must be combined with biochemical irritation that alters the chemical milieu of the nerve root to generate radicular pain.

## TREATMENT

Many models of therapeutic intervention are used in treating low back pain. The focus of treatment has traditionally been based on a physiopathologic hypothesis related to dysfunction of a particular tissue. For example, theories of therapeutic intervention have been based on the disc model, following the work of Mixter and Barr[81] and Cyriax,[90] or the joint model from the field of osteopathy and the influence of Maitland.[59] It is striking that nearly all models of low back intervention have been based on some tissue or group of tissues in the spine.

Does our approach toward low back disorders actually need to be revisited? Waddell[62] points out that low back pain is a "universal, benign, and self-limiting condition, so common in every human being's life, that it could almost be interpreted as a normal occurrence." Failure to embrace this idea may have led to elaborate evaluation and treatment routines for a problem that resolves spontaneously in 80 to 90% of cases. Is it possible that failure to recognize this natural history leads to the conversion of simple low back pain into low back disability? If simple low back pain is treated passively, the problem becomes exaggerated.

It is also important to note the difference between acute low back pain and chronic low back pain syndrome. Waddell[62] notes that

> [A]cute and chronic pain are not only different in time scale but are fundamentally different in kind. Acute pain bears a relatively straightforward relationship to peripheral stimulus, nociception, and tissue damage. There may be some understandable anxiety about the meaning and consequences of the pain, but acute pain, acute disability, and acute illness behavior are generally proportionate to the physical findings. Pharmacologic, physical, and even surgical treatments directed to the underlying physical disorder are generally highly effective in relieving acute pain. In contrast, chronic pain, chronic disability, and chronic illness behavior become increasingly dissociated from their original physical basis, and there may indeed be little objective evidence of any remaining nociceptive stimulus. Instead, chronic pain and disability become increasingly associated with emotional distress, depression, failed treatment, and adoption of a sick role.

All clinicians recognize that chronic pain has the potential to become self-sustaining and is resistant to many therapeutic interventions traditionally used to treat pain. Therefore, the first aspect to consider when initiating therapeutic interventions for the patient with low back pain must clearly be that of separating low back pain from low back disability, and all treatment programs should be based on such a distinction.

The dilemma of diagnosis for activity-related low back disorders complicates the treatment predicament for the clinician. Even though most experts in low back pain agree that we lack the pathologic understanding to arrive at a precise diagnosis, a specific, anatomic diagnosis is usually given anyway. Although this solves an immediate need (the clinician's and patient's uncertainty), the unfortunate result is that many patients are given numerous different diagnoses over the course of their low back pain history, usually based on the bias of the examiner.[61] In fact, terms like disc disease or facet joint syndrome in most cases are actually ambiguous because methods for measuring or corroborating these do not exist. Instead, terms such as simple strain, nonspecific low back pain, or low back pain with leg referral are less ambiguous. In order to judge the efficacy of therapeutic interventions, a simple classification system with nearly universal applicability must be used.

This concept was reinforced by the results of the Quebec Task Force.[61] Of particular concern to the Quebec Workers Health and Safety Commis-

sion was the wide variation in duration and type of treatment from one institution to another for what appeared to be the same condition. They recommended only 11 classifications of activity-related spinal disorders.[61] Can a similar simple system of classification of patients, based on the results of the clinical examination previously discussed, allow us to categorize various treatment techniques into appropriate treatment objectives?

## Classification of Patients

Classification of patients into meaningful, easily understood groupings helps provide direction for therapeutic intervention and rational application of treatment.[91] Perhaps many groupings are possible. However, to be successful a grouping system must have an element of simplicity—that is, it must have nearly universal application across a wide spectrum of clinicians. The more complex a classification system is, the less chance there is that it will demonstrate reliability.

Three categories of patients are evident based on clinical experience:[91]

- Acute injury
- Reinjury
- Chronic pain syndrome

### Acute Injury

In the acutely injured patient, the response to the application of various stresses to the system is proportional to both the time since the injury and the physical trauma of the injury. Acute pain and initial injury bear a relatively straightforward relationship to the stimulus of tissue damage and tissue injury.[62] Because we have no reason to suspect otherwise, the tissues of the low back should have a healing potential like that of any other connective tissue structures in the body. That is, we would expect healing to occur within a framework of 6 to 8 weeks after injury. One tissue in the spine that is anatomically and physiologically different from other tissues of the body is the intervertebral disc. It does not have the same healing potential as other connective tissues in the spine. Perhaps acute injuries that never subside in intensity are truly discogenic.[4]

### Reinjury

Reinjury patients are those who have exacerbations of a previous injury. These patients present with a low back problem that has many similarities to other episodes. They describe that "sore area right over the iliac crest that's acting up again" or state that "my back is getting ready to go out again," or "my back feels stuck again," or "I lifted too much at home this weekend and that central ache is back again." The recurrence of their back problem becomes readily apparent. The initial injury may have occurred 4 years ago and resolved spontaneously. Over the ensuing years they reinjured the same area and it resolved again. They are now seeking medical help because the pain is not completely resolved or the duration of pain is longer than that in past episodes. These patients are not injuring new tissue but are continually stressing an old injury.

### Chronic Pain Syndrome

The third category of patient is the chronic pain syndrome patient. A sense of disquiet is generated by too broad a use of the term chronic pain syndrome, if only because it implies hopelessness and pessimism. Perhaps past approaches to this type of patient have contributed to this. Many patients with symptoms of many months duration can still have treatable low back complaints without significant psychologic components. It must be recognized that the use of the word chronic in the description chronic pain syndrome does not imply a time element. The examining clinician's primary observations in these patients are illness behavior and hopelessness. There is no longer a fairly direct relationship between application of stress (stimulus) and pain response. Chronic pain and chronic disability become increasingly dissociated from the original physical basis.[62] Instead, they become more and more related to anguish, disability, illness behavior, emotional upheaval, and discouragement.

Therefore, after the history and evaluation and perhaps also after a trial course of treatment, the clinician begins to gain a sense of the category of the classification scheme with which the patient most coincides. From this point, a decision must be made about the objectives of treatment for this patient.

## Objectives of Treatment

Why are there so many different ways to treat low back problems? In some ways, treatments for low back problems seem to involve more innovation, ingenuity, and, with some interventions, mysticism than treatments for any other area of the body. Perhaps by considering the objectives of treatment for low back pain, therapeutic intervention can be based on logic and science.

There are four objectives of treatment, and most therapeutic interventions correspond to one or more of these objectives:[91]

- Modulate pain or promote analgesia.
- Generate controlled forces to promote nondestructive movements.
- Enhance neuromuscular efficiency.
- Provide biomechanical counseling.

### Modulating Pain or Promoting Analgesia

Numerous interventions are available to modulate pain. Electromodalities, thermomodalities, and medications are effective means of minimizing the patient's subjective experience of pain. It is essential to recognize that there is a major difference between symptomatic relief and an actual difference in the natural progression of the problem. But it is ethical to treat pain in the appropriate patient, especially in order to move on to a different phase of the rehabilitation process. However, directing the treatment to pain as the primary focus is appropriate for a small, select group of patients, which is discussed later.

### Introducing Nondestructive Forces to Promote Movement

The second objective is to introduce nondestructive forces into the region in order to promote movement. What does this suggest? It is recognized in the current literature that an early return to activity has the most significant impact in the long-term management of low back problems. This objective refers to the ability of the physical therapist to place controlled, nondestructive stresses on the low back region to facilitate and encourage movement by the patient and expedite the patient's return to physical activity. Therefore an evaluation scheme that concentrates on the stresses that reproduce pain is important. This information allows appropriate decision making regarding the application of treatment stresses.

Various techniques are employed. Joint mobilization, soft tissue mobilization, the many different massage techniques, manipulation, traction, muscle energy, strain-counterstrain, stretching, cross friction, myofascial techniques, and spray and stretch are some of the myriad therapeutic interventions available to generate controlled forces in a specific region. The goal of all of these techniques is to generate a state of being that promotes the patient's own active movement.

The difficulty with all of these techniques, and the reason why some people become "disciples" of a particular school of thought, is in explaining the results. When scientifically challenged, it is always difficult to explain why successful clinical results are seen with any one of the techniques. Close inspection, however, reveals that each technique can be explained on the basis of current scientific knowledge by the following mechanisms:

- **Affect fluid dynamics.** Fluid stasis and an altered chemical environment of the tissues that affects the nociceptive system also impede the healing process. It is difficult to find any manual or mechanical technique that does not facilitate tissue fluid movement.
- **Generate afferent input into the central nervous system.** Each technique results in an increase in afferent input into the central nervous system. Although the reflex connections that occur at the central nervous system level are not precisely known, we are aware of two common results:
  - □ Modulation of pain.
  - □ Alteration of the state of muscle contraction. When a change of the patient's movement pattern or lumbar and pelvic postural position is recognized immediately after use of any of the techniques, it is clear that no chemical bonds have been broken in the connective tissue to result in the increase in motion, nor have bones been "put back in place." Instead, the muscle has a new and different resting tension that results in a change in the passive or active motion pattern.
- **Alter connective tissue.** Tissue can be altered only if the force applied is continuous and prolonged; that is, we are altering the chemical bonding of the tissue. Anything less that results in motion changes can occur only as a result of changes in the neuromuscular system.

### Enhancing Neuromuscular Efficiency

The third objective of treatment is to enhance neuromuscular efficiency. As with the second objective, various techniques are used to retrain the neuromuscular system, including progressive resistance exercise programs, stabilization exercises, Feldenkrais, Tai Chi, work hardening, and physical training programs. Training not only alters the muscle tissue but also affects the nervous system.

Why is retraining the neuromuscular system of critical importance?

- Muscles act as shock absorbers in the musculoskeletal system. Training results in increased stiffness of the muscle, which optimizes the ability to attenuate forces converging in the region.
- If the results of our evaluation are to be used to teach the patient patterns of movement to minimize stress, the patient must develop the neuromuscular machinery to carry out this task. Training programs better prepare patients to self-manage their low back problems.

Although the two objectives discussed previously (pain modulation and generation of controlled forces in the region) are important, these passive approaches to the problem must be undertaken with the goal of moving the patient quickly and rapidly toward the objective of enhancing neuromuscular efficiency. The sooner the patient takes this active approach, the better the chance of returning to activity.

### Biomechanical Counseling

Education of the patient is a critical component of any treatment program. The patient and the clinician should recognize that, as with every other human musculoskeletal injury, activity limits must be set. Whether these are limits on frequency, loads, or positions, the fact is that tissue is significantly injured and cannot attenuate stresses with the same effectiveness as normal, uninjured tissue. This is often difficult for patients to accept, because they have expectations for a permanent "cure," but in most situations this is not realistic.

## Matching the Objectives of Treatment to Classification of the Patient

The critical final analysis is deciding which objectives are indicated for a particular patient. Clinical experience suggests that some therapeutic interventions are appropriate for one patient but not for another because the natural course of the problem will not change. Table 3–3[91] provides some guidelines in making these decisions.

**Table 3–3.** MATCHING THE OBJECTIVES OF TREATMENT TO THE PATIENT'S CLASSIFICATION

| | Classification | | |
| Objective | Acute | Reinjury | Chronic |
|---|---|---|---|
| Pain modulation | ** | * | — |
| Generation of forces | ** | * | * |
| Neuromuscular efficiency | — | ** | ** |
| Biomechanical counseling | * | ** | * |

<sup>a</sup> Key: **, strongly indicated and the primary focus of treatment; *, indicated but with recognition that this is not the primary objective; —, not typically indicated.

From DeRosa C, Porterfield JA: A physical therapy model for the treatment of low back pain. Phys Ther 72:261–272, 1992. Reprinted from PHYSICAL THERAPY with the permission of the American Physical Therapy Association.

## Acute Injury

The acutely injured patient, whose history and physical examination suggest injury commensurate with the known response and healing times for musculoskeletal tissue, should be treated with the goals of relieving pain and applying controlled stresses in the involved region to facilitate an early return to activity. Manual techniques are effective as an adjunct to modalities that promote analgesia. These patients also should be given information (biomechanically counseled) about ways to minimize nociceptive stresses for their particular low back injury. Lumbosacral and sacroiliac orthoses can also be used as an adjunct in management during this stage. Figure 3–30 shows two low back orthoses and a third one

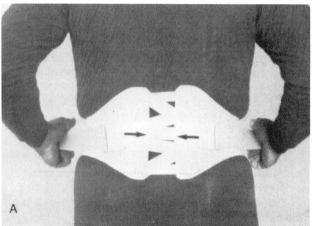
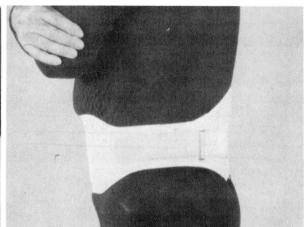
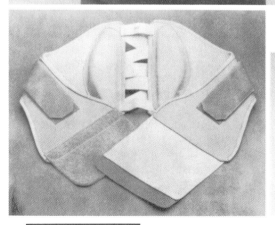
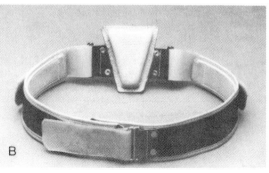

**FIGURE 3–30** ■ (A) Lumbopelvic stabilizer, a lumbar support based on a patented securing and tightening system designed to compress the lumbar tissues into the lamina and spinous processes of the lumbar vertebrae. This support can be tightened as the need arises. (IEM Orthopaedic Systems, P.O. Box 592, Ravenna, OH 44266.) (B) Sacroiliac support, designed to create a posterior to anterior force to the sacrum, a compressive force to the sacral tissues, and a posterior rotary moment to the ilia bilaterally as the support is tightened. (The triangular pad is made of viscoelastic polymer.) (IEM Orthopaedic Systems, P.O. Box 592, Ravenna, OH 44266.)

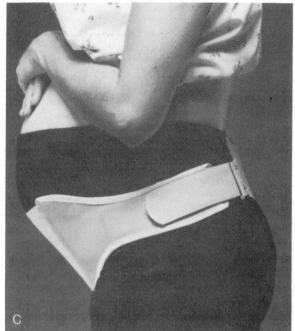

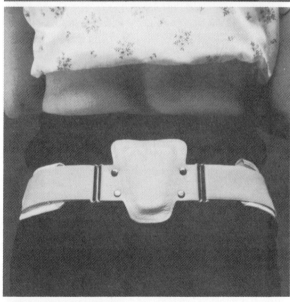

FIGURE 3-30 ■ *Continued* (C) Pregnancy sacroiliac support, a modification of the sacroiliac support made by increasing the anterior width of the belt and adding an elastic panel to the front. The mechanics of the support are the same, that is, to minimize the anterior pelvic tilt and decrease the anterior shear at the lumbosacral unit. All supports are made from leather and a viscoelastic polymer that improves its compatibility with the anatomy. (IEM Orthopaedic Systems, P.O. Box 592, Ravenna, OH 44266.) (From Porterfield JA, DeRosa C: Mechanical Low Back Pain: Perspectives in Functional Anatomy. Philadelphia: WB Saunders, 1990.)

that can be used for management of acute low back pains during pregnancy.

### Reinjury

The reinjury patient must develop the neuromuscular capabilities to help manage his or her problem because there is a high probability of recurrence. Therefore, enhancing neuromuscular efficiency is strongly indicated for these patients. Musculoskeletal health is critical in avoiding reinjury. Biomechanical counseling is important because the limits of the patient's optimal loading zone must be recognized and respected. Use of pain modulation techniques and generation of controlled forces in the region are appropriate only if they promote the patient's activity. The current literature supports an active approach toward rehabilitation.

### Chronic Pain Syndrome

We are beginning to recognize that the patient with true chronic pain syndrome can no longer be treated with an emphasis on pain modulation. Instead, the focus should be on augmenting function and increasing physical activity. These changes not only help modify the attention to pain but also promote well-being and a feeling of self-worth. The treatment program should address the changes that occur logically in any deconditioning syndrome: mobility, endurance, strength, and cardiovascular changes. This is why enhancing neuromuscular efficiency is strongly indicated for these patients. It is especially important to focus on increases in function that can be measured objectively in order to provide positive feedback to the patient.

## SUMMARY

More clinical research is needed to help further our understanding of the proper management of low back disorders. Advances have been made, but in some regards the problem has worsened. Our goals in the future should be a more universally applied, reproducible, and reliable evaluation system and a logical progression of treatment that emphasizes active rehabilitation. Such a plan has been presented. We are beginning to recognize that efficacy of technique depends greatly on the skill of the clinician in administering treatment rather than the technique itself. For this reason, the emphasis in this chapter has been on delineating treatment objectives more clearly and matching these objectives to the appropriate patients.

## CASE STUDY 1

▼Mrs. C.B. is a homemaker with three children who are all over the age of 16. She was referred to physical therapy with the diagnosis of traumatic arthritis of the right sacroiliac joint. The condition began in June of the previous year when she was riding on the back of her son's moped. She was thrown off the moped and landed on her buttocks. She experienced immediate pain on the right side of her pelvis and has been treated for this condition with medication and rest. Her condition has varied in intensity, frequency, and duration. She complains of right buttock pain that often radiates to her right groin and anterior thigh. The pain is worse in the morning, decreases when she has been awake for 2 or 3 hours, and worsens by the end of the day. She estimates 8 out of 10 (10 is the worst pain) on the pain scale, 4 out of 10 (10 is normal preinjury activity) on the activity scale, and 5 out of 10 (10 is major stress) on the stress scale. She has been taking 800 mg of ibuprofen (Motrin) twice a day for the past 3 weeks.

The assessment revealed the following:

*Standing examination:* Normal sagittal plane and frontal plane static structure. Backward bending and side bending to the right reproduced her familiar pain on the right. Overpressure increased the symptoms. A sacral support was placed around the pelvis to assess the patient's response. The patient stated that the force of the support decreased her pain in standing and gave her a sense of decreased pressure.

*Sitting examination:* Positive slouch test in the extreme position, right greater than left. L-4 reflexes were within normal limits.

*Supine lying examination:* Anterior-to-posterior shear of the right sacroiliac region via the long axis of the femur provoked the symptoms. All sensory, motor, and reflex neurologic findings were negative.

*Prone lying examination:* Any posterior-to-anterior shear stresses to the right sacrum or ilium provoked the familiar symptom. Backward bending and side bending stresses were produced by direct posterior-to-anterior pressure to the right lumbosacral. This positive response was reproduced with less posterior-anterior force when the patient rested on her elbows.

*Impression:* Compression-shear injury to the right lumbosacral region.

*Treatment:* The treatment goals were to stabilize the pelvis temporarily, minimize the destructive forces generated in this region during activity and periods of rest via biomechanical counseling, decrease the pain as quickly as possible, and improve painless function.

Treatment was started on the date of evaluation by counseling the patient to rest in a supine position with the femurs and knees flexed for at least two periods of 20 minutes each and to wear the support at all times during weight-bearing activities. The patient was instructed in the use of ice at home to minimize the afferent nociceptive input into the system. Gentle supine side-to-side rocking exercises were recommended to ensure a fluid pressure change that would help decrease the congestion of fluid. She was instructed to call if any abnormal results persisted and was scheduled to return in 3 days for re-evaluation and continued treatment.

On the second visit the patient reported a 30% decrease in the intensity and frequency of pain. Treatment consisted of electrical stimulation of the right lumbopelvic triangle region to enhance fluid dynamics.

Gentle joint mobilization and isometric contraction of the pelvic musculature were performed to stimulate the afferent mechanoreceptors and thereby inhibit the painful stimulus. The patient was counseled to maintain controlled nondestructive forces to the region and continue to wear the sacral support. The treatment progressed for six visits over a period of 2 months. She improved to the point where she did not need to wear the support all the time, only when lifting and carrying. Her morning stiffness and pain had diminished by approximately 70%, and she had pain with prolonged periods of weight bearing. She had to be cautious with lifting and carrying and was restricted by approximately 20% in the amount of work that could be performed. As long as she paced herself and was cognizant of her weight-bearing pattern (directing the force away from the right lumbosacral region), she could function well.

The patient was discharged from our care after 8 weeks of intervention and was instructed to call us if problems arose.

## CASE STUDY 2

▼Dr. M.C. is a 48-year-old obstetrician and gynecologist who has run approximately 30 to 50 miles per week for the past 10 years. He was referred to the rehabilitation center with the diagnosis of degenerative disc disease and sclerosis of the right sacroiliac joint. He had a long history of intermittent pain in the right low back that increased progressively during running and remained a dull ache for about 1 hour after running. The site of pain was the posterior superior iliac spine and it radiated inferiorly and laterally into the midbuttock. Previously the pain was relieved with a non-weight-bearing resting position, but now the discomfort persists even after unweighting the skeleton. This is the reason for seeking professional help. He felt best in the morning; however, the morning stiffness has gradually progressed and by the end of the day his pain is increased. The intensity of his symptom is proportional to his running behavior. He estimates that he is at 8 out of 10 on the pain scale, 9 out of 10 on the activity scale, and 5 out of a 10 on the stress scale.

The assessment revealed the following:

*Standing examination:* Left frontal plane asymmetry (left iliac crest, posterior and anterior superior iliac spine, and greater trochanters all approximately ½ inch low on the left). Backward bending and side bending to the right increased the familiar pain on the right. Calibrated blocks were placed under the right foot to level his pelvis and repeatedly alternated with full equal weight bearing without the correction. This assesses the patient's perception as the weight line is shifted toward the middle of the spine. He felt better on the blocks. Movement testing repeated with the patient on the calibrated blocks showed that it required more range of motion and a greater force to exacerbate his familiar symptoms. This is a positive sign that weight bearing asymmetrically in the frontal plane plays a role in the destructive force(s) of his syndrome.

*Sitting examination:* Negative.

*Supine lying examination:* The only positive finding was a positive figure 4 on the right. This matched the standing assessment, because tightness of the hip joint capsule in flexion, abduction, and external rotation can be compared to tightness in femoral extension during the terminal phases of gait. This tightness translates to increased extension forces at the lumbosacral junction and an anterior rotatory moment of the right ilium. The neurologic assessment was unremarkable.

*Prone lying examination:* All posterior-to-anterior forces on the L-5–S-1 spinous process and the right sacroiliac joint reproduced the familiar pain on the right in the prone examination, which matched the standing examination.

*Impression:* The etiologic diagnosis was that this patient experienced excessive compression and shear loads on the right lumbosacral triangle because of his frontal plane asymmetry. This caused musculoskeletal breakdown of the L-5–S-1 intervertebral disc and right sacroiliac joint, eventually causing symptoms to arise. Leaving the ground during the running gait most likely hastened the tissue breakdown.

*Treatment:* The treatment goals are to balance the weight-bearing pattern in his pelvis and lumbar spine and help him monitor the frequency, intensity, and duration of the loads imparted to this region so that they remain nondestructive. We are also attempting to keep him running as much as possible, because of his love of it and the stress management qualities that he enjoys and to which he is accustomed.

The first phase of rehabilitation was to place a ⅜-inch heel lift below the left leg and a sacral support around his pelvis to stabilize the region. He responded quite well. The second visit consisted of assessing his response to the frontal plane correction and stabilization. He responded favorably to this initial treatment. The second visit included specific mobilization of the sacroiliac region for the purpose of afferent stimulation and fluid movement. The patient felt immediate relief after the mechanical stimulation. He attempted to continue running, and the therapist saw him as necessary and performed mobilization that gave him 4 to 6 days of relief. Eventually, it was clear that running had to be discontinued at this time because we were not reaching our immediate goals of pain relief. He was counseled to discontinue running temporarily, and alternative aerobic activities to meet his needs were discussed. After approximately 4 weeks of controlled alternative activity, his syndrome was under control. After six treatments and alternative activity over a 4-month period he gradually resumed running. We convinced him to spend 1 day a week in the gym to strengthen his trunk muscles instead of the impact loading of aerobics. After 1 year of experimentation, he has lost approximately 30% of his ability to bear weight through this region and has adjusted accordingly and is doing well.

This is an excellent example of the body's gradual progressive changes in response to consistent excessive forces and how one must alter weight bearing to remain active.

## CASE STUDY 3

▼ Mr. C.G. was referred for physical therapy with the diagnosis of herniated nucleus pulposus to the left at the L-5–S-1 segment. The patient is a 51-year-old dock worker for a local trucking industry. Three weeks ago the patient felt "warmth" in his back while lifting freight from the floor onto a pallet. The sensation lasted for approximately 2 hours and then diminished. The next morning he experienced stiffness in the low back region. He continued to work with small amounts of discomfort until the fourth day. The morning stiffness gradually increased to the point that he could not loosen up for approximately 1 hour. On the fourth day, Mr. C.G. sat for 20 minutes on break and then returned to his position and began to unload a truck. He stated that he gradually felt a pain go down his leg into his foot that resulted in numbness on the outside of his left foot. He went home and the leg sensation progressed to a constant ache. He has difficulty sleeping and has not worked in the past 2 weeks. He states that he has complete control of his bowel and bladder. The patient estimates 9 out of 10 on the pain scale, 2 out of 10 on the activity scale, and 7 out of 10 on the stress scale. The patient is presently taking four aceta-minophen–hydrocodone bitartrate (Vicodin) per day and four 800-mg ibuprofen (Motrin) per day with little relief.

The assessment revealed the following:

*Standing examination:* On initial assessment the patient could not stand erect without reproducing his familiar leg pain. He had lost the integrity of his abdominal wall, which significantly altered weight bearing in the sagittal plane. He had approximately 20% of his normal active range of motion, but the quality of that motion was poor. He experienced significant protective guarding. He had a normal frontal plane.

*Sitting examination:* The patient was unable to sit straight and the familiar leg pain was easily reproduced upon raising the left leg. L-4 reflexes were within normal limits.

*Supine lying examination:* The patient had significantly decreased passive left passive hip flexion. He had bilateral figure 4 tests. Straight leg raising on the right at 50 degrees reproduced left buttock and leg pain. On the left it was positive at 20 degrees. Holding this position for approximately 30 seconds reproduced the familiar aching and pain that has kept the patient awake for the past 2 weeks. He explained that his foot "falls asleep." Sensory testing was within normal limits. He had a significantly retarded L-5 and S-1 reflex on the left, grade 2 weakness of the L-5 myotome (extensor hallucis longus), and had lost considerable power with a 15-repetition toe raise test (S-1 gastrocnemius-soleus myotome).

*Prone lying examination:* Initially, he was not able to lie flat on his stomach because this position exacerbated his left leg pain. He had considerable tenderness at the left posterior superior iliac spine and iliac crest at the attachment of the lateral raphe.

*Impression:* Significant neuroforaminal encroachment resulting in L-5–S-1 nerve root involvement.

*Treatment:* The initial goal of treatment was to modulate pain and create a healing environment to ensure a proper beginning of the healing process.

We used 40 minutes of electrical stimulation and ice with the patient lying on the right side. Mobilization of the soft tissue, especially at the left posterior superior iliac spine and iliac crest, was carried out, followed by education about the mechanics of neuroforaminal encroachment. We placed the patient on crutches with a three-point gait. These were to be worn at all times. Gentle active exercise was introduced at the third visit. He began to respond slowly after six treatments. We then suggested to the referring physician the use of epidural steroids. He had the two injections over a period of 2.5 weeks and conservative physical therapy. He had improved sleep and his pain decreased significantly. We then began a physical reconditioning program consisting of gentle active and active resistive therapeutic exercise. The third injection was administered at week 4 and the reconditioning gradually progressed. The intensity, frequency, and duration of the training were monitored closely by trained staff members. At 2½ months after the initial visit, the patient was significantly better in all aspects of his physical life. However, he could not return to his previous job. His employer consented to a gradual return to work (2 weeks at 4 hours per day, 2 weeks at 6 hours per day, and then full return to work). He was given light duty at first, and later the company decided to place him in a different job classification. At re-evaluation 8 months after treatment, his straight leg raising was positive at 45 degrees and his activity level was 7 to 8 out of 10. He will probably never be able to return to lifting because of the weakness in the posterior lateral corner of his intervertebral disc.

# References

1. Spengler DM, Bigos SJ, Martin NA, et al: Back injuries in industry: a retrospective study. 1. Overview and cost analysis. Spine 11:241, 1986.
2. Akeson WH, Murphy RW: Low back pain. Clin Orthop 129:2–17, 1977.
3. National Center for Health Statistics (Series 10, No. 134): Prevalence of Selected Impairment, United States, Hyattsville, MD: Department of Health and Human Services, 1981.
4. Mooney V: Where is the pain coming from? Spine 12:754–759, 1987.
5. Cassidy JD, Wedge JH: The natural history of low back pain and spinal degeneration. *In* Managing Low Back Pain (Kirkaldy-Willis WH, ed). New York: Churchill-Livingstone, 1988, pp 3–15.
6. Benn RT, Wood PHN: Pain in the back: an attempt to estimate the size of the problem. Rheumatol Rehabil 14:121–128, 1975.
7. Kelsey J, White AA: Epidemiology and impact of low back pain. Spine 6:133–142, 1980.
8. McCombe PF, Fairbanks JCT, Cockersole BC, et al: Reproducibility of physical signs in low back pain. Spine 14:908–917, 1989.
9. Nachemson A: The lumbar spine: an orthopaedic challenge. Spine 1:9–21, 1976.
10. White AA, Panjabi MM: Clinical Biomechanics of the Spine. Philadelphia: JB Lippincott, 1978.
11. Buckwalter JA, Pedrini-Mille A, Pedrini V, et al: Proteoglycans of human infant intervertebral disc: electron microscopic and biochemical studies. J Bone Joint Surg [Am] 67:284–294, 1985.
12. Adams P, Eyre DR, Muir H: Biochemical aspects of development and ageing of human lumbar intervertebral discs. Rheumatol Rehabil 16:22–29, 1977.
13. Pearson CH, Happey F, Naylor A, et al: Collagens and associated glycoproteins in the human intervertebral disc: variations in sugar and amino acid composition in relation to location and age. Ann Rheum Dis 31:45–63, 1972.
14. Bushell GR, Ghosh P, Taylor TFK, et al: Proteoglycan chemistry of the intervertebral disks. Clin Orthop 129:115–123, 1977.
15. Pearce RH, Grimmer BJ: The chemical constitution of the proteoglycan of human intervertebral disc. Biochem J 157:753–763, 1976.
16. Taylor JR, Twomey LT: Vertebral column development and its relation to adult pathology. Aust J Physiother 31:83–88, 1985.
17. Twomey LT, Taylor JR: Age changes in the lumbar articular triad. Aust J Physiother 31:106–112, 1985.
18. Pearcy MJ, Tibrewal SB: Lumbar intervertebral disc and ligament deformations measured in vivo. Clin Orthop 191:281–286, 1984.
19. Lemperg RK, Arnoldi CC: The significance of intraosseous pressure in normal and diseased states with special reference to the intraosseous engorgement pain syndrome. Clin Orthop 136:143–156, 1978.
20. Peyron J: Inflammation in osteoarthritis: review of its role in clinical picture, disease progress, subsets and pathophysiology. Semin Arthritis Rheum 11(suppl):115–116, 1981.
21. Bogduk N, Engel R: The menisci of the lumbar zygapophyseal joints. A review of their anatomy and clinical significance. Spine 9:454–460, 1984.
22. Palmoski MJ, Brandt KD: Effects of static and cyclic compressive loading on articular cartilage plugs in vitro. Arthritis Rheum 23:325–334, 1980.

23. Adams MA, Hutton WC: The effects of posture on the role of the apophyseal joints in resisting intervertebral compression force. J Bone Joint Surg [Br] 62:358–362, 1980.

24. Porterfield JA, DeRosa CP: The sacroiliac joint. In Orthopedic and Sports Physical Therapy, 2nd ed. (Gould JA, ed). St. Louis: Mosby–Year Book 1990, pp 553–573.

25. Beal MC: The sacroiliac problem: review of anatomy, mechanics, and diagnosis. J Am Osteopath Assoc 81:667–669, 1982.

26. Bowan V, Cassidy JD: Macroscopic and microscopic anatomy of the sacroiliac joint from embryonic life until the eighth decade. Spine 6:620–628, 1981.

27. Kapandji IA: The Physiology of the Joints, Vol 3. Edinburgh: Churchill-Livingstone, 1974.

28. Lavignolle B, Vital JM, Senegas J, et al: An approach to the functional anatomy of the sacroiliac joints in vivo. Anat Clin 5:169–176, 1983.

29. DeRosa C, Porterfield JA: The Sacroiliac Joint. Berryville, VA: Forum Medicum I-X, 1989.

30. Weisel H: Movements of the sacroiliac joint. Acta Anat 23:80–91, 1955.

31. Sashin D: A critical analysis of the anatomy and the pathological changes of the SI joints. J Bone Joint Surg [Am] 12:891–910, 1930.

32. Sturesson B, Selvik G, Uden A: Movements of the sacroiliac joints: a Roentgen stereophotogrammetric analysis. Spine 14:162–165, 1989.

33. Miller JAA, Schultz AB, Andersson GBJ: Load-displacement behavior of sacroiliac joints. J Orthop Res 5:92, 1987.

34. Walheim GG, Olerud S, Ridde T: Mobility of the pubic symphysis. Measurements by an electromechanical method. Acta Orthop Scand 55:203–208, 1984.

35. Gamble JG, Simmons SC, Freedman M: The symphysis pubis. Clin Orthop Relat Res 203:261–272, 1986.

36. Golighty R: Pelvic arthropathy in pregnancy and the puerperium. Physiotherapy 68:216–220, 1982.

37. Weiss M, Nagelschmidt M, Struck H: Relaxin and collagen metabolism. Horm Metab Res 11:408–417, 1979.

38. Weinstein JN, Rauschning W, Resnick D, et al: Clinical perspectives—part A. In New Perspectives on Low Back Pain (Frymoyer JW, Gordon SL, eds). Park Ridge, IL: American Academy of Orthopedic Surgeons Symposium, 1989, pp 37–57.

39. Bogduk N, Twomey LT: Clinical Anatomy of the Lumbar Spine. New York: Churchill-Livingstone, 1987.

40. Luk KDK, Ho HC, Leong JCY: The iliolumbar ligament: a study of its anatomy, development, and clinical significance. J Bone Joint Surg [Br] 68:197–200, 1987.

41. Bogduk N, Macintosh JE: The applied anatomy of the thoracolumbar fascia. Spine 9:164–170, 1984.

42. Gracovetsky S, Farfan HF, Lamy C: The mechanism of the lumbar spine. Spine 6:249–262, 1981.

43. Gracovetsky S, Farfan HF, Helleur C: The abdominal mechanism. Spine 10:317–324, 1985.

44. Farfan HF: Mechanical Disorders of the Low Back. Philadelphia: Lea & Febiger, 1973.

45. McGill SM, Norman RW: The potential of the lumbodorsal fascia forces to generate back extension moments during squat lifts. J Biomed Eng 10:312–318, 1988.

46. Macintosh JE, Bogduk N: The morphology of the lumbar erector spinae. Spine 12:658–668, 1987.

47. Floyd WF, Silver PHS: Function of the erectores spinae in flexion of the trunk. Lancet 1:133–134, 1951.

48. Kippers V, Parker AW: Posture related to electromyographic silence of erectores spinae during trunk flexion. Spine 7:740–745, 1984.

49. Porterfield JA, DeRosa C: Mechanical Low Back Pain: Perspectives in Functional Anatomy. Philadelphia: WB Saunders, 1990.

50. Nachemson A: The possible role of the psoas muscle for stabilization of the lumbar spine. Acta Orthop Scand 39:47–57, 1968.

51. Parke WW, Watanabe R: Adhesions of the ventral lumbar dura. An adjunct source of discogenic pain? Spine 15:300–303, 1990.

52. Parke WW, Watanabe R: The intrinsic vasculature of the lumbosacral nerve roots. Spine 10:508–515, 1985.

53. Rydevik B, Holm S, Brown MD: Nutrition of the spinal nerve roots: the role of diffusion from the cerebrospinal fluid. Trans Orthop Res Soc 9:276, 1984.

54. MacNab I: The mechanism of spondylogenic pain. In Cervical Pain (Hirsch C, Zotterman Y, eds). Oxford: Pergamon, 1972.

55. McCarron RF, Wimpee MW, Hudkins PG, et al: The inflammatory effect of the nucleus pulposus: a possible element in the pathogenesis of low back pain. Spine 12:760–764, 1987.

56. Payan DG, McGillis JP, Goetzl EJ: Neuroimmunology. Adv Immunol 39:299–323, 1986.

57. Mooney V, Robertson J: The facet syndrome. Clin Orthop 115:149–156, 1976.

58. Feinstein B, Langton JNK, Jameson RM, et al: Experiments on pain referred from deep structures. J Bone Joint Surg [Am] 36:981–997, 1954.

59. Maitland GD: Vertebral Manipulation, 5th ed. London: Butterworths, 1986.

60. Spratt KF, Lehmann TR, Weinstein, JN, et al: A new approach to the low-back physical examination. Spine 15:96–102, 1990.

61. Quebec Task Force on Spinal Disorders: Scientific approach to the assessment and management of activity-related spinal disorders. Spine 12:S1–S59, 1987.

62. Waddell G: A new clinical model for the treatment of low-back pain. Spine 12:632–634, 1987.

63. McCombe PF, Fairbanks JCT, Cockersole BC, et al: Reproducibility of physical signs in low-back pain. Spine 14:909–918, 1989.

64. McNeill T, Warwick D, Andersson GBJ, et al: Trunk strength in attempted flexion, extension and lateral bending in healthy subjects and patients with low back disorders. Spine 5:529–538, 1980.

65. D'Ambrosia RD: Musculoskeletal Disorders: Regional Examination and Differential Diagnosis, 2nd ed. Philadelphia: JB Lippincott, 1986.

66. Rockwood CA, Green DP: Fractures in Adults, 2nd ed. Philadelphia: JB Lippincott, 1984.

67. Tachdjian MO: Pediatric Orthopedics. Philadelphia: WB Saunders, 1972.

68. Gehweiler JA, Osborne RL, Becker RF: The Radiology of Vertebral Trauma. Philadelphia, WB Saunders, 1980.

69. Denis F: The three column spine and its significance in the classification of acute thoracolumbar spinal injuries. Spine 8:817–831, 1983.

70. Chance CQ: Note on a type of flexion fracture of the spine. Br J Radiol. 21:452, 1948.

71. Smith WS, Kaufer H: Patterns and mechanisms of lumbar injuries associated with lap seat belts. J Bone Joint Surg [Am] 51:239–254, 1969.

72. Benson DR: The back: thoracic and lumbar spine. In Musculoskeletal Disorders: Regional Examination and Differential Diagnosis, 2nd ed. (D'Ambrosia RD, ed). Philadelphia: JB Lippincott, 1986, pp 287–366.

73. Frymoyer JW, Krag MH: Spinal stability and instability: definitions, classification, and general principles of management. In The Unstable Spine (Dunsker SB, Schmidek

HH, Frymoyer J, et al, eds). Orlando FL: Grune & Stratton, 1986, pp 1–16.

74. Kirkaldy-Willis WH: Managing Low Back Pain. New York: Churchill-Livingstone, 1983.

75. Hayes MA, Howard TC, Gruel CR, et al: Roentgenographic evaluation of lumbar spine flexion-extension in normal individuals. Abstracts, Federation of Spinal Association Meeting, New Orleans, February 19, 1986.

76. Paris SV: Physical signs of instability. Spine 10:277–279, 1985.

77. Andreoli TE, Carpenter CC, Plum F, et al: Cecil Essentials of Medicine. Philadelphia: WB Saunders, 1986.

78. Goodman CC, Snyder TE: Differential Diagnosis in Physical Therapy. Philadelphia: WB Saunders, 1990.

79. Anderson WAD, Scotti TM: Synopsis of Pathology, 10th ed. St. Louis: CV Mosby, 1980.

80. Yasuma T, Makino E, Saito S, et al: Histological development of the intervertebral disc herniation. J Bone Joint Surg [Am] 68:1066–1072, 1986.

81. Mixter WJ, Barr JS: Rupture of the intervertebral disc with involvement of the spinal canal. N Engl J Med 211:210–215, 1934.

82. Spangfort EV: The lumbar disc herniation: a computer aided analysis of 2504 operations. Acta Orthop Scand [Suppl] 142:1–95, 1972.

83. Saal JA, Saal JS: Nonoperative treatment of herniated lumbar intervertebral disc with radiculopathy—an outcome study. Spine 14:431–437, 1989.

84. Weber H: Lumbar disc herniation: a controlled prospective study with ten years of observation. Spine 8:131–140, 1983.

85. Hitselberger WE, Witten RM: Abnormal myelograms in aysmptomatic patients. J Neurosurg 28:204–206, 1968.

86. Wiesel SW, Tsourmas N, Feffer HL, et al: A study of computer-assisted tomography: the incidence of positive CAT scans in an asymptomatic group of patients. Spine 9:549–551, 1984.

87. Marshall LL, Trethewie ER: Chemical irritation of nerve root in disc prolapse. Lancet 2:230–232, 1973.

88. Ochs S, Worth RM: Axoplasmic transport in normal and pathologic systems. In Physiology and Pathobiology of Axons (Waxman SG, ed). New York: Raven Press, 1978, pp 251–264.

89. Hoyland JA, Freemont AJ, Jayson MIV: Intervertebral foramen venous obstruction: a cause of periradicular fibrosis? Spine 14:558–568, 1989.

90. Cyriax J: Textbook of Orthopaedic Medicine, Vol I. London: Bailliere Tindall, 1978.

91. DeRosa C, Porterfield JA: A physical therapy model for low back disorders. Phys Ther 72:261–272, 1992.

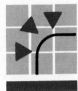

# CHAPTER *Four*

## Shoulder

*MAE L. YAHARA*

## INTRODUCTION

The physical therapist must fully understand the precise, coordinated and synchronous movement of the joints that make up the shoulder complex as these motions permit the hand to be placed in front of the body, where functions can easily be observed.[1] The great mobility available through the shoulder joint complex creates a problem with inherent stability. Therefore, this system relies on dynamic structures (muscle) for increased stability. Effective treatment of shoulder pathology or dysfunction is the result of comprehensive understanding of normal and ab-

normal biomechanics of the four joints that constitute the shoulder complex.

## ANATOMY

### Joints

The shoulder joint complex consists of the scapula, clavicle, and humerus and is generally divided into four articulations: sternoclavicular, acromioclavicular, glenohumeral, and scapulothoracic joints (see Fig. 4–1).[2] A fifth articulation,

159

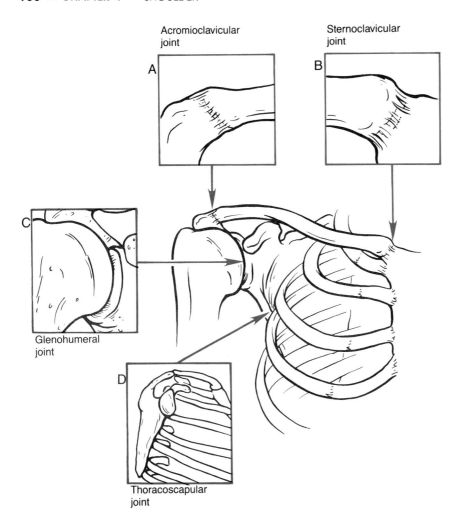

Acromioclavicular
joint

Sternoclavicular
joint

Glenohumeral
joint

Thoracoscapular
joint

**FIGURE 4-1** ■ The shoulder joint complex. (A) Acromioclavicular joint. (B) Sternoclavicular joint. (C) Glenohumeral joint. (D) Scapulothoracic joint.

humerocoracoacromial (commonly known as the coracoacromial arch), is often considered part of the shoulder complex when the area is analyzed functionally (Fig. 4–2).[3]

### Sternoclavicular Joint

The sternoclavicular joint is the only direct bony articulation of the upper extremity with the trunk.[4] It is a saddle-shaped synovial joint. The medial end of the clavicle is separated from the articular surface of the sternal manubrium by an intra-articular disc or meniscus. The disc increases the congruence of the articular surfaces, but it divides the joint into two separate cavities as it attaches superiorly to the clavicle and inferiorly to the manubrium of the sternum (Fig. 4–3).

The motions occurring at the sternoclavicular joint are elevation-depression, protraction-retraction, and rotation. Elevation and depression take place primarily between the disc and the clavicle. The axis is oblique from the sternal end of the clavicle, taking a backward and downward course. Protraction and retraction are primary motions between the disc and the sternum.[5] Therefore, shoulder girdle elevation occurs in an upward and backward direction and depression in a forward and downward direction. Rotation of the clavicle occurs as a spin at the joint and has a range of 30 degrees around its long axis.[6] This rotation occurs after the shoulder has been elevated 90 degrees and is essential for full elevation to be achieved.

The sternoclavicular joint is supported by a strong capsule that is reinforced anteriorly and posteriorly by the sternoclavicular ligaments. These serve to limit protraction and retraction of the clavicle (see Fig. 4–3). The right and left clavicles are connected by an interclavicular ligament that crosses over the sternal notch. The costoclavicular ligament adds further stability to

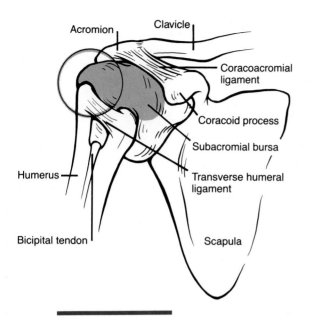

**FIGURE 4–2** ■ The coracoacromial arch.

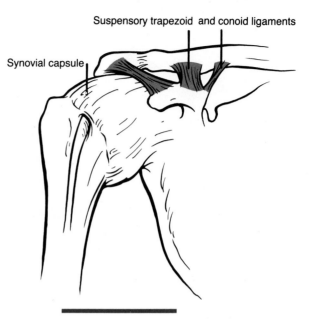

**FIGURE 4–4** ■ Acromioclavicular joint.

this joint by attaching the inferior surface of the clavicle to the superior surface of the first rib, thus limiting excessive rotation, elevation, and depression.

## Acromioclavicular Joint

The small concave facet on the acromion process of the scapula articulates with the small convex facet on the lateral end of the clavicle to form the acromioclavicular joint. In this plane, synovial joint motion is limited. In general, the literature concurs that the primary movement of the scapula at the acromioclavicular joint is scapular rotation.[7,8]

The capsule of the acromioclavicular joint is weak and its integrity is maintained by the reinforcing ligaments. Superior and inferior support is provided by the acromioclavicular ligaments.

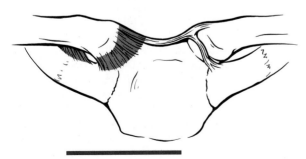

**FIGURE 4–3** ■ Sternoclavicular joint.

The clavicle is held firmly to the coracoid process of the scapula by the coracoclavicular ligament. This ligament is divided into a medial portion, the trapezoid, and a lateral portion, the conoid. (Fig. 4–4). These ligaments limit separation of the clavicle and scapula during movement.

## Scapulothoracic Articulation

The articulation between the scapula and the thorax cannot be considered a true anatomic joint because it lacks the usual joint characteristics. However, it warrants discussion because the movement of the concave anterior surface of the scapula on the convex rib cage is intimately related to movements at the sternoclavicular, acromioclavicular, and glenohumeral joints.[9] The scapular movements from rest on the posterior thorax are elevation-depression, abduction-adduction (protraction-retraction), and upward-downward rotation (Fig. 4–5). Muscular attachments also determine scapular position. The joint effect of acromioclavicular and sternoclavicular motions is to permit scapular rotation so that the glenoid cavity may face forward and upward or downward, as called for by the motion.

## Glenohumeral Joint

This joint is classified as a ball-and-socket synovial joint; the large convex head of the humerus articulates with the smaller, shallow, con-

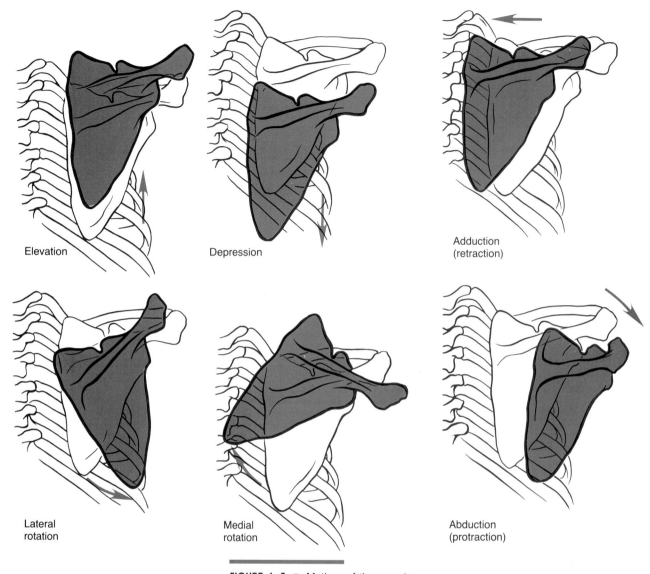

Elevation

Depression

Adduction
(retraction)

Lateral
rotation

Medial
rotation

Abduction
(protraction)

**FIGURE 4–5** ■ Motions of the scapula.

cave glenoid fossa of the scapula. The articular surfaces are deepened by the glenoid labrum, a fibrocartilaginous rim that surrounds the fossa. (Fig. 4–6). The glenohumeral joint is capable of a large range of movement: flexion-extension, abduction-adduction, and internal-external rotation (Fig. 4–7). Circumduction at the glenohumeral joint is a combination of flexion, external rotation, abduction, extension, adduction, and internal rotation to produce a circular movement of the hand in space (Fig. 4–8).

The capsule surrounding this joint is twice the size of the humeral head.[10] Its size and relative weakness permit large excursions of movement. Ligamentous and muscular attachments maintain the integrity of the capsule and the humeral

head in the glenoid fossa. The coracohumeral ligament passes obliquely downward and laterally from the coracoid process to the greater tuberosity. It counteracts the downward pull of gravity on the arm and limits external rotation and extension. The glenohumeral ligaments (Fig. 4–9) are divided into superior, middle, and inferior portions. They are extremely important in resisting downward and anterior displacement of the humeral head.

### Humerocoracoacromial Joint

This joint is also known as the coracoacromial arch and is not a true joint. It consists of the acromion and the coracoacromial ligament. The

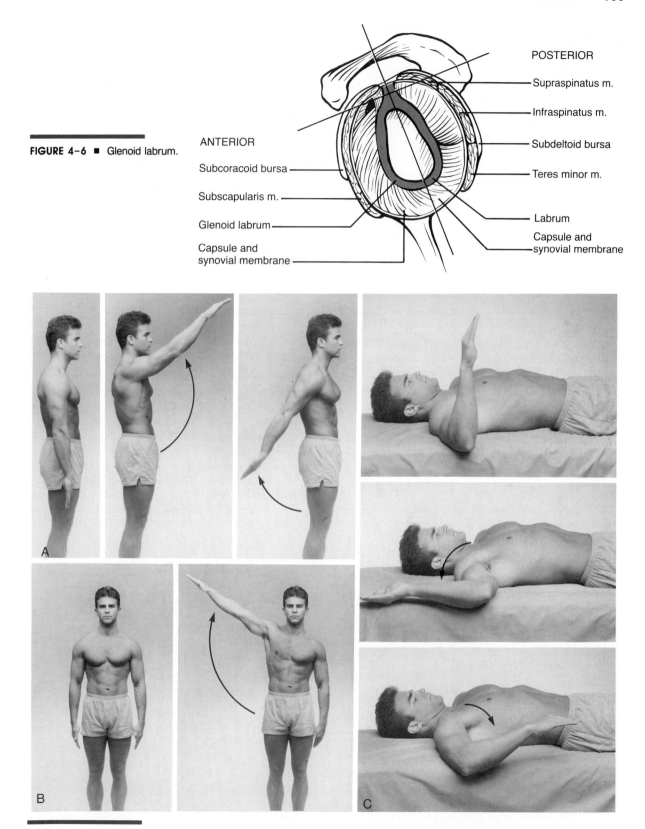

**FIGURE 4-6** ■ Glenoid labrum.

POSTERIOR

Supraspinatus m.

Infraspinatus m.

Subdeltoid bursa

Teres minor m.

Labrum

Capsule and
synovial membrane

ANTERIOR

Subcoracoid bursa

Subscapularis m.

Glenoid labrum

Capsule and
synovial membrane

**FIGURE 4-7** ■ Range of motion of the shoulder. (A) Neutral, flexion-extension, hyperextension. (B) Neutral, abduction. (C) Neutral, external rotation, internal rotation.

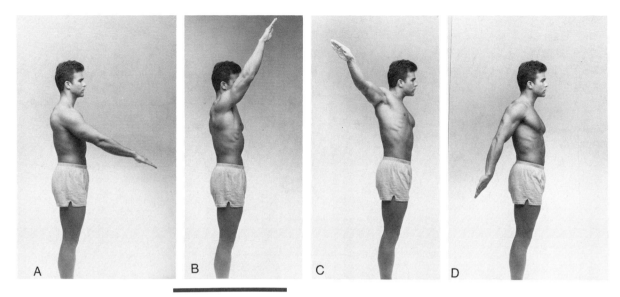

**FIGURE 4-8** ■ Circumduction of the shoulder joint complex.

humerocoracoacromial joint protects the humeral head and its overlying muscles, tendons, and bursae from direct trauma by forming an archway for these structures to glide through as the arm is moved overhead (see Fig. 4–2).

## Muscles

The muscles of the shoulder joint complex are most easily understood if analyzed in a functional categorization, related to the origin and insertion of tendons:

- Scapulohumeral muscles originate from the scapula and attach to the humerus. They are the subscapularis, teres major, teres minor, supraspinatus, infraspinatus, coracobrachialis, and deltoideus (Fig. 4–10A).
- Axioscapular muscles originate on the axial skeleton and attach to various portions of the scapula. They are the trapezius (upper, middle, and lower fibers), serratus anterior, rhomboideus major, rhomboideus minor, pectoralis minor, and levator scapulae (Fig. 4–10B).

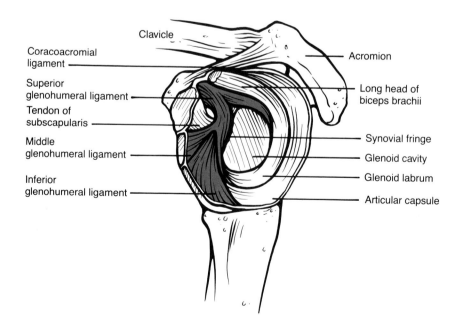

Clavicle
Coracoacromial ligament
Superior glenohumeral ligament
Tendon of subscapularis
Middle glenohumeral ligament
Inferior glenohumeral ligament
Acromion
Long head of biceps brachii
Synovial fringe
Glenoid cavity
Glenoid labrum
Articular capsule

**FIGURE 4-9** ■ Glenohumeral ligaments (superior, middle, inferior).

■ Muscles traversing from the axial skeleton to the humerus (axiohumeral) include the latissimus dorsi and the pectoralis major (Fig. 4–10C).

■ Finally, the scapuloradial muscle (biceps brachii) and the scapuloulnar muscle (triceps) are also important to shoulder function (Fig. 4–10D).

The actions of these muscle groups are discussed in depth in the section on biomechanics.

## Bursae

In the shoulder complex there are 10 bursae located between adjacent structures where motion is required.[2] These include the subscapular, subacromial, subdeltoid, subcoracoid, coracobrachialis, infraspinatus, latissimus dorsi, teres major, pectoralis major, and subcutaneous acromial bursae (Fig. 4–11).

Those with the most clinical significance are

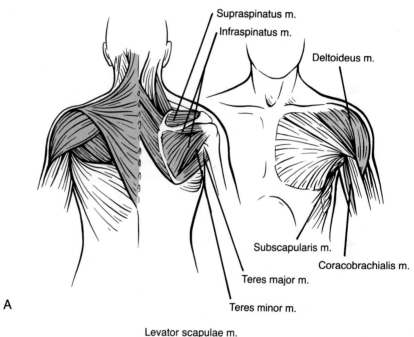

**FIGURE 4-10** ■ (A) Scapulohumeral muscles (subscapularis, teres major and minor, supraspinatus, infraspinatus, coracobrachialis, deltoideus). (B) Axioscapular muscles (trapezius—upper, middle, lower fibers; serratus; rhomboideus; pectoralis minor; levator scapulae). *Illustration continued on following page.*

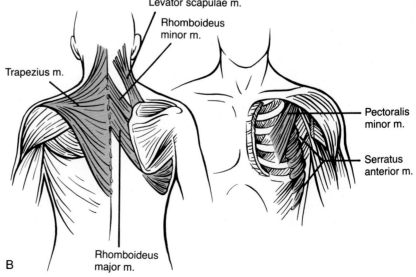

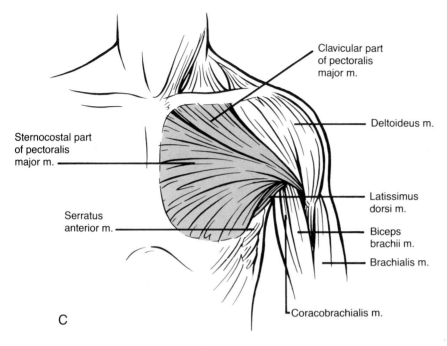

Clavicular part of pectoralis major m.

Deltoideus m.

Sternocostal part of pectoralis major m.

Latissimus dorsi m.

Biceps brachii m.

Brachialis m.

Serratus anterior m.

Coracobrachialis m.

C

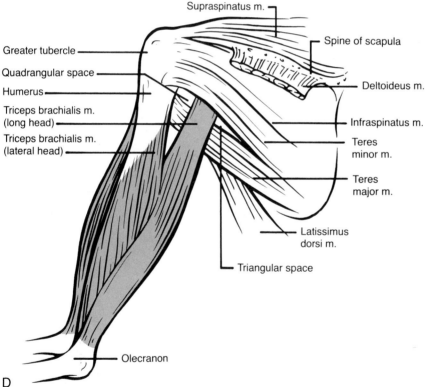

Supraspinatus m.

Spine of scapula

Greater tubercle

Quadrangular space

Deltoideus m.

Humerus

Triceps brachialis m. (long head)

Infraspinatus m.

Triceps brachialis m. (lateral head)

Teres minor m.

Teres major m.

Latissimus dorsi m.

Triangular space

Olecranon

D

**FIGURE 4–10** ■ *Continued* (C) Axiohumeral muscles (latissimus and pectoralis major). (D) Scapuloradial (biceps), scapuloulnar (triceps).

the subscapular, subacromial, and subdeltoid bursae. The subscapular bursa sits between the tendon of the subscapularis and the underlying joint capsule communicating with the synovial cavity. The subacromial bursa lies between the inferior surface of the acromion and the joint capsule. It usually extends under the coracoacromial ligament. Friction reduction on the supraspinatus tendon as it passes under the coracoacromial arch is its primary function. Like the

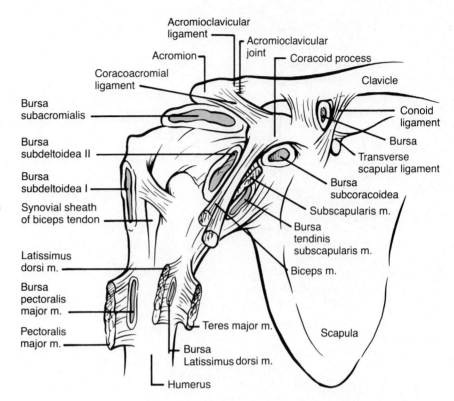

Acromioclavicular
ligament
Acromioclavicular
joint
Acromion
Coracoid process
Coracoacromial
ligament
Clavicle
Bursa
subacromialis
Conoid
ligament
Bursa
subdeltoidea II
Bursa
Transverse
scapular ligament
Bursa
subdeltoidea I
Bursa
subcoracoidea
Synovial sheath
of biceps tendon
Subscapularis m.
Bursa
tendinis
subscapularis m.
Latissimus
dorsi m.
Biceps m.
Bursa
pectoralis
major m.
Teres major m.
Scapula
Pectoralis
major m.
Bursa
Latissimus dorsi m.
Humerus

**FIGURE 4–11** ■ Bursae at the shoulder joints.

subacromial bursa, the subdeltoid bursa does not communicate with the synovial cavity but is extensive between the deep surface of the deltoid and the joint capsule. This bursa functions to reduce friction between the deltoid and the capsule.

## Nerves

Nerve fibers to the shoulder originate from the fifth, sixth, and seventh cervical nerve roots. The peripheral nerves include the axillary, suprascapular, subscapular, and musculocutaneous. Because the nerves are supplied by many sources, the innervation patterns are variable and denervation of the joint is difficult.[9] Figure 4–12 demonstrates sensory distribution patterns for the upper extremity. Table 4–1 details the muscles about the shoulder, their actions, and their nerve supply.

## Blood Supply

Vascularity of the shoulder complex is most important when considering the blood supply to

the rotator cuff tendons and possible causes of dysfunction. The infraspinatus and teres minor are supplied principally by the posterior humeral circumflex and suprascapular arteries. The anterior portion of the cuff (supraspinatus) is supplied primarily by the anterior humeral circumflex artery and occasionally by the thoracoacromial, suprahumeral, and subscapular arteries. The supraspinatus muscle superiorly is supplied by the thoracoacromial artery (Fig. 4–13). Rothman and Parke[11] identified congenital areas of hypovascularity in the rotator cuff that affect nutrition and potentially subject these tendons to degeneration.

## BIOMECHANICS

The four major articulations of the shoulder complex act in concert to provide this joint with its range of motion. This section first examines the kinematics of this joint complex. Kinematics is the description of motion regardless of the forces causing the movement.[12] To analyze motion more completely, the kinetics or the actions of muscles and the resultant forces on the joints are presented. Finally, implications of faulty or pathomechanics complete this section.

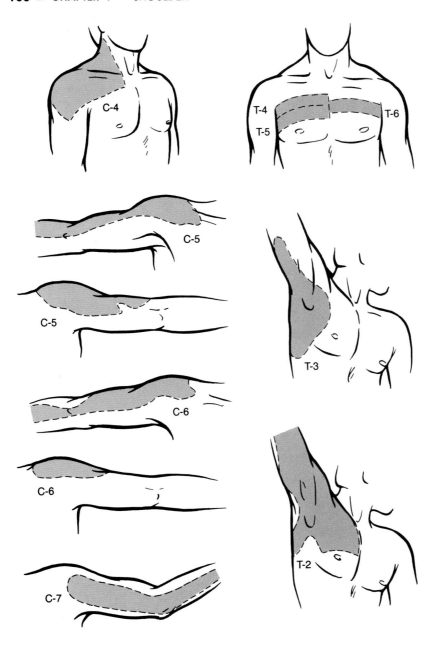

**FIGURE 4–12** ■ Sensory distribution pattern of the upper extremity.

## Kinematics

Shoulder elevation is described as movement of the humerus away from the thorax in any plane. Flexion is elevation in the sagittal plane and abduction occurs in the frontal plane. A more functional description of elevation was proposed by Johnston in 1937.[13] He described forward elevation in the plane of the scapula, midway between forward flexion and abduction, because the scapula is oriented at an angle ap-

proximately 30 to 45 degrees anterior to the frontal plane (Fig. 4–14). The rationale for this functional description is that the inferior portion of the glenohumeral joint capsule is not twisted and the deltoid and supraspinatus are optimally aligned for elevation of the arm. Therefore, there is less chance for impingement of the subacromial tissues. Shoulder rotation about the long axis of the humerus is another functionally important motion that can be performed in varying degrees of elevation. Other motions available at the shoulder include backward elevation or ex-

**Table 4-1.** MUSCLES ABOUT THE SHOULDER: THEIR ACTIONS AND NERVE SUPPLY (INCLUDING NERVE ROOT DERIVATION)

| Action | Muscles Performing Action | Nerve Supply | Nerve Root Derivation |
|---|---|---|---|
| Forward flexion | 1. Deltoid (anterior fibers) | Circumflex (axillary) | C-5, C-6 (posterior cord) |
| | 2. Pectoralis major (clavicular fibers) | Lateral pectoral | C-5, C-6 (lateral cord) |
| | 3. Coracobrachialis | Musculocutaneous | C-5, C-6, C-7 (lateral cord) |
| | 4. Biceps (when strong contraction required) | Musculocutaneous | C-5, C-6, C-7 (lateral cord) |
| Extension | 1. Deltoid (posterior fibers) | Circumflex (axillary) | C-5, C-6 posterior cord) |
| | 2. Teres major | Subscapular | C-5, C-6 (posterior cord) |
| | 3. Teres minor | Circumflex (axillary) | C-5, C-6 (posterior cord) |
| | 4. Latissimus dorsi | Thoracodorsal | C-6, C-7, C-8 (posterior cord) |
| | 5. Pectoralis major (sternocostal fibers) | Lateral pectoral | C-5, C-6 (lateral cord) |
| | | Medial pectoral | C-8, T-1 (medial cord) |
| | 6. Triceps (long head) | Radial | C-5, C-6, C-7, C-8, T-1 (posterior cord) |
| Horizontal adduction | 1. Pectoralis major | Lateral pectoral | C-5, C-6 (lateral cord) |
| | 2. Deltoid (anterior fibers) | Circumflex (axillary) | C-5, C-6 (posterior cord) |
| Horizontal abduction | 1. Deltoid (posterior fibers) | Circumflex (axillary) | C-5, C-6 (posterior cord) |
| | 2. Teres major | Subscapular | C-5, C-6 (posterior cord) |
| | 3. Teres minor | Circumflex (axillary) | C-5, C-6 (brachial plexus trunk) |
| | 4. Infraspinatus | Suprascapular | C-5, C-6 (brachial plexus trunk) |
| Abduction | 1. Deltoid | Circumflex (axillary) | C-5, C-6 (posterior cord) |
| | 2. Supraspinatus | Suprascapular | C-5, C-6 (brachial plexus trunk) |
| | 3. Infraspinatus | Suprascapular | C-5, C-6 (brachial plexus trunk) |
| | 4. Subscapularis | Subscapular | C-5, C-6 (posterior cord) |
| | 5. Teres minor | Circumflex (axillary) | C-5, C-6 (posterior cord) |
| | 6. Long head of biceps (if arm externally rotated first, trick movement) | Musculocutaneous | C-5, C-6, C-7 (lateral cord) |
| Adduction | 1. Pectoralis major | Lateral pectoral | C-5, C-6 (lateral cord) |
| | 2. Latissimus dorsi | Thoracodorsal | C-6, C-7, C-8 (posterior cord) |
| | 3. Teres major | Subscapular | C-5, C-6 (posterior cord) |
| | 4. Subscapularis | Subscapular | C-5, C-6 (posterior cord) |
| Medial rotation | 1. Pectoralis major | Lateral pectoral | C-5, C-6 (lateral cord) |
| | 2. Deltoid (anterior fibers) | Circumflex (axillary) | C-5, C-6 (posterior cord) |
| | 3. Latissimus dorsi | Thoracodorsal | C-6, C-7, C-8 (posterior cord) |
| | 4. Teres major | Subscapular | C-5, C-6 (posterior cord) |
| | 5. Subscapularis (when arm is by side) | Subscapular | C-5, C-6 (posterior cord) |
| Lateral rotation | 1. Infraspinatus | Suprascapular | C-5, C-6 (brachial plexus trunk) |
| | 2. Deltoid (posterior fibers) | Circumflex (axillary) | C-5, C-6 (posterior cord) |
| | 3. Teres minor | Circumflex (axillary) | C-5, C-6 (posterior cord) |
| Elevation of scapula | 1. Trapezius (upper fibers) | Accessory C-3, C-4 nerve roots | Cranial nerve XI |
| | 2. Levator scapulae | C-3, C-4 nerve roots Dorsal scapular | C-3, C-4 C-5 |
| | 3. Rhomboid major | Dorsal scapular | (C-4), C-5 |
| | 4. Rhomboid minor | Dorsal scapular | (C-4), C-5 |
| Depression of scapula | 1. Serratus anterior | Long thoracic | C-5, C-6, (C-7) |
| | 2. Pectoralis major | Lateral pectoral | C-5, C-6 (lateral cord) |
| | 3. Pectoralis minor | Medial pectoral | C-8, T-1 (medial cord) |
| | 4. Latissimus dorsi | Thoracodorsal | C-6, C-7, C-8 (posterior cord) |
| | 5. Trapezius (lower fibers) | Accessory C-3, C-4 nerve roots | Cranial nerve XI C-3, C-4 |
| Protraction (forward movement) of scapula | 1. Serratus anterior | Long thoracic | C-5, C-6 (C-7) |
| | 2. Pectoralis major | Lateral pectoral | C-5, C-6 (lateral cord) |
| | 3. Pectoralis minor | Medial pectoral | C-8, T-1 (medial cord) |
| | 4. Latissimus dorsi | Thoracodorsal | C-6, C-7, C-8 (posterior cord) |
| Retraction (backward movement) of scapula | 1. Trapezius | Accessory | Cranial nerve XI |
| | 2. Rhomboid major | Dorsal scapular | (C-4), C-5 |
| | 3. Rhomboid minor | Dorsal scapular | (C-4), C-5 |

*Table continued on following page*

■■■■■■ **Table 4-1.** MUSCLES ABOUT THE SHOULDER: THEIR ACTIONS AND NERVE SUPPLY (INCLUDING NERVE ROOT DERIVATION) *Continued*

| Action | Muscles Performing Action | Nerve Supply | Nerve Root Derivation |
|---|---|---|---|
| Lateral (upward) rotation of inferior angle of scapula | 1. Trapezius (upper and lower fibers) | Accessory<br>C-3, C-4 nerve roots | Cranial nerve XI<br>C-3, C-4 |
| | 2. Serratus anterior | Long thoracic | C-5, C-6, (C-7) |
| Medial (downward) rotation of inferior angle of scapula | 1. Levator scapulae | C-3, C-4 nerve roots<br>Dorsal scapular | C-3, C-4<br>C-5 |
| | 2. Rhomboid major | Dorsal scapular | (C-4), C-5 |
| | 3. Rhomboid minor | Dorsal scapular | (C-4), C-5 |
| | 4. Pectoralis minor | Medial pectoral | C-8, T-1 (medial cord) |
| Flexion of elbow | 1. Brachialis | Musculocutaneous | C-5, C-6, (C-7) |
| | 2. Biceps brachii | Musculocutaneous | C-5, C-6 |
| | 3. Brachioradialis | Radial | C-5, C-6, (C-7) |
| | 4. Pronator teres | Median | C-6, C-7 |
| | 5. Flexor carpi ulnaris | Ulnar | C-7, C-8 |
| Extension of elbow | 1. Triceps | Radial | C-6, C-7, C-8 |
| | 2. Anconeus | Radial | C-7, C-8, (T-1) |

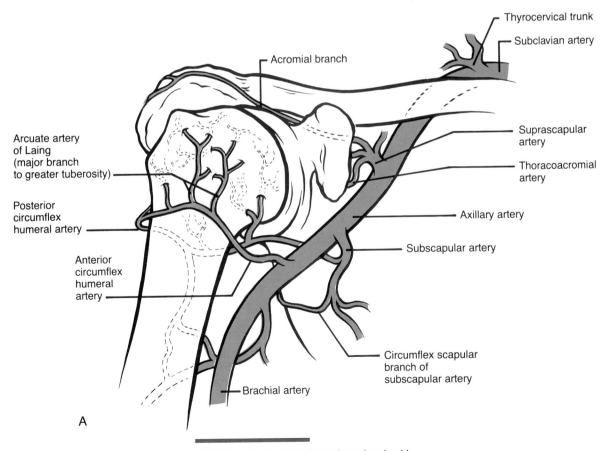

**FIGURE 4-13** ■ Arterial supply to the shoulder.

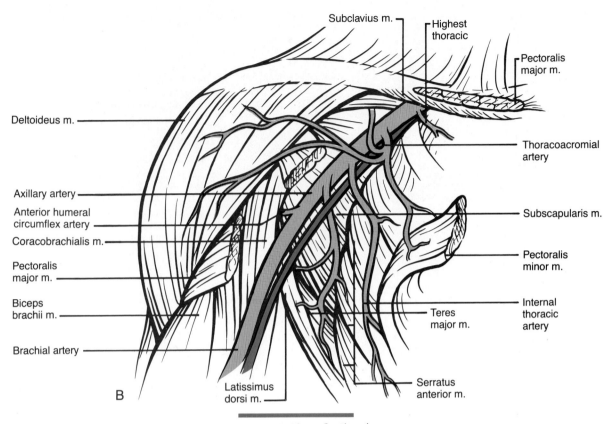

Subclavius m.
Highest thoracic
Pectoralis major m.
Deltoideus m.
Thoracoacromial artery
Axillary artery
Anterior humeral circumflex artery
Subscapularis m.
Coracobrachialis m.
Pectoralis major m.
Pectoralis minor m.
Biceps brachii m.
Internal thoracic artery
Teres major m.
Brachial artery
B
Latissimus dorsi m.
Serratus anterior m.

**FIGURE 4–13** ■ *Continued*

tension in the sagittal plane, and adduction, the action of bringing the humerus closer to the side of the body (see Fig. 4–7). Horizontal or transverse plane motion is usually measured from a

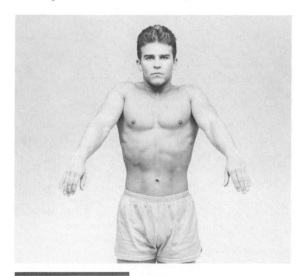

**FIGURE 4–14** ■ Forward flexion of the arm in the scapular plane.

starting position of 90 degrees of humeral abduction and is called horizontal flexion or adduction as the arm is drawn across the body, and horizontal extension or abduction as the arm crossed over the body is brought out to the side (Fig. 4–15).

The three types of surface motion (arthrokinematic motions) at the glenohumeral joint are rolling, gliding, and rotation. Rolling occurs when various points on a moving surface break contact with various points on a stationary surface. In gliding, one point on a moving surface makes contact with multiple points on a stationary surface. Both of these motions produce a significant change in the contact area between the joint surfaces. Rotation occurs when one or more points on a moving surface make contact with one point on the stationary surface (Fig. 4–16). All three of the surface motions occur at the glenohumeral joint, but not in equal proportion. In 1976, Poppen and Walker[14] studied the instant centers of rotation of the glenohumeral joint during scapular plane elevation of normal and abnormal subjects. The results suggested that the normal, primary surface joint motion is rotation

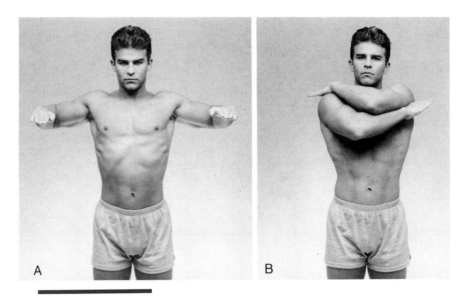

**FIGURE 4-15** ■ Range of motion of the arm. (A) Abduction. (B) Horizontal adduction.

at the glenohumeral joint and that significantly greater excursion in either rolling or gliding occurs in the presence of shoulder injury. This indicates a need to evaluate the arthrokinematics at the glenohumeral joint and establish the normal rotatory surface motions.

Saha's theory of shoulder rotation describes posterior gliding of the humeral head with internal rotation and anterior gliding with external rotation.[15] Kummel demonstrated that the anterior capsule must be extensible for external rotation to occur.[16] Thus, manual mobilization techniques glide the humeral head to stretch the opposing soft tissue and permit it to glide anteriorly and posteriorly.

Because full shoulder function requires synchronous movements from the sternoclavicular, acromioclavicular, and scapulothoracic joints in addition to the glenohumeral joint, their motions (previously described in the section on arthrology) should be reviewed in preparation for the comprehensive shoulder complex evaluation.

## Scapulohumeral Rhythm

Interaction of the joints that permits elevation of the hand overhead is complex and variable. It has been described as scapulohumeral rhythm. In the first 30 degrees of humeral abduction, the scapula moves only slightly compared to the humerus. As abduction proceeds, the scapula rotates laterally and the sternoclavicular joint elevates, causing motion at the acromioclavicular joint. Rotation of the acromioclavicular joint

occurs around the longitudinal axis of the clavicle as the coracoclavicular ligaments pull on the clavicle's inferior aspect. The humerus must also rotate laterally before 90 degrees to prevent the

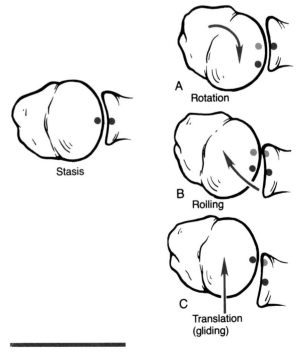

**FIGURE 4-16** ■ Surface motion at the glenohumeral joint. (A) Rotation. (B) Rolling. (C) Translation or gliding. (Redrawn from Nordin M, Frankel VH: Basic Biomechanics of the Musculoskeletal System, 2nd ed. Philadelphia: Lea & Febiger, 1989, Figure 12-7.)

greater tuberosity of the humerus from imping-ing on the inferior portion of the acromion pro-cess. Many authors have attempted to describe a ratio of humeral to scapular motion during hu-meral or upper extremity elevation.[6,14,17-20] Dif-ferences in ratios may be due to variation in measurement technique, plane of arm elevation measured, and anatomic variations among indi-viduals. "In general, most would concede that the range of scapular motion does not exceed 60 degrees, while that of the glenohumeral joint does not exceed 120 degrees."[12]

## Kinetics

The study of kinetics deals with forces that produce, arrest, or modify motions of bodies.[4] The orthopaedic physical therapist is concerned with the forces exerted by gravity, muscles, fric-tion, and external resistance. Application of these forces leads to joint compression and distraction as well as pressure on soft tissues. When one understands how and to what degree these forces act on the shoulder, manipulation of these forces to restore function is possible.

Forces are vector quantities with magnitude and direction. Analysis of forces at the shoulder joint is difficult for three reasons:

■ Muscles acting on the humerus must act simultaneously with other muscles to avoid a dislocating force, a factor of inherent instabil-ity.
■ A single muscle may span and affect several joints simultaneously. The latissimus dorsi originates on the chest wall and inserts on the humerus, thus spanning the scapulothoracic, acromioclavicular, and glenohumeral joints.
■ The position of the arm alters muscle function as it causes the available range of motion to vary.[21]

The joint reaction force at the glenohumeral joint has been demonstrated by Poppen and Walker[22] to equal 90% of body weight at 90 degrees of abduction. Maximum shear force across the glenohumeral joint occurred at 60 de-grees of abduction.

When studying shoulder muscle function dur-ing movement, origin and insertion cannot be used to determine muscle action. Muscle actions are often coupled with active and passive stabi-lizing forces. Many of the muscles acting across the shoulder are short and attach to the upper end of the humerus, which limits leverage. Movement of the scapulae increases the force of

arm movements and, by tilting the glenoid cavity in the desired direction, increases the range of motion of the upper extremity.

For instance, as the arm is abducted, the del-toid and supraspinatus are the prime movers at the shoulder joint. This abduction is accompa-nied by an upward rotation of the glenoid cavity brought about by the combined action of the serratus anterior and the upper and lower trape-zius. If unopposed, the translatory component of the deltoid and supraspinatus forces would make the humeral head move into the coracoacromial arch and impinge on the subacromial structures (Fig. 4-17). The rotator cuff muscles (infraspina-tus, teres minor, subscapularis) act during abduc-tion to compress the humeral head into the glenoid fossa. In addition, to accomplish full ab-duction the humerus must rotate externally, an action involving the infraspinatus and teres minor.

The upper portion of the trapezius muscle is the primary elevator of the shoulder girdle. However, the levator muscles of the scapula and the rhomboids are capable of producing eleva-tion if the trapezius is weakened or paralyzed. Depression of the shoulder girdle occurs without direct muscle pull as the tension in the elevators is released. If additional shoulder girdle depres-sion is necessary, as in crutch walking or pushing up from a chair, the lower trapezius and latissi-mus dorsi act together with the pectoralis major to accomplish these tasks.

Protraction and retraction can be described as the forward and backward movement of the scapula on the rib cage. Protraction occurs as the serratus anterior at the scapula and the pectoralis major on the humerus contract simultaneously. Retraction is a combined action of the trapezius and rhomboids. The upward and downward ro-tary actions counteract one another. The tend-ency for the upper trapezius and rhomboids to elevate the scapula is checked by the depressor action of the lower trapezius and the weight of the arm.

To implement the first 90 degrees of shoulder flexion, the anterior and middle deltoid muscles act together with the supraspinatus, pectoralis major, coracobrachialis, and both heads of the biceps. The actions of all muscles except the del-toid cease to function after 90 degrees. The rota-tor cuff muscles serve a similar synergistic force couple action during this motion.

Muscles involved in adduction and extension of the shoulder are similar but vary in propor-tion. The adductor and extensors of the shoulder are the latissimus dorsi, pectoralis major (axiohu-meral), teres major, posterior deltoid, and long

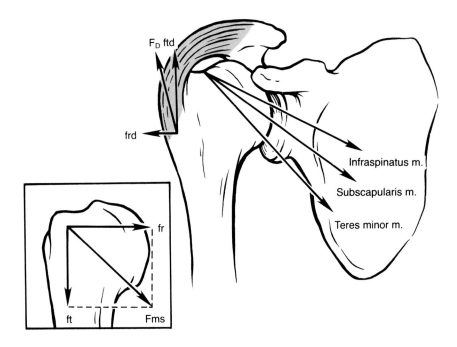

**FIGURE 4-17** ■ Force couple of the rotator cuff and the deltoid.

head of the triceps. The latissimus and the pectoral muscles are firmly fixed on the trunk, and the teres major requires synergistic action of the rhomboids to stabilize the scapula. The scapula would rotate without the action of these muscles. When extension continues past midline into hyperextension, the action of the pectoralis declines and that of the posterior deltoid increases.

The muscles responsible for isolated external rotation of the humerus are the infraspinatus and teres minor. The subscapularis, teres major, latissimus dorsi, and pectoralis major contribute to isolated internal rotation.

## Pathomechanics

Because of the extensive mobility, lack of stability, and high function of the shoulder complex, it is frequently dysfunctional and commonly treated by the orthopaedic physical therapist. Shoulder rehabilitation restores normal kinematics and kinetics to this complex. Therefore, knowledge of the normal state is essential to developing an effective treatment protocol for shoulder dysfunction.

Several static factors contribute to the stability of the glenohumeral joint:

■ Adequate size of the glenoid fossa. The longitudinal diameter of the fossa must be more than 75% of the longitudinal diameter of the humeral head.

■ Posterior tilt of the glenoid fossa
■ Humeral head retroversion
■ Intact capsule and glenoid labrum[23]

Equilibrium factors act to create dynamic stability:

■ Force of the prime movers
■ Force of gravity
■ Force of the compressors (rotator cuff) and stabilizers (synergists)
■ Equal and opposite forces of friction and joint reaction force.[6] Any disruption of dynamic stability alters the center of rotation of the humeral head and causes excessive excursion of the head in the glenoid fossa.

In some patients the kinematics of the joint may appear normal in that full motion is available but the strength of the motion and arthrokinematics are not. This occurs when the serratus anterior is not functioning normally, allowing the trapezius to rotate the scapula upward so that full abduction is still possible but is weakened. In flexion, if the trapezius is weak, the serratus can produce full but weakened motion.[4]

## EVALUATION

Data obtained in examining the patient guide clinical problem solving, a main objective of the evaluation process. It should be a continuous process independent of specific treatment philosophies. Rothstein and Echternach developed a generic model for evaluations, the hypothesis-oriented algorithm for clinicians, outlined in Figure 4–18.[24] This section presents and analyzes the subjective and objective examination of the patient with shoulder dysfunction.

## Subjective Evalution

The history taken by the therapist is extremely important because it determines the direction of the objective examination. A description of the patient's initial and current symptoms helps the examiner to understand the nature of the complaint and the severity of the condition. Valuable information can be ascertained about the onset and sequential behavior of the symptoms. A sudden onset suggests a need to identify the mechanism of injury. If the onset is more gradual, the examiner must question the patient about previous and current activities, including type, frequency, duration, intensity, and skill level. In addition, environmental conditions, equipment used in sport or labor, level of conditioning, and symptoms elsewhere in the body must be investigated. The impact of posture on the symptoms is elucidated by questioning about the irritability of the condition in response to positions for sleeping, sitting, standing, and particular movements. Information about medications, inactivity, or other factors that increase or decrease the symptoms is also helpful in determining the appropriate level of aggressiveness to be used in the objective examination (see Shoulder Evaluations chart).

In this subjective section of the examination, the past history of shoulder problems or musculoskeletal dysfunction should be examined. Previous response to injury or surgery may explain the current symptoms. In addition, systemic sources of shoulder girdle area pain or paresthesia, such as diabetes mellitus, cardiac ischemia, or gallbladder, gastric, hepatic, and/or cervical spine problems must be ruled out.[25]

Remember that shoulder lesions are commonly perceived by the patient as arm pain, usually involving the C-5 dermatome. Many patients incorrectly perceive the upper trapezius region as the shoulder and the location of symptoms referred from the cervical spine.

Several conditions respond typically to rest and activity. Most tendonitis conditions are aggravated by movement and relieved by rest. Capsular tightness is commonly described as a painful limitation of movement into abduction

and external rotation. Acute bursitis may be painful at rest. Instability is often noted in specific positions, especially abduction and external rotation. It is important that the examiner understand the relationships between dysfunction and subjective information provided by the patient.

## Objective Evaluation

### Observation

With a thorough history and a good understanding of anatomy and biomechanics, the therapist can proceed to determine the patient's objective problems. The examination begins with observation of the total patient, including static and dynamic states. The examiner observes the patient's standing posture from anterior, posterior, and lateral perspectives. The position of the head, neck, and trunk is noted.

Upper thoracic kyphosis may limit the available range of motion of the upper extremity at the shoulder. It alters the resting position of the scapula and changes the starting position for sagittal plane movement of the glenohumeral joint (Fig. 4–19A and B).[26]

Shoulder girdle contour may be observed for any structural deformities. A subluxed or dislocated glenohumeral joint can be identified by a prominent acromion angled laterally, a depressed scapula, and a slightly abducted humerus (Fig. 4–20). Separation of the acromioclavicular joint is indicated by an abrupt stair-step appearance of the clavicle above the acromion (Fig. 4–21).[27] Protracted shoulders; winged scapulae (Fig. 4–22); or visible atrophy of the trapezius, deltoid, supraspinatus, or infraspinatus may be observed, indicating other pathologies (Fig. 4–23). These symptoms require more detailed analysis. The presence of surgical scars and their location, size, color, and closure should be recorded. By observing the patient during gait, the presence or absence of the normal rhythmic tandem motion of the arms can be evaluated.

### Joint Clearing

At this point, if the examiner suspects that the symptoms present in the shoulder region may be referred from another joint or the viscera, appropriate evaluation of that joint by the therapist or referral to another practitioner for systemic evaluation is appropriate. Several authors suggest upper quarter screening or clearing examinations in the presence of shoulder pathology.[28] These

## HYPOTHESIS-ORIENTED ALGORITHM FOR CLINICIANS

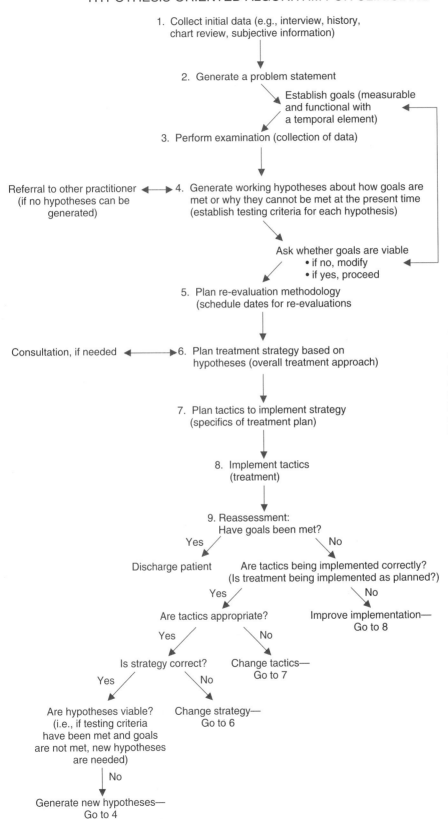

FIGURE    4–18 ■ Hypothesis-oriented algorithm for clinicians. (Modified from Rothstein JM, Echternach JL: Hypothesis-oriented algorithm for clinicians. Phys Ther 69:1388–1394, 1986.)

# SHOULDER EVALUATIONS

Date: _____

Name: _____    Age: _____

Doctor: _____    Diagnosis: _____

Occupation requirements: _____

_____

_____

Activities: _____

_____

_____

Date of injury: _____    Date of Surgery: _____

Type of surgery: _____

X-ray findings: _____

Medications: _____

_____

Allergies: _____

Past medical history: _____

_____

_____

Previous shoulder problems and treatment: _____

_____

_____

Specific Patient Problems: 1. _____
(pain, limitation of
motion, limits                      2. _____
of activity)
                                    3. _____

Sleeping Position: _____

Posture/Description (scars, etc.): _____

_____

_____

PASSIVE RANGE OF MOTION: (circle involved side)    Position: _____

|  | Left | Right |
|---|---|---|
| Flexion | | |
| Extension | | |
| Abduction | | |
| Adduction | | |
| Horizontal adduction | | |
| External rotation | | |
| Internal rotation | | |

| Joint mobility (glenohumeral) | Left | Right |
|---|---|---|
| Anterior glide | | |
| Posterior glide | | |
| Inferior glide | | |

| Joint mobility | Left | Right |
|---|---|---|
| (Scapulothoracic) | | |
| (Acromioclavicular) | | |
| (Sternoclavicular) | | |

ACTIVE RANGE OF MOTION:

|  | Left | | Right | |
|---|---|---|---|---|
|  | Sitting | Supine | Sitting | Supine |
| Flexion | | | | |
| Extension | | | | |
| Abduction | | | | |
| Adduction | | | | |
| Horizontal adduction | | | | |
| External rotation | | | | |
| Internal rotation | | | | |

| MANUAL MUSCLE TEST: | Left | Right | Pain |
|---|---|---|---|
| Biceps (C5–6) | | | |
| Musculocutaneous | | | |
| Triceps (C6–7) | | | |
| Radial | | | |
| Anterior deltoid (flex.) | | | |
| (C5–6) axillary | | | |
| Middle deltoid (abd.) | | | |
| (C5–6) axillary | | | |
| Posterior deltoid (ext.) | | | |
| (C5–6) axillary | | | |
| External rotation (C5–6) | | | |
| Suprascapular, axillary | | | |
| Internal rotation (C5–7) | | | |
| Pectoral, axillary | | | |
| Thoracodorsal, subscap- | | | |
| ular | | | |
| Middle trapezius | | | |
| (C3–4) accessory | | | |
| Upper trapezius | | | |
| (C3–4) accessory | | | |
| Lower trapezius | | | |
| (C3–4) accessory | | | |
| Rhomboids (C-5) | | | |
| Dorsal scapular | | | |
| Adduction (int. rot.) | | | |
| (C5–6) | | | |
| Horizontal adduction | | | |
| (C5–6) | | | |
| Serratus anterior | | | |
| (C5–7) long thoracic | | | |

Sensory tests (arm dermatomes, nerves): _____

_____

_____

Palpation: _____

_____

_____

Special Tests: _____

_____

_____

Problems: _____

_____

_____

Short-term goals: _____

_____

_____

Long-term goals: _____

_____

_____

Treatment plan: _____

_____

_____

_____

_____

Date to return to M.D.: _____

_____

Physical therapist's signature

---

clearing tests include cervical spine range of motion; sensory, reflex, and motor tests for the cervical nerve roots; vascular pulses and thoracic outlet screening tests; and peripheral joint motion and muscle testing. It is beyond the scope of this chapter to describe these tests in detail. Refer to Chapter 1 and the reference list for more information.

## Active Range of Motion

Active motion testing reveals the patient's willingness and ability to move the joint. It provides the examiner with information that can be used to assess the effectiveness or progression of treatment. Goniometric measurements are recorded with the patient sitting and supine for both the involved and uninvolved shoulders. The examiner observes substitution patterns, painful arcs, and specific muscle weakness. The motions tested include flexion; extension; abduction; adduction; horizontal abduction and adduction; internal and external rotation of the glenohumeral joint; elevation, depression, protraction, and retraction of the scapulothoracic articulation; and elevation of the limb in the scapular plane.

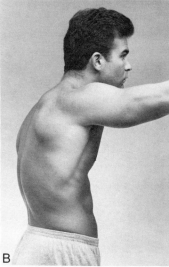

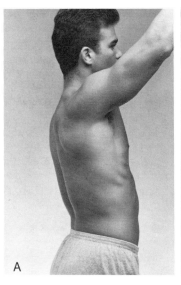

A     B

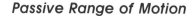

**FIGURE 4–19 ■** (A) Normal thoracic kyphosis and full shoulder flexion. (B) Increased kyphosis and reduced shoulder flexion.

Lack of motion or a painful arc of motion can be diagnostically significant. Kessel and Watson[29] reported that a painful arc may indicate a subacromial disorder because the 60 to 120 degree arc of motion in abduction is the phase in which the greater tuberosity and overlying structures clear the coracoacromial arch (Fig. 4–24). Excessive scapular elevation and rotation may occur in the presence of limited glenohumeral motion (Fig. 4–25). However, the cause of that restriction must be investigated.

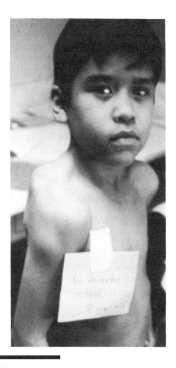

**FIGURE 4–20 ■** Subluxed glenohumeral joint. (From Rockwood CA, Green DP: Fractures, 2nd ed. Philadelphia: JB Lippincott, 1984.)

### Passive Range of Motion

Passive motion is divided into two types: physiologic and accessory. Physiologic movements include flexion, extension, and abduction. Accessory movements are the motions at the joint surface described in the section on kinematics. Accessory motions are not under voluntary control but are necessary for normal motion to occur in the shoulder complex.[30]

Assessment of physiologic passive motion provides information on joint flexibility without muscular influence. However, if passive motion is restricted in the direction opposite to the active restriction, there may be muscle or contractile tissue (tendon, tendoperiosteal) involvement. If the muscles about the shoulder are in spasm, the results of passive testing are limited. If active and passive motions are restricted in the same direction, noncontractile structures such as the joint capsule, bursa, ligaments, or neurovascular structures may be involved.[31] Goniometric measurements are recorded with the patient sitting and supine. Excessive motion may be available, suggesting instability.

Cyriax[32] emphasizes the importance of the "end feel" and pain resistance sequence in determining the nature and severity of the problem. Table 4–2 summarizes Cyriax's findings.

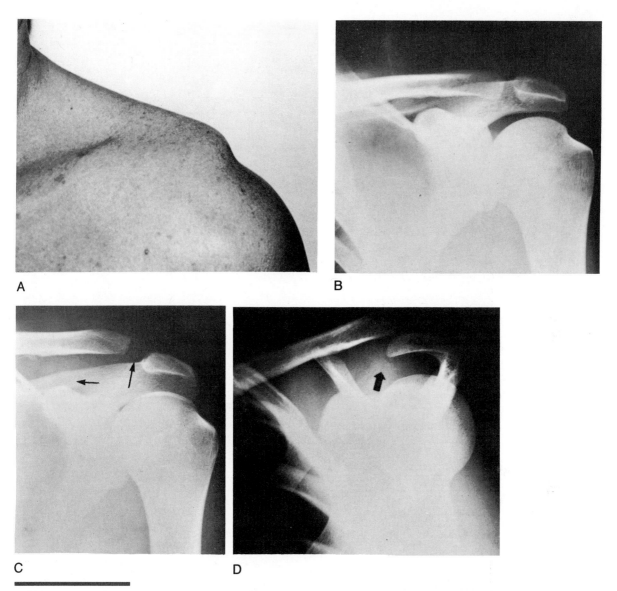

FIGURE 4-21 ■ (A) Acromioclavicular separation. (From Rockwood CA, Matsen FA: The Shoulder. Philadelphia: WB Saunders, 1990.) (B) Patient supine. (C) Patient standing with 4 pounds suspended from the wrist. (D) Lateral view of the acromioclavicular joint showing complete separation. (From O'Donoghue DH: Treatment of Injuries to Athletes, 4th ed. Philadelphia: WB Saunders, 1984.)

Accessory motion tests have been described by many authors[30,32-34] and are summarized in Table 4-3 along with their pathologic implications. It is beyond the scope of this chapter to describe these specific techniques. These tests determine the integrity of the ligaments and joint capsules. Their motions must be recorded as normal, hypomobile, or hypermobile and compared to those of the uninvolved limb.

## Palpation

The shoulder joint complex should be palpated for swelling, cutaneous temperature, sensation, pulses, crepitus, and point tenderness. The opposite shoulder may serve as a control for the examiner and introduce the patient to the process. The presence of crepitus about the shoulder joints is suggestive of irregular articular surfaces,

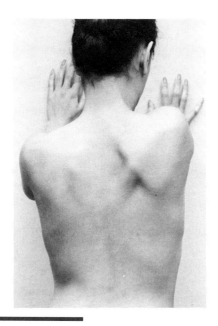

**FIGURE 4-22** ■ Winged scapula. (From Rockwood CA, Matsen FA: The Shoulder. Philadelphia: WB Saunders, 1990.)

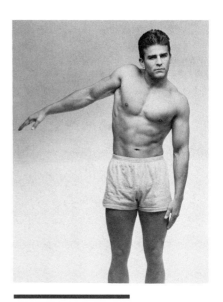

**FIGURE 4-24** ■ The "painful arc" range.

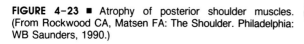

**FIGURE 4-23** ■ Atrophy of posterior shoulder muscles. (From Rockwood CA, Matsen FA: The Shoulder. Philadelphia: WB Saunders, 1990.)

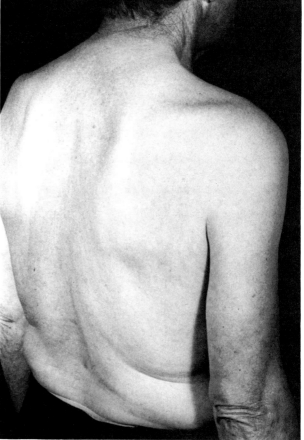

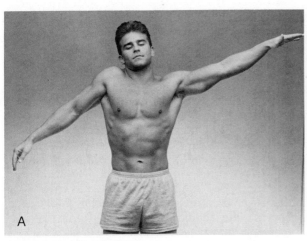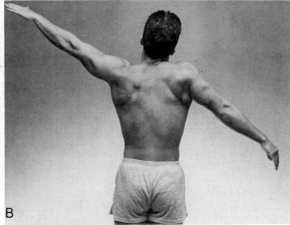

**FIGURE 4–25** ■ Excessive scapular elevation and rotation resulting from restricted glenohumeral motion. (A) Anterior. (B) Posterior.

**Table 4–2.** END FEEL

| End Feel | End-Range Sensation | Treatment Guidelines |
| --- | --- | --- |
| Tissue approximation | The limiting factor of joint movement feels "soft" and pressure at the initial end of range of motion easily yields more range | Probably easily rehabilitated and full movement restoration will be rapid |
| Capsular | There is a linear relationship between distance and resistance. The initial end of range of motion can be increased, but resistance is greater and the amount of range increase is smaller. | The capsule can be stretched over a period of time, dependent on how firm the capsular end feel is and the chronicity of symptoms |
| Bone-on-bone | An abrupt end feel occurs that does not yield more range from the initial end range when pressure is applied; unyielding | Small chance of increasing the present range of motion. Manipulation under anesthesia or surgical intervention most likely needed |
| Springy block | When end range is reached, there is a rebound felt. Intra-articular meniscal displacement is the usual cause. | Traction is the only alternative to allow the intra-articular block to move out of the path of movement |
| Spasm | A rapid abrupt stop of the movement with muscle tension apparent. Spasm end feel will many times vary the range. Avoidable with increases or decreases in speed of movement | Spasm is secondary to irritation. Check muscle unit and joint structures. Treat for inflammation |
| Empty | When moving through the range of motion, no resistance is felt regarding the joint surfaces, but at a point in the range the client will voluntarily contract the muscles and stop further movement: an abrupt, unexpected stop of movement | This end feel can indicate major problems in tissue around and serving the joint. It can also be of psychological origin. Usually the end range does not vary with speed of movement as it does with spasm end feel |

From Gould JA III, Davies GA: Orthopaedic and sports rehabilitation concepts. *In* Orthopaedic and Sports Physical Therapy, Vol. 2 (Gould JA III, Davies GA, eds). St. Louis: CV Mosby, 1985, Table 8–1.

tenosynovitis of the biceps tendon, or an in-flamed subacromial bursa according to Clancy.[35] Joint effusion and/or increased temperature may be suggestive of an active inflammatory response. Cutaneous sensation testing involves testing for the ability to distinguish light touch and pin prick in both the dermatomes of the upper quarter and areas supplied by the peripheral nerves (see Fig. 4–12). The circulation of the upper extremity can be palpated at the brachial artery just medial to the biceps, at the axillary artery in the axilla with firm pressure, and at the radial artery on the palmar surface of the distal radius. The criteria for circulation of the upper extremity are strength and speed of the palpable beat.

Palpation for point tenderness may be directed to the least suspected painful areas first to avoid irritating the structure and limiting the examination.

The rotator cuff tendons of the supraspinatus, infraspinatus, and teres minor insert on the greater tuberosity of the humerus. These tendons can be palpated by passively placing the hu-merus in internal rotation, extension, and horizontal adduction (Fig. 4–26). This position brings the insertion out from under the acromion. The subdeltoid bursa overlies this area and must be considered when differentiating the pain elicited through palpation. The subscapularis tendon insertion on the lesser tuberosity may be palpable with the humerus in extension and external rotation. The bicipital groove lies between the greater and lesser tuberosities and houses the biceps tendon. This tendon and its surrounding sheath are sensitive and require minimal pressure during palpation. The subacromial bursa lies inferior to the acromion, lateral to the bicipital groove, and beneath the deltoid. It is palpated with the hu-merus in passive extension. The muscles about the shoulder complex should be palpated for any abnormalities in gross structure or tenderness to pressure.

In addition, Travell and Simons describe trigger points in muscles that refer pain to the shoulder region in predictable patterns.[36] These muscles include but are not limited to the sca-lenus (Fig. 4–27), subclavius (Fig. 4–28), levator

---

**Table 4–3.** ASSESSMENT OF ACCESSORY MOVEMENTS OF THE SHOULDER JOINT AND THEIR PATHOLOGICAL IMPLICATIONS

| Accessory Movement | Implication |
|---|---|
| **Glenohumeral Joint** | |
| Lateral traction (movement of the head of the humerus away from the glenoid cavity) | Hypomobility of the shoulder joint |
| Posterior glide (posterior movement of the head of the humerus within the glenoid cavity) | Restricted flexion |
| Anterior glide (anterior movement of the head of the humerus within the glenoid cavity) | Restricted abduction and external rotation |
| Posterior shear (posterior movement of the head of the humerus with the arm in 90° of shoulder flexion) | Restricted flexion |
| Caudal glide (inferior movement of the head of the humerus within the glenoid cavity) | Hypomobility of the shoulder joint (results in a compromised subacromial space) |
| **Sternoclavicular Joint** | |
| Cranial glide | Restricted depression |
| Caudal glide | Restricted elevation |
| Ventral glide | Restricted protraction |
| Dorsal glide | Restricted retraction |
| **Acromioclavicular Joint** | |
| Cranial glide | Restricted abduction |
| Caudal glide | Restricted adduction |
| Ventral glide | Restricted flexion/abduction |
| Dorsal glide | Restricted extension/abduction |
| Combined cranioventral glide | Restricted external rotation |
| Combined caudodorsal glide | Restricted internal rotation |

From Halbach J, Tank R: The shoulder. *In* Orthopaedic and Sports Physical Therapy, Vol. 2 (Gould JA III, Davies GA, eds). St. Louis: CV Mosby, 1985, Table 21–1.

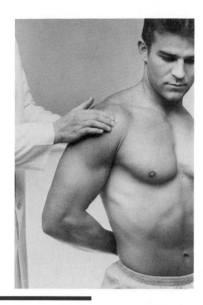

**FIGURE 4-26** ■ Palpation of the bursa and rotator cuff.

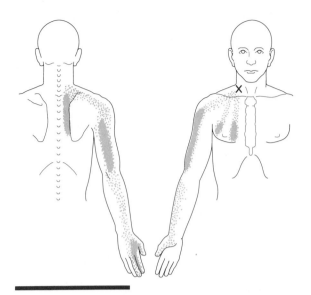

**FIGURE 4-27** ■ Trigger points of the scalene muscles. (From Travell FP, Simons DJ: Myofascial Pain and Dysfunction: The Trigger Point Manual. Baltimore: Williams & Wilkins,1983.)

scapulae (Fig. 4–29), subscapularis (Fig. 4–30), supraspinatus (Fig. 4–31), teres major and minor (Fig. 4–32), and latissimus dorsi (Fig. 4–33).

### Resisted Motions

Manual muscle tests for the shoulder girdle musculature are described by Kendall and McCreary[37] and Daniels and Worthingham.[38] To obtain objective, reliable data the results should be recorded for the specific positions in the reference texts, the grade given for the effort (normal to zero or five to zero) should be standardized, and the pain should be described on a 10-point scale. The resisted tests are also part of the neurologic evaluation because they test the motor branches of spinal nerves. If weakness is present, the deep tendon reflexes of the upper limb should be tested to add more information about the neurologic status of the region. These include the biceps, triceps, and brachioradialis reflexes (Fig. 4–34A–C).

## Special Tests

Several tests are available for further examination of a suspected lesion in the shoulder complex. Their inclusion in the examination depends on the findings in the preceding parts of the assessment. They are subsequently discussed in terms of the condition a positive test indicates and a negative test rules out.

### Bicipital Tendinitis

In 1931 Yergason described a test for bicipital tendinitis.[39] The test is positive when pain is elicited on the anteromedial portion of the shoulder as the examiner resists supination of the forearm with the patient's arm at the side and the elbow flexed 90 degrees (Fig. 4–35). Lippman's test displaces the tendon from side to side through palpation.[40] The examiner palpates the tendon in the bicipital groove with the patient standing with the arm at the side. A positive test is pain on palpation (Fig. 4–36). The reverse of this was described by de Anquin, who palpated the groove while rotating the humerus internally and externally (Fig. 4–37).[25] Ludington's test requires the patient to grasp his or her head and forcibly perform an isometric contraction into elbow flexion. Pain is positive[41] (Fig. 4–38). Hawkins and Kennedy describe the straight arm test in which pain may be elicited with resisted humeral flexion with an extended elbow (Fig. 4–39).[42] Because the biceps tendon is generally tender, the Yergason test and the straight arm test of Hawkins and Kennedy are favored.

### Transverse Humeral Ligament

The integrity of the humeral ligament across the bicipital groove is tested by a maneuver de-

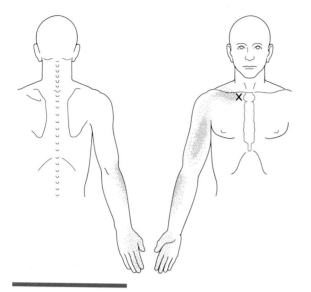

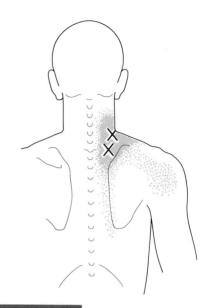

**FIGURE 4-28** ■ Trigger points of the subclavius muscle. (From Travell FP, Simons DJ: Myofascial Pain and Dysfunction: The Trigger Point Manual. Baltimore: Williams & Wilkins, 1983.)

**FIGURE 4-29** ■ Trigger points of the levator scapulae muscle. (From Travell FP, Simons DJ: Myofascial Pain and Dysfunction: The Trigger Point Manual. Baltimore: Williams & Wilkins, 1983.)

scribed by Booth and Marvel.[25] The patient's arm is abducted and rotated externally with the examiner's fingers placed along the bicipital groove. As the arm is rotated internally, a positive sign is the tendon snapping in and out of the groove (Fig. 4–40). Rupture of this ligament would create excessive movement of the biceps tendon and be a cause of inflammation.

### Rotator Cuff

Complete rupture of the supraspinatus, of the rotator cuff, is suspected when a drop arm test is positive. The patient is unable to lower the arm slowly and smoothly from a position of 90 degrees of passive abduction by the therapist. The patient's hand is held in a palm-down position. Pain and lack of motor control constitute a positive test (Fig. 4–41).

Rotator cuff impingement under the coracoacromial arch is tested in a number of different positions. Neer and Welsh's test consists of resisted forward flexion with the arm rotated internally. They suggest that this pain is relieved by injection of lidocaine (Xylocaine) under the acromion (Fig. 4–42).[43] Hawkins and Kennedy described a similar maneuver in forward flexion at 90 degrees with the examiner resisting internal rotation (Fig. 4–43).[42] Clancy feels the test is performed better by having the patient move into the flexed and internally rotated position from 90 degrees of abduction[35] Often, the patient may have described one of these positions of impingement in giving a subjective history. If straight plane manual muscle tests have not implicated the rotator cuff, these tests may be valuable.

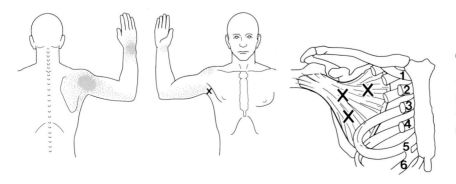

**FIGURE 4-30** ■ Trigger points of the subscapularis muscle. (From Travell FP, Simons DJ: Myofascial Pain and Dysfunction: The Trigger Point Manual. Baltimore: Williams & Wilkins, 1983.)

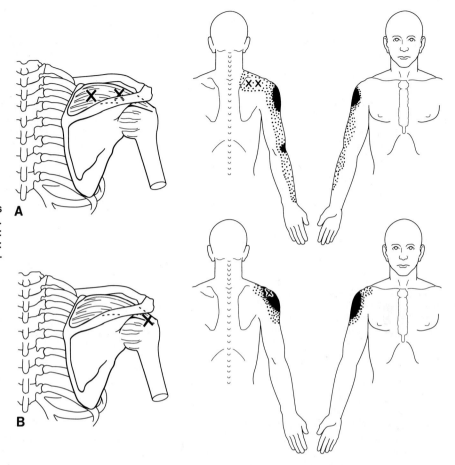

**FIGURE 4–31** ■ Trigger points of the supraspinatus muscle. (From Travell FP, Simons DJ: Myofascial Pain and Dysfunction: The Trigger Point Manual. Baltimore: Williams & Wilkins,1983.)

A

B

## Glenoid Labrum Tear

With the patient standing or supine, the examiner or patient takes the patient's arm into full abduction as the humeral head is forced anteriorly. The arm is externally rotated, potentially causing subluxation of the glenohumeral joint. The humeral head is then repositioned by adducting the arm horizontally. A "clunk" sensation may be suggestive of the humerus rolling over a labral tear (Fig. 4–44).[44] This is a common finding in patients who demonstrate excessive mobility at the glenohumeral joint and report vague shoulder symptoms.

## Glenohumeral Subluxation (Dislocation)

The test for anterior glenohumeral subluxation or potential dislocation is called the apprehension test because the patient's arm is placed in a posi-

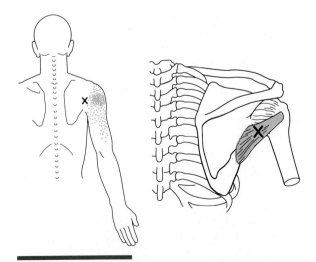

**FIGURE 4–32** ■ Trigger points of the teres major and minor muscles. (From Travell FP, Simons DJ: Myofascial Pain and Dysfunction: The Trigger Point Manual. Baltimore: Williams & Wilkins,1983.)

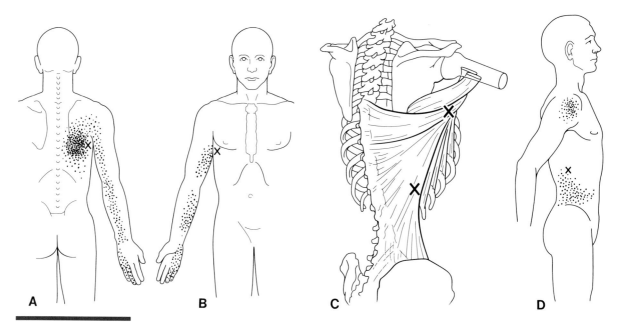

**FIGURE 4-33** ■ Trigger points of the latissimus dorsi muscle. (From Travell FP, Simons DJ: Myofascial Pain and Dysfunction: The Trigger Point Manual. Baltimore: Williams & Wilkins, 1983.)

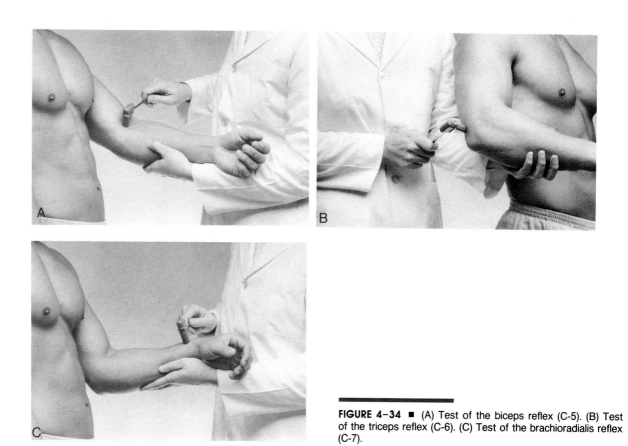

**FIGURE 4-34** ■ (A) Test of the biceps reflex (C-5). (B) Test of the triceps reflex (C-6). (C) Test of the brachioradialis reflex (C-7).

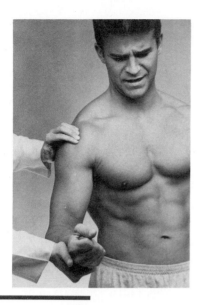

**FIGURE 4-35** ■ Yergason's test for biceps tendinitis.

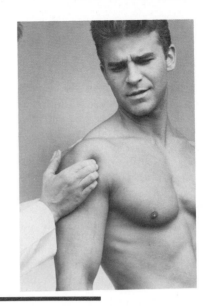

**FIGURE 4-36** ■ Lippman's test for biceps tendinitis.

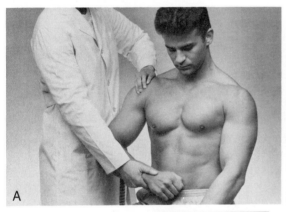

A

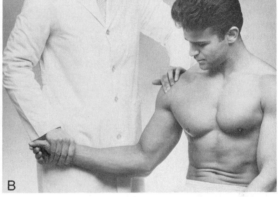

B

**FIGURE 4-37** ■ De Anquin's test for biceps tendinitis.

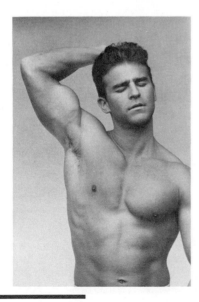

**FIGURE 4-38** ■ Ludington's test for biceps tendinitis.

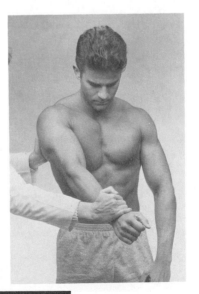

**FIGURE 4-39** ■ Hawkins and Kennedy's test for biceps tendinitis.

tion of abduction and external rotation, producing an apprehensive or fearful look as the patient anticipates subluxation (Fig. 4–45). Apprehension testing for posterior instability may also be done by placing the patient in a relaxed supine position while the examiner provides a posteriorly transmitted force to the humeral head with the arm in various angles of flexion and internal rotation (Fig. 4–46).[43]

## Thoracic Outlet

Testing for proximal compression of the subclavian artery, vein, and/or brachial plexus involves placing the patient in several positions that may provoke compression of these structures.

In 1927 Adson and Coffey described a test to evaluate the role of the anterior scalene muscle in compression of the subclavian artery as it passes between the scalene muscles.[45] Adson and Coffey stipulated hyperextension and rotation of the head toward the affected side with a deep breath hold. The examiner monitors the radial pulse of the affected extremity as it rests at the patient's side (Fig. 4–47). Obliteration or slowing of the pulse rate indicates a positive test.

A test to implicate the space between the first rib and clavicle as the site of neurovascular compression was described by Falconer and Weddell in 1943.[46] The patient is asked to retract and depress the shoulders from a relaxed position, often described as the exaggerated military posture. Again, the radial pulse is monitored for

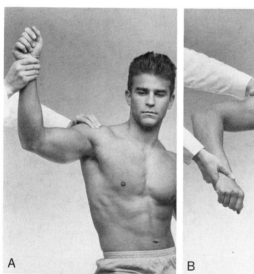
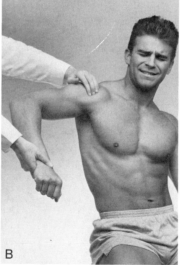

**FIGURE 4–40** ■ Booth and Marvel's test for integrity of the transverse humeral ligament.

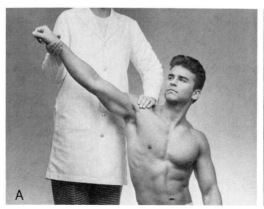
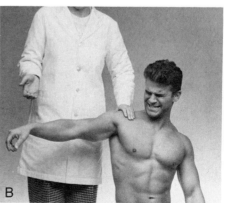

**FIGURE 4–41** ■ Drop arm test.

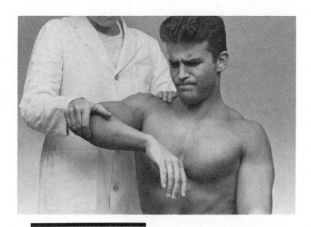

**FIGURE 4–42** ■ Impingement sign (Neer and Walsh).

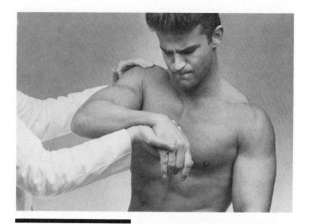

**FIGURE 4–43** ■ Impingement sign (Hawkins and Kennedy).

**FIGURE 4–44** ■ Clunk test/maneuver for glenoid labrum tear. (A) The upper extremity is internally rotated. (B) The glenoid head drops during internal rotation and can be palpated by the therapist.

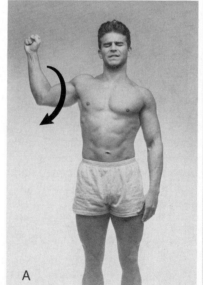

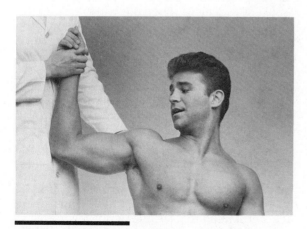

**FIGURE 4–45** ■ Apprehension sign for anterior-inferior subluxation or dislocation.

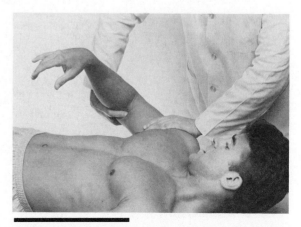

**FIGURE 4–46** ■ Apprehension sign for posterior instability of the glenohumeral joint.

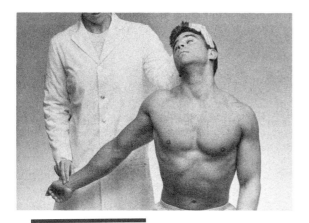

**FIGURE 4-47** ■ Adson maneuver for thoracic outlet.

obliteration (Fig. 4-48). Also, the onset of symptoms indicates a positive test.

A third test, described in 1945 by Wright, monitors pulse and symptom changes as the affected arm is moved into an abducted position, called the hyperabduction maneuver.[47] Between 0 and 90 degrees of abduction the subclavian vessels and plexus may be stretched around the coracoid process; above 90 degrees, the costoclavicular space narrows (Fig. 4-49).

The fourth provocative maneuver was initially described by Roos in 1982 and involves a 3-minute elevated arm test.[48] The patient sits or stands with arms abducted to 90 degrees and the elbows flexed to 90 degrees. The patient is asked to maintain this position for 3 full minutes while

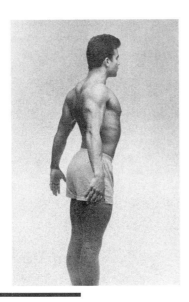

**FIGURE 4-48** ■ Military posture test for thoracic outlet.

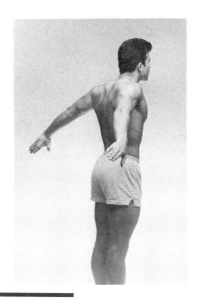

**FIGURE 4-49** ■ Hyperabduction maneuver test for thoracic outlet.

alternately opening and closing the hands to make fists. Inability to complete the 3-minute test and/or onset of symptoms constitutes a positive test (Fig. 4-50).

The therapist must be aware that a positive provocation test alone does not indicate the presence of thoracic outlet syndrome. Further documentation of blood flow or neurologic changes is necessary.

### Isokinetic Evaluation

Data from isokinetic testing at the shoulder are difficult to interpret because no true normative data have been established. Studies have used different testing devices, inconsistent methodology, and varied positions of the patients. The results of isokinetic tests are most helpful for bilateral comparison. However, this comparison does not account for differences in dominance. The various isokinetic devices allow testing of specific joint motions or diagonal patterns. Several reports on isokinetic testing of the shoulder have appeared.[49-57] Continued research is needed in this area as therapists strive for improved methods of objective documentation of progress.

### Functional Biomechanics

Studies of the individuals performing tasks or sports may provide valuable information about the contribution of technique to the development of shoulder pathology. Several authors

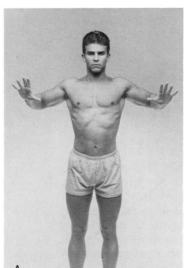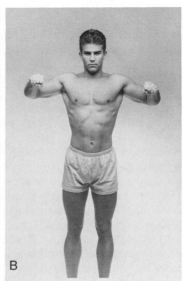

**FIGURE 4-50** ■ Three-minute elevated arm test for thoracic outlet.

have studied pathomechanics of overuse syndromes.[58-61]

## DIFFERENTIAL DIAGNOSIS

Many different pathologies affect the shoulder joint complex. In this section, common shoulder pathologies are defined and the etiologies or potential mechanisms of injury analyzed. In addition, clinical features of these disorders and descriptions of possible surgical interventions are presented. Understanding the possible pathologies and clinical presentations allows the examiner to take the subjective and objective data from the examination and categorize them to develop a treatment plan.

## Adhesive Capsulitis ("Frozen" Shoulder)

*Adhesive capsulitis* and *frozen shoulder* are two of the terms commonly used to describe a painful and stiff shoulder joint. Although this entity was described in the medical literature as early as 1872,[62] it was not until 1945 that Neviaser discovered the thickening and tightness of the joint capsule of adhesive capsulitis.[63] Before this, practitioners described the stiffness as being associated with other conditions such as tendinitis or bursitis.

Adhesive capsulitis is a chronic capsular inflammation with fibrosis of the capsule.[64] The etiology of the condition is unknown, but it is theorized that there are two types: primary idiopathic and secondary. Primary adhesive capsulitis is spontaneous; an unknown stimulus creates histologic changes in the joint capsule that are different from the changes caused by immobilization or aging.[65] In contrast, secondary adhesive capsulitis is always preceded by an episode of trauma or immobilization, voluntary or involuntary, as a result of pain or systemic disease (especially diabetes).[66-69] The incidence of adhesive capsulitis is higher among females and persons in the age range of 40 to 60. It develops more commonly in the nondominant arm.[70,71]

Clinical manifestations of primary and secondary adhesive capsulitis are the same. The patient describes an acute onset of pain that is not relieved by rest. Pain is usually the primary complaint during the first few weeks and can disturb sleep. As the condition proceeds, pain at rest subsides and restricted, painful movement becomes the primary complaint. The pain is usually diffuse over the deltoid and/or C-5 dermatome. Medical attention is usually sought because of the subsequent loss of motion and diminished function in activities of daily living (e.g., grooming, dressing).[72]

Objective examination findings vary with the stage or irritability of the condition. In the acute stage, the patient exhibits guarded motion and protective muscle spasm during range-of-motion testing (an empty end feel). Later, in the subacute stage, motion restriction with a capsular end feel predominates. As described by Cyriax,[31] a capsular pattern of restriction occurs; external rotation is more limited than abduction, which is more limited than internal rotation. In this pattern accessory motions are also limited, especially anterior and inferior glide of the glenohumeral joint. Disuse atrophy may be present; however, resisted motions are generally strong and pain free. Despite the presence of pain in the C-5 dermatome, neurologic tests are generally negative.

Adhesive capsulitis cannot be identified by x-ray examination, but radiographs of the shoulder are used to rule out other conditions. Arthrography can be used diagnostically because it can reveal shoulder volume reduction of as much as 50% and loss of the axillary recess, confirming a tight, thickened capsule.[65] Binder et al. noted that although this test is diagnostic, the arthrogram provides no information about the type of onset or extent of recovery.[73]

Surgical intervention in adhesive capsulitis is rare. Physical therapy is the treatment approach of choice. Although often lengthy, a slow progressive exercise program can reduce the symptoms of adhesive capsulitis without the trauma of a closed reduction manipulation. The exercise program is complemented by pain reduction modalities and a home exercise program. Occasionally, manipulation of the glenohumeral joint under general anaesthesia is performed. However, this procedure is controversial because of the trauma to tissues.[74,75]

## Bursitis

Bursitis of the shoulder girdle is a primary condition only in patients with rheumatoid arthritis, gout, and pyrogenic infections.[76] It appears that the intimate relationship between the subacromial and subdeltoid bursae and the rotator cuff tendons makes the bursa more susceptible to secondary shoulder injury, trauma, or overuse. Calcium salt (calcific tendinitis) extrudes from the tendon and irritates and eventually ruptures the bursa.[77] This causes the bursal inflammation in rotator cuff pathology.

The patient with an acutely inflamed bursa usually has a history of severe pain at rest, especially at night. Both active and passive ranges of motion are limited but passive motion is not limited in a capsular pattern. End feel is empty. In the early stages, palpation reveals severe tenderness and a spongy swelling. The acute pain may resolve within a few days, and subsequent treatment is sought if pain persists or motion remains limited.

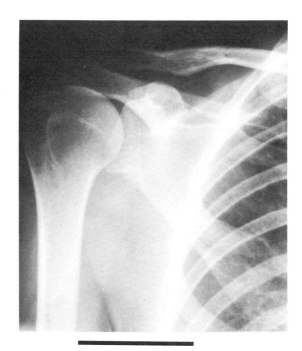

**FIGURE 4–51** ■ Calcific tendon.

Radiographs can reveal the calcium deposits in the tendon and also rule out other causes of the pain (Fig. 4–51). Surgical intervention is reserved for chronic cases with significant fibrosis and thickening. The subacromial space can be decompressed with removal of the bursa through arthroscopy. The technique is discussed in the next section. Physical therapy protocols are designed to reduce pain and inflammation, increase motion, and restore the patient to full activities of daily living.

## Rotator Cuff Pathology

### Tendinitis or Impingement Syndrome

Tendons of the rotator cuff are subject to inflammation as a result of direct blows, excessive tensile forces, or repetitive microtrauma.[78] Activities requiring repetitive or sustained use of the arms overhead often predispose the rotator cuff tendons to injury. There are two reasons for this biomechanical trauma: (1) mechanical impingement of the subacromial structures against the anterior acromion and coracoacromial ligament when the arm is lifted overhead, especially in abduction and flexion with the arm internally rotated, and (2) hypovascularity of the rotator cuff tendons in this region. As the inflamed tendons are continually subjected to impingement, metabolism is altered and the tendons' consistency is changed by scarring and swelling. This further limits the size of the coracoacromial arch and contributes to the impingement cycle. The bursa and other tendons (i.e., long head of the biceps) may also become inflamed. The shape of the acromion or osteophyte formation on the acromion can also contribute to the impingement by limiting the subacromial space. A fall on an outstretched arm can cause the force to be transmitted through the humeral head in a rapid abduction movement. This mode of trauma can disrupt the rotator cuff.

Neer describes three progressive stages of impingement syndrome.[79] The first stage is characterized by edema and hemorrhage and the patient describes a dull ache of the shoulder after activity. The pain may progress and occur during activity. As this stage progresses, pain may occur after activity and interfere with activities of daily living. Physical examination reveals a painful arc of active abduction, pain-free passive range of motion, strong but painful resisted abduction (supraspinatus) and/or external rotation (infraspinatus, teres minor), and tenderness to palpation over the greater tuberosity and anterior edge of the acromion process. Jobe and Moynes suggest the ability to isolate the supraspinatus in the "empty can" position (Fig. 4–52).[80] Painful active or resisted motions incriminate the tendon. Special tests for impingement (see Figs. 4–42 and 4–45) are also positive at this stage. The physician can inject lidocaine into the subacro-

mial space to differentiate impingement from other shoulder pathology.[43]

Chronic inflammation or repeated overuse in the impingement position (flexion, internal rotation) can lead to the second stage, in which fibrosis and thickening of the tendons and bursa occur. The signs and symptoms of the first stage increase in intensity and there is more limitation of passive range of motion. The limitation incriminates the noncontractile bursa according to Cyriax.[31] According to Hawkins and Kennedy,[42] there may also be a catching sensation with the reversal of elevation or extension. Scar tissue entrapment beneath the acromion may cause the catching sensation.

Patients with a long history of refractory tendinitis may have significant tendon degeneration. The physical findings in this third stage of impingement include visible atrophy of the supraspinatus, infraspinatus, and deltoideus; greater active than passive rotation limitations; weak abduction and external rotation; and a positive drop arm test.

Radiographs in the early stages of impingement or rotator cuff tendinitis are negative. In the later stages, cystic changes at the greater tuberosity, sclerotic changes or osteophyte formation on the underside of the acromion, or acromioclavicular joint changes may be visible.[81]

Conservative management involves physical therapy to evaluate accessory motion, weakness of the rotator cuff, and supporting musculature and inflammation. Modalities to control pain and inflammation are necessary in the acute stages, with progression to an exercise program to restore normal function of the shoulder joint complex.

Surgical intervention is reserved for cases of impingement in which conservative measures have failed. Surgical decompression of the subacromial space alleviates the pain of impingement. Procedures include one or more of the following: coracoacromial ligament resection, anterior acromioplasty, distal clavicle resection, and acromioclavicular joint inferior osteophyte resection.[81] These surgeries may be performed as open or arthroscopic procedures.[82-84]

## Rotator Cuff Tears

Impingement may cause tendon degeneration and progression to a complete tear, referred to as an attritional or degenerative tear. An acute injury such as a fall on an outstretched arm or an abduction movement of high force and velocity can also tear the rotator cuff.

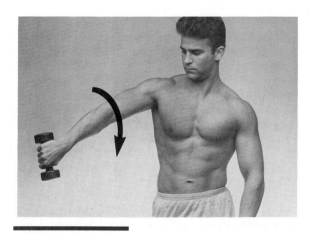

FIGURE 4–52 ■ "Empty can" position as described by Jobe.

Clinically, the patient presents with a significant limitation of active motion, particularly abduction. The glenohumeral rhythm is altered extensively. The drop arm test may be positive. Passive motion is not significantly limited unless the condition is chronic or extremely painful. Weakness in abduction and external rotation is also evident in most patients.

Radiographs of the shoulder may be negative; however, arthrography and magnetic resonance imaging can confirm the diagnosis of rotator cuff defect.

Surgical exposure of the region best reveals the extent of defect. Rotator cuff tears may be classified as full-thickness tears (entire vertical thickness), pure transverse ruptures, pure vertical rents or longitudinal splits paralleling the direction of the cuff fibers, tears with retraction, and massive avulsions. To visualize the tear, the deltoid is detached and the subacromial bursa removed. Occasionally, the tear may be repaired with tendon-to-tendon sutures. More commonly, the cuff is avulsed from the greater tuberosity and drill holes are placed in it to reapproximate the cuff.

Physical therapy is common postoperatively. A period of immobilization follows the surgical procedure. The time varies depending on the surgeon's preference. Gradual passive to active mobilization follows with strengthening and function at the end of the rehabilitation process.

## Biceps Tendon Pathology

### Tendinitis

The biceps tendon has two heads: the long head originates from the glenoid labrum at its superior aspect, arches over the head of the humerus, and descends into the bicipital groove; the short head arises from the coracoid process and joins the belly of the biceps muscle above the elbow joint (Fig. 4–53). The long head is a common site of tendinitis because of its intraarticular placement and its enclosure in a sheath of synovium.[78] Tendinitis causes inflammation by tissue changes similar to those of the rotator cuff impingement. In addition, the biceps is a stabilizer and decelerator in the throwing motion.[85]

Subjectively, the patient complains of shoulder and arm pain. The stage of the injury determines the symptoms and clinical signs. Blazina and coworkers described a system of categorizing tendinitis ranging from early or mild changes to severe ones[86] (Fig. 4–54). A painful arc with active motion is present. Passive motion may be pain free unless other noncontractile tissue such as the bursa is involved. Tendinitis is differentiated from rotator cuff pathology by palpation of the bicipital groove. In tendinitis the bicipital groove is more tender than the greater tuberosity or supraspinatus tendon. Tests described for bicipital tendinitis can be used for further isolating the bicipital tendon (see Figs. 4–35 through 4–39). Radiographs are not diagnostic for this condition but can reveal other causes of the pain. Arthroscopic examination can be used to determine the grade of tendinitis and to decompress the coracoacromial arch if impingement is present. If the biceps tendon is severely attenuated, tenodesis (surgical fixation) may be necessary.[87,88]

The role of the physical therapist is to control the pain and inflammation, examine and correct biomechanical faults, and restore strength and function to maximal capacity.

### Biceps Tendon Ruptures

The long head of the biceps can rupture in traumatic injuries.[89] Athletes most commonly experience an avulsion of the long head of the biceps from the glenoid labrum. In gymnastics and throwing sports the rupture occurs as the biceps head contracts violently, usually eccentrically. In the older individual, chronic impingement can also rupture the tendon. Surgical repair is usually the treatment of choice. An arthrotomy of the shoulder is conducted, and sufficient healing time must be allowed before stressing the structure with exercise.

### Subluxation of the Biceps Long Head

The long head of the biceps is maintained in the bicipital groove on the humerus by the transverse humeral ligament. Overloading the arm in abduction and external rotation may cause this ligament to rupture, resulting in subluxation of the biceps tendon. In cases in which an injury has not occurred, the shape of the groove may predispose the patient to develop this condition. The test for subluxation is described under Glenohumeral Subluxation (Dislocation) (see Fig. 4–40). In these cases, the patient presenting with anterior shoulder pain frequently complains of a snapping sensation when the arm is moved rapidly from internal to external rotation. Crepitus may be noted. A surgical procedure described by Odonohue consists of tenode-

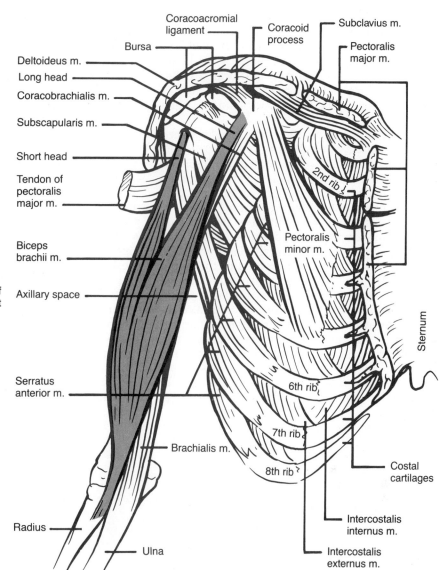

**FIGURE 4–53** ■ Origin of biceps tendon, long and short heads.

### TENDINITIS STAGING

**0**= No pain

**1**= Pain occurs only after participation in sports or physical activity

**2**= Pain appears when beginning activity, disappears after warming up, but reappears after the activity is completed

**3**= Pain occurs during and after the activity and is severe enough to prevent participation

**4**= Pain is constant and limits the activities of daily living

**FIGURE 4–54** ■ Blazina staging of tendinitis. (Data from Blazina ME, Kerlan RK, Jobe FW, et al: Jumper's knee. Orthop Clin North Am 4:665–678, 1973.)

sis of the origin and suturing of the tendon into the groove.[90]

If conservative management is attempted, the therapist must counsel the patient about activities that could cause subluxation of the biceps tendon, for example, throwing.

## Glenohumeral Joint Pathology

### Dislocation

The relative absence of bone stability and the large, redundant capsule render the glenohumeral joint particularly susceptible to dislocation.[91] In complete dislocations, the head of the humerus actually passes through the capsular restraint and rests beside the glenoid (Fig. 4–55). The majority (95%) of dislocations occur in an anterior-inferior direction and are located either under the coracoid process (subcoracoid) or under the anterior aspect of the glenoid (subglenoid).[92]

The mechanism of this injury is usually forced external rotation when the arm is abducted. The greater tuberosity is levered against the acromion process and the coracoacromial ligament, tearing the inferior glenohumeral ligament, anterior capsule, and possibly the glenoid labrum.[92] Immediate recognition of this condition is possible because of the characteristic position of the arm, with a prominent acromion, displaced humeral head, and sharp contour compared to the opposite limb. Before reduction, a neurovascular examination is done to identify brachial plexus and/or axillary artery involvement. Several techniques are available for relocating the joint, including the Hippocrates, Kocher, Stimson, and Milch techniques.[93] Radiographs are typically obtained before and after reduction to assess the potential complications of fracture of the anterior glenoid rim, Hill-Sachs compression fracture of

the posterior humeral head, and fracture of the greater tuberosity.[94] Another lesion associated with acute dislocation is the Bankart lesion, which is an avulsion of the anterior capsule and labrum resulting from the glenoid and rotator cuff tear.

The orthopedic literature reflects large variation in the management of initial glenohumeral dislocations. The duration of strict immobilization after reduction varies from a few days to 8 weeks.[95–98] This variation may account for the high recurrence rate of dislocation or subluxation (50 to 60%). Age is also a factor: 80% of those under age 20 but only 15% of those over age 50 have recurrences.[99]

Surgery is rarely the treatment of choice after initial dislocation. Therefore, it is discussed in the next section.

Posterior dislocations of the glenohumeral joint are more rare. The mechanism of injury is most commonly a position of forced adduction with internal rotation in some degree of elevation. Immobilization followed by rehabilitation is the treatment of choice for initial dislocations in this direction.[100]

Rehabilitation after initial dislocation, either anterior or posterior, involves muscular re-educa-

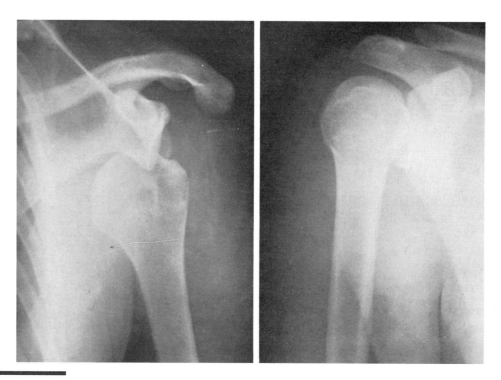

**FIGURE 4–55** ■ Glenohumeral dislocation. (From O'Donoghue DH: Treatment of Injuries to Athletes, 4th ed. Philadelphia: WB Saunders, 1984.)

tion to avoid the positions of injury. As strength and neuromuscular control improve, the shoulder is gradually worked into more stressful positions.

## Subluxations and Instability

A subluxation occurs at the glenohumeral joint when the humerus slips over the glenoid rim but spontaneously relocates without any external force other than instantaneous muscle contraction.[101] After a complete dislocation for which there was inadequate or unsuccessful rehabilitation, patients are often unable to control the instability. This is also common in those with a congenitally shallow glenoid fossa. Subluxations and instability may occur in an anterior, posterior, or combined direction.

An individual with chronic subluxations and shoulder instability presents with vague shoulder pain and a history of participation in an activity in which the mechanism of injury is apparent (e.g., throwing, volleyball, swimming backstroke). The apprehension test is usually positive and there is tenderness anteriorly or posteriorly at the origin or insertion of the inferior glenohumeral ligament.

X-ray examination is usually used to rule out fracture or Hill-Sachs lesion. Special tests such as magnetic resonance imaging (Fig. 4–56) or ar-

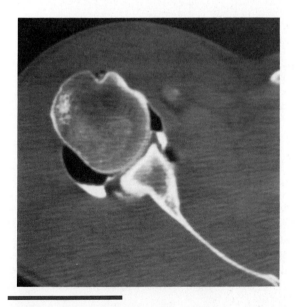

**FIGURE 4–56 ■** Arthrogram with computed tomographic scan of posterior disruption, glenoid labrum tear and associated subperiosteal bone formation. (From Pappas AM: Injuries of the shoulder complex and overhand throwing problems: *In* Clinical Sports Medicine [Grana WA, Kalenak A, eds]. Philadelphia: WB Saunders, 1991.)

throgography combined with computed tomography (Fig. 4–57) can be used to determine the presence of a Bankart lesion or rotator cuff involvement. Surgery is indicated only when conservative management such as a rigorous physical therapy regimen has failed. Several surgical procedures are used to stabilize the glenohumeral joint. Procedures that attempt to restore the normal anatomy of the glenohumeral joint tend to reduce the range of motion minimally. For anterior instability, the Bankart repair involves exposing the capsule and suturing the labrum and capsule back to the glenoid rim. In addition, a capsular imbrication may be performed to stabilize a stretched or lax capsule. This is done in a deltopectoral arthrotomy. A Bankart lesion may also be repaired arthroscopically by staple or suture capsulorrhaphy.[102] Capsulorrhaphy is also the treatment of choice for a posteriorly unstable shoulder. Other open procedures used to stabilize the glenohumeral joint with anterior subluxation shorten or advance the subscapularis tendon (Putti-Platt and Magnuson-Stack) or increase bone stability at the anterior rim of the glenoid with a bone graft or transfer of the coracoid process (Bristow-Helfet and Eben-Hybbinette).[103-105] Many surgeons modify or use combinations of these procedures.[106]

Gradual restoration of range of motion after immobilization begins the rehabilitation process. In general, some loss of external rotation is expected. Strengthening and proprioceptive activities progress as the patient gains function.

## Labral Tears

Tears of the glenoid labrum can result from the shear forces on the glenohumeral joint produced in cases of capsular hypermobility or through traction stress of the biceps tendon at its attachment on the superior labrum.[107] The traction injuries to the labrum from the biceps tendon appear to be the result of high deceleration forces applied to slow the rate of elbow extension during throwing.[107]

The patient may have symptoms of "popping" or "catching" in the joint during quick movements. Pain is usually more evident at the extremes of motion, especially active motion. There is often associated joint hypermobility, and the "clunk" test previously described may be positive. Arthrography with computed tomographic scan, magnetic resonance imaging, and arthroscopy are helpful in confirming the diagnosis. Surgical intervention involves removal, suturing, or stapling of the torn tissue. In cases of hyper-

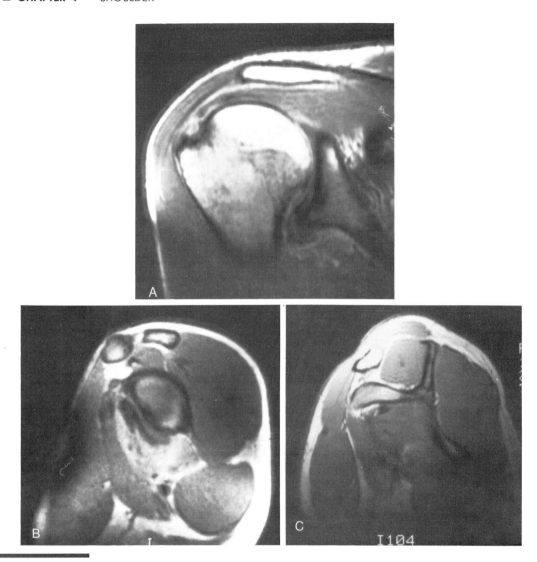

**FIGURE 4–57** ■ Magnetic resonance image of shoulder. (From Pappas AM: Injuries of the shoulder complex and overhand throwing problems. *In* Clinical Sports Medicine [Grana WA, Kalenak A, eds]. Philadelphia: WB Saunders, 1991.)

mobility, reconstructive procedures may also be necessary.

## Osteoarthritis

Osteoarthritis of the glenohumeral joint occurs on the humeral head and glenoid, sites of significant joint reaction force (90 degrees of abduction). Radiographic findings include marginal osteophytes, asymmetric cartilage wear, and subchondral bone sclerosis (Fig. 4–58).

In severe cases in which pain is unrelenting, the treatment of choice is prosthetic replacement. Prosthetic development for the shoulder has progressed because arthrodesis (surgical ankylosis) failed to produce satisfactory results. Total shoulder replacement prostheses are of two types: constrained and unconstrained. The constrained prosthesis has a fixed fulcrum and is designed to minimize the need for strong deltoid and rotator cuff muscles. With the unconstrained prosthesis only the cartilage is replaced; all other structures are repaired.[108] Postoperative management is discussed in case history form at the end of this chapter.

## Rheumatoid Arthritis

Shoulder dysfunction is common in many of the rheumatic diseases, including ankylosing

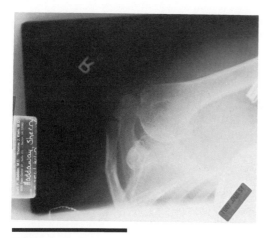

**FIGURE 4–58** ■ Osteoarthritis glenohumeral joint.

spondylitis, systemic lupus erythematosus, polymyalgia rheumatica, polymyositis, dermatomyositis, Reiter's syndrome, and gout. Patients who have received high doses of corticosteroids may develop aseptic necrosis (death of the bone) of the humeral head.[109]

Rheumatoid arthritis is a systemic inflammatory disease characterized by progressive deterioration of the joints. As the disease progresses, cartilage and bone erosion, capsular scarring, atrophy, and contracture occur.[109]

Characteristic x-ray findings in rheumatoid arthritis include juxta-articular osteoporosis, uniform narrowing of the joint space, marginal erosions, and subchondral cysts.[110] The primary clinical manifestations at the shoulder are joint pain and tenderness to palpation, effusion, warmth, and stiffness. These inflammatory characteristics lead to progressive atrophy and dysfunction.

Physical therapy includes pain and inflammation control, maintenance of muscle tone, and maintenance of range of motion.

Surgical options include synovectomy, acromionectomy/acromioplasty, total shoulder arthroplasty, and arthrodesis.

## Acromioclavicular Joint Pathology

### Acromioclavicular Separations

The term acromioclavicular separation is commonly used to describe various degrees of ligamentous sprain at the acromioclavicular joint. Typically, the mechanism of injury is a downward-directed force applied to the edge of

the acromion process because of a fall onto the shoulder with the arm adducted or onto an outstretched hand.

The severity of the injury is classified as mild, moderate, or severe. In mild sprains, the acromioclavicular ligament is stretched but not disrupted. Clinically, the individual has localized pain and swelling over the acromioclavicular joint with minimal restriction of movement initially. The clavicle is not visibly elevated and the joint is relatively stable. In moderate or second-degree sprain, the acromioclavicular ligament is disrupted significantly and the coracoclavicular ligament is stretched. Greater tenderness and swelling are observed with mild elevation of the clavicle relative to the acromion process, and there is significantly greater initial restriction of shoulder range of motion. In severe or third-degree sprain, both the acromioclavicular and coracoclavicular ligaments are ruptured, there is obvious elevation of the clavicle, and the individual is forced to support his or her arm as the pain and tenderness are also significantly increased.[27]

X-ray examination is necessary to rule out fractures and to grade the degree of injury (Fig. 4–59). The method of clinical management is controversial, but first-degree separations are commonly treated for inflammation and early mobilization is advocated, whereas second- and third-degree sprains may either be managed conservatively with a sling or an acromioclavicular splint (Fig. 4–60) for 3 to 6 weeks or surgically repaired.[111] Rehabilitation follows either course of care. Isometric exercises of the shoulder musculature with the arm at the side can begin early. Gradual passive and active assistive range-of-motion exercises are begun as soon as healing and pain permit. Strengthening initially below 90 degrees of flexion and abduction progresses to full range-of-motion exercises and eventual functional activities. Potential complications include inability to regain full range of motion and development of arthritic changes in the joint that eventually cause impingement syndrome.

### Acromioclavicular Joint Degeneration

Osteoarthritic changes are more common in the acromioclavicular joint than in the glenohumeral joint. Restricted glenohumeral joint mobility often leads to excessive movement of the acromioclavicular joint and subsequent degeneration.[112] Osteophytes and sclerosis of the soft tissue may be visible upon x-ray examination. The

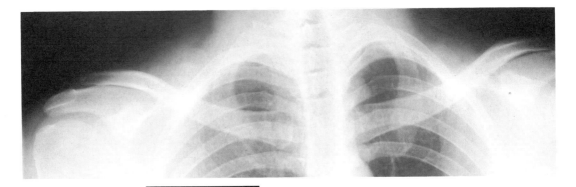

FIGURE 4-59 ■ Acromioclavicular separation (third degree).

joint may be tender to palpation and active and passive range-of-motion exercises may be painful. Surgical intervention may include arthroscopic acromioplasty and partial acromionectomy.

## Sternoclavicular Joint Pathology

### Joint Sprains

The sternoclavicular joint may be injured by a direct force to the sternum or an indirect force resulting from a fall on an outstretched arm. The majority of ligamentous disruptions cause anterior subluxations or dislocations. The grading system for disruption of this ligament and the clinical signs are similar to those for acromioclavicular joint sprains. Immobilization with a sling for 3 to 6 weeks allows healing. Progressive mobilization and strengthening within pain limitations are the treatments of choice. In cases of chronic instability, surgical fixation may be necessary.

### Muscle Strains

Primary muscle strains are less common at the shoulder joint. These strains involve primarily the deltoideus, pectoralis major and minor, latissimus dorsi, and rotator cuff muscles. The mechanism of injury typically involves force overload, as in moving or throwing a heavy object, or activities exceeding the work capacity of the muscle, as in increasing the frequency of activity. Muscle strains are graded as mild, moderate, and severe. Increasing disruption of muscle fibers causes greater loss of tensile force of the muscle. Severe muscle strains are classified as complete ruptures if there is loss of muscle function. The majority of mild and moderate strains are managed conservatively with rest, anti-inflammatory measures, and progressive mobilization and strengthening. Complete ruptures may require surgical repair.

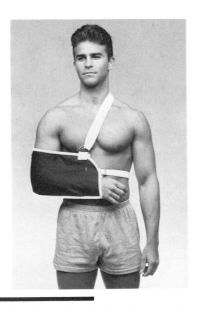

FIGURE 4-60 ■ Acromioclavicular separation splint.

### Fractures

Most fractures of the shoulder joint complex occur because of direct trauma. The structures most commonly fractured are the clavicle, scapula, and humerus.

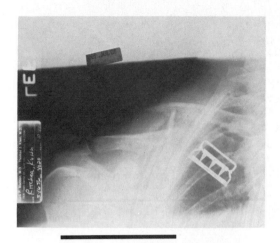

**FIGURE 4-61** ■ Clavicle fracture.

**Clavicular Fractures.** A fall on the lateral aspect of the shoulder or, less commonly, onto an outstretched arm may cause a fracture of the clavicle.[113] The bone usually breaks in its mid-portion.[114] Clavicular fracture is common in children and is usually reduced satisfactorily with immobilization by a figure-of-8 bandage holding the shoulders upward and backward. In adults, the fracture fragments must be maintained in good opposition (Fig. 4-61). The reduction position is the same as the position used in children unless open reduction is required. The immobilization period varies from 2 to 6 weeks depending on healing time. Factors influencing healing time include severity of the trauma, bone loss, infection, the bone that is fractured, effectiveness of immobilization, age, general health, and activity level.[115] The glenohumeral joint may be mobilized progressively from passive to active as healing permits.

**Scapular Fractures.** Fractures of a portion of the scapula are rare and are most commonly caused by a direct blow to the area. Displacement of the fragments is even more uncommon because the scapula is encased in a heavy muscular envelope.[114] Fractures of the body and spine are usually minimally displaced and do not require reduction. Fractures of the neck do not require anatomic reduction unless there is severe angulation of the articular surface, predisposing the glenohumeral joint to subluxation or dislocation (Fig. 4-62).[116] A stress fracture of the coracoid process or acromion may occur when there is excess demand on the bone. An avulsion fracture of a portion of the rim of the glenoid may accompany glenohumeral subluxation and dislocation.

**Humeral Fractures.** Fractures of the proximal half of the humerus can affect shoulder girdle function. These fractures can involve the humeral head, greater tuberosity, neck, and shaft. Osteochondral (involving the bone and its overlying cartilage) fractures of the humeral head are caused by direct contact of the humeral head against the glenoid. The most common example is the Hill-Sachs lesion (Fig. 4-63) that accompanies an anterior dislocation of the glenohumeral joint. The greater tuberosity may fracture in a direct fall onto the shoulder (Fig. 4-64). In these cases, if the fragment is not displaced, minimal immobilization is necessary and passive exercise is initiated early to avoid joint stiffness. If the fracture is the result of an avulsion or if the fragment is displaced, it is commonly reduced by internal screw fixation. The procedure often requires acromioplasty to allow adequate clearance during abduction.[117] Postoperative immobilization is usually for 3 to 6 weeks.

Fracture of the humeral neck is often the result of a fall onto an outstretched arm (Fig. 4-65) and occurs most commonly in elderly people. If the fragments are not displaced, the arm is stabilized in a sling but may be removed from the sling frequently for exercise. If the fragments are displaced but do not require open reduction, the arm is held tightly to the chest with a sling and

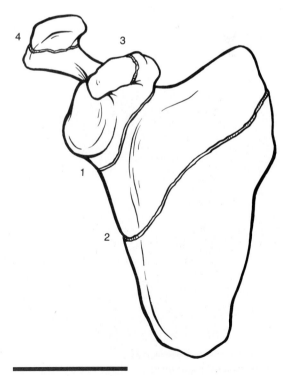

**FIGURE 4-62** ■ Portions of scapula (bone, spine, back).

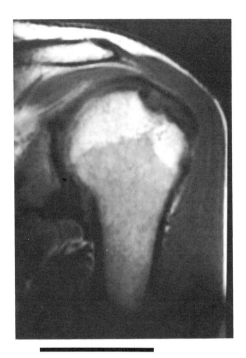

FIGURE 4-63 ■ Hill-Sachs lesion.

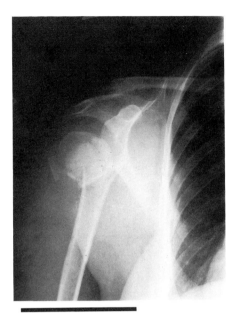

FIGURE 4-65 ■ Fractured humeral neck.

swathe for 2 to 4 weeks. In cases of open reduction, plates or intramedullary rods may be placed in the bone; the severity of the procedure and fracture dictates the immobilization time.

Fractures of the humeral shaft may result from a direct blow or a twisting force. Those resulting from a twisting force are spiral fractures (Fig. 4-66). Although uncommon, a spiral fracture may occur during a throwing action because of the torque produced as the arm is forcibly rotated internally just before ball release.[118]

It is not uncommon for prolonged immobilization after humeral fracture to create significant joint stiffness of all the articulations of this complex. Therefore, early passive range-of-motion exercise is necessary to prevent scarring.

Bone tumors may involve the humerus and are potential causes of pathologic fractures (Fig. 4-67). The more common benign tumors include unicameral bone cysts, osteochondromas, giant cell tumors, and chondroblastomas. Primary malignant bone tumors arise in the humerus less frequently. Metastatic carcinoma from primary sites such as the breast, kidney, prostate, and lung frequently involves the humerus.[114]

## Myofascial Dysfunction

Myofascial dysfunction may be the diagnosis applied to chronic shoulder girdle pain or dysfunction. Reynolds characterizes the syndrome in this region in terms of absence of articular signs, significant loss of range of motion, swelling, or crepitus.[119] Neurologic tests, radiographs, and imaging studies are generally normal. The muscles of the shoulder girdle have exquisite point

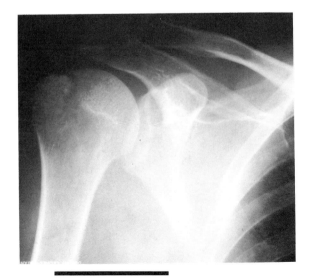

FIGURE 4-64 ■ Greater tuberosity fracture.

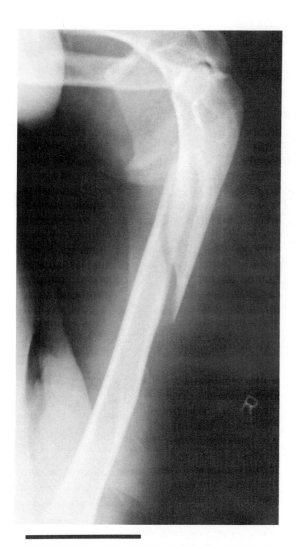

**FIGURE 4-66** ■ Spiral fracture of the humeral shaft.

tenderness upon palpation and often have palpable fibrous bands. These bands are called trigger points. The patient generally has a history of progressive spread of pain, exacerbations and remissions that may be related to physical activity or emotional stress, and failure of conventional therapy to provide relief.

Travell and Simons describe severe perpetuating factors that can be controlled: postural stress, constriction of muscles (a tight brassiere strap or heavy shoulder strap), and structural inadequacies such as scoliosis.[36]

Yunus et al. attempted to differentiate between myofascial syndrome and primary fibromyalgia.[120] The primary difference is the systemic nature of fibromyalgia, in which multiple anatomic sites are symptomatic with no underlying cause. Myofascial dysfunction usually affects only one area.

Treatment of trigger points is designed to release the restriction through pressure, massage, release techniques, stretching, heat, ultrasound, and transcutaneous electrical stimulation. In addition, postural retraining is essential.

## Thoracic Outlet Syndrome

In thoracic outlet syndrome, or more appropriately thoracic inlet syndrome,[121] upper quarter pain arises from nerve and/or vascular compression in the superior triangle opening of the thorax. There is controversy in the medical profession regarding the frequency of its occurrence.[122-124] Investigators cite a high rate of recurrence of symptoms after surgical repairs to relieve the pressure.

The onset of symptoms in this disorder is commonly insidious with trauma to the shoulder girdle. Middle-aged women are affected most frequently,[125] and the symptoms include pain, tingling and numbness, heaviness, and temperature and skin changes of the neck, upper extremity, and hand. Functional activities that provoke symptoms include overhead activities for short periods of time, such as hair styling, or static postures such as those used in needlework or carrying a handbag or briefcase.

Primary and secondary etiologies of thoracic outlet syndrome are described by Jager et al.[126] The primary causes are compression resulting from soft tissue abnormality including, but not limited to, a cervical rib, malunion of the clavicle, anomalous fibromuscular bands of the scalene muscles, and Pancoast's tumor of the apex of the lung. Secondary thoracic outlet syndrome occurs in the absence of any anatomic variation and is the direct result of traumatic variation in cervicothoracic posture. Special tests for this condition were described under Thoracic Outlet (see Figs. 4–47 through 4–50).

The majority of patients are managed conservatively by posture correction. This involves stretching soft tissue restrictions, strengthening weak muscle groups, and modifying posture. Surgical intervention is required if conservative measures fail or if the cause is a bone abnormality or tumor. Occasionally, muscle is excised to free the thoracic inlet. As mentioned earlier, surgical success is not high and surgery is a last resort.

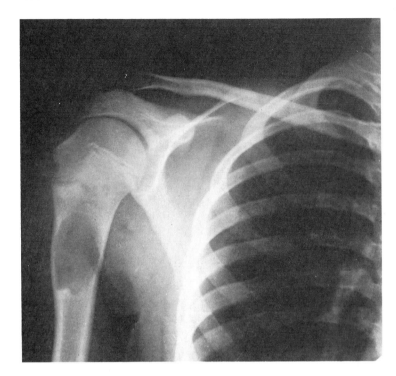

**FIGURE 4-67** ■ Bone tumor. (From Gartland JJ: Fundamentals of Orthopaedics, 4th ed. Philadelphia: WB Saunders, 1987.)

## TREATMENT

### General Principles

Fractures and surgical repairs require the shoulder complex to be immobilized for a period of time to permit healing. This immobilization causes stiffness of the periarticular connective tissues and weakness of the surrounding musculature. There has been abundant research on the histologic, biochemical, and mechanical changes that result from immobilization.[127,128] These include loss of extensibility of capsule, ligaments, tendon, and fascia secondary to aberrant cross-linking of fibers; deposition of fibrofatty infiltrates; breakdown of hyaline cartilage on the articular surfaces; and atrophy and adaptive length changes in muscles. Thus, movement must take place as soon as healing permits.[129]

A thorough understanding of the stages of soft tissue healing helps the clinician use progressive exercise to reduce the deleterious effects of immobilization and promote the patient's functional return to activity. Connective tissue heals through formation of scar tissue after an initial inflammatory response and proliferation of ground substance and collagen protein in the area.[78] The inflammatory and proliferative stages last approximately 14 days. After 2 weeks the organization stage continues until the tissue approaches its pretrauma state. Stress to the tissues during this later stage determines the orientation of the collagen fibers. Randomly organized fibers produce a firm scar that limits motion; fibers reoriented in the direction of normal motion do not limit motion.[130,131]

The specific design of therapeutic intervention requires a thorough understanding of the biomechanics of the shoulder mechanism during normal motion and identification of the disrupted biomechanics and specific mechanics the patient attempts to regain. The joint and muscle interactions have been outlined in earlier sections of this chapter and must also be considered in designing the therapeutic regime. Activity-specific mechanics are described in the literature concerning function and activities of daily living, sports, and industry, work, or task demands. These activities must be analyzed and conditioning in the deficit components used to enable the patient to return to full independent activities.

### Therapeutic Procedures

#### Restoration of Passive Range of Motion

Joint mobilization, a form of passive joint movement in which oscillatory, distractive, arti-

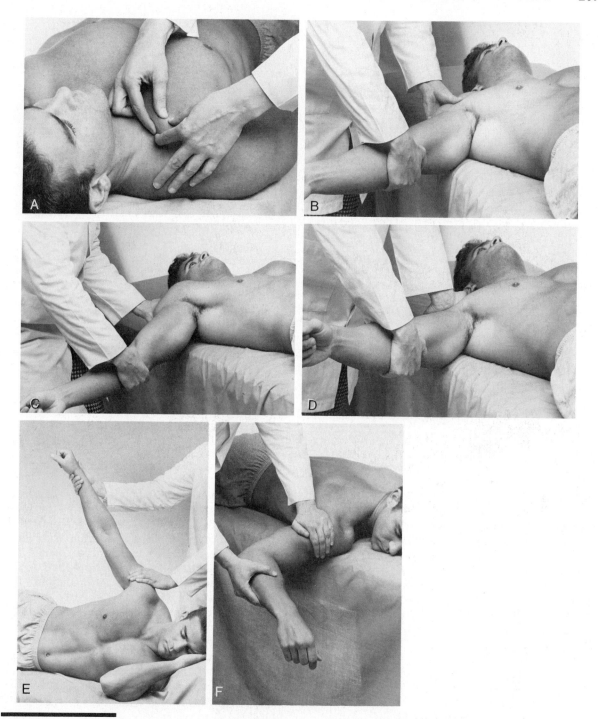

**FIGURE 4–68**  ■  Specific mobilizations of shoulder joint. (A) Joint play at acromioclavicular joint. (B) Cranial-to-caudal force at glenohumeral joint. (C) Posterior-to-anterior force at glenohumeral joint. (D) Anterior-to-posterior force at glenohumeral joint. (E) Caudal glide in abduction. (F) Scapular abduction or lateral glide. *Illustration continued on following page*

culatory, and manipulative techniques are used to restore normal arthrokinematics (the intimate mechanics of joint surfaces) and osteokinematics (the movement of bones), is an integral part of the rehabilitation program.[132] Mobilization techniques are also effective in modulating pain by enhancing mechanoreceptor stimulation within the joint.[133] The direction of the force applied to

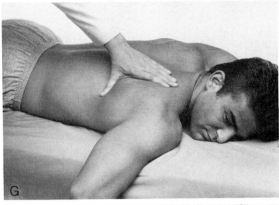

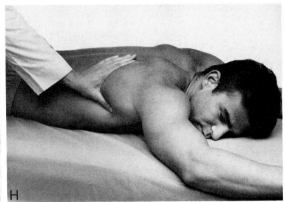

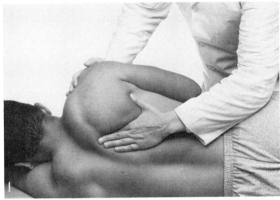

FIGURE 4–68 ■ *Continued* (G) Scapular rotation. (H) Restriction of scapular movement during glenohumeral elevation. General scapular movement, side lying.

the joint is determined during the evaluation of joint mobility (Fig. 4–68). Forces are applied within the patient's tolerance and tissue resistance or end feel. Table 4–3 lists the specific mobilizations performed at the shoulder joints. The specific mobilization techniques are described in more detail elsewhere.[30,33,134,135]

Flexibility or stretching exercises restore length to shortened muscles and reduce trigger point irritability in the muscle, thus improving passive range of motion. A muscle stretches more easily if it has been warmed before stretching. This may be accomplished with heating modalities or mild exercise.[136] Stretching exercises require an understanding of the joint biomechanics, lines of muscle pull, and tissue characteristics.

## Restoration of Active Range of Motion

As passive mobility is established, the patient begins to work on active motion and strengthening exercises. Initially, the patient attempts to restore active motion with normal biomechanics. It is typical for a patient to achieve full range of motion at the shoulder joint by allowing one

joint to compensate for another less functional joint.

Use of neuromuscular electrical stimulation and electromyographic biofeedback in the initial stages of active motion is helpful for muscle re-education and establishing normal kinetics.[137] Active assisted motion in cardinal planes and functional patterns, as in proprioceptive neuromuscular facilitation, eases the patient into greater degrees of effort. In the early stages of rehabilitation, the patient may perform the initial stage of strengthening exercises—isometrics. The type of injury or surgery and the patient's healing characteristics determine readiness for this form of intervention. Injured tissues can be protected by splinting or positioning to allow other supporting muscles to begin the strengthening process.

## Restoration of Strength

When normal passive and active motion is achieved, a strengthening program that concentrates on deficiencies found in the evaluation process is emphasized. The therapist should constantly re-evaluate and reassess the patient while

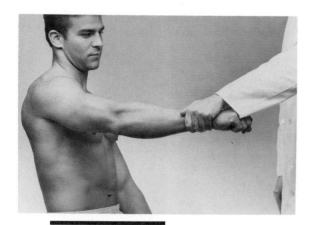

FIGURE 4–69 ■ Manual resistance exercise.

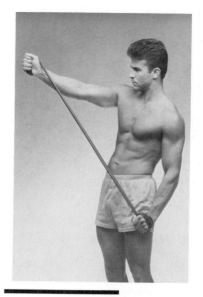

FIGURE 4–70 ■ Surgical tubing exercise.

aggressively but safely guiding the patient to maximal function.

Principles of strengthening include specificity, overload, and trainability. Specificity refers to exercises that isolate particular muscles or muscle groups,[61,138] as well as the type of exercise needed for particular activities. One must analyze whether the functional activities require aerobic or anaerobic efforts; whether the contractions are concentric, eccentric, isometric, or combination of the three types; and which joint positions determine the muscle action. Overload refers to methods used to improve the muscle physiologically: frequency, intensity, and duration of exercise. To increase strength significantly, the muscle must be gradually overloaded. In the early stages of rehabilitation, the strengthening program typically involves daily exercises with light resistance for large numbers of repetitions. In the more advanced stages, the intensity can be increased, the duration shortened, and the

frequency of exercise altered. Trainability concerns the rate of progression from one stage of strengthening to the next. This is influenced by the patient's previous physical condition; an individual whose muscles have atrophied for a long period of time takes longer to train initially but may then make rapid gains. The strengthening required should be altered accordingly.

Many types of resistance training programs are available. Manual resistive exercises direct the activity through manual feedback and intensity is based on the patient's response (Fig. 4–69). Progressive resistance training includes use of surgical tubing or similar resistive material (Fig. 4–70), dumbbells, machines, body weight (Fig. 4–71), ergometers, and functional activities (Fig.

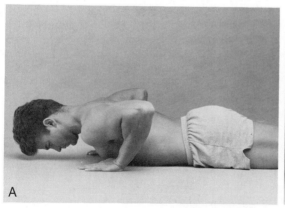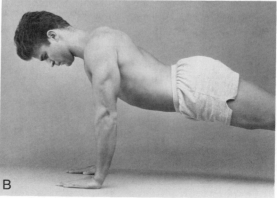

FIGURE 4–71 ■ Body weight resistance exercise.

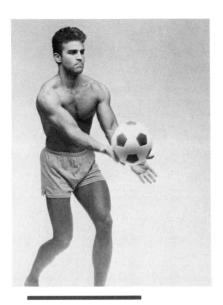

**FIGURE 4-72** ■ Functional activities.

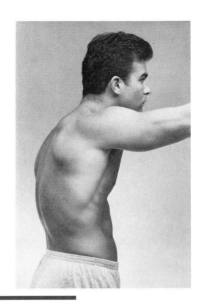

**FIGURE 4-73** ■ Forward head with rounded shoulders, protracted and elevated scapulae, and tight pectoralis.

4-72). Isokinetic training devices utilize constant speed of exercise with accommodating resistance. These exercise devices provide several modes of exercise: passive, isometric, isotonic, and variations in isokinetic resistance sequences. The regimens include concentric-concentric, concentric-eccentric, eccentric-concentric, passive-concentric, and passive-eccentric programs. These devices also provide exercises within controlled ranges of motion.

### Posture and the Shoulder

Posture and its impact on the shoulder and function must be dealt with throughout the rehabilitation process. Posture should be analyzed in standing, sitting, sleeping, and activities of daily living. The upper quarter of the body consists of the head, cervical spine, thorax, and upper extremities. Positions of the components influence the positions of the related parts, and this relationship becomes altered in deviations. It is difficult to solve a rotator cuff tendinitis problem if the static and dynamic postural examination reveals a forward head position with rounded shoulders, protracted and elevated scapulae, and tight pectoralis minor (Fig. 4-73). Strengthening the rotator cuff in this position exacerbates the problem. The relief resulting from cortisone injection or rest and modalities is only temporary if postural dysfunction is not corrected.

In addition to making static and dynamic pos-

tural changes, the patient must avoid activities that perpetuate the shoulder pathology. These include carrying a briefcase, suitcase, or handbag in the affected arm's hand or with a strap on the affected shoulder; sleeping on the shoulder with the hand elevated; and "testing" the shoulder constantly with arm circles or activities that cause pain.

### SUMMARY

The patient must continue to perform exercises and alter the activities of daily living to avoid motions that expose the shoulder to reinjury. In the noncompliant patient, chronic conditions of shoulder dysfunction and instability can arise that are painful and reduce function. Therefore, both the patient and the patient's family must be educated in an appropriate long-term exercise program, modified work and recreational activities, and self-care techniques. In this way, the patient can function maximally with little or no pain after the conclusion of formal rehabilitation.

### CASE STUDY 1

▼ The patient was an 18-year-old male high school senior who presented with a diagnosis of bilateral rotator cuff tendinitis-impingement syndrome. He had a 3-month history of pain with a gradual onset. He received a cortisone injection 1 month previously with temporary reduction of symptoms. His primary activity was weight training. He was not consistent with a

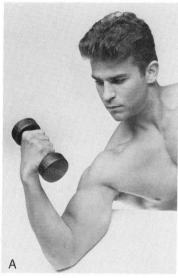
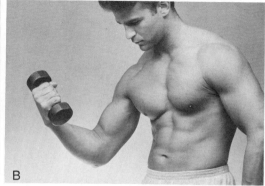

**FIGURE 4-74** ■ Biceps exercises.

**FIGURE 4-75** ■ Triceps exercises.

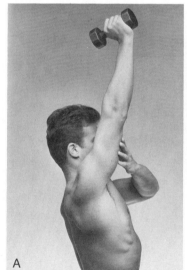

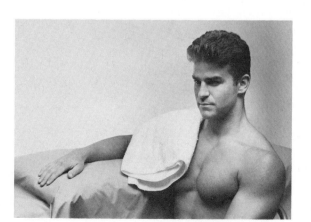

**FIGURE 4-76** ■ Moist heat applied in slight flexion and abduction.

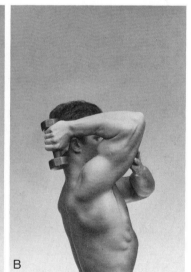

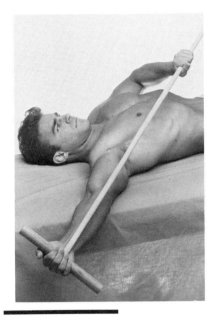

FIGURE 4–77 ■ Stretch of pectoralis muscle.

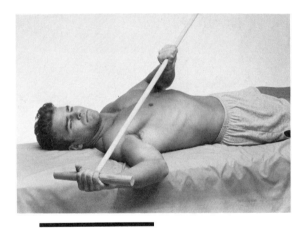

FIGURE 4–78 ■ Stretch of subscapularis muscle.

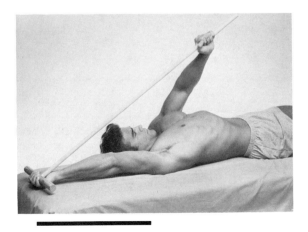

FIGURE 4–79 ■ Stretch of latissimus dorsi muscle.

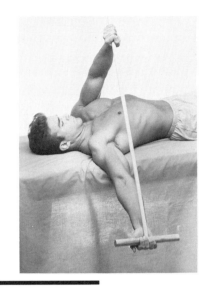

FIGURE 4–80 ■ Stretch of anterior shoulder capsule.

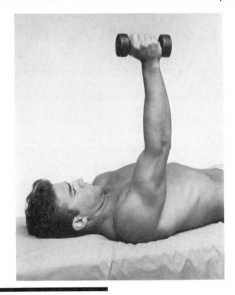

FIGURE 4–81 ■ An example of strengthening exercise.

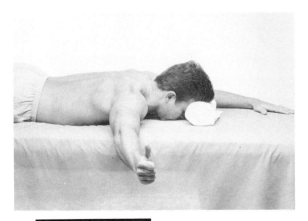

FIGURE 4–82 ■ Biofeedback for posture retraining.

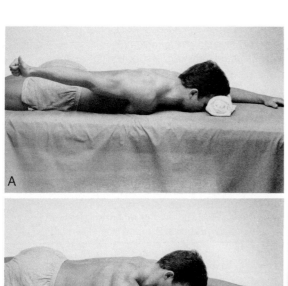

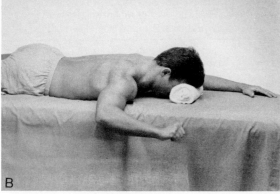

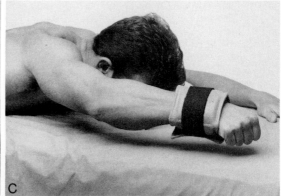

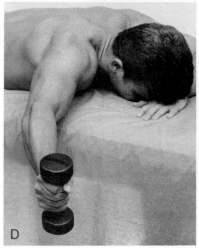

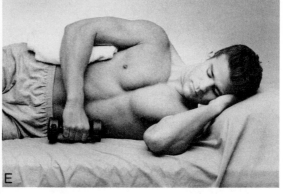

**FIGURE 4-83** ■ Rotator cuff strengthening program.

warm-up and stretching program before or after his weight training routine, which consisted of several chest press positions, military press, lat pulls, and work on biceps and triceps. He was currently taking a 2-week dose of nonsteroidal anti-inflammatory medication. He was taking no other medications. Past medical history was insignificant.

Examination revealed a well-developed anterior musculature and proportionately less developed posterior muscle groups. Posturally, he had moderately round shoulders and forward head. The scapula appeared elevated and abducted. Passive motion was pain free; however, tightness was noted in the pectoralis minor,

biceps brachii, and subscapularis. There was a painful arc in active flexion and abduction between 90 and 130 degrees of motion. Resisted external rotation and abduction were painful with the arm in a neutral position. Resisted elbow flexion with the shoulder flexed 80 degrees was also painful. The patient was unable to perform the motions suggested by Blackburn et. al. to isolate the posterior cuff muscles.[138] On manual testing, the middle and lower trapezius and the serratus anterior were weak compared to the anterior muscles: pectoralis, anterior deltoideus, upper trapezius, and levator scapulae. The impingement sign was positive.

Assessment of problem areas in this case revealed

postural, flexibility, strength, training, and technique errors that predisposed the young man to the development of impingement tendinitis of the rotator cuff and biceps tendons. Our short-term goal was to reduce inflammation. The long-term goal was to return the patient to his activity of choice in a progressive manner in order not to aggravate the condition.

The patient was given a thorough explanation of the relationship of his current posture to the development of tendinitis. He immediately began a period of rest from overhead weight training and activities of daily living. He was advised about shoulder care to minimize aggravation of the condition. We encouraged continuation of the remainder of his weight training program and modified biceps and triceps exercises (Figs. 4–74 and 4–75).

Modalities in physical therapy included phonophoresis of the anterior and posterior cuff in the positions recommended by Cyriax.[31] This was followed by moist heat with the patient in a position of slight flexion and abduction to ensure adequate vascular supply to the subacromial structures (Fig. 4–76). Exercises included stretching of tight musculature and the anterior capsule (Figs. 4–77 to 4–80). Strengthening exercises for the anterior serratus and middle and lower trapezius were begun to help restore the normal biomechanical muscle balance of the region (Figs. 4–81 and 4–82). Postural training and respositioning exercises were also initiated and continued (see Fig. 4–82).

As symptoms subsided over a 3-week period, the patient was progressed through a rotator cuff strengthening program (Fig. 4–83A–E). Care was taken to begin in a position consistent with the plane of the scapula in isokinetic training.

When the patient was free of pain with active and resisted motions and we were comfortable with his technique for continuing the strength progression (8 weeks after the initial evaluation), we accompanied him to his health club to organize a new upper body regimen and review proper technique, frequency, intensity, duration, and warm-up and cool-down techniques.

## CASE STUDY 2

▼The patient was a 60-year-old man with a significant history of osteoarthritis of the left shoulder. He was seen in the hospital 1 day after total shoulder replacement with an unconstrained Neer prosthesis. The operative report showed that the patient had an intact rotator cuff, the surgical approach was deltopectoral (the

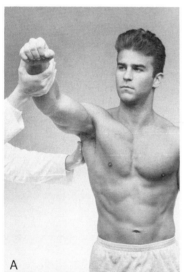
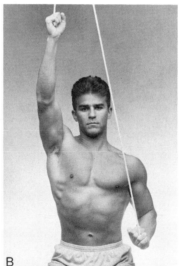
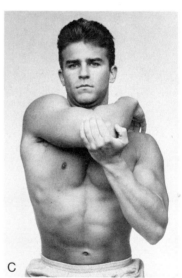
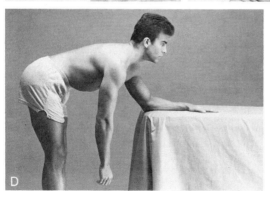

**FIGURE 4–84 ■** Active assistive exercises. (A) Manual assistance. (B) Mechanical assistance. (C) Patient's assistance. (D) Pendulum exercise.

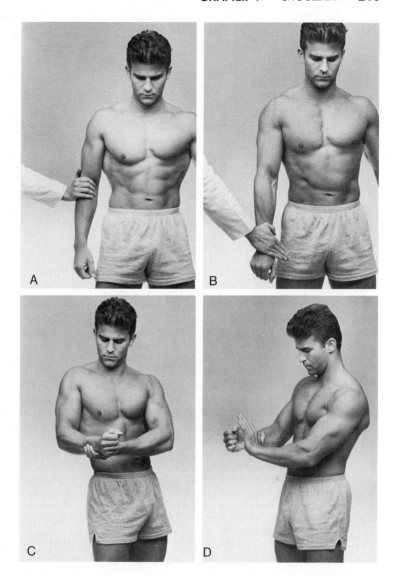

**FIGURE 4–85** ■ Isometric exercises. (A) Abduction. (B) Flexion. (C) External rotation. (D) Internal rotation.

deltoid was not taken down), and a partial anterior acromionectomy was performed.

The patient's first visit was an educational session regarding the rehabilitation process. Because the shoulder would be immobilized with a sling and swathe for the first 5 to 7 days, the patient was reminded not to roll onto that arm at night or attempt to use the arm for repositioning in bed. The patient was also advised to expect three types of discomfort in the rehabilitation process: (1) incisional for the first 5 to 7 days, (2) at the extremes of motion during exercise, and (3) fatigue of the muscles that would gradually resolve through strengthening exercises. The patient was instructed in elbow and hand range-of-motion exercises to be performed when the sling was removed over the next several days for hygiene.

The patient returned for outpatient physical therapy on the sixth postoperative day. Initial exercise consists of passive and active assisted routines as illustrated in Figure 4–84A–D. Isometric exercises were initiated on day 10 after surgery as illustrated in Figure 4–85A–D. Active exercises were begun 2 weeks after surgery, and by approximately 12 weeks maximum active motion was achieved: abduction 140 degrees, flexion 150 degrees, and external rotation 40 degrees. The patient continued motion and strengthening exercises using rubber tubing at home. By approximately 5 months after surgery, the patient had regained a significant amount of function as evidenced by his activities of daily living.

## CASE STUDY 3

▼The patient was a 28-year-old man whose primary recreational activity was volleyball. Although he never experienced a frank dislocation, the right glenohumeral

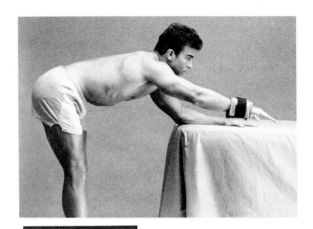

**FIGURE 4-86** ■ Free weight progressive resistance exercise.

joint had experienced multiple subluxation episodes beginning 3 years previously. The two most recent injuries were 2 weeks and 1 year previously. Both injuries involved a spiking motion of abduction and external rotation. There was intense pain and a sense that the arm became numb for a short period of time. The patient typically applied ice and stopped playing. He could generally return to playing in 1 to 2 weeks. He modified his activity by decreasing the frequency and intensity of play. At the time we saw him, the patient was to attempt a rehabilitation program as a conservative effort before surgery. An arthrogram with computed tomographic scan had shown no rotator cuff tear but suggested an inferior glenoid labrum tear (Bankart's lesion) and possibly a tear of the inferior glenohumeral ligament. The medical history was insignificant. The affected arm was dominant and had "loose" joints but no other symptomatic areas.

deus and infraspinatus area. Postural examination revealed no significant abnormalities. Active motion in straight planes was equal bilaterally but was noted to be excessive compared to normal. Passive motion testing with the patient supine revealed 125 degrees of external rotation at 90 degrees of abduction on the right compared to 115 degrees on the left. This motion also made the patient apprehensive about subluxation. Resisted manual muscle testing suggested weakness of one grade of the right infraspinatus, supraspinatus, and middle deltoideus (G/N or 4/5). The middle and lower trapezius muscles were weak bilaterally. The clunk test for glenoid labrum tear was positive. There was no palpable tenderness about the shoulder girdle. Accessory motions bilaterally were hypermobile.

Our treatment approach with this patient was to restore maximum strength and kinesthesia to the right

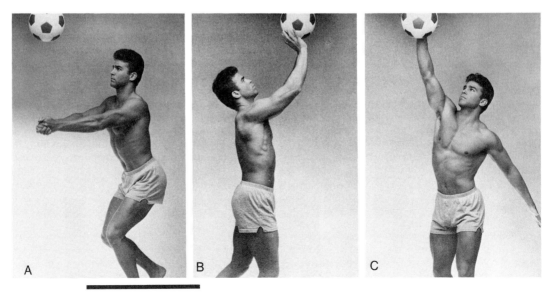

**FIGURE 4-87** ■ Volleyball specific drill. (A) Setting low. (B) Setting high. (C) Spike.

shoulder as a means of avoiding or preparing for surgery. We initiated a multifaceted program including isokinetics, resistance with proprioceptive neuromuscular facilitation patterns for the glenohumeral and scapulothoracic joints, free weight progressive resistance exercises, stabilization and kinesthesia training with body weight through the arm, and activity-specific drills for technique and timing. See Figures 4–86 and 4–87 for examples and progression. Within the first 2 weeks of treatment, the patient was given an isokinetic evaluation of the shoulder rotators. This revealed only an eccentric deficit in the right external rotators from midrange to 70 degrees of internal rotation. In addition, because this was his dominant arm, we would expect it to perform better overall than the left arm. Unfortunately, the literature does not provide the exact proportion, although there are several activity-specific profiles.[50]

Over the course of 6 weeks, the patient noted an overall improvement in strength and joint position sense of the right shoulder. He returned to volleyball competition as he had continued to practice all other aspects of the game except overhand serve and spike. He did well for 6 months and then experienced a subluxation. He eventually went on to arthroscopic repair of the Bankart lesion and inferior glenohumeral ligament.

## References

1. Kelly DL: Kinesiological Fundamentals of Motion Description. Englewood Cliffs, NJ: Prentice-Hall, 1971.
2. Gray H: Anatomy of the Human Body, 29th ed. Philadelphia: Lea & Febiger, 1973.
3. Carmichael SW, Hart DL: Anatomy of the shoulder joint. J Orthop Sports Phys Ther 6(4):225–228, 1985.
4. Brunnstrom S: Clinical Kinesiology (revised by LD Lehmkuhl and LK Smith). Philadelphia: FA Davis, 1983.
5. Dempster WT: Mechanism of shoulder movement. Arch Phys Med Rehabil 46A:49, 1965.
6. Inman VT, Saunders M, Abbott LC: Observations on the function of the shoulder joint. J Bone Joint Surg [Am] 26:1, 1944.
7. Morris J. Joints of the shoulder girdle. Aust J Physiother 24(2), 1978.
8. Reference deleted
9. Bateman, JE: The Shoulder and Neck. Philadelphia: WB Saunders, 1971.
10. Rothman RH, Marvel JP, Heppenstall RB: Anatomic considerations in the glenohumeral joint. Orthop Clin North Am 6:341–352, 1975.
11. Rothman RH, Parke WW: The vascular anatomy of the rotator cuff. Clin Orthop 41:176–186, 1965.
12. Soderburg G: Kinesiology: Application to Pathological Motion. Baltimore, Williams & Wilkins, 1986.
13. Johnston TB: The movements of the shoulder joint: a plea for the use of the "plane of the scapula" as the plane of reference for movements occurring at the humeroscapular joint. Br J Surg 25:252–260, 1937.
14. Poppen NK, Walker PS: Normal and abnormal motion of the shoulder. J. Bone Joint Surg [Am] 58:195–201, 1976.
15. Saha AK: Theory of Shoulder Mechanism: Descriptive and Applied. Springfield, IL: Charles C Thomas, 1961.
16. Kummel BM: Spectrum of lesions of the anterior capsular mechanism of the shoulder. Am J Sports Med 7:11, 1979.
17. Saha AK: Mechanics of elevation of glenohumeral joint. Acta Orthop Scand 44:668–678, 1973.
18. Doody SG, Freedman L, Waterland JC: Shoulder movement during abduction in the scapular plane. Arch Phys Med Rehabil 51:595–604, 1970.
19. Bagg DS, Forrest WJ: A biomechanical analysis of scapular rotation during arm abduction in the scapular plane. Am J Phys Med Rehabil 67:238, 1988.
20. Freedman L, Munro RR: Abduction of the arm in the scapular plane: scapular and glenohumeral movements: A roentgenographic study. J Bone Joint Surg [Am] 48:1503, 1966.
21. Zuckerman JD, Matsen FA: Biomechanics of the shoulder. In Basic Biomechanics of the Musculoskeletal System (Nordin M, Frankel VH, eds), 2nd ed. Philadelphia: Lea & Febiger, 1989.
22. Poppen NK, Walker PS: Forces at the glenohumeral joint in abduction. Clin Orthop 135:165–170, 1978.
23. Saha AK: Dynamic stability of the glenohumeral joint. Acta Orthop Scand 42:491–505, 1971.
24. Rothstein JM, Echternach JL: Hypothesis-oriented algorithm for clinicians. Phys Ther 66:1388–1394, 1986.
25. Booth RE, Marvel JP: Differential diagnosis in shoulder pain. Orthop Clin North Am 6:353, 1975.
26. Bowling RW, Rockar PA, Erhard R: Examination of the shoulder complex. Phys Ther 66:1867, 1986.
27. Allman FL: Fractures and ligamentous injuries of the clavicle and its articulations. J Bone Joint Surg [Am] 49:774–784, 1967.
28. Moran CA, Saunders SR: Evaluation of the shoulder: a sequential approach. In Physical Therapy of the Shoulder (Donatelli RA, ed), 2nd ed. New York: Churchill-Livingstone, 1991.
29. Kessel L, Watson M: The painful arc syndrome. J Bone Joint Surg [Br] 49:2, 1977.
30. Maitland GD: Peripheral Manipulation. Boston: Butterworths, 1977.
31. Cyriax JH: Textbook of Orthopaedic Medicine: Diagnosis of Soft Tissues Lesions, 5th. ed. Baltimore: Williams & Wilkins, 1970.
32. Cyriax JH: Illustrated Manual of Orthopaedic Medicine. London: Butterworths, 1983.
32. Kaltenborn FM: Manual Therapy for the Extremity Joints: Specialized Tests, Techniques, and Joint Mobilization, 2nd ed. Oslo: Olaf Norlis Borkhandel, 1976.
34. Mennell JM: Joint Pain: Diagnosis and Treatment Using Manipulative Techniques. Boston: Little, Brown, 1964.
35. Clancy WG: Shoulder problems in overhead-overuse sports. Am J Sports Med 7(2):138, 1979.
36. Travell J, Simons DJ: Myofascial Pain and Dysfunction: The Trigger Point Manual. Baltimore: Williams & Wilkins, 1983.
37. Kendall FP, McCreary EK: Muscles: Testing and Function, 3rd ed. Baltimore, Williams & Wilkins, 1983.
38. Daniels L, Worthingham C: Muscle Testing, 4th ed. Philadelphia: WB Saunders, 1980.
39. Yergason RM: Supination sign. J Bone Joint Surg 13:160, 1931.
40. Lippman RK: Frozen shoulder: periarthritis, bicipital tenosynovitis. Arch Surg 47:283, 1943.
41. Ludington NA: Rupture of the long head of the biceps tendon cubiti muscle. Ann Surg 77:358, 1923.

42. Hawkins RJ, Kennedy JC: Impingement syndrome in athletes. Am J Sports Med 8:151–158, 1980.
43. Neer CS II, Welsh RP: The shoulder in sports. Orthop Clin North Am 8:583, 1977.
44. Zarin A, Andrew J, Carson M: USOC: Injuries to the Throwing Arm. Philadelphia: WB Saunders, 1985.
45. Adson AW, Coffey JR: Cervical rehabilitation. Ann Surg 85:839, 1927.
46. Falconer MA, Weddell G: Costoclavicular compression of the subclavian artery and vein. Lancet 2:539, 1943.
47. Wright JS: The neurovascular syndrome produced by hyperabduction of the arms. Am Heart J 29:1, 1945.
48. Roos DB: The place for scalenectomy and first rib resection in thoracic outlet syndrome. Surgery 92:1077, 1982.
49. Davies G: A Compendium of Isokinetics in Clinical Usage. La Crosse: S & S Publishers, 1984.
50. Hinton RY: Isokinetic evaluation of shoulder rotational strength in high school baseball pitchers. Am J Sports Med 16:274, 1988.
51. Alderink GJ, Kuck DJ: Isokinetic shoulder strength of high school and college age baseball pitchers. J Orthop Sports Phys Ther 7:163, 1986.
52. Soderberg GJ, Blaschak MJ: Shoulder internal and external rotation peak torque production through a velocity spectrum in differing positions. J Orthop Sports Phys Ther 8:518, 1987.
53. Connelly-Maddux RE, Kibler WB, Uhl T: Isokinetic peak torque and work values for the shoulder. J Orthop Sports Phys Ther 1:264, 1989.
54. Cook EE, Gray VL, Savinar-Nogue E, et al: Shoulder antagonist ratios: a comparison between college level baseball pitchers and non pitchers. J Orthop Sports Phys Ther 8:451, 1987.
55. Reid DC, Salboe L, Burnham R: Current research of selected shoulder problems. *In* Physical Therapy of the Shoulder (Donatelli R, ed). New York: Churchill-Livingstone, 1987.
56. Ivey FM, Calhoun JH, Rusche K, et al: Isokinetic testing of shoulder strength: normal values. Arch Phys Med Rehabil 66:384, 1985.
57. Coleman AE: Physiological characteristics of major league baseball players. Phys Sports Med 10:51, 1982.
58. Richardson AB, Jobe FW, Collins JR: The shoulder in competitive swimming. Am J Sports Med 8:159, 1980.
59. Jobe FW: Shoulder problems in overhead-overuse sports: thrower problems. Am J Sports Med 7:139, 1979.
60. Pappas AM, Zawacki RM, Sullivan TJ: Biomechanics of pitching. Am J Sports Med 13:216–222, 1985.
61. Moynes DR, Perry J, Antonelli: DJ, et al: Electromyography and motion analysis of the upper extremity in sports. Phys Ther 66:1905–1911, 1986.
62. Wadsworth C: Frozen shoulder. Phys Ther 66(12):1878, 1986.
63. Neviaser JS: Adhesive capsulitis of the shoulder: a study of the pathological findings in periarthritis of the shoulder. J Bone Joint Surg 27:211–222, 1945.
64. Neviaser RJ: Painful conditions affecting the shoulder. Clin Orthop 173:63–69, 1983.
65. Rizk TE, Pinals RS: Frozen shoulder. Semin Arthritis Rheumatol 11:440–452, 1982.
66. Bruckner FE, Nye CJ: A prospective study of adhesive capsulitis of the shoulder ("frozen shoulder") in a high risk population. Q J Med 50:191–204, 1981.
67. Jayson MI: Frozen shoulder adhesive capsulitis. Br Med J [Clin Res] 283:1005–1006, 1981.
68. Lequesne M, Dang N, Bensasson M, et al: Increased association of diabetes mellitus with capsulitis of the shoulder and shoulder hand syndrome. Scand J Rheumatol 6:53, 1977.
69. Bridgman JF: Periarthritis of the shoulder and diabetes mellitus. Ann Rheum Dis 31:69, 1972.
70. Kay NR: The clinical diagnosis and management of frozen shoulders. Practitioner 225:164–167, 1981.
71. Neviaser RJ: Painful conditions affecting the shoulder. Clin Orthop 173:63–69, 1983.
72. Grey RG: The natural history of "idiopathic" frozen shoulder. J Bone Joint Surg 60:564–1978.
73. Binder AI, Bulgen DY, Hazleman BL, et al: Frozen shoulder: an arthographic and radionuclear scan assessment. Ann Rheum Dis 43:365–369, 1984.
74. Post M, ed: The Shoulder: Surgical and Nonsurgical Management. Philadelphia: Lea & Febiger, 1978.
75. Helbig B, Wagner P, Dohler R: Mobilization of frozen shoulder under anaesthesia. Acta Orthop Belg 49:267–274, 1983.
76. Neviaser RJ: Lesions of the biceps and tendinitis of the shoulder. Orthop Clin North Am 11:343–348, 1980.
77. Simon WJ: Soft tissue disorders of the shoulder: frozen shoulder, calcific tendinitis, and bicipital tendinitis. Orthop Clin North Am 6:521–539, 1975.
78. Curwin S, Stanish WD: Tendinitis: Its Etiology and Treatment, Lexington, MA: Collamore Press, 1984.
79. Neer CS: Impingement lesions. Clin Orthop 173:70–77, 1983.
80. Jobe FW, Moynes DR: Delineation of diagnostic criteria and a rehabilitation program for rotator cuff injuries. Am J Sports Med 10(6):336–339, 1982.
81. Hawkins RJ, Abrams JS: Impingement syndrome in the absence of rotator cuff tear. Orthop Clin North Am 18(3):377, 1987.
82. Neer CS II: Anterior acromioplasty for the chronic impingement syndrome in the shoulder: a preliminary report. J Bone Joint Surg [Am] 54:41–50, 1972.
83. Ellman J: Arthroscopic sub-acromial depression. Orthop Trans 9(1):48, 1985.
84. Hawkins RJ, Brock RM, Abrams JS, et al: Acromioplasty for impingement with an intact rotator cuff. J Bone Joint Surg [Br], 70:795–797, 1988.
85. Blackburn TA: Throwing injuries to the shoulder. *In* (Donatelli RA, ed). Physical Therapy of the Shoulder, 2nd ed. New York: Churchill-Livingstone, 1991.
86. Blazina M, Kerlan RK, Jobe FW, et al: Jumper's knee. Orthop Clin North Am 4:665–678, 1973.
87. Penny JN, Welsh RP: Shoulder impingement syndromes in athletes and their surgical management. Am J Sports Med 9:11–15, 1981.
88. Dines D, Warren RF, Inglis AE: Surgical treatment of lesions of the long head of the biceps. Clin Orthop, 164:165–171, 1982.
89. Del Pizzo W, Norwood LA, Jobe RW, et al: Rupture of the biceps tendon in gymnastics: a case report. Am J Sports Med, 6:283–286, 1978.
90. Odonohue DH: Subluxing biceps tendon in the athlete. J Sports Med 1:20–29, 1973.
91. Gordon EJ: Diagnosis and treatment of common shoulder disorders, Med Trial Tech Q 28:25–73, 1981.
92. De Palma AF, Flannery GF: Acute anterior dislocations of the shoulder. J Sports Med 1:6–15, 1973.
93. Henry JH: How I manage dislocated shoulder. Physician Sports Med 12(8):65–69, 1984.
94. Hume EL: Disorders of the shoulder. *In* Fundamentals of Orthopaedics (Gartland JJ, ed). Philadelphia: WB Saunders, 1987, pp 228–230.

95. Rowe CR: Factors related to recurrences of anterior dislocation of the shoulder. Clin Orthop 20:21, 1961.

96. Hastings DE: Recurrent subluxation of the glenohumeral joint. Am J Sports Med 9:352, 1981.

97. Aronen JG, Regan K: Decreasing the incidence of first time anterior shoulder dislocations with rehabilitation. Am J Sports Med 12:283, 1984.

98. Simonet WT, Cofield RJ: Prognosis in anterior shoulder dislocation. Am J Sports Med 12:19, 1984.

99. Rockwood CA: Dislocations about the shoulder. In Fractures (Rockwood CA, Green DP, eds). Philadelphia: JB Lippincott, 1975.

100. Hawkins RJ, Koppert G, Johnston G: Recurrent posterior instability of the shoulder. J Bone Joint Surgery [Am] 66:169–174, 1984.

101. Perry J: Normal upper extremity kinesiology. Phys Ther 58(3):265, 1978.

102. Gross RM: Arthroscopic shoulder capsulorraphy: does it work? Am J Sports Med 17:495, 1989.

103. Miller LS, Donahue JR, Good RP, et al: The Magnuson-Stack procedure for treatment of recurrent glenohumeral dislocations. Am J Sports Med 12:133–137, 1984.

104. Shively J, Johnson J: Results of modified Bristow procedure. Clin Orthop 187:150–153, 1984.

105. Paavolainen P, Bjorkenheim JM, Ahovuo J, et al: Recurrent anterior dislocations of the shoulder: results of the Eden-Hybbinette and Putti-Platt operations. Acta Orthop Scand 55:556–560, 1984.

106. Lombardo SJ, Keklan RK, Jobe FW, et al: The modified Bristow procedure for recurrent dislocation of the shoulder. J Bone Joint Surg [Am] 58:256–261, 1976.

107. Carson WG, McLeod WD, Andrews JR: Glenoid labrum tears in relation to the biceps tendon. Am J Sports Med 13:337–341, 1985.

108. Cofield RJ: Unconstrained total shoulder prostheses. Clin Orthop 173:97, 1983.

109. Gibson KR: Rheumatoid arthritis of the shoulder. Phys Ther 66(12):1920–1929, 1986.

110. Martel W: Roentgenographic features of the rheumatic diseases. In Primer on the Rheumatic Diseases, 8th ed. (Ordnan GP, Schumacher HR, eds). Atlanta: Arthritis Foundation, 1983, pp 174–183.

111. Glick JM, Milburn LJ, Haggerty JG, et al: Dislocated acromioclavicular joint: follow up study of 35 unreduced AC dislocations. Am J Sports Med 5:264–270, 1977.

112. Bateman JE: The Shoulder and Neck, 2nd ed. Philadelphia: WB Saunders, 1978.

113. Adams JC: Outline of Fractures, Including Joint Injuries, 9th ed. London: Churchill-Livingstone, 1987.

114. Gartland JJ: Fundamentals of Orthopaedics, 4th ed. Philadelphia: WB Saunders, 1987.

115. Cruess RL: Healing of bone, tendon and ligament. In Fractures in Adults (Rockwood CA, Green DP, eds). Philadelphia: JB Lippincott, 1984, p 147.

116. Pappas AM: Injuries of the shoulder complex and overhand throwing problems. In Clinical Sports Medicine (Grana WA, Kalenak A, eds). Philadelphia: WB Saunders, 1991, p 352.

117. Turek SL: Orthopaedics: Principles and Their Applications, 4th ed. Philadelphia: JB Lippincott, 1980.

118. Pappas AM: Injuries of the shoulder complex and overhand throwing problems. In Clinical Sports Medicine (Grana WA, Kalenak A, eds). Philadelphia: WB Saunders, 1991, p 353.

119. Reynolds MD: Myofascial trigger points in persistent posttraumatic shoulder pain. South Med J 77:1277, 1984.

120. Yunus MB, Kalyan-Roman UP, Kalyan-Roman K: Primary fibromyalgia syndrome and myofascial pain: clinical features and muscle pathology. Arch Phys Med Rehabil 69:451, 1988.

121. Howell JW: Evaluation and management of thoracic outlet syndrome. In Physical Therapy of the Shoulder, 2nd ed. (Donatelli RA, ed). New York: Churchill-Livingstone, 1991.

122. Johnson DA: Posture and cervicobrachial pain syndromes. J Am Med Assoc 159:1507, 1955.

123. Hadler NA: Medical Management of the Regional Musculoskeletal Diseases. Orlando, FL: Grune & Stratton, 1984.

124. Williams HT, Carpenter NJ: Surgical treatment of the thoracic outlet compression syndrome. Arch Surg 113:850, 1978.

125. McGough EC, Pearce MB, Byrne JP: Management of thoracic outlet syndrome. J Thorac Cardiovasc Surg 77:169, 1979.

126. Jager SH, Read R, Smullens S, et al: Thoracic outlet syndrome: diagnosis and treatment. In Rehabilitation of the Hand (Hunter J, Mackin E, Bell J, et al, eds). St. Louis: CV Mosby, 1984.

127. Akeson WH, Amiel D, Woo S: Immobility effects on synovial joints: the pathomechanics of joint contractures. Biorheology 17:95, 1980.

128. Woo S, Matthews JV, Akeson WH, et al: Connective tissue response to immobility: correlative study of biomechanical and biomechanical measurements of normal and immobilized rat knees. Arthritis Rheum 18:257, 1975.

129. Frank C, Akeson WH, Woo SL, et al: Physiology and therapeutic value of passive joint motion. Clin Orthop 185:113–125, 1984.

130. Frank C, Woo S, Amiel D, et al: Medial collateral ligament healing: a multidisciplinary assessment in rabbits. Am J Sports Med 11:379, 1983.

131. Arnoczkey S, Curwin S: Healing constraints, revascularization, and rehabilitation concerns. Presented at the Sports Physical Therapy Conference, Lake Tahoe, NV, 1990.

132. Dorland's Illustrated Medical Dictionary. Philadelphia: WB Saunders, 1977.

133. Frank C, Akeson WH, Woos S, et al: Physiology and therapeutic value of passive joint motion. Clin Orthop 185:113, 1984.

134. Donatelli RA: Mobilization of the shoulder. In Physical Therapy of the Shoulder, 2nd ed. (Donatelli RA, ed). New York: Churchill-Livingstone, 1991.

135. Saunders DH: Evaluation, Treatment, and Prevention of Musculoskeletal Disorders. Edina, MN: Educational opportunities, 1985, pp 233–238.

136. Michlovitz SL: Thermal Agents in Rehabilitation. Philadelphia, FA Davis, 1986.

137. Baker LL, Parker K: Neuromuscular electrical stimulation of the muscles surrounding the shoulder. Phys Ther 66(12):1930–1937, 1986.

138. Blackburn TA, McLeod WD: EMG analysis of posterior rotator cuff exercises. Athletic Training 25(1):40–45, 1990.

## Bibliography

Calliet R: Shoulder Pain, 3rd ed. Philadelphia: FA Davis, 1991.

Fowler P: Shoulder problems in overhead-overuse sports: swimmer problems. Am J Sports Med 7(2):141, 1979.

Hoppenfeld S: Physical Examination of the Spine and Extremities. Norwalk, CT: Appleton-Century-Crofts, 1976.

Neer CS, Watson RC, Stanton FJ: Recent experience in total shoulder replacement. J Bone Joint Surg 64(3):3119–3137, 1982.

Poppen NK, Walker PS: Forces at the glenohumeral joint in abduction. Clin Orthop 135:165, 1978.

Rathburn JB, MacNab I: The neurovascular pattern of the rotator cuff. J Bone Joint Surg [Br] 52:540–553, 1970.

Simon ER, Hill JA: Rotator cuff injuries: An update. J Orthop Sports PT 10(10), 1989.

Soderberg GL: Kinesiology. Baltimore: Williams & Wilkins, 1986.

Steindler A: Kinesiology of the Human Body. Springfield, IL: Charles C Thomas, 1966.

# CHAPTER

# *Five*

## Elbow

### SUSAN W. STRALKA / JILL G. BRASEL

## ANATOMY

Treatment of pathologic conditions of the elbow requires a complete understanding of the anatomy and kinesiology of the joint. The stability of the joint requires a combination of joint geometry and congruity, capsuloligamentous integrity, and intact balance of the musculature.[1]

Laboratory investigations have shown that 50% of elbow stability results from its bone configuration and the remaining 50% from the joint capsule medial and lateral configurations.[2]

One must know the normal anatomy of the elbow to understand the pathology and to be able to determine proper treatment. As described by Reid and Kushner, the elbow joint is a unique, multifaceted articulation between the capitulum and trochlea of the distal end of the humerus and the radial head and olecranon with the proximal radius and ulna.[3] The elbow comprises three separate joints. The ulna and the humerus form a hinge joint that allows flexion and extension of the elbow through a range of 0 to 160 degrees. The gliding joint is the radiohumeral joint, which allows flexion and extension of the forearm and pronation and supination of the radius. The third joint is the proximal radioulnar joint, which permits rotational motion of the radius around the ulna.

The joint capsule of the elbow is a thin, transparent structure that is reinforced by the radial (lateral) and ulnar (medial) collateral ligaments and reinforced anteriorly by the brachialis tendon and posteriorly by the triceps tendon. The anterior fibers attach proximally above the coronoid and radial fossae, distally to the anterior portion of the coronoid fossa and medially and laterally to the annular ligament. Posteriorly, its attachment is superior to the olecranon fossa and along the medial and lateral margins of the trochlea.[3] The anterior capsule is taut in extension and lax in flexion.

Other structures around the elbow are the synovial membrane (synovium), which lines the joint capsule, and the synovial tissue between the capitulum and the radial head. Morrey described the synovial tissue as a fold of tissue that forms the "meniscus" of the radiohumeral joint.[4] This synovial lining secretes synovia, which lubricates the joint surfaces. The "fat pad" is located between the synovium and the capsule and is the site of effusion. Because of the close relationships of the components of this complex synovial joint, injury to any part often affects other parts.

The ligaments of the elbow (lateral and medial collateral ligaments) resist and prevent excessive movements in adduction or abduction and provide sites for musculocutaneous attachments. According to Morrey, the ligaments consist of specialized thickenings of the medial and lateral capsule that form collateral ligament complexes.[4] The medial collateral ligament complex is composed of anterior, posterior, and transverse parts (Fig. 5–1). Valgus stability is provided by the medial collateral ligament, anterior capsule, and bone configuration of the elbow in extension.

Morrey described the lateral ligament complex as consisting of the radial collateral ligament, the lateral ulnar collateral ligament, the accessory lateral collateral ligament, and the annular ligament[4] (Fig. 5–2). This complex has a rather inconsistent pattern compared to the medial ligament complex.

The main muscles acting on the elbow joint are the triceps, biceps, and brachialis. The flexor group of muscles (biceps and brachialis) crosses the anterior aspect of the joint to insert into the base of the coronoid process of the ulna and into the bicipital tuberosity of the radius. The bicipital aponeurosis is a broad band of tissue composed of the anterior, medial, and distal muscle fasciae that is palpable medially when the elbow is flexed to 90 degrees. This broad band reinforces the attachment of the biceps. The biceps acts as a major flexor of the elbow and also as a supinator. Morrey states that the brachialis has the largest cross-sectional area of the elbow flexors but has a mechanical disadvantage because it crosses so close to the axis of rotation.[4] The brachialis has fibers that insert into the capsule and it assists in retracting the capsule during elbow flexion.[5]

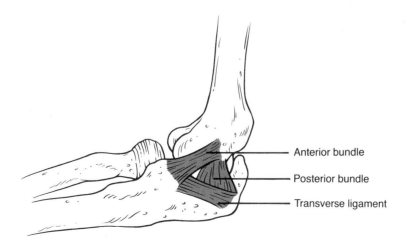

Anterior bundle

Posterior bundle

Transverse ligament

**FIGURE 5–1** ■ Medial collateral ligament including the anterior and posterior bundles and the transverse ligament.

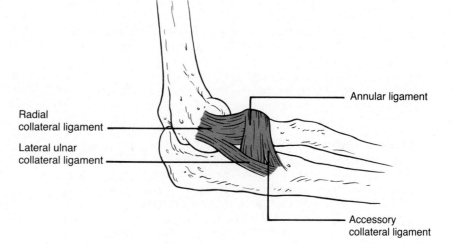

**FIGURE 5–2** ■ Radial or lateral collateral ligament.

The triceps is the main muscle on the posterior aspect of the joint. Two of its three heads originate from the posterior aspect of the humerus, and the third, long head, originates from the infraglenoid tuberosity. All three heads blend in the midline of the humerus to form a common muscle that attaches through a tendon to the tip of the olecranon. Like the biceps, the triceps has a layer of fascial reinforcement distally. The primary function of the triceps at the elbow is to extend the elbow. According to Basmajian and DeLuca, the medial head of the triceps seems to be the most consistent in its action on the extension mechanism of the elbow.[6] The long and lateral heads provide extra strength for extension but are only minimally active in low-power movements. The strength of the triceps is reinforced when the elbow and shoulder are extended simultaneously. Smith described the triceps fascia as being similar to the fascia expansions of the knee.[7] Thus, during elbow extension the synovium is pulled away, avoiding impingement.

Other muscle groups around the elbow are the supinator and pronators. The supinator, is characterized by its absence of tendinous tissue and its complex attachment (three sets above and below the elbow). The supinator allows the radius to rotate around the ulna and is best tested with the elbow in 90 degrees of flexion to rule out biceps and prevent shoulder substitution. Morrey states that the supinator is weaker than the biceps in comparison to its function as a supinator.[4] The pronator teres and pronator quadratus are the pronators of the elbow and allow the radius to rotate around the ulna.

# EVALUATION

## Observation

The three articulations (humeroulnar, humeroradial, and radioulnar) of the elbow and the soft tissues surrounding them should be examined.

### Carrying Angle

A normal carrying angle is present at the elbow along the longitudinal axis in anatomic position with the arm extended. This angle normally is approximately 5 degrees in men and 10 to 15 degrees in women.[8] An increased carrying angle (cubitus valgus) can be caused by a lateral epicondylar fracture that damages the epiphysis, which may also lead to delayed ulnar nerve palsy. A decreased carrying angle (cubitus varus), also called a gunstock deformity, is often caused by trauma, such as a supracondylar fracture in a child that results in malunion or growth retardation of the epiphyseal plate. Carrying angles should be bilaterally symmetric.

### Swelling

Localized swelling is most often seen as a specific mass confined to a limited area. It is generally contained within the joint capsule or bursa and does not extravasate into nearby tissue.

## Palpation

### Bone Palpation

Check for pain, swelling, temperature elevation, and crepitation with elbow range of motion. Crepitation may indicate synovial or bursal thickening, or it may be secondary to fracture or osteoarthritis.

**Medial epicondyle.** It is covered by the wrist flexors and is often fractured in children.[8]

**Medial supracondylar line of the humerus.** Palpate linearly for any excess bone that may trap the median nerve and cause symptoms of compression of the nerve.

**Olecranon.** Elbow flexion exposes the olecranon from its fossa; it is covered by the olecranon bursa and triceps tendon.

**Lateral epicondyle.** It is prominent but smaller than the medial epicondyle.

**Radial head.** Palpate with the patient's arm abducted and elbow flexed to 90 degrees. It is found in a depression about 1 inch distal to the lateral epicondyle and just posteromedial to the wrist extensor muscle group. The radial head rolls under the palpating fingers with slow pronation and supination.

The capitulum and the radial notch in which the radial head lies are not palpable. Pain in this area may indicate synovitis or osteoarthritis of the radial head itself.

### Soft Tissue Palpation

Four clinical zones (described by Hoppenfeld[8]) are used in examining the soft tissue surrounding the elbow. Throughout the examination, position the patient's elbow near 90 degrees of flexion with slight shoulder abduction to make the structures more accessible for palpation.

ZONE I—MEDIAL ASPECT

**Ulnar nerve.** Palpate between the medial epicondyle and the olecranon process. Gently check to see if it can be displaced from the groove as it is rolled under the index and middle fingers. Scar tissue buildup, which can cause nerve compression leading to paresthesias in the ulnar distribution of the hand, may feel like a thickening in this area.

**Wrist flexor-pronator group.** This group comprises the pronator teres, flexor carpi radialis, palmaris longus, and flexor carpi ulnaris. These muscles originate from the medial

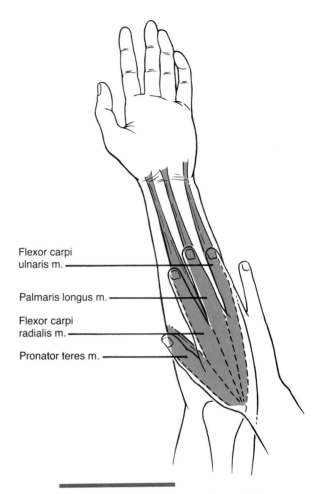

Flexor carpi ulnaris m. ——

Palmaris longus m. ——

Flexor carpi radialis m. ——

Pronator teres m. ——

**FIGURE 5-3** ■ Wrist flexors and pronators.

epicondyle as a common tendon, then split and continue into the forearm (Fig. 5–3). An easy way to remember the order of the muscles is to place one hand on the opposite forearm with the thenar eminence on the medial epicondyle and spread the fingers down the forearm. The thumb represents the pronator teres, the index finger the flexor carpi radialis, the middle finger the palmaris longus, and the ring finger the flexor carpi ulnaris. Check for tenderness, which may be due to strains caused by flexion-pronation activities such as tennis, golf, and using a screwdriver. Note that the palmaris longus bisects the anterior aspect of the wrist. To palpate it, have the patient flex the wrist and appose the tips of the thumb and little finger. This muscle is absent in about 70% of the population and is found unilaterally in many people.[8] Its absence does not hinder function. It is frequently used as a tendon graft for traumatized flexor tendons.

**Medial collateral ligament.** It runs from the medial epicondyle to the medial aspect of the ulna's trochlear notch. It stabilizes the humeroulnar articulation. It cannot be palpated directly, but the area in which it lies should be checked for tenderness caused by sprains resulting from forced valgus stress.

**Supracondylar lymph nodes.** Palpate at the medial supracondylar line. These nodes may be enlarged if the hand or wrist is infected.

### ZONE II — POSTERIOR ASPECT

**Olecranon bursa.** It is not distinctly palpable. If olecranon bursitis is present, the area feels boggy and thick. Explore the areas along the posterior ulnar border for rheumatoid nodules.

**Triceps.** The long head crosses both the glenohumeral joint and the elbow, so the triceps is a two-joint muscle. It lies subcutaneously on the posteromedial aspect of the arm. The lateral head lies on the posterolateral aspect. The medial head is deep and lies under the long head, but it can be palpated at the distal end of the humerus. Check the triceps aponeurosis for tenderness or defects secondary to trauma at the proximal end of the olecranon process.

### ZONE III — LATERAL ASPECT

**Wrist extensors.** Three muscles make up the wrist extensor group: brachioradialis, extensor carpi radialis longus (ECRL), and extensor carpi radialis brevis (ECRB). They are often called the "extensor wad" or the "mobile wad of three."[8] The brachioradialis originates from the lateral supracondylar ridge and is easily identifiable on the anterolateral aspect of the arm. This is the only muscle in the body that extends from the distal end of one bone to the distal end of another. Although anatomically it is part of the wrist extensor group, it functions as an elbow flexor.

   **ECRL and ECRB.** Resisted wrist ~~flexion~~ ext. makes these muscles more prominent for palpation just proximal to the second and third metacarpals.

**Lateral collateral ligament.** This rope-like structure extends from the lateral epicondyle to the side of the annular ligament. After a strain resulting from sudden varus stress, this ligament is tender.

**Annular ligament.** This ligament is attached to the lateral collateral ligament and encircles the radial head and neck, holding them in place as they articulate with the ulna.

### ZONE IV — ANTERIOR ASPECT

**Cubital fossa.** This is a triangular space bordered by the brachioradialis laterally and the pronator teres medially. The base is defined by an imaginary line drawn between the two humeral epicondyles. The structures that pass through the fossa, from lateral to medial, are the biceps tendon, brachial artery, median nerve, and musculocutaneous nerve. To palpate the biceps tendon, which lies just medial to the brachioradialis, have the patient resist elbow flexion and forearm supination. The medial expansion of the biceps tendon crosses the wrist flexor group. A biceps tendon ruptures when the elbow has been forcibly ~~flexed~~ ext. against strong resistance. The antecubital fossa becomes tender and the tendon is not palpable. The muscle forms a bulbous swelling in the upper arm.

**Brachial artery.** The pulse of the brachial artery can be palpated directly medial to the biceps tendon.

**Median nerve.** The median nerve is a tubular structure just medial to the brachial artery. Its course passes through the pronator teres as it enters the forearm on the way to the hand.

**Musculocutaneous nerve.** This nerve is just lateral to the biceps tendon and provides sensation in the forearm. A hyperextension injury leading to a sprain in the anterior joint capsule can cause tenderness in this area. The nerve is not palpable.

## Range of Motion

**Flexion.** Normal range of motion is 135+ degrees. Elbow flexion is normally limited by muscles, primarily the biceps brachii, on the anterior aspect of the arm.

**Extension.** The range of motion in normal extension has a bony end feel when the olecranon fossa meets the olecranon. Range of motion is normally zero, but many women can hyperextend the elbow as much as 5 degrees.

**Supination.** Normal range of motion is 85 to 90

degrees and is best tested with 90 degrees of elbow flexion and the arm held next to the body to prevent substitution. Supination is limited by the degree to which the radius can rotate over the ulna.

**Pronation.** Normal pronation has the same bone limitation as supination. It is tested in the same position as supination and should be 90 degrees from neutral.

## Neurologic Examination

Perform muscle tests, reflex tests, and sensation tests.

### Muscle Tests

Perform manual muscle tests on the elbow flexors and extensors and the forearm supinators and pronators to assess C-5 to T-1, as shown in the following chart.

### Reflex Tests

■ Biceps reflex—C-6
■ Brachioradialis reflex—C-6
■ Triceps reflex—C-7

By testing these three reflexes, the integrity of the nerve supply to the elbow can be further assessed.

### Sensation Tests

Sensation in the area surrounding the elbow is controlled by four nerve supplies (Fig. 5–4):

■ C-5: sensory branches of axillary nerve—lateral arm
■ C-6: sensory branches of musculocutaneous nerve—lateral forearm
■ C-8: antebrachial cutaneous nerve—medial forearm
■ T-1: brachial cutaneous nerve—medial arm

# MUSCLE TESTS

| | | |
|---|---|---|
| Flexion | Brachialis | Musculocutaneous nerve C5-6 |
| | Biceps | |
| | Brachioradialis | Radial nerve C-6 |
| | Supinator | Radial nerve C-6 |
| Extension | Triceps | Radial nerve C-7 |
| | Anconeus | |
| Supination | Biceps | Musculocutaneous nerve C5-6 |
| | Supinator | Radial nerve C-6 |
| Pronation | Pronator teres | Median nerve C-6 |
| | Pronator quadratus | Anterior interosseous branch of median nerve C-8, T-1 |
| | Flexor carpi radialis | Median nerve C-7 |

## Special Tests

**Ligament tests.** To assess the integrity of the medial and lateral collateral ligaments, varus and valgus stress tests may be performed.

**Tinel's sign.** Tapping the area of the ulnar nerve in the groove between the olecranon and the medial epicondyle elicits a tingling sensation down the forearm if a neuroma is present. The area may also be tender normally.

**Tennis elbow test.** The pain of tennis elbow may be reproduced at the site of the common extensor origin. Resistance to wrist ex-

tension is applied after the patient has made a fist and extended the wrist.

## Examination of Related Areas

The wrist, shoulder, and cervical spine can refer symptoms to the elbow. Shoulder and wrist pathology may refer pain into the elbow because there are two-joint muscles crossing the elbow (both wrist flexors and extensors and biceps brachii and triceps). Pain may be referred into the elbow area from a herniated cervical disc or os-

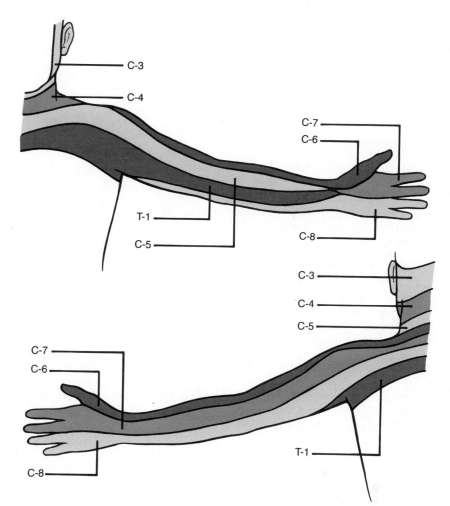

**FIGURE 5–4** ■ Dermatome chart of the upper limb.

teoarthritic changes in the cervical spine. Pain precipitated by physical exertion and relieved by rest, specifically in the left arm and elbow, may suggest angina.

After any examination, the patient should be warned of the possibility of exacerbation of symptoms as a result of the evaluation.

## FRACTURES AND DISLOCATIONS OF THE ELBOW IN ADULTS

### Distal Humeral Fractures

Because of the congruence of the joint, the relationship of the ligaments and muscles to the articular surface, and the sensitivity of the joint capsule and soft tissue to trauma, distal humeral fractures are difficult to treat. According to Bryan and Morrey, the results of operative treatment with internal fixation are almost invariably disappointing, with most patients experiencing limitation of motion.[9]

### Extra-articular Fractures

Extension fractures are most commonly caused by a fall on the outstretched hand.[9] Displacement of the proximal fragment may result in damage to nerves or blood vessels, and proximal posterior displacement of the distal fragment may occur because of the pull of the triceps muscle. Flexion injuries are less common and occur most often in elderly people because of a fall; younger people react more quickly and instinctively to protect themselves in a fall. This fracture is potentially unstable and becomes an intra-articular fracture as the fracture line extends across the supracondylar columns. The brachial artery and the median and radial nerves are at risk.

## Intra-articular Fractures

Unlike extra-articular injuries, these fractures frequently require open reduction and internal fixation. Intra-articular fractures of the distal humerus include T and Y condylar, lateral and medial condylar, capitular, and trochlear fractures.

## Complications

Serious complications are often associated with distal humeral fractures. They include loss of motion, which is probably the most common, nerve injury, malunion, nonunion, instability, vascular injury, and myositis ossificans.

Factors leading to decreased motion are

- Soft tissue fibrosis and scarring (surgical trauma, prolonged immobilization, and damage to the anterior capsule also contribute to soft tissue fibrosis)
- Development of myositis ossificans
- Articular malalignment
- Excessive callus formation
- Improper placement of internal fixation

Malunion and excessive callus formation, usually involving the supracondylar bone and fossa, may compromise the characteristic close fit of this joint.

Insult to all three nerves can occur, either because of the trauma or during manipulation or surgery. Tardy ulnar nerve palsy is classically associated with increased valgus angulation at the elbow, especially after lateral type II condylar fractures as described by Milch.[10] Usual symptoms include paresthesia, atrophy, paralysis of some motor function, pain, and anesthesia.

Myositis ossificans occurs most commonly after fracture-dislocations, especially with radial head involvement. This is discussed earlier, but it is important to emphasize that early active motion is unlikely to contribute to the development of this complication, whereas aggressive passive motion or massage often leads to myositis ossificans.

## Olecranon Fractures

Olecranon fractures are generally classified as displaced, nondisplaced, or comminuted. They result primarily from a direct fall on the elbow or a hyperextension force that also dislocates the joint. Soft tissue swelling is present posteriorly, proximal to the olecranon. Although uncommon, tendon rupture may occur as the triceps contracts to decelerate a fall on the outstretched hand, leaving flecks of bone avulsed from the olecranon in the soft tissues.

## Radial Head Fractures

Radial head fractures account for approximately one third of all fractures about the elbow and for about 18% of all elbow trauma, making them the most common elbow injury in adults.[11] Most radial head fractures are caused by a fall on the outstretched hand with the elbow partially flexed and the forearm supinated. Radial head fractures are commonly classified in three categories described by Mason and Shutkins:[12]

- Type I—undisplaced
- Type II—displaced (a marginal fracture, often a single fragment, with displacement of more than 3 cm)
- Type III—comminuted

Morrey described a type IV radial head fracture with elbow dislocation that occurs in about 10% of patients with radial head fractures and is treated differently from other types[4] (see Elbow Dislocations).

### Type I Fractures

Type I fractures are typically immobilized for 2 to 3 weeks, although more recently early motion has been instituted to allow faster return of function and greater end motion. Displacement after early motion, however, has led to some treatment failures.

### Type II Fractures

Radial head resection in type II fractures is justified, although it is not necessarily preferable to nonoperative treatment. Radial head resection is recommended if 30% of the head is involved and displacement is greater than 2 to 3 mm and causes significant loss of range of motion (30 degrees or more).

### Type III Fractures

Type III fractures are usually severe injuries involving the capsule, ligaments, and capitulum. Complete radial head excision is usually recommended rather than removal of only the more displaced fragments. Results are variable, and many patients do not regain full extension, flexion, supination, or pronation. Few attempts have been made to compare different treatment methods, but persistent rehabilitation, including complete upper extremity weight training and continual range-of-motion efforts, has produced good results in our patients.

## Elbow Dislocations

### Fracture-Dislocations

Radial head fractures occur in approximately 10% of elbow dislocations (type IV), and the reverse is also true.[13] Treatment involves immediate reduction of the dislocation and treatment of the fractured radial head based on the degree of severity. Early excision of the radial head is usually performed to avoid the development of myositis ossificans. McLaughlin emphasized that if surgery is necessary it should be done within 24 hours of injury.[14] The outcome of type IV fracture-dislocations appears to be related to the period of immobilization. If immobilization continues longer than 4 weeks, 15 to 30 degrees loss of extension and 25 to 30 degrees loss of rotation may be expected. Early motion, beginning by the sixth day after surgery, has improved the outcome, resulting in approximately 10 to 140 degrees of extension in most patients.

### Dislocation Without Fracture

Falls on an outstretched hand are responsible for most dislocations (Fig. 5–5). Less common mechanisms of injury include direct trauma and motor vehicle accidents. Dislocations are classified as posterior, anterior, recurrent, and divergent. Posterior dislocations are by far the most frequent. Recurrent dislocations result from insufficient healing of the capsular and ligamentous restraints, primarily the posterolateral capsule, which allows dislocation with forces much less than those responsible for the initial injury. In divergent dislocations the radius becomes displaced from the ulna, with concomitant dislocation of the humeroulnar joint. This is associated with severe trauma and is a rare injury.

Treatment of elbow dislocations in adults should be focused on prompt restoration of the articular alignment of the elbow without causing further damage. Neurovascular complications and associated musculoskeletal injuries must not be overlooked. Early return to functional activity is the goal and is achieved by careful prereduction evaluation.

Results of treatment of uncomplicated dislocations are excellent. More than half of patients have satisfactory results, with no more than 15 degrees loss of flexion or extension, minimal

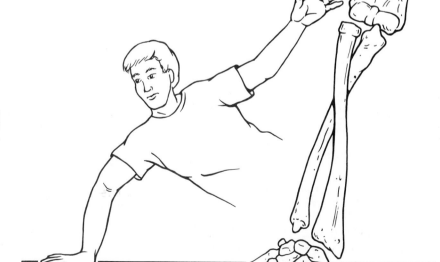

**FIGURE 5–5** ■ The mechanism of extension injury in radial head fractures is a fall on an outstretched hand.

pain, and normal stability. Approximately 15% of patients with dislocations may have complications;[13] however, continued improvement for at least 6 months is usual and some patients continue to improve for as long as 18 months. The elbow is usually immobilized in 90 degrees of flexion, which is the most stable position, for 3 to 5 weeks. More progressive rehabilitation may improve extension; otherwise, limited extension is the most common post-traumatic finding. Fortunately, instability of varus or valgus stress is rare after treatment. Neurologic problems occur in almost 20% of patients with dislocations; the ulnar nerve is most susceptible to injury.[13]

# FRACTURES AND DISLOCATIONS OF THE ELBOW IN CHILDREN

Fractures in children differ from those in adults because of the child's greater potential for bone remodeling. Children's bones are more malleable, but adults have a thicker periosteum, which helps to stabilize the reduction and decrease displacement. Nonunion is rarely a problem in children, but angular and rotational deformities are frequent.

## Distal Humeral Fractures

Fractures of the distal humerus in children are most often supracondylar or involve a single condyle. Table 5–1 shows the incidences of different types in 713 elbow fractures in children reviewed by Boyd and Altenberg.[15]

■■■■■ **TABLE 5–1.** DISTAL HUMERAL FRACTURES IN CHILDREN

| Type of Fracture | Number | Percent |
| --- | --- | --- |
| Supracondylar | 465 | 65.4 |
| Condylar | | 25.3 |
|   Lateral condyle | 124 | |
|   Medial epicondyle | 33 | |
|   Medial condyle | 23 | |
| Radial neck | 34 | 4.7 |
| Monteggia's | 16 | 2.2 |
| Olecranon | 12 | 1.6 |
| T condylar | 6 | 0.8 |

Data from Christensen JB, Telford IR: Synopsis of Gross Anatomy. Philadelphia: JB Lippincott, 1988.

Several factors complicate the treatment of distal humeral fractures in children: strong flexor and extensor muscle groups attached to the medial and lateral condyles, respectively, tend to rotate and displace the immature condyle. Treatment consists of accurate reduction and alignment of the fracture surfaces and use of wires for internal fixation. Nonunion is common after a single condyle fracture; malunion also occurs, causing changes in the carrying angle of the elbow.

## Supracondylar Fractures

Supracondylar and intercondylar fractures of the distal humerus constitute 50 to 65% of all fractures about the elbow in children.[16] The left arm is fractured more often than is the right because it is used for protection and guarding when falling. It has been reported that 98% of these fractures occur with the arm extended and the wrist dorsiflexed.

Treatment methods vary according to fracture types, but regardless of the method of treatment, Canale states that obtaining satisfactory roentgenograms to determine fracture reduction is of utmost importance.[16] The goal of any treatment method should be anatomic restoration of the humerus and resolution of any complications, with normal alignment and function. The first priority of treatment is to assess for compromised neurovascular structures and splint in a position that presents the least risk to the neurovascular structures. After the initial assessment, treatment is chosen according to the type of fracture. Choices include splinting of minimally displaced or angulated fractures, closed reduction of moderately displaced fractures with minimal to moderate swelling, traction for fractures that are severely displaced and swollen, closed reduction and percutaneous pinning for fractures that can be reduced easily but are unstable, and open reduction with pinning and splinting for open fractures and fractures with significant neurovascular compromise.

Complications, such as neurapraxia, associated with supracondylar fractures are reported to occur in 3 to 22% of patients.[16] Brachial artery injury occurs in 10% and in some cases resolves spontaneously after the fracture is reduced. Other vascular compromises, such as Volkmann's ischemia, are rare but must be considered. A frequent complication of supracondylar fractures in children is malunion with a resultant cubitus varus deformity.

## Lateral Condylar Fractures

Fracture of the lateral condyle of the humerus is the most common distal humeral epiphyseal fracture in children. According to Canale, most of these fractures occur in children approximately 6 years of age.[16]

Regardless of the classification of lateral condylar fractures, most treatment recommendations are based on the amount of displacement. For undisplaced fractures, Beaty and Wood recommend close observation with serial casting and roentgenograms for 6 to 8 weeks.[17] If any amount of displacement occurs, open reduction and internal fixation are indicated. Beaty and Wood reported union of all 32 lateral condylar fractures treated with open reduction and internal fixation and nonunion in 4 of 14 fractures (28.5%) treated by closed methods.[17] Four patients with unrecognized and untreated fractures had nonunions at long-term follow-up, with cubitus valgus deformity, weakness, loss of elbow motion, and occasional pain; three had tardy ulnar nerve palsy.

## Radial Head and Neck Fractures

A fall on the outstretched arm produces a valgus thrust at the elbow, causing radial neck fracture with or without medial avulsion injuries to other structures. O'Brien divided these fractures into three types according to the degree of angulation:[18]

**Type 1,** 0 to 30 degrees
**Type 2,** 30 to 60 degrees
**Type 3,** more than 60 degrees

In children between the ages of 4 and 14 years, radial head and neck fractures constitute 4 to 7% of all elbow fractures and dislocations.[19] The radial neck is fractured more frequently than the radial head. Fractures of the head and neck of the radius may be isolated injuries or complications of other fractures and dislocations. Reports in the literature indicate that the following principles should be considered when treating these fractures in children:

■ Closed treatment generally gives better results than open reduction.
■ If open reduction is necessary, use as little internal fixation as possible.
■ Treat promptly.

■ Do not use transcapitular wires.
■ Do not immobilize the fracture for more than 3 weeks.

If open reduction is necessary because of severe displacement, internal fixation should be performed within 5 to 7 days after the injury because myositis ossificans has been reported after delayed surgical treatment.

Complications after open reduction include loss of motion, premature physeal closure, nonunion of the radial neck, avascular necrosis of the radial head, radioulnar synostosis, and injury to the posterior interosseous nerve. Fractures with angulation of more than 45 degrees that is unreduced usually result in limited pronation and supination.[16] According to Wenge, loss of 20 degrees of supination or up to 40 degrees of pronation is not disabling when it occurs at a young age.[19] Poor results occur when loss of forearm rotation is more than 40 degrees. Loss of elbow flexion and extension has been reported to be less frequent in children than in adults; loss of extension in children is usually from 30 to 35 degrees.[19]

## Elbow Dislocations

Dislocations of the elbow account for 6 to 8% of elbow injuries in children.[16] Because of the weakness of the growth plate, epiphyseal injuries occur more frequently than dislocations. Spontaneous reduction of traumatic elbow dislocations is not uncommon, especially if the coronoid process is avulsed. Elbow dislocations in children are most often posterior (Fig. 5–6) but may be anterior, medial, or lateral. Canale[16] reports that, regardless of the type, most dislocations can be reduced closed.[16] Reduction with the patient under general anesthesia is recommended within 6 hours of injury. The reduction should be confirmed roentgenographically, especially if an associated fracture is present. After satisfactory reduction of a posterior dislocation, the elbow is immobilized in 90 degrees or more of flexion to allow the triceps to tighten posteriorly and act as a splint to prevent the ulna from slipping. As in adults, joint stiffness is the most common complication. Letts et al. recommended that a child's elbow should not be immobilized for longer than 3 to 4 weeks and that immobilization should be followed by physical therapy for elbow exercise.[16a]

Because fractures in adults and children are treated either conservatively, with a splint or

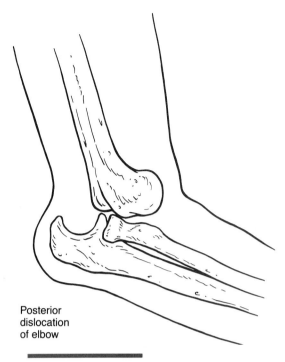

Posterior
dislocation
of elbow

**FIGURE 5–6** ■ Posterior dislocation of the elbow.

cast, or surgically, with internal fixation, each rehabilitation program is different. General treatment guidelines are discussed in the section on therapeutic intervention.

## CONGENITAL ANOMALIES

Congenital anomalies, especially congenital radial head dislocations and congenital radioulnar synostosis, may be confused with acute injuries. Congenital radial head dislocations may be distinguished from traumatic dislocations on the basis of radiographs. In patients with traumatic dislocations, the shapes of the radius and ulna are normal. The congenitally dislocated radial head is dome shaped rather than trumpet shaped. Also, the radius is longer than normal and the ulna has a concave appearance rather than a slightly convex appearance. The capitulum may be hypoplastic or absent. Congenital dislocations are most often anterior (50%) or posterior (40%) and rarely are lateral (10%).[20] Most congenital dislocations are bilateral, and they are often associated with other congenital anomalies. Some pain may be present with congenital dislocations, but most patients have minimal functional limitations.

Congenital radioulnar synostosis may be associated with rotational hypermobility of the wrist, distal ulnar subluxation, radial shaft bowing, and radial head subluxation.

## DISORDERS OF MUSCLES, TENDONS, AND LIGAMENTS ABOUT THE ELBOW

### Tendinitis or Epicondylitis

#### Lateral Epicondylitis

Most commonly involved is the extensor carpi radialis brevis (ECRB) tendon. It has proximal attachments to the lateral collateral ligament and often to the annular ligament, in addition to the lateral epicondyle of the humerus. The extensor carpi radialis longus (ECRL) and brachioradialis attach above the epicondyle, rather than the common extensor tendon insertion, and are less commonly involved. The ECRB is stretched over the radial head when the elbow is extended and fully pronated.[21] This fulcrum effect may partially explain its susceptibility to chronic inflammation at or near its attachment. In addition, the ECRB must attenuate increased stresses in the position of wrist flexion and ulnar deviation with the elbow extended and the forearm pronated. This is the same as the backhand position in tennis. At the point of contact, the extensor muscles must contract to stabilize the wrist and grip the racquet firmly. This repetitive muscle contraction, chronically overloading the ECRB in its most vulnerable position, leads to fatigue and microtrauma. Although the etiology of lateral epicondylitis is often unrelated to sports (any activity causing repeated, gradual stresses to the wrist extensors, primarily the ECRB, can lead to the acute or chronic overuse syndrome), this condition commonly is called tennis elbow, a term adopted in the late 1800s when the prevalence of lateral epicondylitis increased with greater participation in tennis. It is more prevalant in those over 35 years of age. The same stresses are applied, but with aging the tendons are less able to attenuate forces and decreased levels of glycosaminoglycans (GAG) lead to decreased extensibility.[21] The inflammatory response is an attempt to increase the rate of tissue production to compensate for the increased rate of tissue microdamage. If rehabilitation is not initiated early, treatment is more difficult and return to sport or activity is delayed.

## EVALUATION

*Onset* is usually gradual and is related to increased activity of the wrist extensors, such as grasping, pulling weeds, hammering, and tennis backhand. Occasionally a direct blow to the lateral epicondyle may initiate the inflammation of the soft tissues. Initial symptoms include a dull ache at rest, which may escalate to sharp pain during activity.

*Active movement* is generally painless, but with severe involvement pain may be felt during active wrist flexion with the elbow extended because of stretching of the ECRB.

*Passive movement,* including full wrist ~~exten~~ *flex.* ~~sion~~ with ulnar deviation, forearm pronation, and elbow extension, should reproduce the pain.

*Resisted movement* (wrist extension) with the elbow extended reproduces the pain.

*Joint play* should be full and painless.

*Palpation* elicits exquisite tenderness over the lateral epicondyle and occasionally tenderness in the muscle belly.

*Temperature* may be slightly elevated over the epicondyle.

*Inspection* is insignificant.

## TREATMENT

The goals are to restore normal, pain-free use of the extremity and to prevent recurrence, which is common when proper stresses are not applied to the tendon. Improper stresses result in formation of scar tissue during healing. Thus, the treatment objectives are as follows:

1. Resolve inflammatory process.
2. Encourage proper maturation of scar tissue and collagen formation to allow extensibility and the ability of the tendon to attenuate tensile stresses.
3. Restore normal strength and extensibility of the musculotendinous unit.

### Acute Lateral Epicondylitis

Patients with acute symptoms may have pain referred into the forearm and hand and occasionally into the lateral brachial aspect of the arm, pain at rest, and muscle spasm in response to stress with passive or resistive movement. Treatment of these patients involves progression to the chronic state by resolving the acute inflammation as follows:

1. Ice—two or three times a day over the site of inflammation.

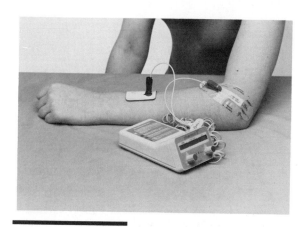

**FIGURE 5–7** ■ Iontophoresis over the lateral epicondyle for treatment of the local inflammatory process.

2. Rest—wrist immobilization (resting splint or cock-up splint). Immobilize wrist, hand, and fingers but not the elbow. Restrict activities requiring grasping, pinching, or fine finger movements, such as carpentry, tennis, or knitting.

3. Gentle active wrist flexion–forearm pronation with elbow extension stretching, in addition to general wrist and forearm range of motion, two or three times a day. The patient's brace must be removed for these exercises.

Modalities such as iontophoresis or phonophoresis may help resolve the inflammatory process (Fig. 5–7).

### Chronic Lateral Epicondylitis

1. The appropriate level of activity is determined, restricting heavy activities that stress the tendon.

2. Ultrasound assists in the resolution of inflammatory exudates by increasing the local blood flow (Fig. 5–8). A water medium may be necessary for conduction because of the uneven contour of the epicondyle.

3. Deep transverse friction massage is effective for tendinitis, generally because of the mechanically induced hyperemia and its influence on tissue maturation. Friction massage works faster with shoulder rotator cuff tendinitis because of the hypovascularity of the supraspinatus tendon, which is usually not the case at the elbow, but mechanical stimulus is necessary to promote proper orientation of immature collagen along the lines of stress, parallel to the muscle fibers. It is important for the patient to perform transverse friction massage properly because longitudinal

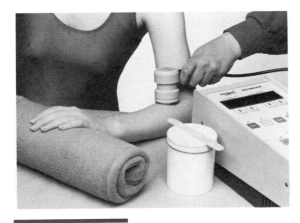

FIGURE 5-8 ■ Ultrasound used to resolve inflammatory exudates by increasing local blood flow. Phonophoresis may also be utilized.

massage or stress may cause continued rupture of fibers at the lesion site.

4. Local anti-inflammatory agents (phoresor, phorophoresis) may produce dramatic results and temporary benefit, but do not have a lasting effect on the pathologic factors.

5. Strength and mobility should be restored and the patient should gradually resume activities. Optimize tissue extensibility after ultrasound and friction massage by gently stretching into elbow extension, forearm pronation, ulnar deviation, and wrist and finger flexion. Stretching should be slow, gentle, and painless. The stretching should be continued before the activity that exacerbates the problem (e.g., tennis, gardening, carpentry (Fig. 5–9). Transverse friction massage may also help before activity. The muscles have undergone reflex inhibition and disuse atrophy. Strengthening is necessary to protect the tendon against high-strain passive loading. Many methods are available, from standard dumbbells to elastic bands (Theraband), weighted rubber balls (Plioballs), and ropes with hanging weights. Strength exercises should be comprehensive, including wrist extension and flexion, pronation, and supination and radial and ulnar deviation (Figs. 5–10 to 5–14). Both concentric and eccentric loadings should be used.

6. The patient should be taught preventive measures, including proper attire in inclement weather, proper technique and conditioning, and limiting activity after the muscles begin to fatigue. It is important not to work through the pain; otherwise, the severity of the tendinitis may increase.

In tennis players, a poor backhand stroke is a frequent cause of the problem. Typically, players who develop poor backhand technique use the elbow and wrist extensors as the power source rather than the shoulder external rotators, which professional players use.[11] The arm should begin in a position of shoulder adduction and internal rotation and elbow flexion to about 70 degrees. Tennis elbow patients often do not adduct and internally rotate the shoulder and may not pronate the forearm, which places great strain on the elbow. Other ways to relieve the strain on the elbow include trying to hit the ball in the center of the racket, keeping the elbow and wrist

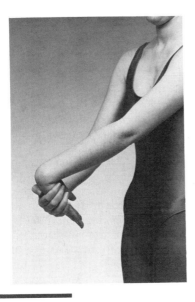

FIGURE 5-9 ■ Wrist extensor stretching for the treatment of lateral epicondylitis.

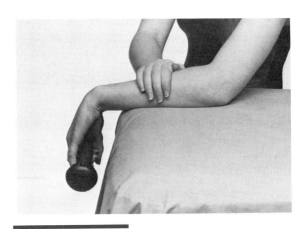

FIGURE 5-10 ■ Start position for wrist extensor strengthening starting with a stretch and working both concentrically and eccentrically.

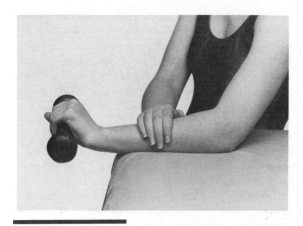

**FIGURE 5–11** ■ End position for wrist extension dumbbell exercises.

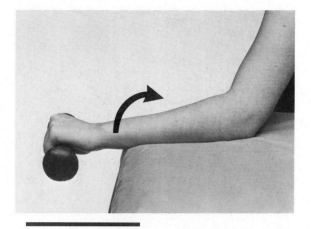

**FIGURE 5–13** ■ Dumbbell strengthening for supination.

immobile with the bony prominence toward the ground when contact is made with the ball, using a relaxed grip before ball impact, and exerting maximal pressure upon impact.[11,22] The less experienced player must learn not to grip the racket tightly through all phases of the stroke, because this places a continuous load on the extensor muscles of the forearm.[22] Using the largest grip handle that the player can grasp firmly lessens the tendency to supinate the wrist rather than readjust hand position.

Besides the tennis backhand, excessive net play can be harmful, but flexing the elbow to 70 degrees helps counteract this. Increased top spin, or "wrist curl," forehands also increase the activity of the wrist extensors. A light racket may be helpful.[11]

Counterforce bracing is designed to diminish the overload forces that lead to or prolong tennis elbow. Snyder-Mackler and Epler reported that the Aircast tennis elbow band caused a greater decrease in electromyographic function of the ECRB and the extensor digitorum communis than did a standard tennis elbow band.[23] These bands, worn over the proximal forearm, can help relieve pain during activity.

### Medial Epicondylitis

Medial epicondylitis, which is less common than lateral epicondylitis by a ratio of 7:1, is often referred to as golfer's elbow.[21] It occurs characteristically with wrist flexor activity and active pronation, as in baseball pitching, golf swings, or the pull-through phase of swimming strokes. It occurs most often in middle-aged patients involved in these sports or in occupations that require a strong hand grip and an adduction movement of the elbow.

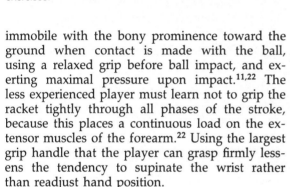

**FIGURE 5–12** ■ Dumbbell strengthening for pronation.

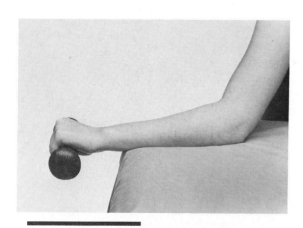

**FIGURE 5–14** ■ Dumbbell exercise for radial and ulnar deviation.

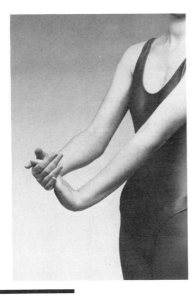

FIGURE 5-15 ■ Wrist flexor stretching for treatment of medial epicondylitis.

The primary muscles involved are the pronator teres and flexor carpi radialis and occasionally the palmaris longus, flexor carpi ulnaris, and flexor digitorum superficialis. Compression neurapraxia of the ulnar groove causes similar symptoms.

Stretches should be performed with the elbow extended and wrist and fingers dorsiflexed (Fig. 5-15). The muscles to be strengthened, as in lateral epicondylitis, should include elbow flexors, extensors, forearm pronators and supinators, and wrist flexors in particular. Inclusion of eccentric training is important.

## Triceps Tendinitis

Triceps tendinitis occurs at the attachment of the triceps to the olecranon. Typically, it flares up after sudden severe strain as the arm is fully extended (javelin throwers) or with sudden snapping of elbow extension as in the end phase of the crawl or backstroke in swimming. Pain is reproduced by resisting elbow extension from a starting position of elbow flexion and forearm supination.

## Bursitis

The olecranon bursa lies between the superior olecranon and the skin. It may become inflamed because of trauma, inflammatory disease such as gout, or, most often, prolonged pressure. Students, carpenters, desk workers, and others whose tasks involve constant pressure on the elbow often have olecranon bursitis. Infection must be ruled out by the physician. Cortisone injections and protective padding are treatments of choice. Relative rest is advisable unitl the inflammatory process subsides.

## Postimmobilization Capsular Tightness

Capsular restriction at the elbow is usually seen after immobilization. Less frequently it is caused by arthritis (inflammatory or rheumatoid arthritis more often than traumatic arthritis). Elbow immobilization, usually in 90 degrees of flexion, is common in the management of humeral shaft fractures, supracondylar fractures, Colles' fractures, and elbow dislocations.

### Treatment

Most capsular restrictions are managed as chronic conditions because the period of immobilization after injury allows the acute inflammatory process to subside. Treatment of acute capsulitis should be designed to decrease pain and to guard the muscle. Ice, superficial heat, and electrical stimulation are beneficial in decreasing pain, guarding the muscle, and gently increasing the range of motion.

For chronic capsulitis, ultrasound should be used over tight capsular tissues before or during capsular stretching with joint play movements. Progression to prolonged stretches is allowed as tolerated and strengthening activities are increased.

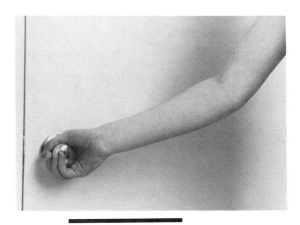

FIGURE 5-16 ■ Doorknob stretch.

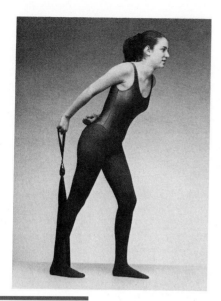

FIGURE 5-17 ■ Theraband triceps-strengthening exercise.

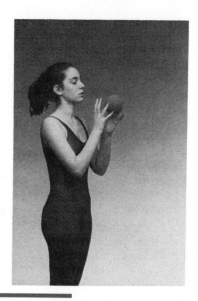

FIGURE 5-19 ■ Rebounding with 2- to 3-pound Plioball overhead.

Use of a dynamic extension splint should also be considered. We have found low-load dynamic splints (Dynasplint) to be especially effective in resolving flexion contractures. It can be placed on the arm immediately after treatment to maintain gains in range of motion or it can be used as a night splint, slowly increasing the tension to tolerance. The prolonged splinting should be painless. If soreness lasts longer than 2 hours or

the following day, the tension should be decreased.

Exercises to increase elbow extension include the following:

■ Doorknob stretch (Fig. 5-16).
■ Triceps strengthening exercise. Stabilize shoulder while patient performs active extension with Theraband and/or dumbbells (Fig. 5-17).
■ Hanging from bar, using hand helper by Theraband for assistance (Fig. 5-18).
■ Rebounding or throwing with 2- to 3-pound Plioballs overhead (Figs. 5-19 and 5-20).
■ With patient supine, elbow in a stretched position of extension, and ice or superficial heat over anterior musculature and joint capsule before and after treatment, use of Theraband tied around wrist and to the table or of a small Velcro wrist weight (Fig. 5-21).
■ Contraction-relaxation muscle inhibition techniques (Fig. 5-22).
■ Passive mode, slow oscillations with Kincom or other available robotic dynamometer (Fig. 5-23).

Exercises to increase elbow flexion include the following:

■ Gravity-assisted active flexion in supine position. Shoulder flexed to 90 degrees, with 2- to 3-pound Velcro wrist weight (Fig. 5-24).
■ Contraction-relaxation, gentle stretching (Fig. 5-25).

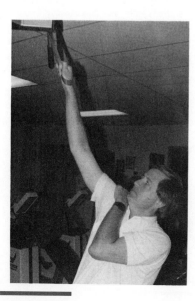

FIGURE 5-18 ■ Hanging from bar, using hand helper by Theraband for assistance.

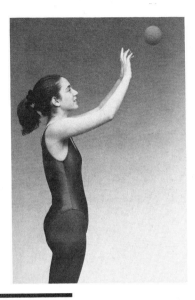

**FIGURE 5–20** ■ Throwing with 2- to 3-pound Plioball overhead.

- Self-stretching while prone on elbows (Fig. 5–26).
- Rebounding with 2- to 3-pound Plioballs with emphasis on catching (Fig. 5–27).

## Biceps Brachii Muscle Rupture

Rupture rarely occurs in the substance of the biceps brachii muscle unless the muscle has been lacerated. Usually, ruptures occur at the musculotendinous or tendo-osseous juncture. Function of the biceps is difficult to predict after a substance rupture caused by a laceration because of

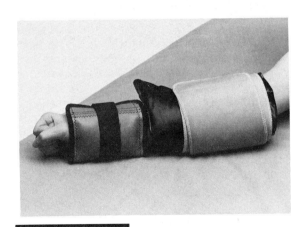

**FIGURE 5–21** ■ Utilization of ice packs and wrist Velcro weights over anterior musculature and joint capsule after treatment.

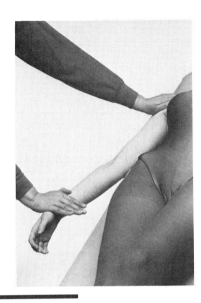

**FIGURE 5–22** ■ Contraction-relaxation muscle inhibition techniques for extension.

the loss of muscle-generated tension. According to Phillips, the ability of a muscle to generate tension and contractility after an untreated sharp laceration is approximately 50% and after repair of the laceration is 66%.[24] Scar tissue fills in the defect and myoneural function is limited if the scar tissue is binding.

A widely accepted nonsurgical way to manage biceps brachii muscle ruptures is placing the arm in a Velpeau bandage with the elbow flexed 90 degrees or more for 3 to 6 weeks until healing is secured. If surgery is necessary to close the biceps lesion, it is desirable to limit the number of adhesions of the muscle to the skin by making an anterolateral incision parallel to the lateral

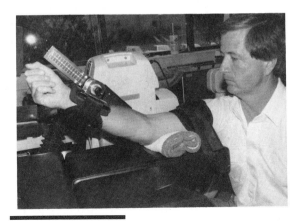

**FIGURE 5–23** ■ Passive mode, slow oscillations with Kincom or other robotic dynamometer.

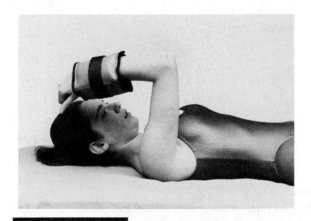

FIGURE 5-24 ■ Gravity-assisted active flexion in supine position. Shoulder flexed to 90 degrees, 2- to 3-pound Velcro wrist weight.

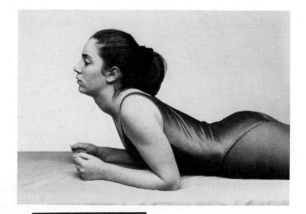

FIGURE 5-26 ■ Self-stretch while prone on elbows.

aspect of the biceps and then suturing the ruptured muscle with interrupted mattress sutures of medium-size nonabsorbable material.

## Proximal Tendon Rupture

Gilcreest reported that more than 50% of biceps brachii ruptures occur through the tendon of the long head and are located within the proximal part of the intertubercular groove or within the shoulder.[25]

Treatment of ruptures of the proximal biceps tendon has been, for the most part, based on clinical observations (Figs. 5-28 and 5-29) and

determined by the age and activity level of the patient. Generally accepted guidelines are that conservative treatment is appropriate for ruptures in middle-aged and older patients and that surgical repair is needed for younger, more athletic patients (B.B. Phillips, personal communication, 1992). Neer,[26] Hawkins and Kennedy,[27] and Dines et al.[28] recommended conservative treatment for middle-aged patients because of their clinical observations that the ruptures caused little loss of strength and because surgical repair has a 30% failure rate.[1-3] Neviaser and Neviaser suggested surgical repair for all healthy, vigorous athletes to restore as much power as possible; they did not indicate a specific age group.[29] Postacchini noted that surgical repair improved the

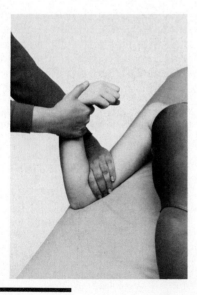

FIGURE 5-25 ■ Contraction-relaxation, gentle stretching for flexion.

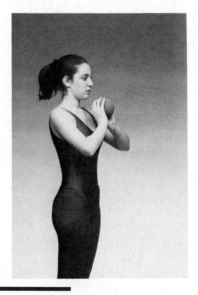

FIGURE 5-27 ■ Rebounding with 2- to 3-pound Plioball with emphasis on catching.

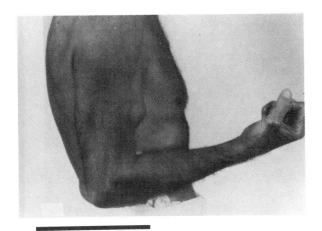

**FIGURE 5-28** ■ Proximal biceps rupture, involved arm.

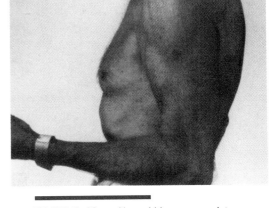

**FIGURE 5-29** ■ Normal biceps musculature.

power of elbow flexion and forearm supination and reduced or abolished the cosmetic defect in 12 patients with complete ruptures.[30] According to Watson-Jones, surgical repair of a rupture of the long head of the biceps is not necessary but is usually desirable for both functional and cosmetic reasons.[31]

Few objective data have been reported to substantiate these clinical impressions used as guidelines for treatment. Soto-Hall and Stroot used a tensiometer to test an unspecified number of patients with biceps ruptures.[32] For recent ruptures, they found 20% loss of elbow flexion power and 17% weakness in shoulder abduction in external rotation. For late ruptures, there was no appreciable weakness. Warren used a Cybex isokinetic dynamometer to evaluate 10 patients 2 years after biceps tendon rupture. He found no statistically significant loss of elbow flexion but found approximately 10% loss of strength in forearm supination.[33] Mariani et al. tested 27 patients with a torque cell dynamometer and found statistically significant differences between surgical

and nonsurgical groups only in elbow flexion and forearm supination strength.[34]

We compared the results of nonoperative and operative treatment of biceps tendon ruptures in middle-aged patients to determine the validity of these observations. Subjective evaluation, clinical evaluation, and objective testing were used. Of 25 patients with an average age of 69 years who were evaluated subjectively (19 personally and 6 by telephone) at an average of 7.9 years after injury, only one had any complaint related to the biceps tendon: a 73-year-old woman who was dissatisfied with the cosmetic defect. Despite their age, these patients continue to be active; nine still participate in sports activities including golf, tennis, handball, and weightlifting. Clinical examination and objective testing of 19 patients (average age 67.2 years) showed little difference between those treated surgically (7 patients) and those treated without surgery (12 patients) (Table 5-2). Manual muscle testing also showed no significant differences between the two groups (Table 5-3). The functional result after rupture

**■■■■■ Table 5-2.** CLINICAL EXAMINATION

| Observation | With Tenodesis (n = 7) | Without Tenodesis (n = 12) |
|---|---|---|
| Impingement | 4 (57%) | 7 (58%) |
| Bicipital groove tenderness | 1 (14%) | 5 (42%) |
| Normal range of motion | 5 (71%) | 5 (42%) |
| Manual muscle testing | | |
|   Shoulder abduction in external rotation | 4/5 strength | 4/5 strength |
|   Forearm supination | 4/5 strength | 4/5 strength |
| Cybex average deficit | 10.3% (range 0-20%) | 6.1% (range -46-36%) |

From Phillips B, et al: Ruptures of the proximal biceps tendon in middle-aged patients. Ortho Rev 22 (3), 1993.

■■■■ **Table 5–3.** MANUAL MUSCLE TESTING

| Grade | Forearm Supination of Involved Extremity | |
| | *With Tenodesis* | *Without Tenodesis* |
| --- | --- | --- |
| Normal | 3 | 5 |
| Good + | 2 | 1 |
| Good | 1 | 4 |
| Good − | 1 | 2 |

appears to be more closely related to rehabilitation than to the treatment method.

We had hoped to determine whether surgery was indicated for younger patients and athletic older patients. However, there were almost no younger people with biceps tendon ruptures and few of the ruptures in older patients were caused by athletic activity. Our results indicate that the middle-aged and older patients with biceps tendon ruptures function quite well in activities of daily living, whether they are treated nonoperatively or operatively. All 25 of our patients were satisfied with the functional results related specifically to biceps function, and only one was dissatisfied with cosmetic results. Whether surgical repair is indicated for young, athletic patients could not be answered by this study. It appears, however, that conservative treatment is appropriate for biceps tendon ruptures in middle-aged and older patients unless pain or limitation of function dictates surgical intervention for associated shoulder disorders.

## SPORTS-RELATED INJURIES IN CHILDREN

Elbow injuries in young children are usually traumatic and result in fractures and dislocations, whereas during the adolescent years most elbow problems are caused by overuse, especially in adolescents involved in repetitive throwing activities.[16] Four types of injuries that result from throwing are common in adolescents:[16]

■ Traction apophysitis of the medial epicondyle
■ Avulsion of the medial epicondyle
■ Osteochondrosis of the capitulum
■ Osteochondritis dissecans of the capitellum

These injuries occur through a valgus stress mechanism in which the medial collateral ligament may be stretched, causing apophysitis or avulsion of the medial epicondyle. On the lateral side the valgus stress produces compression, which may cause osteochondrosis or osteochondritis dissecans of the capitulum or even secondary changes in the radial head.

## Acute Valgus Stress Syndrome

In young athletes who throw, repetitive valgus stress and flexor forearm muscle pull can produce a stress fracture through the medial epicondylar epiphysis. Physical signs of this syndrome include decreased range of motion, usually more than 15 degrees, and tenderness over the medial epicondyle. Progressive pain and decreases in throwing distance and accuracy are also indicative of acute valgus stress syndrome. Adams[35] originally described these injuries as "Little League" elbow, and the term has become common, although many argue that most children with these overuse problems develop then when they are older than Little League age. Whether the problems begin in Little League and cause symptoms later is unknown. Regardless of the age at which the injury occurs, chronic repetitive valgus stress from throwing-type activities produces orthopaedic problems in adolescent athletes.

## Medial Epicondylar Fracture

Fractures of the medial epicondyle are caused by more forceful valgus stress, usually resulting from a fall or a violent muscular contracture. This fracture is usually through the epiphyseal plate, and the child complains of pain and tenderness over the medial epicondyle with inability to extend the elbow completely (Fig. 5–30).

## Medial Epicondylitis and Avulsion of the Medial Epicondyle

The early treatment of medial epicondylitis and stress lesions of the child's elbow consists of reduction of activity until the acute symptoms resolve. Intermittent use of an ice pack helps decrease pain (Fig. 5–31). After the acute symptoms resolve, the child begins a stretching and strengthening program for the musculature around the elbow and shoulder. It is often necessary to obtain video studies for evaluation and to make changes as necessary to ensure that

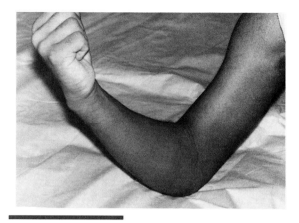

FIGURE 5–30 ■ Sixteen-year-old baseball pitcher with inability to extend arm fully.

proper biomechanics are observed. The child is encouraged to ice the elbow after sporting events.

## Chronic Injuries

Osteochondritis and osteochondritis dissecans of the capitulum have been subjects of much discussion and confusion. Are they really different entities, and does it really matter? Osteochondrosis is generally thought to occur because of avascularity of the capitulum, usually when the child is about 10 years old; fragmentation of the entire capitulum and mild (10 to 15 degree)

flexion contracture occur. The condition is sometimes bilateral and often causes secondary changes in the radial head. Osteochondrosis of the capitulum can generally be treated with rest, stretching exercises, and moderation of sports activities to exclude throwing. Osteochondritis dissecans of the capitellum is thought to be caused by trauma, avascularity, or a recalcitrant form of osteochondrosis. It usually occurs in adolescents, involves a discrete focal area of the capitulum, and causes lack of elbow extension. Because it sometimes involves multiple joints, some authors have suggested that osteochondritis dissecans is a variant of multiple epiphyseal dysplasia. The treatment of osteochondritis dissecans of the capitulum generally consists of observation.

Repetitive stress from throwing in adolescent athletes has been reported to involve significant risk of permanent injury. Why these injuries can occur in the nondominant arm or in adolescents who have no history of participation in throwing sports is unexplained.

## ARTHROSCOPY OF THE ELBOW

Arthroscopy of the elbow has been reported to improve exposure with less surgical trauma than traditional surgical methods (Fig. 5–32). Andrews and Carson reported that 85% of results of 12 arthroscopic elbow procedures were good.[36] Removal of loose bodies is the most common indication for elbow arthroscopy, but Miller has

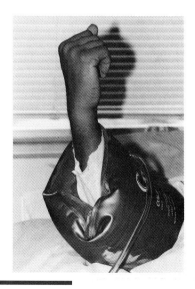

FIGURE 5–31 ■ Sixteen-year-old baseball pitcher using intermittent ice to decrease pain after treatment.

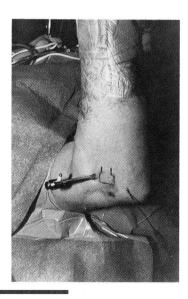

FIGURE 5–32 ■ Portal sites during arthroscopic débridement.

also found arthroscopy useful in the following situations:[37]

■ Evaluation and removal of loose bodies
■ Evaluation and treatment of osteochondritis dissecans of the capitulum
■ Evaluation and treatment of chondral or osteochondral lesions of the radial head
■ Excision of osteophytes from the humerus and olecranon
■ Partial synovectomy, especially in rheumatoid disease
■ Débridement or lysis of adhesions about the elbow in post-traumatic or degenerative disease
■ Evaluation of the painful elbow when other diagnostic tests are inconclusive

Complications of elbow arthroscopy are rare. According to the Arthroscopy Association of North America, in 1569 procedures only three complications occurred.[37] Reported complications of elbow arthroscopy include infection, tourniquet problems, instrument breakage, and neurovascular damage. Neurovascular complications are most frequent.

### Treatment

Rehabilitation is begun early after arthroscopy of the elbow to avoid complications. The following is the Campbell Clinic protocol for physical therapy after arthroscopic removal of loose bodies from the elbow (P.L. Head, PT, ATC, personal communication, 1992):

**1 to 3 days after surgery**

■ Pain and edema control
■ Education of the patient
■ Gentle active movement in dressing after splint removal
■ Emphasis on hand, wrist, and shoulder exercises

**4 to 7 days after surgery (wound care as needed)**

■ Active exercise (gentle range of motion) continued
■ Gentle contraction-relaxation exercises for elbow
■ Progressive resistive exercises for elbow
■ Active pronation and supination
■ Scar mobilization

**7 to 14 days after surgery**

■ Active and passive range-of-motion exercises
■ Gentle ballistic stretching and end range-of-motion exercises to stretch capsule and fire mechanoreceptor

■ Increased progressive resistive exercise (1 to 3 pounds weight)
■ Increased repetitions (three sets of 15 to 20 repetitions, then advance amount of weight)
■ Mobilization, if needed, of radioulnar, radiohumeral, and ulnohumeral joints
■ Emphasis on functional use of involved upper extremity

**2 to 4 weeks after surgery**

■ Advance all exercises, repetitions, and weight (3 to 10 pounds) after assessment of soft tissue and range of motion

**4 to 6 weeks after surgery**

■ Progress to interval throwing or to sports-specific activity as condition of joint and soft tissues allows
■ Theraband exercises
■ Simulation of sports activity
■ Interval throwing program
■ Maintenance of range of motion
■ Flexibility program
■ Strength maintenance program
■ Assessment of biomechanics of sports activity

Ice may be used before (if needed) and always after exercise.

## COMPLICATIONS AFTER INJURY

### Reflex Sympathetic Dystrophy Syndrome

Common injuries that may require immobilization of the elbow are certain upper extremity fractures (humeral shaft, Colles, supracondylar) and elbow dislocations. These injuries may lead to reflex sympathetic dystrophy syndrome (RSDS), resulting in a painful, restricted extremity.[38] RSDS has been divided into three stages[39]:

■ Stage 1—acute
■ Stage 2—dystrophic
■ Stage 3—atrophic

Nerve trauma is often associated with RSDS, especially after Colles' fractures. The most severe manifestation of RSDS is shoulder-hand syndrome, for which rehabilitation is usually lengthy and difficult.

The pathophysiology of RSDS is not well understood. It has been postulated that both peripheral and central mechanisms may lead to sympathetic dysfunctions. Neuropeptides have been implicated in causing inflammation and maintaining the sympathetic symptoms.

As defined by Schutzer and Gossling, RSDS is an excessive response manifested by four characteristics:[40]

- Intense prolonged pain
- Vasomotor disturbances
- Delayed functional recovery
- Various associated trophic changes

Clinical symptoms include

- Pain
- Swelling
- Pitting edema
- Tenderness
- Bluish skin color with shiny red discoloration
- Restricted movement

These symptoms may appear alone or in combination during various stages of the disorder. The widespread disturbance of central autonomic regulation is thought to be due to vasospasm of small arterioles and capillaries, causing the bluish appearance and coolness to touch of the extremity.[41] The edema is caused by outflow from the capillaries of plasma and fibrin. Osteopenic changes caused by the altered blood flow are often visible on roentgenograms. Stiffness of the elbow, wrist, hand, or shoulder is caused by tissue ischemia that results in fibrin deposition and fibrosis in the soft tissues.

### Treatment

Treatment consists of early recognition, early intervention by physical therapy, tricyclic agents, anti-inflammatory agents, and nerve blocks. Early diagnosis and early treatment to break the cycle while it is reversible are key to successful treatment. Physical therapy treatment of RSDS of the upper extremity and elbow consists of early recognition, pain and edema control, desensitization exercises, weight-bearing activities, stiffness prevention, and functional activities. Because of the severity of this disorder, psychologic support is often necessary.

## ✷ Myositis Ossificans

Trauma to the elbow joint can initiate a cellular reaction, such as edema, inflammation, and fibroplasia.[42] Three interchangeable terms have been used to describe bone formation around a joint or muscle:[43]

- Ectopic bone ("out of place")
- Heterotopic bone ("other place")

### Myositis ossificans ("ossified inflammatory muscle")

This discussion of myositis ossificans is limited to bone formation in muscle, most commonly after a severe contusion of the thigh muscles or a fracture-dislocation of the elbow. Extreme inflammatory reactions may be seen in myositis ossificans, and in a rehabilitation program this must be considered and the therapy adapted to avoid causing additional tissue reaction.

Myositis ossifications can also result from extremely aggressive attempts to mobilize the joint or from early massage of the brachialis (if contusions are present) and often results in permanent restriction of motion, extension more than flexion. According to Kessler and Hertling, stretching the anterior capsule rather than the brachialis muscle for a capsular restriction greatly decreases the likelihood of myositis ossificans forming.[21] To avoid contributing to the problem, the physical therapist must recognize the two common conditions leading to myositis ossificans. First, during the evaluation, determine the cause of the restriction, distinguishing between capsular and muscular restriction of elbow range of motion. Limitation of extension more than flexion with an elastic end feel suggests muscular restriction. A capsular pattern (flexion more than extension) and capsular end feel suggest a capsular restriction.

### Treatment

Stretch tight elbow flexors vigorously in agreement with the attending physician and in cases of persistent restriction. Use gentle techniques, emphasizing active exercise, self-active and passive stretches, and prolonged stretching devices such as the low-load dynamic splint. Second, evaluate for signs of brachialis inflammation by palpating for a hematoma or excessive tenderness over the distal brachialis muscle belly. If these signs are present, avoid vigorous mobilization. Note that a local temperature rise persisting more than 24 hours may indicate the need to decrease the intensity of the stretching program. Thermistor readings should be recorded before and after treatments to document this.

## ✷ Volkmann's Ischemic Contracture

Volkmann's ischemic contracture is the most incapacitating complication that can follow a fracture or dislocation of the elbow. According to

Stewart of the Campbell Clinic (M.J. Stewart, personal communication, 1992), traumatic injuries of the elbow joint, whether by direct contusion or transmitted from the hand, always involve tearing of the capsule and ligamentous structures, which produces an inflammatory reaction that can lead to arterial ischemia or Volkmann's contracture. According to Mubarak and Hargens, Volkmann's contracture refers to the end stage of an ischemic injury to the muscles and nerves of a limb, with obstruction of arterial blood supply and venous return.[37a] This is often associated with supracondylar fractures because of the tendency to produce hemorrhage beneath the deep fascia. In the early period of immobilization after elbow injury, frequent observation and prompt action to relieve any impairment of circulation are necessary. If impaired circulation is unrecognized, muscular fibrosis and atrophy develop, leading to permanent contracture. Depending on the severity of the lesion, necrosis occurs in the flexor muscles, median and ulnar nerves, and skin. Extensive scar tissue frequently replaces the necrotic muscle, leading to permanent contracture.

According to Segelov, the symptoms of Volkmann's contracture are clear and definite:[38]

■ Severe pain in the forearm muscles that are being starved of blood (this pain disappears later as all sensation is lost)
■ Limited and extremely painful finger movement
■ Purple discoloration of the hand with prominent veins
■ Initial paresthesia followed by loss of sensation
■ Loss of radial pulse and later loss of capillary return
■ Pallor, anesthesia, and paralysis

Surgical intervention is often necessary for patients with established Volkmann's contracture. The dead and contracted muscle must be excised, with rearrangement of the viable musculature to allow as much function as possible.

## TREATMENT

Each rehabilitation program must be individualized to meet the special needs of the patient. An injury leads to a sequence of physiologic responses. The role of the physical therapist is to reduce the severity of these physiologic effects, decrease the healing time, and enhance the rehabilitation without causing deleterious effects (Figs. 5–33 and 5–34). According to Harrelson,

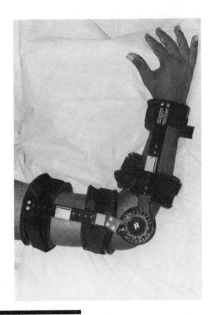

FIGURE 5–33 ■ Braces allowing different degrees of range of motion during rehabilitation.

a rehabilitation program should include the following goals:[44]

■ Decrease pain
■ Decrease inflammatory response to trauma
■ Return full, pain-free range of motion
■ Decrease effusion
■ Return muscle strength, power, and endurance (Fig. 5–35)
■ Regain full, asymptomatic function (Fig. 5–36)

Remember that proper use of exercise can expedite healing and waiting too long to start exercise can result in permanent loss of range of motion.

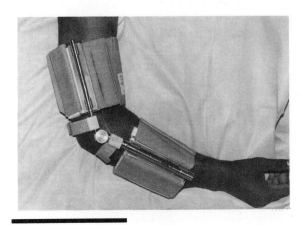

FIGURE 5–34 ■ Dynasplint used to gain elbow extension during rehabilitation.

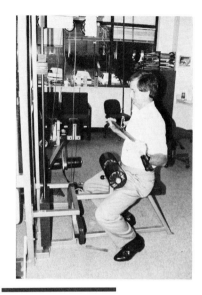

**FIGURE 5-35** ■ Return to normal strength.

Caution must be observed in rehabilitating the elbow. Too vigorous a program can cause a flare-up of the inflammatory condition. In a comprehensive rehabilitation program after elbow trauma, pain and swelling must be treated initially; otherwise additional soft tissue problems may develop.

Generally, acute inflammatory conditions around the elbow are treated with cold applications because cold minimizes acute edema and hemorrhage and acts as an analgesic. Researchers such as Schmidt et al.[45] and Rippe and Grega[46] recommend cold for acute inflammation. In the subacute and chronic stages, heat is used to in-

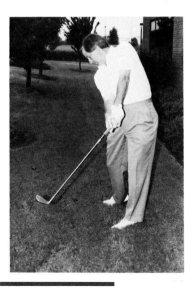

**FIGURE 5-36** ■ Full asymptomatic range.

crease blood flow and reabsorption of exudates. The rationale for using heat for adhesions and contracted tissue is that, in combination with stretching, it can alter viscoelastic properties and make tissue more extensible. However, others have recommended the use of ice rather than heat because heat was found to aggravate edema formation and prolong recovery time of acute orthopaedic injuries.

In in vitro studies, Dyson and Suckling found that ultrasound accelerates the inflammatory and repair processes and can be used in healing.[47] They postulated that the effects of low-intensity ultrasound in healing tissue are nonthermal.

Transcutaneous electrical nerve stimulation has been successful in relieving pain around the elbow. The relief often persists beyond the period of treatment. Mannheimer and Lampe reported its use to reduce pain and increase range of motion after fracture of the olecranon treated with open reduction and internal fixation.[48] We have used transcutaneous nerve stimulation in treating RSDS of the elbow. The pain and self-imposed immobilization of the elbow result in increased edema and inflammation, and the stimulation has been successful in improving motion and decreasing symptoms. Reports of successful management of RSDS in children by transcutaneous electrical nerve stimulation suggest that a normal balance of sympathetic nervous system activity may be restored and other symptoms relieved. Gersh discusses the use of TENS for pain management.[49] Numerous other electrical modalities have been used to provide analgesia, including high-voltage stimulation, interferential stimulation, and low-voltage stimulation. It is beyond the scope of this chapter to discuss all of these.

Scar tissue formation may be divided into four stages: inflammation, granulation, fibroplastic, and maturation. It is important during the inflammatory stage of scar tissue formation to allow the tissue to rest for 48 hours and avoid increasing the inflammation and hemorrhage. During the granulation stage capillary bleeding is important because fibroblasts need nutrients to survive. During the fibroplastic stage the gap is closed with immature scar.

Mismanagement or use of excessive traction can weaken the portion of the scar that is closing the wound and result in increased scarring and adhesions. According to many sources, new scar tissue is capable of being modified and treatment can change the length and bulk of the scar tissue. Arem and Madden reported that new scar tissue can be stretched by gentle and persistent treatment.[50] Friction massage reportedly affects collagen fiber orientation. Its use during rehabilitation stimulates the ligament or tendon to orient the fibers longitudinally without stressing the tissue, and it can help improve the extensibility of tissue.[54] Cooper reports that friction massage is ideal for overuse conditions such as tennis elbow and golfer's elbow.[51]

Elbow range of motion is often limited after biceps laceration because of the formation of two types of scar tissue: intramuscular (within the muscle) and intermuscular (between the muscle and adjacent structures). Intramuscular scar tissue adhesions form between the fasciculi of the muscle, limiting passive lengthening or active shortening of the muscle. Intramuscular adhesions in the biceps brachii usually limit active elbow flexion and active and passive elbow extension. Treatment must be started early for prevention.

For most patients with elbow injuries, appropriate use of modalities and other agents, along with exercise, improves function and decreases symptoms. Knowledge of the complex anatomic structures about the elbow and the conditions and injuries that occur in this joint is mandatory for proper rehabilitation. The patient must be evaluated carefully to determine the specific condition or injury, the physiologic status, and the goals of rehabilitation. Early intervention is the key to a successful outcome.

## CASE STUDY 1

▼A patient sustained bilateral radial head fractures and a humeroulnar dislocation of the right elbow in a fall from a ladder onto his elbows. He was treated postoperatively in physical therapy for approximately 11 months. Surgery involved bilateral radial head resections and open reduction of the right humeroulnar joint. According to the literature, most patients never regain more than 20 degrees of extension after fracture-dislocations of the radial head. The rehabilitation of this patient illustrates the importance of patience, perseverance, and determination in attaining treatment goals, especially range of motion.

### EVALUATION

Three weeks after surgery, the patient had active assisted range of motion of the left elbow of −12 degrees of extension, 118 degrees of flexion, 85 degrees of pronation, and 22 degrees of supination. Shoulder and wrist ranges of motion were normal. There was minimal swelling over the proximal radius, and he had pain with supination and pronation. Because of the severity of the injury, the right elbow was immobilized in 90 degrees of flexion for 5.5 weeks. At that time he had 130 degrees of flexion, 30 degrees of supination, 45 degrees of pronation, and a 75-degree flexion contracture. All other ranges of motion of the right upper

extremity were normal, but indurated edema about the elbow joint persisted. Active movement was painful. Strength was not assessed at this time.

### TREATMENT GOALS

Short-term goals included decreasing pain and edema before exercise sessions and increasing range of motion on the left by 75% and on the right by approximately 30%. Long-term goals were discussed and determined by the patient and therapist. The goals were for the patient to regain as much range of motion as possible, to regain normal strength bilaterally, and to return to playing golf, in which he was proficient, scoring an average of 73 to 75 per game.

### INITIAL TREATMENT AND ASSESSMENT

Initially, treatment was focused on gaining range of motion gently, using modalities to increase myofascial and joint extensibility, and decreasing pain and edema. The left elbow was treated with moist heat and ultrasound over the anterior joint capsule and biceps tendon, during which a Theraband was placed around the patient's wrist and secured to a table leg to add a prolonged, passive extension stretch (Fig. 5–37). Active resisted range of motion and proprioceptive neuromuscular facilitation techniques were used to increase extension. Massage was used with caution over the distal biceps brachii insertion and anterior aspect of the elbow.

Ultrasound was applied to the posterior aspect of the elbow and the distal triceps tendon. After this, joint mobilization techniques, plus active stretching and contraction-relaxation or proprioceptive neuromuscular facilitation, were used to assist in flexion. Ultrasound and/or massage was applied over the interosseous membrane, in addition to myofascial spray-and-stretch techniques, before working on supination. An especially effective joint mobilization technique was used to increase pronation: ulnar-triquetral joint mobilization as described by Kessler and Hertling.[21] The Baltimore Therapeutic Exercise pronation-supination attachment

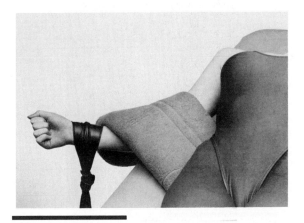

**FIGURE 5–37 ■** Patient receiving moist heat and prolonged passive extension with Theraband.

was used with minimal resistance for pronation-supination range of motion. Treatment was always followed by use of ice packs or JOBST cold intermittent compression with the elbow placed on a slight stretch for extension.

Initial treatment of the right elbow differed slightly. Because of the chronic edema that restricted range of motion, treatment started with high-voltage pulsed galvanic stimulation, using four electrodes placed around the elbow, along with moist heat over the biceps brachii. The patient tolerated a 10-pound weight resting over his wrist during application of modalities while stretching into extension.

A home program of active-assisted range-of-motion exercises for elbow flexion, extension, and forearm pronation and supination was performed twice daily. A Dynasplint was used for extension of the right elbow.

This basic routine was used before cautious stretching three times a week for 4 months and twice a week for another 5 months. For the right elbow, the attending physician approved vigorous stretching into extension after 1 month of therapy.

## RESULTS OF INITIAL TREATMENT

Three weeks after the beginning of therapy, the left elbow had nearly full extension (−5 degrees), 111 degrees of flexion, 80 degrees of pronation, and 65 degrees of supination. Therapy was then concentrated on flexion and supination, and the full home program for the left elbow was continued.

Four weeks after initiation of treatment, the right elbow had gained 30 degrees of extension. Flexion decreased from 130 to 115 degrees, probably because of the use of the low-load dynamic splint during sleep, and pronation and supination both improved significantly. The primary goal was to increase extension range of motion.

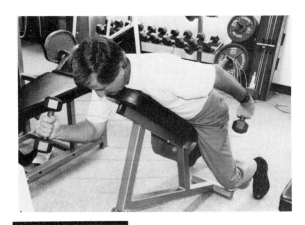

**FIGURE 5-39** ■ Alternating composite flexion and extension of the upper extremities.

By the 12th week of therapy, the right elbow had gained 56 degrees of extension. Of these 56 degrees, 30 degrees were gained in the first month, 18 degrees in the second, and 8 degrees in the third. Range of motion at this time was −18 degrees of extension. One degree was gained each month for 3 months. The physician then administered a cortisone-lidocaine injection before therapy over adhesions at the triceps tendon, which were causing great pain with extension. Six degrees of extension were gained in the following month and 1 degree in the next month. Thus, at a time when progress toward range of motion appeared to level off, consistent efforts by both the patient and therapist led to a remarkable improvement and functionally acceptable result of −7 degrees of active extension.

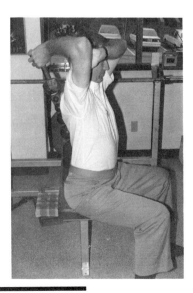

**FIGURE 5-38** ■ Triceps strengthening with dumbbell.

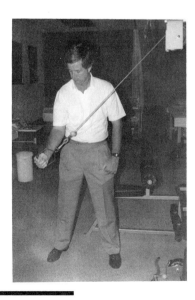

**FIGURE 5-40** ■ Cable pulley exercise for shoulder and elbow extension and wrist extension stabilization.

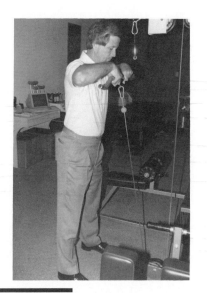

**FIGURE 5–41** ■ Rowing exercise strengthening wrist flexion and ulnar deviation and pronation.

## FOLLOW-UP TREATMENT

During rehabilitation, strength training was instituted, beginning with the yellow Theraband and 2-pound dumbbells and progressing to the use of full free weights, cable pulleys, and pushups. Dumbbell exercises were performed for biceps, triceps, supinators, pronators, and wrist extensors and flexors (Figs. 5–38 to 5–41). Cable pulleys in proprioceptive neuromuscular facilitation patterns were used for grip strength and overall strengthening of the upper extremity. Barbell overhead triceps exercises, biceps curls, and bench

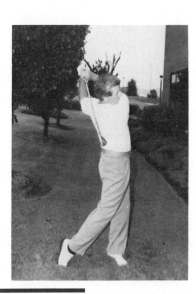

**FIGURE 5–42** ■ Patient in full swing after rehabilitation.

**Table 5–4.** ACTIVE ASSISTED RANGE OF MOTION OF ELBOW AND FOREARM

|  | Right | | Left | |
|---|---|---|---|---|
|  | 5.5 weeks | 11 months | 3 weeks | 11 months |
| Extension | −75° | −7° | −12° | 0° |
| Flexion | 130° | 135° | 118° | 142° |
| Supination | 30° | 85° | 22° | 80° |
| Pronation | 45° | 90° | 85° | 90° |

presses also were done. Latissimus dorsi pull-down bar exercises were used for strengthening and prolonged extension stretching. Additional stretching techniques used for elbow extension and flexion were passive mode Kincom, tossing and catching 2- and 3-pound plioballs, and wrist-assist Theraband self-helped passive extensions.

When the patient returned to playing golf several months before discharge, he had pain and localized swelling bilaterally over the medial epicondyles because of the instability created in the forearm by the absence of the radial heads and annular ligaments. Iontophoresis with cortisone and lidocaine was effective in treating this. He also found neoprene elbow braces helpful while playing golf (Fig. 5–42).

### ASSESSMENT OF REHABILITATION PROGRAM

This patient regained full extension and pronation, with 5 to 10 degrees lag of supination and flexion in the left elbow. He regained 7 degrees to 135 degrees of elbow extension and flexion, with full pronation and supination on the right (Table 5–4). He has normal strength bilaterally, as determined by manual muscle test procedures, and has returned fully to the activities of daily living, including golf. He now scores an average of 72 to 74 for 18 holes and has played in two proamateur tournaments. He faithfully continues a home strengthening and flexibility program. He attributes greater stability of the medial aspect of the forearm, especially the wrist flexor and pronator groups, to his strengthening program.

The key to this successful result was persistence and unwillingness to accept an unsatisfactory result at apparent plateaus in treatment. Research has shown that range of motion after this type of injury continues to improve for 1 to 1.5 years after the injury.

## CASE STUDY 2

▼ A 49-year-old female patient was referred to physical therapy with a diagnosis of lateral epicondylitis and arthritis in her left elbow (Figs. 5–43 and 5–44). She had received treatment from several physicians, physical therapists, a ''sports trainer,'' and an acupuncture therapist because of pain and loss of motion.

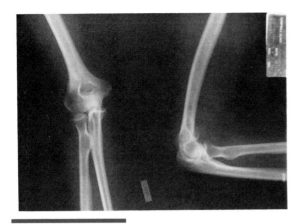

**FIGURE 5–43** ■ Radiograph of patient showing arthritic changes.

## EVALUATION

The patient came to physical therapy with ongoing complaints of pain and decreased range of motion in her left elbow. She reported that the pain began 3 years earlier when she "strained" her elbow while water skiing. Past treatments had included several cortisone injections, a countertension brace, modalities, joint mobilization, massage, nonsteroidal anti-inflammatory drug therapy, and acupuncture. The patient reported that these treatments had provided only temporary relief of the pain and no improvement in range of motion.

On evaluation, she had 114 degrees of active elbow flexion and −18 degrees of active elbow extension. A hard end feel was noted with end-range passive flexion and extension. Pronation and supination were

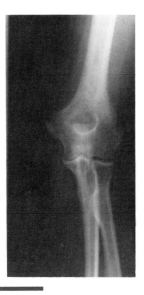

**FIGURE 5–44** ■ Radiograph of patient showing arthritic changes.

within normal limits, as were shoulder and wrist ranges of motion. Minimal swelling was noted in the medial and posterior aspects of the joint, along with increased tone in the forearm musculature. The patient reported pain at rest and with active and passive flexion and extension. Strength was not evaluated at the time.

## TREATMENT GOALS

Short-term goals included decreasing pain and swelling to allow for an increase in function of the left upper extremity and increasing range of motion to −10 degrees of extension and 125 degrees of flexion. Long-term goals were to regain full range of motion, compared to the uninvolved elbow, and full, painless function of the left upper extremity. The patient wished to be able to resume golf and water skiing without limitations. The length of time since the injury and its effect on the prognosis were discussed with the patient.

## INITIAL TREATMENT AND ASSESSMENT

Initial treatment included the use of moist heat and ultrasound applied to the antecubital fossa to increase the extensibility of the anterior capsule and biceps tendon. A passive stretch into elbow extension was provided manually by the therapist during ultrasound treatment. This was followed by soft tissue mobilization of the biceps, biceps tendon, and forearm musculature and by joint mobilization techniques. Active and passive range-of-motion exercises were used in conjunction with contraction-relaxation techniques to increase both flexion and extension. Treatments concluded with ice and elevation to decrease pain and edema.

## FOLLOW-UP TREATMENT

After three physical therapy sessions, the elbow pain had decreased slightly but no gains were made in range of motion. The patient was asked to bring in the radiographs from her referring physician. These showed a large loose body in the posterior aspect of the joint and ossification in the medial aspect. In consultation with one of our orthopaedists, it was determined that arthroscopic removal of the loose body and release of the anterior capsule might be more beneficial than conservative management in meeting the established goals.

Approximately 1 month after the initial evaluation, the patient underwent arthroscopic removal of the loose body (1.5 cm in diameter) from the posterior aspect of the joint (Fig. 5–45); a small incision was needed posteriorly to allow its removal. The anterior joint capsule was released and the joint was cleansed of several smaller loose bodies.

Physical therapy was resumed 5 days after arthroscopy, with emphasis on pain and edema control and gentle active range-of-motion exercises. As the incision healed and edema decreased, the previously described physical therapy program was resumed and strength training was begun. Multiangle isometric exercises were used for both biceps and triceps to in-

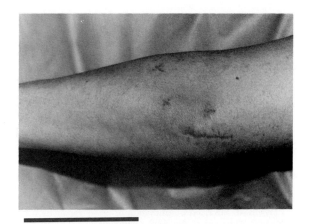

**FIGURE 5-45** ■ Incision after arthroscopic examination.

crease strength in the new ranges of flexion and extension. Strengthening progressed to the use of Theraband and free weights for biceps, triceps, pronators, supinators, and wrist flexors and extensors.

The patient continued with a supervised therapy program for 5 weeks and was then discharged with a home strengthening and range-of-motion program.

### ASSESSMENT OF REHABILITATION PROGRAM

The patient regained full extension and 134 degrees of flexion (compared to 140 degrees in the uninvolved elbow). She reported a significant increase in pain-free functional use of her left upper extremity after rehabilitation. The patient continues with a daily home strengthening program and reports no problems 2 months after arthroscopic surgery.

The success of this patient's rehabilitation can be attributed primarily to good communication between the therapist and the orthopaedist. After reviewing the patient's radiographs, it was obvious that the goals of rehabilitation could not be met with conservative management alone. This case study also illustrates the importance of treatment based on the physical therapist's evaluation of the patient, rather than on the diagnosis provided by the physician. By using our skills in conjunction with those of the physician, the patient will reap the rewards of a successful rehabilitation program.

## REFERENCES

1. Sisk TD, Wright PE II: Arthroplasty of shoulder and elbow. *In* Campbell's Operative Orthopaedics, 8th ed. (Crenshaw AH, ed). St. Louis: Mosby Year Book, 1992, Vol II, p 651–654.
2. Morrey BF, An KN: Articular ligament contribution to stability of the elbow. Am J Sports Med 11:315–319, 1983.
3. Reid DC, Kushner S: The elbow region. *In* Orthopaedic Physical Therapy (Donatelli R, Wooden MJ, eds). New York: Churchill-Livingstone, 1989, p 179–181.
4. Morrey BF: Anatomy of the elbow joint. *In* The Elbow and Its Disorders (Morrey BF, ed). Philadelphia, WB Saunders, 1985, p 19–22.
5. Pauly JE, Rushing JL, Schering LE: An EMG study of muscles crossing the elbow joint. Anat Rec 1:42, 1967.
6. Basmajian JV, DeLuca CJ: Muscles Alive, 5th ed. Baltimore: Williams & Wilkins, 1985, p 281–285.
7. Smith FS: Anatomy of the elbow region. *In* (Smith FS: Surgery of the Elbow, 2nd ed.) Philadelphia: WB Saunders, 1972, p 31.
8. Hoppenfeld S: Physical Examination of the Spine and Extremities. New York: Appleton-Century-Croft, 1976, p 36–40.
9. Bryan RS, Morrey BF: Fracture of the distal humerus. *In* The Elbow and Its Disorders (Morrey BF, ed). Philadelphia: WB Saunders, 1985, p 302–339.
10. Milch H: Fracture and fracture-dislocation of the humeral condyle. J Trauma 4:592–595, 1964.
11. Conwell HE: Injuries to the Elbow. Ciba Clin Symp 21(2):35–62, 1969.
12. Mason JA, Shutkins NM: Immediate active motion in the treatment of fractures of the head and neck of the radius. Surg Gynecol Obstet 76:731–740, 1943.
13. Linscheid RL: Elbow dislocations. *In* The Elbow and Its Disorders (Morrey BF, ed). Philadelphia: WB Saunders, 1985, p 414–432.
14. McLaughlin HL: Some fractures with a time limit. Surg Clin North Am 35:553–557, 1985.
15. Boyd HB, Altenberg AR: Fractures about the elbow in children. Arch Surg 49:213–222, 1944.
16. Canale ST: Fractures and dislocations. *In* Operative Pediatric Orthopaedics (Canale ST, Beaty JH, eds). St. Louis: Mosby Year Book, 1991, p 963–975.
16a. Letts M, Locht R, Wiens J: Monteggia fracture-dislocations in children. J Bone Joint Surg 67B:724–727, 1985.
17. Beaty JH, Wood AB: Lateral condyle fractures: long-term results. Presented at the Annual Meeting of the American Academy of Orthopaedic Surgeons, Las Vegas, January 18, 1985.
18. O'Brien PI: Injuries involving the proximal radial epiphysis. Clin Orthop 41:51–57, 1965.
19. Wenge JH: Fracture of the neck of the radius in children. *In* The Elbow and Its Disorders (Morrey BF, ed). Philadelphia: WB Saunders, 1985, p 237–239.
20. Karasiek D, Burke DL JR, Gross G: Trauma to the elbow and forearm. Semin Roentgenol 26:318–332, 1991.
21. Kessler RM, Hertling D: Management of Common Musculoskeletal Disorders. Philadelphia: Harper & Row, 1983, pp 311–328.
22. Nagler W, Johnson E, Gardner R: The pain of tennis elbow. Current Concepts Pain Analg, 1985.
23. Snyder-Mackler L, Epler M: Effects of standard air cast tennis elbow bands, and integrated electromyography of forearm extensor musculature proximal to the bands. Am J Sports Med 17:278–281, 1989.
24. Phillips BB: Traumatic disorders. *In* Campbell's Operative Orthopaedics, 8th ed. (Crenshaw AH, ed). St. Louis: Mosby Year Book, 1992, vol III, p 1924–1933.
25. Gilcreest EL: Dislocation and elongatoin of the long head of the biceps brachii. Ann Surg 104:118–126, 1936.
26. Neer CS II: Impingement lesions. Clin Orthop 173:70–77, 1983.
27. Hawkins RJ, Kennedy JC: Impingement sign in athletes. Am J Sports Med 8:151–158, 1980.
28. Dines D, Warren RF, Ingles AE: Surgical treatment of lesions of the long head of the biceps. Clin Orthop 164:165–171, 1982.
29. Neviaser TJ, Neviaser RJ: Lesions of the long head of the biceps. AAOS Instr Course Lect 30:250–257, 1981.

30. Postacchini R: Rupture of the rotator cuff of the shoulder associated with rupture of the tendons of the long head of the biceps. Ital J Orthop Traumatol 12:137–149, 1986.
31. Watson-Jones R: Fractures and Joint Injuries, 5th ed., vol II. Baltimore: Williams & Wilkins, 1976, p 532–533.
32. Soto-Hall R, Stroot JH: Treatment of ruptures of the long head of the biceps brachii. Am J Orthop 60:192, 1960.
33. Warren RF: Lesions of the long head of the biceps tendon. AAOS Instr Course Lect 34:204–209, 1985.
34. Mariani EM, Cofield RH, Askew J, et al: Rupture of the tendon of the long head of the biceps brachii: surgical versus non-surgical treatment. Clin Orthop 228:233–239, 1988.
35. Adams JE: Injury of the throwing arm: a study of traumatic changes in the elbow joints of boy baseball players. Calif Med 102:127–131, 1965.
36. Andrews JR, Carson WG: Arthroscopy of the elbow. Arthroscopy 1:97–107, 1985.
37. Miller RH III: Arthroscopy of upper extremity. *In* Campbell's Operative Orthopaedics, 8th ed. (Crenshaw AH, ed) St. Louis: Mosby Year Book, 1992, vol III, p 1865–1891.
37a. Mubarak SJ, Hargens AR: Compartment Syndrome and Volkmann's Contracture. Philadelphia: WB Saunders, 1981, pp183–193.
38. Segelov PM: Complications of Fractures and Dislocations. St. Louis: Mosby Year Book, 1990, p 40–42.
39. Wyndell H: Reflex sympathetic dystrophy. *In* Plastic Surgery (Marj J, Little JW, eds). Philadelphia: WB Saunders, 1940, vol VII, p 4884.
40. Schutzer SF, Gossling HR: The treatment of reflex sympathetic dystrophy. J Bone Joint Surg [Am] 66:625–629, 1984.
41. Jaeger SH, et al: Nerve injury. Comp Mgt Neurogenic Pain Syn 2(1):223, 1986.
42. Ingles AE: The rehabilitation of elbow athletic injury. AAOS Instr Course Lect 40:45–49, 1991.
43. Coventry MB: Ectopic ossification about the elbow. *In* The Elbow and Its Disorders (Morrey BF, ed). Philadelphia: WB Saunders, 1985, p 464–471.
44. Harrelson GL: Introduction to rehabilitation. *In* Physical Rehabilitation of the Injured Athlete (Andrews JR, Harrelson GL, eds). Philadelphia: WB Saunders, 1991, p 165–195.
45. Schmidt KL, Ott VR, Rocher G, et al: Heat, cold, and inflammation. Rheumatology 38:391, 1979.
46. Rippe B, Grega GJ: Effects of isoprenaline and cooling on histamine-induced changes of capillary permeability of the rat. Acta Physiol Scand 103:252–262, 1978.
47. Dyson M, Suckling J: Simulation of tissue repair by ultrasound: a survey of the mechanisms involved. Physiotherapy 64(4):105–108, 1978.
48. Mannheimer JS, Lampe GW: Clinical Trancutaneous Electrical Nerve Stimulation. Philadelphia: FA Davis, 1984, p 400–403.
49. Gersh MR: TENS for management of pain and sensory pathology. *In* Electrotherapy for Rehabilitation (Gersh MR, ed). Philadelphia: FA Davis, 1992, p 149–196.
50. Arem AJ, Madden SW: Effects of stress on healing wounds. J Surg Res 20:93–97, 1976.
51. Cooper M: The use of modalities in rehabilitation. *In* Physical Rehabilitation of the Injured Athlete (Andrews JR, Harrelson GL, eds). Philadelphia: WB Saunders, 1991, p 136–146.

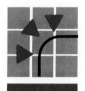

# Hand and Wrist

## JANNA L. JACOBS

## INTRODUCTION

The hand and wrist are a part of the upper quarter or upper extremity complex. Therefore, injury or disease involving the hand and wrist affects the remainder of the upper extremity. The function of the upper extremity complex (the shoulder, elbow, and forearm) is to place the hand in space to allow it to perform a specific task. If the hand or wrist is injured or diseased, it functions at a lower level, performing fewer and less complicated tasks. Therefore, the more proximal joints of the shoulder girdle and elbow do not place the hand in space as frequently or as adeptly, and stiffness may result. The converse is also true; injury and disease of the proximal upper extremity can cause hand and wrist dysfunction.

To be able to differentiate between proximal and distal dysfunction in the upper extremity, the practitioner must be knowledgeable about the anatomy and biomechanics of the hand and wrist, injuries and diseases that commonly afflict the distal upper extremity, and evaluation procedures and rehabilitation protocols specific to the symptoms identified. This chapter is designed to provide this information.

## ANATOMY

### Surface Anatomy

The hand and wrist are described as having volar (palmar) and dorsal surfaces and radial (thumb side) and ulnar borders. The palm has three designated regions (from the radial side to the ulnar side): the thenar, midpalm, and hypothenar regions (Fig. 6-1). The thenar region (or thenar eminence) is the fleshy area proximal to the thumb; intrinsic musculature contributes to the contour of the area. The hypothenar region (or hypothenar eminence) is the fleshy area on the ulnar side of the palm, proximal to the small finger; this fleshy contour is also a result of underlying intrinsic muscles. The remainder of the palm constitutes the midpalm region.

Other landmarks on the palmar surface of the hand are the creases of the hand (proximal to distal): the wrist, thenar, and proximal and distal palmar creases. The digital creases are the palmar digital, proximal interphalangeal, and distal interphalangeal creases. These creases divide the segments of the digits. Each digit, with the exception of the thumb, has three segments, the proximal, middle, and distal phalanges. The thumb has only two segments, the proximal and distal phalanges. The digits are termed the thumb and the index, middle (or long), ring, and small fingers.

### Skeletal Anatomy

The hand consists of 27 bones. These include the 8 carpal bones, 5 metacarpal bones, and 14 phalanges. Figure 6-2 shows the bones of the hand and wrist.

The carpus consists of seven major carpal bones: the trapezium, trapezoid, scaphoid, lunate, hamate, capitate, and triquetral. The eighth carpal bone, the pisiform, is a sesamoid bone. It lies volar to the triquetral and does not play a major role in the carpal complex.

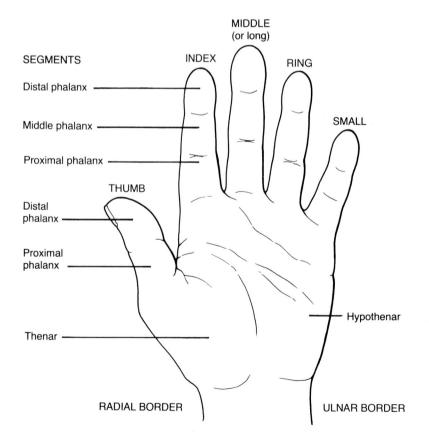

SURFACE ANATOMY
(palmar surface)

**FIGURE 6-1 ■** Hand surfaces, borders, and regions.

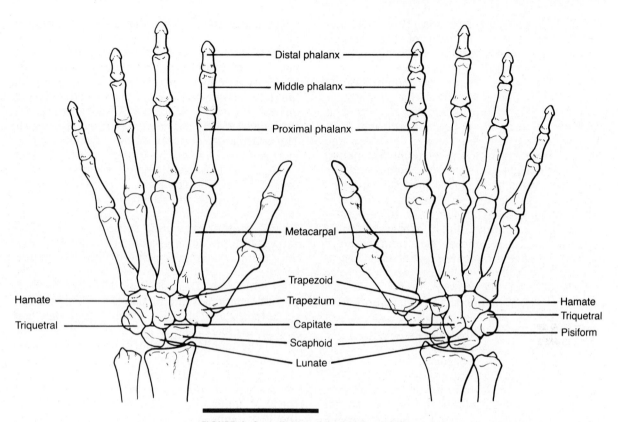

**FIGURE 6-2** ■ Bones of the hand and wrist.

The carpal bones are arranged in two transverse rows: the proximal row, moving ulnarly, consists of the scaphoid, lunate, and triquetral; the distal row includes the trapezium, trapezoid, capitate, and hamate. The structural anatomy of the proximal row conforms to that of the distal row and the radius to permit mobility of its members. The proximal articulating surface of the proximal row is concave in shape and covered by cartilage, providing a congruent surface to join with the forearm bone anatomy. The distal row of the carpal bones articulates with the five metacarpal bones of the hand. This row is more rigid in construction than the proximal row. The capitate acts as the key member of the row, firmly linked to the rigid second and third metacarpal bones. The entire carpus has a volarly curved shape, providing a channel through which tendons, nerves, and vessels pass.

Navarro et al present another analysis of carpal anatomy.[1-4] Rather than two transverse rows, they describe the carpus in terms of three longitudinal columns: the radial, central, and ulnar columns (Fig. 6-3). The radial or lateral column consists of the scaphoid and trapezium. The lu-

nate, trapezoid, capitate, and hamate make up the central column. The ulnar or medial column consists of the triquetral and pisiform. Biomechanically, the central column acts as the pivot point between the radius and the central meta-

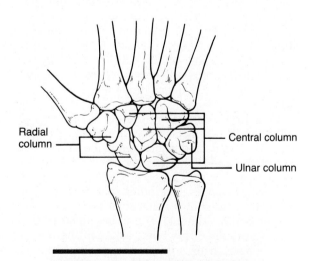

**FIGURE 6-3** ■ Navarro carpal column theory.

carpals in flexion and extension. Thus, dysfunction of the lunate, the base of the column, disrupts the column's stability. The radial column serves as the supporting base of the thumb and is responsible for its independent motion. Scaphoid dysfunction interferes with the stability of this column. The fifth metacarpal is supported by the ulnar column, which permits the rotation of that metacarpal. In this column concept, the proximal row acts as the pivot point for motion at the radiocarpal and midcarpal joints and the central column is more mobile than the others.

Another description of the carpus involves only two longitudinal columns, a force-bearing column and a control column. Weber[4] describes the force-bearing column as the "central core of the wrist" and the ulnar portion of the wrist as the "control column." This concept is derived from analysis of the contours of the bone surfaces, ligamentous support, and kinematics of the forearm, carpus, and metacarpals.

The radius and ulna are proximal to the carpus; however, the carpus articulates directly only with the radius. The ulna does not articulate directly with the proximal row; in fact, it is separated from the carpus by an articular disc. The distal end of the ulna (the head) is concave except for a lateral or ulnar projection, the styloid process. The radial or medial aspect of the ulnar head articulates with the radius, forming the distal radioulnar joint. The medial convex articulating surface of the radius that receives the ulnar head is referred to as the ulnar notch. The radioulnar joint permits rotation about its axis; this rotation of approximately 175 degrees constitutes supination and pronation. The distal end of the radius is a convex surface that articulates with the carpus. Both the distal radius and ulna are covered by cartilage. An important part of the distal radioulnar structure is the triangular fibrocartilage complex (TFCC). This complex, which includes the articular disc separating the ulna from the carpus, is described in the following as part of the ligamentous anatomy of the wrist.

Distal to the carpus are the other 19 bones of the hand: the 5 metacarpals and 14 phalanges. The metacarpals and phalanges make up the five rays of the hand. The first ray, the thumb, is the shortest and comprises the thumb metacarpal and two phalanges. The other four rays, varying in length, consist of a metacarpal and three phalangeal bones. Although the index metacarpal is the longest metacarpal bone, as a unit the middle ray is longest. This is due to the greater length of its proximal and middle phalanges. These length

relationships influence the hand's functional mobility.

Other joints of the hand are designed to facilitate functional mobility. In addition to the wrist joint just described, there are 17 mobile joints in the hand (Fig. 6–4). The joints of the thumb include the carpometacarpal (CMC), metacarpophalangeal (MP), and interphalangeal (IP) joints. The articulating surfaces of the carpometacarpal joint are provided by the trapezium and the first metacarpal. This saddle joint is important because it permits complex movements, significantly enhancing the functional abilities of the hand. The other joints, the MP and IP joints, are formed by the articulating surfaces of the metacarpal and proximal phalanx and the proximal and distal phalanges, respectively. The index, middle, ring, and small fingers share the same joint structures. These include the carpometacarpal, MP, proximal interphalangeal (PIP), and distal interphalangeal (DIP) joints. The index and middle carpometacarpal joints have no clinically detectable mobility, the fourth or ring finger carpometacarpal joint has only a few degrees of motion, and the fifth joint is very mobile. The metacarpal–proximal phalanx articulation forms the MP joints, the proximal-middle phalanges the PIP joints, and the middle-distal phalanges the DIP joints.

The curves or arches of the hand, shown in Figure 6–5, also contribute to its function. There are two transverse arches, the carpal and metacarpal arches, and a longitudinal arch. The transverse arches are apparent at the levels of the distal carpus and the metacarpal heads. The relative positions of the fixed and mobile stuctures of the carpus and hand form these arches. The longitudinal arch consists of the metacarpals and phalanges. They can be affected by various conditions, such as nerve impairment, and therefore can provide diagnostic information. Even when they are not directly affected, these arches must be preserved during the rehabilitation process.

## Fibrous Anatomy

The fibrous anatomy includes the ligaments, aponeuroses, and fasciae. The fibrous structures provide support and stability to bones and joints, fixation of the skin, containment or partitioning of structures from one another, guidance and restraint of joint motion, guidance of tendon motion, and protection—all of which contribute to optimal function of the hand and wrist unit.

An intricate ligamentous structure binds the

JOINTS

BONES

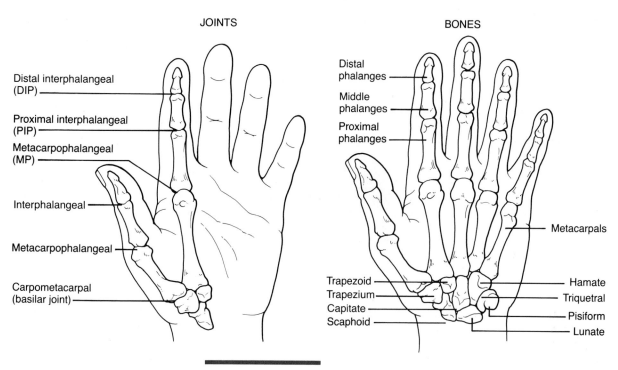

Distal interphalangeal (DIP)

Proximal interphalangeal (PIP)

Metacarpophalangeal (MP)

Interphalangeal

Metacarpophalangeal

Carpometacarpal (basilar joint)

Distal phalanges

Middle phalanges

Proximal phalanges

Metacarpals

Trapezoid
Trapezium
Capitate
Scaphoid

Hamate
Triquetral
Pisiform
Lunate

**FIGURE 6-4** ■ Bones and joints of the hand.

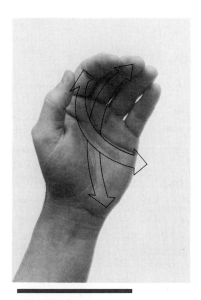

**FIGURE 6-5** ■ Arches of the hand.

carpus to its distal and proximal articulations. Dorsally, the dorsal radiocarpal ligament and the radial and ulnar collateral ligaments bridge the carpus with the radius and ulna (Fig. 6–6); the volar radiocarpal ligament and the ulnocarpal ligaments bind the volar aspect of the carpus (Fig. 6–7). The radial and ulnar collateral ligaments also serve to connect the carpus to the forearm, and the dorsal and volar radioulnar ligaments connect the radius and ulna. The term *triangular fibrocartilage complex,* introduced by Palmar,[5] describes the ligamentous complex of the distal radius and ulna and carpus. It consists of the dorsal and volar radioulnar ligaments, ulnar collateral ligament, ulnocarpal meniscus (meniscus homologue), articular cartilage of the ulna, and sheath of the extensor carpi ulnaris (Fig. 6–8). The TFCC is a stabilizer of the radioulnar joint and carpus and is a cushion for the ulna. Other volar wrist ligaments include the radiocapitate, radiotriquetral, ulnolunate, ulnotriquetral, radioscaphoid, and transverse carpal ligaments.[6–9]

There are numerous intercarpal ligaments. Some of the more important ligaments include, volarly, the capitotriquetral, scaphotrapezium, scapholunate, and volar intercarpal ligaments. Located dorsally are the lunate-triquetral, scapholunate interosseous, and deltoid ligaments.[3,6–9]

In this extensive list, the key ligaments of the wrist are the volar radiocarpal, radiocapitate, radiotriquetral (largest ligament of the wrist), radioscaphoid, ulnolunate, ulnotriquetral, and dorsal radiocarpal ligaments. These volar ligaments are

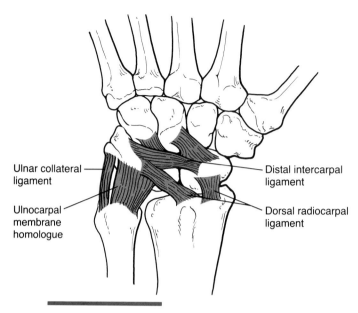

Ulnar collateral ligament

Ulnocarpal membrane homologue

Distal intercarpal ligament

Dorsal radiocarpal ligament

**FIGURE 6–6 ■** Dorsal radius, ulna, and carpal ligaments.

much stronger than their dorsal counterparts, which contributes to greater wrist stability in flexion than extension.[6–9]

A ligament-like structure of the wrist, the flexor retinaculum, lies distal to the radial joint. It spans across the carpal gutter and transforms it into a tunnel through which flexor tendons and the median nerve pass (Fig. 6–9). The flexor retinaculum or transverse carpal ligament provides the extrinsic flexor tendons with a pulley mechanism that maximizes the line of pull of the tendons. It has been observed that disruption of the

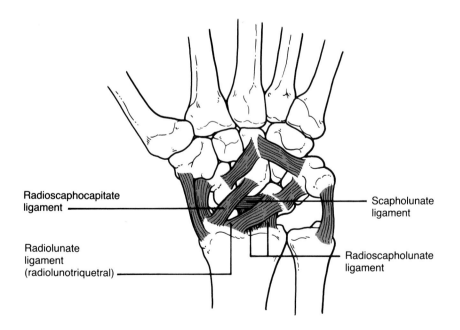

Radioscaphocapitate ligament

Radiolunate ligament (radiolunotriquetral)

Scapholunate ligament

Radioscapholunate ligament

**FIGURE 6–7 ■** Volar (palmar) radius, ulna, and carpal ligaments.

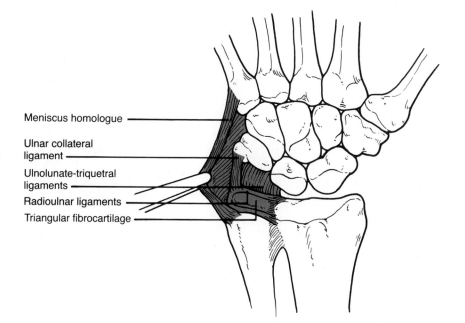

**FIGURE 6-8** ■ The triangular fibrocartilage complex.

Meniscus homologue

Ulnar collateral ligament

Ulnolunate-triquetral ligaments

Radioulnar ligaments

Triangular fibrocartilage

flexor retinaculum results in ''bowstringing'' of the tendons,[10-12] which decreases grip strength. The transverse carpal ligament is also the villain in carpal tunnel syndrome, a condition in which the median nerve is compressed as the carpal tunnel narrows.

This complex ligamentous structure provides support and stability for the radius, ulna, and carpal complex. The volar wrist ligaments are the primary stabilizers of the proximal segment of the joint. Stabilization of the distal row is provided mainly by the capitotriquetral and radiocapitate ligaments. The ligaments control the motion of the wrist joint, allowing greater motion in its central portion and less in the radial aspect of the joint. Most injuries of the wrist are sus-

tained as a result of falls on an outstretched hand. The structures most commonly involved in these injuries are the radius, scaphoid, and lunate. Because motion at the wrist is, in part, dependent on the ligamentous structures about the joint, ligamentous disruption can interfere with the functional mechanics of the joint. Flexion and extension of the wrist, a hinge joint, take place between the proximal and distal carpal rows and at the radius and ulna. The average ranges of motion at the wrist are 80 degrees into flexion and 70 degrees extension, 20 degrees of radial deviation, and 30 degrees of ulnar deviation.[13] Radial deviation occurs with an ulnar shift of the proximal row, whereas a radial shift of the proximal row yields ulnar deviation. The distal

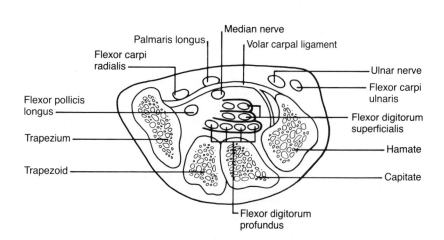

**FIGURE 6-9** ■ Anatomy of the carpal tunnel.

Palmaris longus

Flexor carpi radialis

Median nerve

Volar carpal ligament

Flexor pollicis longus

Trapezium

Trapezoid

Ulnar nerve

Flexor carpi ulnaris

Flexor digitorum superficialis

Hamate

Capitate

Flexor digitorum profundus

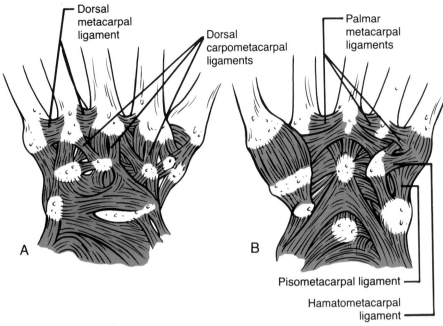

Dorsal
metacarpal
ligament

Dorsal
carpometacarpal
ligaments

Palmar
metacarpal
ligaments

Pisometacarpal ligament

Hamatometacarpal
ligament

**FIGURE 6–10** ■ (A) Dorsal carpometacarpal ligaments; (B) palmar carpometacarpal ligaments.

row moves opposite to the proximal row in both deviations.[3,4,6,7,9,14,15]

The ligaments located at the carpometacarpal level are the dorsal and palmar carpometacarpal ligaments (Fig. 6–10A and B). These ligaments provide support and stability to the carpometacarpal joints.

The MP, PIP, and DIP joints of the digits have similar ligamentous structures (Fig. 6–11). The radial and ulnar collateral ligaments provide lateral support and stability to the joints. They also contribute to flexion contractures of the digital joints. At the MP joint, the collateral ligaments are placed under tension when the joint is flexed. Conversely, the collateral ligaments of the IP joints are under tension when the joints are extended. It is important to consider this when immobilizing the digits. The preferred position for immobilization is with the MP joints at 60 to 70 degrees of flexion and the IP joints in near to full extension. Of course, injury or surgical procedures may not indicate this position. Volarly, the anterior capsule is thickened and referred to as the volar plate; only a thin capsular component exists dorsally. At the MP joints, the deep transverse intermetacarpal ligament connects the volar plates. It extends from the radial aspect of the second metacarpal head to the ulnar aspect of the fifth metacarpal head. The ligament manifests different characteristics on each digit. These characteristics permit varying degrees of stability and mobility of each of the joints within each digit. This variety in digit stability and mobility contributes to the optimal functional capabilities of the hand.

A portion of the flexor retinacular system extends beyond the wrist to the digits. This portion consists of fibrous sheaths or pulleys. The finger pulleys are located palmarly in the digits. Two types of retinacular pulleys are the annular pul-

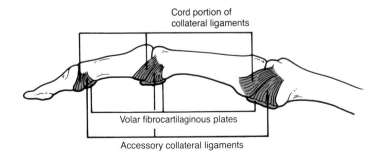

Cord portion of
collateral ligaments

Volar fibrocartilaginous plates

Accessory collateral ligaments

**FIGURE 6–11** ■ Ligamentous structures of the digital joints.

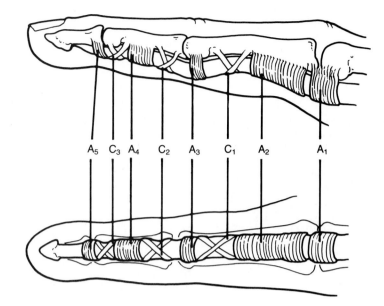

**FIGURE 6–12 ■** Digital pulley system.

leys and cruciate ligaments (Fig. 6–12). Each of the four digits has five annular and three cruciate pulleys; the thumb has three pulleys (two annular and one oblique). The pulleys maintain the tendons in proper alignment to the axis of the digit, preventing anterior-posterior and lateral shifts. A common phenomenon that occurs with loss of pulleys is bowstringing. Inadequate line of pull results (Fig. 6–13), causing decreased range of motion and strength of flexion. The $A_2$ and $A_4$ pulleys are the major ones in the system. These pulleys contribute significantly to grip strength.[10,12]

The synovial sheaths are deep to the fibrous sheaths in the digits and wrist (Fig. 6–14). The tendon sheaths are synovial sheaths through which the flexor tendons glide. They reduce or eliminate frictional forces that would result as the tendon moved across bone.

The tendons are made of specialized fibrous tissue that transmits the action of the muscle into action of the joints. The sliding of the tendon through the tendon sheaths transmits this motion. This action is optimized by synovial fluid that surrounds the tendons, minimizing friction in the tendon sheath system and providing a source of nutrition to the tendons. As nutritional and vascular conditions surrounding the flexor tendons vary, the following levels or zones have been identified[10-12] (Fig. 6–15):

■ **Zone 1**—the area between the insertion of the flexor digitorum profundus (FDP) on the distal

phalanx and the flexor digitorum superficialis on the middle phalanx.
■ **Zone 2**—the area bordered distally by the insertion point of the flexor digitorum superficialis and proximally by the proximal end of the $A_1$ pulley.
■ **Zone 3**—the area of the palm bordered by the proximal end of the $A_1$ pulley and the distal edge of the transverse carpal ligament.
■ **Zone 4**—the carpal tunnel itself. The transverse carpal ligament spans this area.
■ **Zone 5**—a large area. Distally, it is marked by the proximal edge of the transverse carpal ligament and proximally by the flexor musculotendinous junctions.

It is important to point out that the nutritional and vascular differences of these zones influence the surgical and therapeutic management of tendon injuries at the various levels. Therefore, the clinician must be knowledgeable about these details.

The superficial palmar fascia is also part of the fibrous skeleton of the hand. It consists of the superficial palmar fasciae, the palmar compartments, and the deep palmar and dorsal aponeuroses (Fig. 6–16). The superficial palmar fascia spans from the flexor retinaculum to the base of the digits and is divided into three segments: central, lateral, and medial. The central, triangular portion provides a roof for the compartment that houses the flexor tendons and neurovascular bundles. The lateral palmar fascia (thenar apo-

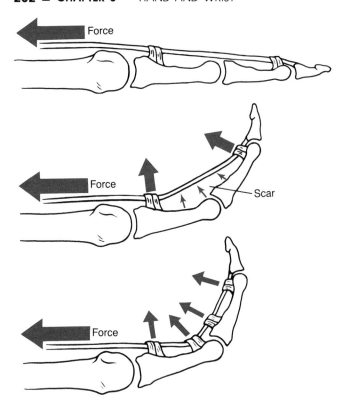

FIGURE 6-13 ■ Bowstringing of tendon.

FIGURE 6-14 ■ Synovial sheaths and bursae.

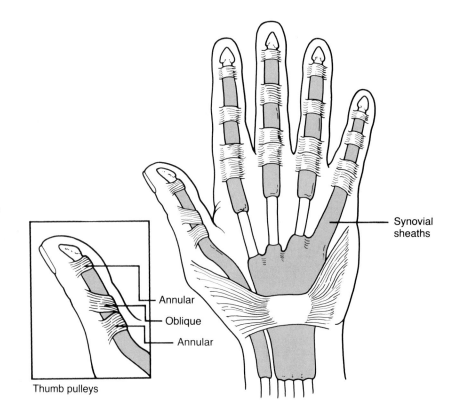

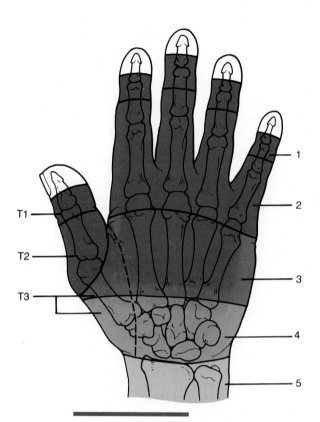

**FIGURE 6-15** ■ Flexor tendon zones.

neurosis) covers the thenar muscles; the medial palmar fascia (hypothenar aponeurosis) covers the hypothenar musculature. Blood vessels pass through this tissue to supply the skin. Fibrous fasciculi extend from this palmar fascia and attach to the overlying palmar skin. These fibrous connections act to tether the skin to the underlying superficial palmar fascia, to allow little skin shifting during grasp. The fasciculi also section off subcutaneous fat into masses. By contrast, the dorsal cutaneous and subcutaneous tissues are lax and mobile, permitting comfortable, unrestrained flexion of the joints. Lymphatic vessels, veins, and sensory nerves pass through the dorsal cutaneous and subcutaneous tissue.[8] This accounts for the marked lymphedema frequently seen on the dorsum of the hand.

The deep palmar aponeurosis covers the palmar aspect of the metacarpals and interosseous muscles. It is connected to the superficial palmar fasciae by the fascial septa, forming the palmar compartments. These palmar compartments correspond to the segments of the superficial palmar fasciae. The midpalmar space contains the long flexor tendons and their sheaths, the

superficial palmar arch, and the digital nerves and vessels. Within the thenar compartment are the four thenar muscles and the flexor pollicis tendon and its sheath. The hypothenar compartment houses the three hypothenar muscles.

The dorsal aponeurosis spans across the metacarpals and carpus. The superficial dorsal fascia lies dorsally over the extensor tendons. The deep dorsal fascia, underlying the extensor tendons, is located in a gliding space. An area of the deep fascia of the hand and distal forearm has been identified as the dorsal transverse carpal ligament. This ligament is specialized in that it consists of compartments in which certain extensor tendons are contained (Fig. 6–17A and B). There are six extensor compartments, which house the following tendons (from radial to ulnar): (1) abductor pollicis longus and extensor pollicis brevis, (2) extensor carpi radialis longus and brevis, (3) extensor pollicis longus, (4) extensor indicis proprius and the extensor digitorum communis tendons, (5) extensor digiti minimi, and (6) extensor carpi ulnaris. These compartments are covered dorsally by the extensor retinaculum or dorsal annular ligament.[16-19]

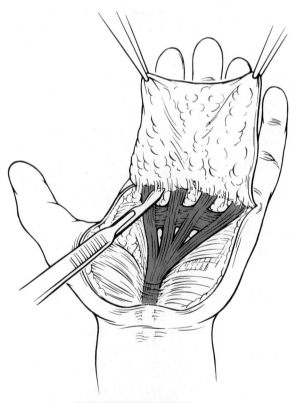

**FIGURE 6-16** ■ Palmar fascia.

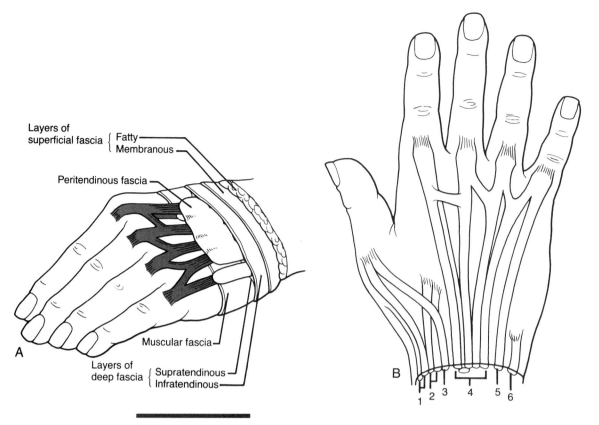

Layers of superficial fascia { Fatty — Membranous —

Peritendinous fascia —

Muscular fascia —

A

Layers of deep fascia { Supratendinous — Infratendinous —

B

1 2 3 4 5 6

**FIGURE 6-17** ■ (A) Dorsal fascia; (B) dorsal extensor compartments.

## Muscles

The musculature of the hand is divided into two categories: intrinsic and extrinsic. The intrinsic muscles reside within the hand itself; both the origin and insertion are inside the bounds of the hand. The extrinsic musculature originates outside the hand. A delicate balance is maintained between the intrinsics and extrinsics, and any disruption of this balance can greatly affect the function of the hand and wrist as a unit, as discussed later.

### Extrinsic Musculature

Twenty extrinsic muscles power the movements of the wrist and hand. These motions of the forearm and wrist include supination-pronation, flexion-extension, and radial-ulnar deviation (Fig. 6–18A to H). The motions of the fingers and thumb provided by the extrinsic musculature are flexion, extension, and hyperextension of the fingers (Fig. 19A–C) and flexion,

extension, palmar abduction, and radial abduction of the thumb (Fig. 6–20A to E). In order to understand why each muscle produces a particular motion, the therapist must have a thorough knowledge of muscle origins, insertions, actions, and nerve innervations. The references for this information are Gray[20] and Warfel.[21]

#### FOREARM MUSCLES

**Biceps Brachii.** The biceps brachii has two points of origin, the short head from the coracoid process of the scapula and the long head from the supraglenoid tuberosity of the scapula. The muscle spans the anterior surface of the humerus. It inserts into the radial tuberosity and into the origins of forearm flexors via the lacertus fibrosus. The biceps brachii flexes the elbow and supinates the forearm. It is innervated by the musculocutaneous nerve (C-5, C-6).

**Supinator.** The supinator originates from the lateral epicondyle of the humerus. Insertion is on the lateral and anterior upper third of the radius. This muscle supinates the forearm. The supinator

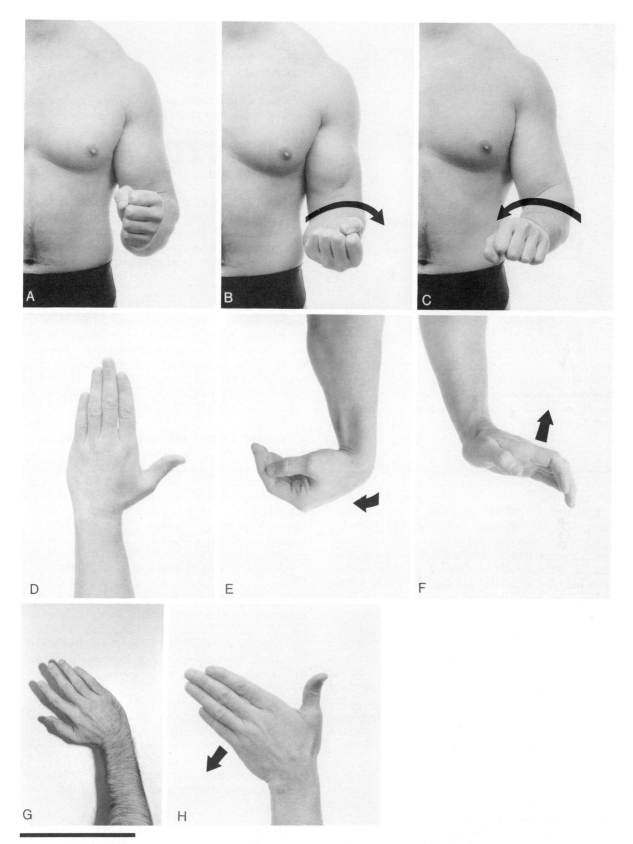

**FIGURE 6–18** ■ (A) Forearm neutral position; (B) forearm supination; (C) forearm pronation; (D) wrist neutral; (E) wrist flexion; (F) wrist extension; (G) wrist radial deviation; (H) wrist ulnar deviation.

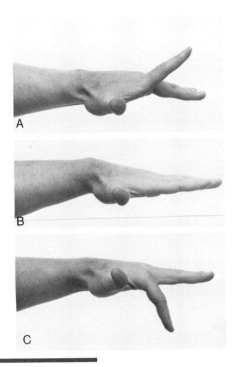

FIGURE 6-19 ■ (A) Digital hyperextension; (B) digital extension; (C) digital flexion.

is innervated by the deep branch of the radial nerve (C-5, C-6).

**Pronator Teres.** The pronator teres originates from both the humerus and ulna. The humeral head arises from the medial epicondylar ridge of the humerus, the ulnar head from the medial side of the coronoid process of the ulna. It inserts into the middle of the lateral surface of the radius. The pronator teres pronates the forearm and assists in flexion of the elbow. Its innervation is provided by the median nerve (C-6, C-7).

**Pronator Quadratus.** This muscle originates from the distal fourth of the volar surface of the ulna and inserts laterally into the distal fourth of the volar surface of the radius. Pronation of the forearm is the sole motion of the pronator quadratus. The anterior interosseus branch of the median nerve (C-6, C-7) innervates this muscle.

WRIST MUSCLES

Many muscles act on the wrist, some inserting at or about the wrist and others at the digital level. Several of the muscles provide motion in more than one plane. Examples are the flexor and extensor carpi ulnaris, which act to deviate

the wrist ulnarly as well as to flex or extend the wrist with other muscles.

**Flexor Carpi Radialis (FCR).** The flexor carpi radialis flexes and radially deviates the wrist because it originates from the medial epicondyle of the humerus and inserts into the base of the second and third metacarpal bones. It is innervated by the median nerve (C-6).

**Palmaris Longus (PL).** This muscle also originates from the medial epicondyle of the humerus and inserts into the transverse carpal ligament and palmar aponeurosis. The palmaris longus flexes the wrist. It is innervated by the median nerve (C-6).

**Flexor Carpi Ulnaris (FCU).** The flexor carpi ulnaris has two points of origin. The humeral head arises from the medial epicondyle of the humerus and the ulnar head from the olecranon. Its insertion spans the pisiform, hamate, and base of the fifth metacarpal. The FCU flexes and ulnar-deviates the wrist. The ulnar nerve (C-8, T-1) innervates this muscle.

**Extensor Carpi Radialis Longus (ECRL).** The ECRL originates from the lower third of the lateral supracondylar ridge of the humerus and lateral intermuscular septum. The muscle inserts dorsally to the base of the second metacarpal. It extends and radially deviates the wrist. The extensor carpi radialis longus is innervated by the radial nerve (C-6, C-7).

**Extensor Carpi Radialis Brevis (ECRB).** The extensor carpi radialis brevis originates on the lateral epicondyle of the humerus and the intermuscular septum and inserts dorsally into the base of the third metacarpal. The muscle extends and radially deviates the wrist. It receives its innervation from the posterior interosseus branch of the radial nerve (C-6, C-7).

**Extensor Carpi Ulnaris (ECU).** The ECU extends and ulnar-deviates the wrist. The muscle originates from the lateral epicondyle of the humerus and the posterior border of the ulna and inserts into the ulnar aspect of the fifth metacarpal. The extensor carpi ulnaris is also innervated by the posterior interosseus branch of the radial nerve (C-7).

**Abductor Pollicis Longus (APL).** The abductor pollicis longus contributes to radial deviation of the wrist because it inserts into the radial

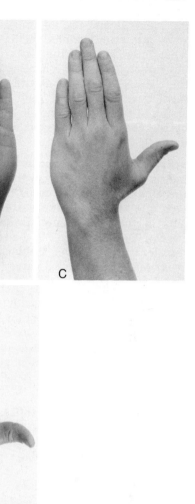

**FIGURE 6–20** ■ (A) Thumb flexion; (B) thumb extension; (C) thumb radial abduction; (D) thumb adduction; (E) thumb palmar abduction.

aspect of the base of the first metacarpal and originates from the posterior surface of the ulna, the interosseus membrane, and middle posterior surface of the radius. Its innervation is from the posterior interosseus branch of the radial nerve (C-7).

EXTRINSIC MUSCLES ACTING ON THE DIGITS

**Flexor Digitorum Superficialis (FDS).** The flexor digitorum superficialis has three heads: the humeral head arises from the medial epicondyle of the humerus, the ulnar head from the coronoid process of the ulna, and the radial head from the oblique line of the radius. The muscle divides into four tendons that insert into the radial and ulnar aspects of the volar surfaces of the middle phalanges of the index, middle, ring, and small fingers. This muscle flexes the PIP joints of these fingers. Secondarily, this muscle

assists in flexion of the MP joints of the respective fingers, as well as the wrist. It is innervated by the median nerve (C-7, C-8, T-1).

**Flexor Digitorum Profundus (FDP).** The FDP arises from the medial and anterior surface of the ulna, the medial side of the coronoid process, and interosseus membrane. This muscle also splits into four tendons, each of which inserts into the volar surface of the distal phalanx of the index, middle, ring, and little fingers. The muscle flexes the DIP joints of the fingers and assists in flexion of the PIP joints and wrist. It has dual innervation; the index and middle fingers are innervated by the anterior interosseus branch of the median nerve (C-8, T-1) and the ring and small fingers by the ulnar nerve (C-8, T-1).

**Extensor Digitorum Communis (EDC).** This muscle originates from the lateral epicondyle of the humerus and the intermuscular septa. It divides into four tendons that insert into the extensor mechanism of the digits. (A more detailed description of this mechanism appears later in the chapter.) The EDC extends the MP joints of the index, middle, ring, and small fingers and assists in wrist extension. The EDC is innervated by the posterior interosseus branch of the radial nerve (C-7).

**Extensor Indicis Proprius (EIP).** The extensor indicis proprius arises from the dorsal surface of the ulna and the interosseus membrane and inserts into the dorsal surface of the proximal phalanx of the index finger. Extension of the MP joint of the index finger is the sole action of this muscle. It is innervated by the posterior interosseus branch of the radial nerve (C-7).

**Extensor Digiti Minimi (EDM).** This muscle arises from the lateral epicondyle of the humerus and the intermuscular septum and inserts into the dorsal surface of the proximal phalanx of the small finger. The extensor digiti minimi extends the MP joint of the small finger. The posterior interosseus branch of the radial nerve (C-7) innervates the EDM.

**Flexor Pollicis Longus (FPL).** The flexor pollicis longus, having a wide base of origin, arises from the volar surface of the radius, the interosseus membrane, and medial aspect of the coronoid process of the ulna. It inserts volarly into the base of the distal phalanx of the thumb. The muscle flexes the IP joint of the thumb and assists in flexion of the MP joint, as well. It is innervated by the anterior interosseus branch of the median nerve (C-8, T-1).

**Abductor Pollicis Longus (APL).** The abductor pollicis longus originates from the dorsal surface of the ulna, the interosseus membrane, and dorsal surface of the middle third of the radius. It inserts into the radial aspect of the base of the first metacarpal. This muscle radially abducts the thumb ray. Innervation is by the posterior interosseus branch of the radial nerve (C-7).

**Extensor Pollicis Brevis (EPB).** The origin of this muscle is the dorsal surface of the radius and interosseus membrane. It inserts into the base of the proximal phalanx of the thumb. The extensor pollicis brevis extends the MP joint of the thumb. It is innervated by the posterior interosseus branch of the radial nerve (C-7).

**Extensor Pollicis Longus (EPL).** The extensor pollicis longus originates at the middle third of the dorsal ulna and the interosseus membrane and inserts dorsally into the base of the distal phalanx of the thumb. It has multiple functions: extension of the IP and MP joints of the thumb and retroposition of the thumb metacarpal. It is innervated by the posterior interosseus branch of the radial nerve (C-7).

### Intrinsic Musculature

The hand has 19 intrinsic muscles. These muscles complement the motions of the extrinsics and provide abduction and adduction of the fingers (Fig. 6–21A and B) and opposition or anteposition of the thumb (Fig. 6–22).

**Lumbrical Muscles.** The four lumbrical muscles all originate on the FDP tendons. The first two lumbricals arise from the radial side of the

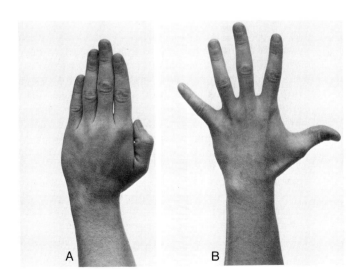

**FIGURE 6–21** ■ (A) Finger adduction; (B) finger abduction.

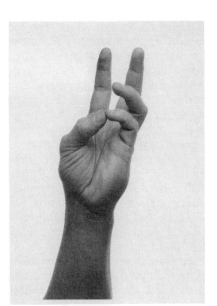

**FIGURE 6-22** ■ Opposition (anteposition).

index and middle fingers, the third from the ulnar aspect of the middle and the radial aspect of the ring fingers, and the fourth from the ulnar aspect of the ring and radial aspect of the small fingers. They insert into the extensor mechanism (described under Extensor Tendon Injuries). The lumbricals extend the IP joints and, secondarily, flex the MP joints of the fingers. The index and middle lumbricals are innervated by the median nerve (C-8, T-1) and the ring and small lumbricals by the ulnar nerve (C-8, T-1).

**Interosseous Muscles.** There are seven interosseous muscles, four dorsal and three palmar. Each dorsal interosseus has two heads that arise from the adjacent sides of the metacarpals. They insert into the metacarpal heads, the first from the radial aspect of the index, the second and third from the radial and ulnar aspects, respectively, of the middle finger, and the fourth from the ulnar aspect of the ring finger. The dorsal interossei abduct the index, ring, and small fingers away from the middle finger. The palmar interossei originate from the metacarpals, the first from the ulnar aspect of the second metacarpal, the second from the radial aspect of the fourth metacarpal, and the third from the radial aspect of the fifth metacarpal. The insertion of these muscles is into the base of the proximal phalanges, the first into the ulnar aspect of the index proximal phalanx and the second and third into the radial aspect of the proximal phalanges of the ring and small fingers, respectively. The

palmar interossei adduct the index, ring, and small fingers toward the middle finger. The interosseous muscles, as a group, flex the MP joints and extend the IP joints of the index, middle, ring, and small fingers. These muscles are innervated by the ulnar nerve (C-8).

**Adductor Pollicis.** The adductor pollicis brevis has two heads. The oblique head's volar origin spans the trapezium, trapezoid, and capitate, as well as the bases of the second and third metacarpals; the transverse head arises from the volar surface of the third metacarpal. The muscle inserts into the ulnar aspect of the base of the proximal phalanx of the thumb. It functions to adduct the thumb metacarpal to the second metacarpal. It also assists in opposition or anteposition of the thumb. It is innervated by the ulnar nerve (C-8).

### HYPOTHENAR MUSCLES

**Abductor Digiti Minimi.** This muscle originates from the pisiform and tendon of the flexor carpi ulnaris and inserts into the ulnar aspect of the base of the proximal phalanx of the small finger. The abductor digiti minimi abducts the small finger and assists in flexing its MP joint. Innervation is from the ulnar nerve (C-8).

**Flexor Digiti Minimi.** The flexor digiti minimi arises from the hamate and transverse carpal ligament. It inserts into the ulnar aspect of the base of the proximal phalanx of the small finger. This muscle flexes the MP joint of the small finger. It is innervated by the ulnar nerve (C-8).

**Opponens Digiti Minimi.** Originating from the hamate and the transverse carpal ligament, the opponens digiti minimi courses distally to insert into the ulnar aspect of the fifth metacarpal. This muscle flexes the metacarpal joint of the small finger and opposes the finger toward the thumb. It is innervated by the ulnar nerve (C-8).

### THENAR MUSCLES

**Abductor Pollicis Brevis.** The abductor pollicis brevis originates from the transverse carpal ligament and the scaphoid and trapezium. It inserts into the radial aspect of the base of the proximal phalanx of the thumb. The muscle functions to abduct the thumb metacarpal palmarly. Innervation is by the median nerve (C-6, C-7).

**Opponens Pollicis.** This muscle arises from

the transverse carpal ligament and the trapezium. It inserts radially into the palmar surface of the first metacarpal. It opposes or antepositions the thumb metacarpal. The opponens pollicis is innervated by the median nerve (C-6, C-7).

**Flexor Pollicis Brevis.** The flexor pollicis brevis consists of a superficial and a deep portion. The superficial portion originates from the transverse carpal ligament; the deep portion arises from the ulnar aspect of the first metacarpal. Both portions insert into the base of the proximal phalanx of the thumb. This muscle flexes and opposes the metacarpal of the thumb. The two portions of the muscle have different innervations; the superficial portion by the median nerve (C-6, C-7) and the deep portion by the ulnar nerve (C-8).

---

## Nerves

An effective practitioner must be knowledgeable about the anatomy, function, and dysfunction of the peripheral nervous system to implement a thorough evaluation and deliver effective treatment. The median, ulnar, and radial nerves supply the motor and sensory components of the hand. The arrangement of the nerves is similar to that of the blood vessels. Frequently, the nerves and arteries are located side by side. Knowing the path of each of the nerves and their order of innervation permits identification of the level of injury or compression and tracking of the recovery pattern.

### Median Nerve

The lateral and medial cords of the brachial plexus form the median nerve (Fig. 6–23). Therefore, the contributing spinal nerves are C-5, C-6, C-7, C-8, and T-1.

The median nerve enters the forearm at the level of the pronator teres muscle. It innervates the pronator teres, flexor carpi radialis, palmaris longus, and flexor digitorum superficialis. It passes under and follows the flexor digitorum superficialis (within the muscle sheath) and continues distally over the anterior surface of the forearm. In the area of the cubital fossa, a branch splits from the median nerve, forming the anterior interosseus nerve (AIN). The AIN lies ulnar to the median nerve and courses distally to innervate the flexor pollicis longus, flexor digitorum profundus of the index and middle fingers, and the pronator quadratus. The AIN

terminates over the distal radius. The remaining, larger portion of the median nerve courses distally with flexor digitorum superficialis tendons and passes deep to the flexor retinaculum through the carpal tunnel, along with the tendons of the flexor digitorum superficialis and flexor digitorum profundus. In the palm, the median nerve passes below the palmar aponeurosis. At this point, the nerve splits into numerous branches innervating various muscles, joints, skin, and vessels.[11,22,23]

Volarly, five muscles are innervated by the median nerve. The abductor pollicis brevis, opponens pollicis, and superficial head of the flexor pollicis brevis receive innervation, totally or in part, from the recurrent motor branch of the median nerve. The lateral two lumbricals are innervated by the palmar digital branches. The palmar skin, joints, and vessels of the thumb, index finger, middle finger, and radial half of the ring finger are also supplied by palmar digital nerves. The radial two thirds of the palm receives cutaneous innervation from the median nerve. Dorsally, the digital branches of the median nerve provide sensory innervation to the distal half of the index finger, middle finger, and radial half of the ring finger (Fig. 6–24).[11,22,23]

Patients present with compression syndromes of the proximal and distal portions of the median nerve. Proximally, the median nerve can be compressed at the head of the pronator teres muscle, the lacertus fibrosis, and the arcade formed by the heads of the flexor digitorum superficialis muscle.[23–25] Distally, the carpal tunnel is a common site of compression (Fig. 6–25) and is frequently involved in cumulative trauma disorders or repetitive strain injuries in industry.

### Ulnar Nerve

The ulnar nerve comes from the medial cord in the brachial plexus (Fig. 6–26). It receives contributions from C-8 and T-1 spinal nerves.

The ulnar nerve enters the forearm posterior to the medial epicondyle. It passes deep to the intermuscular septum and the flexor carpi ulnaris, providing innervation to that muscle and the ulnar half of the flexor digitorum profundus. The ulnar nerve enters the distal forearm along with the ulnar artery between the flexor digitorum superficialis and profundus muscles radially and the flexor carpi ulnaris muscle ulnarly. The ulnar nerve courses over the volar carpal ligament but volar to the transverse carpal ligament. It passes between the pisiform and the hook of the hamate. These anatomic structures form Guyon's

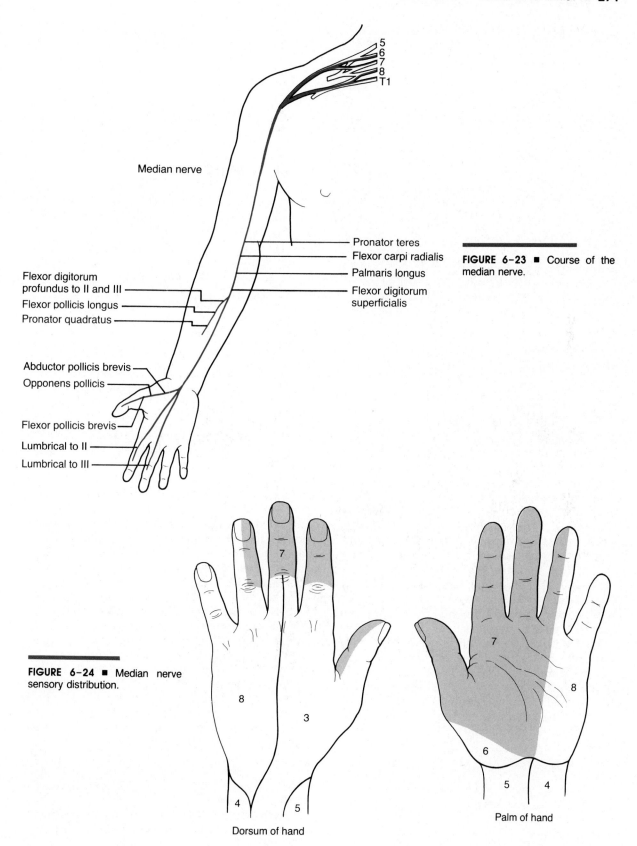

Median nerve

Pronator teres
Flexor carpi radialis
Palmaris longus
Flexor digitorum superficialis

Flexor digitorum profundus to II and III
Flexor pollicis longus
Pronator quadratus

Abductor pollicis brevis
Opponens pollicis

Flexor pollicis brevis
Lumbrical to II
Lumbrical to III

**FIGURE 6-23** ■ Course of the median nerve.

**FIGURE 6-24** ■ Median nerve sensory distribution.

Dorsum of hand

Palm of hand

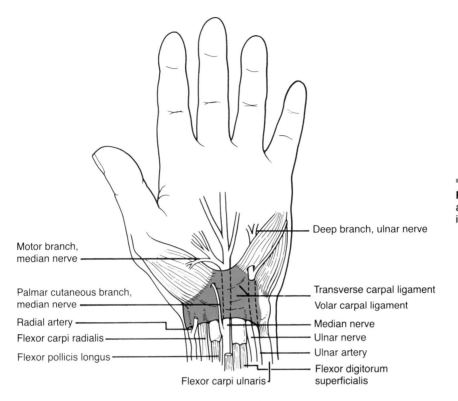

Motor branch,
median nerve

Palmar cutaneous branch,
median nerve

Radial artery

Flexor carpi radialis

Flexor pollicis longus

Flexor carpi ulnaris

Deep branch, ulnar nerve

Transverse carpal ligament

Volar carpal ligament

Median nerve

Ulnar nerve

Ulnar artery

Flexor digitorum
superficialis

**FIGURE 6-25** ■ Carpal tunnel anatomy. Carpal tunnel is shown in color.

canal (Fig. 6-27). Upon exiting the canal, the ulnar nerve divides into superficial and deep branches. The superficial branch innervates the palmaris brevis and provides sensory branches to the palmar surface of the small finger and ulnar half of the ring finger (Fig. 6-28). The superficial branch may also communicate with the median nerve. The deep branch of the ulnar nerve supplies the remaining intrinsic muscles of the hand: the abductor digiti minimi, flexor digiti minimi, opponens digiti minimi, the ulnar two lumbricals, all seven interosseous, the adductor policis, and the deep head of the flexor pollicis brevis. Dorsally, the dorsal cutaneous and dorsal digital branches of the ulnar nerve provide sensation to the entire ulnar third of the dorsum of the hand and digits.[11,22,23]

The ulnar nerve may also be compressed proximally and distally. Proximal compression may occur in the intermuscular septum or cubital tunnel and distally in Guyon's canal.[22-24]

### Radial Nerve

The radial nerve is a continuation of the posterior cord of the brachial plexus (Fig. 6-29). It consists of portions of C-5, C-6, C-7, C-8, and T-1 spinal nerves.

The radial nerve enters the forearm at the lateral epicondyle. It innervates the brachioradialis and extensor carpi radialis longus muscles. The radial nerve then divides into two branches, the superficial branch and the posterior interosseus nerve (PIN). The superficial branch of the radial nerve passes over the dorsal carpal ligament, enters the hand, and divides at Lister's tubercle and the radial styloid. The PIN continues distally, innervating the extensor carpi radialis brevis, and passes through and innervates the supinator. The posterior interosseus nerve also innervates the extensor digitorum communis, extensor digiti minimi, extensor carpi ulnaris, abductor pollicis longus, extensor pollicis longus and brevis, and extensor indicis proprius, in that order. The PIN terminates at the wrist and provides innervation to that joint. Distally, the radial nerve does not provide any motor innervation in the hand, only dorsal sensory innervation. The various branches of the superficial radial nerve supply the radial two thirds of the dorsum of the hand, the entire dorsum of the thumb, and the dorsum of the index, long, and the radial half of the ring fingers from MP to PIP joint level (Fig. 6-30).[11,22,23]

The radial nerve can be compressed proximally as it passes through the two heads of the supi-

continues on to join the ulnar artery, forming the superficial palmar arch. The superficial palmar arch lies at approximately the midmetacarpal level and forms the common digital arteries. These arteries course distally toward the fingers. At the metacarpophalangeal joints the common digital arteries split to form the proper volar digital arteries. The latter travel the length of the fingers, forming branches that supply the flexor tendons, the vincula (Fig. 6–33). The superficial palmar arch supplies vessels to the middle, ring, and small fingers and to the ulnar aspect of the index finger.[11]

The branch of the radial artery deep to the volar carpal ligament courses posterior to the thumb metacarpal, passes under the abductor pollicis longus and extensor pollicis longus and brevis tendons, and re-enters the palm between the two heads of the first dorsal interosseous muscle. In the palm, the radial artery joins the ulnar artery to form the deep palmar arch. The deep palmar arch supplies the thumb and radial half of the index finger. It also gives rise to the volar metacarpal arteries.[11]

The ulnar artery enters the wrist lateral to the pisiform bone under the volar carpal ligament. Distal to the pisiform the ulnar artery branches into two vessels. One branch travels distally, joining the radial artery to form the superficial palmar arch. The other branch, the deep palmar branch, courses ulnarly and deep and reverses its direction to pass under the superficial branch of the ulnar nerve at about the level of the fifth metacarpal base. At the metacarpal base, the ulnar nerve joins the radial artery to form the deep palmar arch.[11]

The radial and ulnar arteries also provide circulation dorsally. The branch of the radial artery that passes posteriorly before re-entering the palm branches to travel ulnarly, proximal to the insertions of the extensor carpi radialis longus and brevis tendons. This vessel joins a branch of the ulnar artery, the dorsal carpal branch, to form the dorsal carpal arterial arch. The arterial arch branches to form the dorsal metacarpal arteries, which provide distal blood supply. At the metacarpal heads these arteries split to form the dorsal digital arteries. The dorsal carpal branch of the ulnar artery also gives rise to vessels that supply the carpal bones.[11]

The terminal branches previously described contribute to a rich network of arterioles and capillaries in the hand. This network supplies the osseous, fibrous, dermal, and connective tissues of the hand. The vascular network consists of shunting mechanisms between the arterioles and

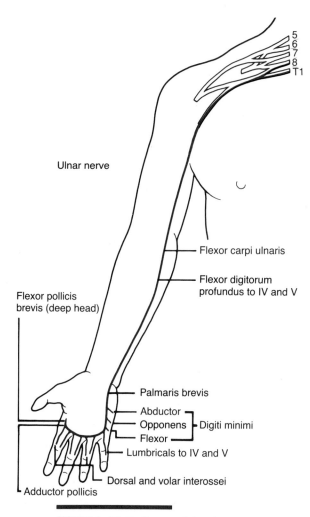

**FIGURE 6–26** ■ Course of the ulnar nerve.

Labels on figure:
Ulnar nerve
Flexor carpi ulnaris
Flexor digitorum profundus to IV and V
Flexor pollicis brevis (deep head)
Palmaris brevis
Abductor
Opponens — Digiti minimi
Flexor
Lumbricals to IV and V
Dorsal and volar interossei
Adductor pollicis
5 6 7 8 T1

nator muscle (the arcade of Frohse), by fibrous bands at the radial head and by fascia extending from the ECRB muscle (Fig. 6–31).[22–24] Distally, the superficial radial nerve can be compressed where it passes under the fascia of the brachioradialis.

## Blood Supply

The radial and ulnar arteries course through the forearm to supply blood to the hand (Fig. 6–32). The radial artery, located to the radial side of the forearm and hand, branches off into the superficial palmar branch just before entering under the volar carpal ligament. This superficial branch of the radial nerve courses over the volar carpal ligament and passes between the opponens pollicis and the abductor pollicis brevis. It

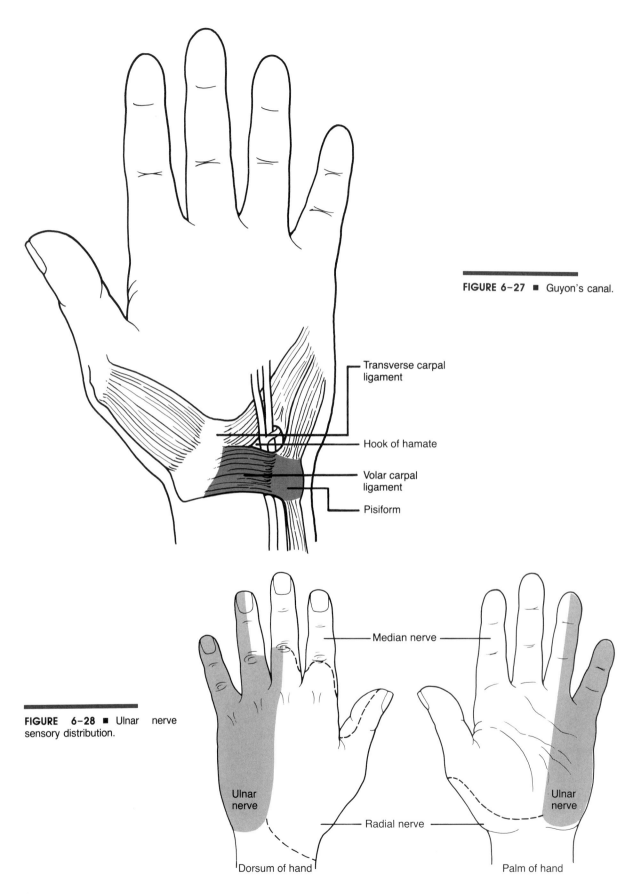

FIGURE 6-27 ■ Guyon's canal.

Transverse carpal ligament

Hook of hamate

Volar carpal ligament

Pisiform

FIGURE 6-28 ■ Ulnar nerve sensory distribution.

Median nerve

Radial nerve

Ulnar nerve

Ulnar nerve

Dorsum of hand

Palm of hand

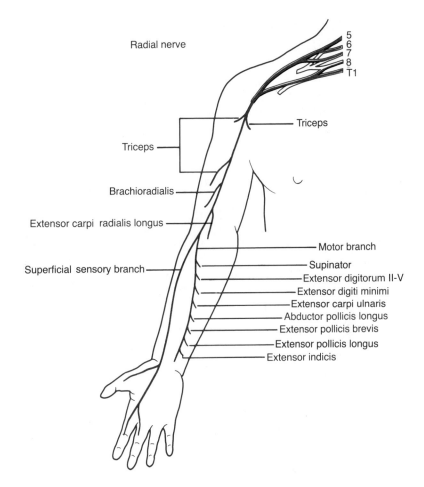

**FIGURE 6-29** ■ Course of the radial nerve.

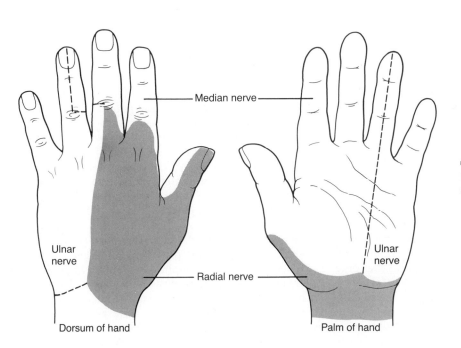

**FIGURE 6-30** ■ Radial nerve sensory distribution.

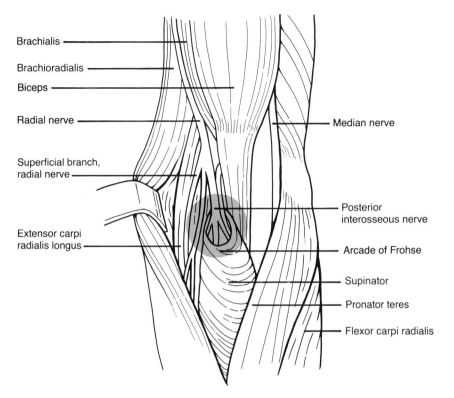

Brachialis

Brachioradialis

Biceps

Radial nerve

Superficial branch, radial nerve

Extensor carpi radialis longus

Median nerve

Posterior interosseous nerve

Arcade of Frohse

Supinator

Pronator teres

Flexor carpi radialis

**FIGURE 6-31** ■ Radial nerve compression at the arcade of Frohse (highlighted area).

venules, as well as direct arteriovenous anastomoses.[8]

The venous system of the hand consists of two portions, the superficial and the deep venous systems. The superficial veins lie in the superficial fascia and are concentrated on the dorsum of the hand. Venous flow from the superficial system becomes continuous with the cephalic and basilic veins dorsally and with the median antebrachial vein volarly. The deep venous system contains venous arches that correspond to the superficial and deep palmar arches of the arterial system. Venous flow from the deep venous system enters the venae comites, the deep venous system of the forearm. The lymphatic system mimics the venous system design.[8]

## EVALUATION

Evaluation of the hand and wrist is based on a detailed anatomic analysis of the complex skeletal, muscular, neural, arterial, and venous structures. The evaluation process should be organized and standardized to enable the practitioner to be comprehensive and objective. If only one extremity is involved, it is important to compare the involved to the uninvolved extremity or the "abnormal" to the "normal." In addition, practitioners should be encouraged to examine the joints above and below the area of dysfunction to differentiate local pathology from referred pain.

## History

Initially, a history should be taken from the patient to obtain information that is to be considered in differential diagnosis and treatment. Age, hand dominance, occupation, and avocations are general categories of questions. More significant information includes the duration of the present condition or date of injury; the mechanism of injury; conditions in which the injury occurred; treatment to date; other medical problems that may affect symptoms, response to treatment, or prognosis (rheumatoid arthritis, vascular or collagen disease); and medications being taken. The patient should be questioned about current and previous functional status: what problems or limitations are being experienced in personal care, activities of daily living, or his or her job. If there are complaints of pain, the type of pain sensation, time and pattern of occurrence, duration and frequency, factors that

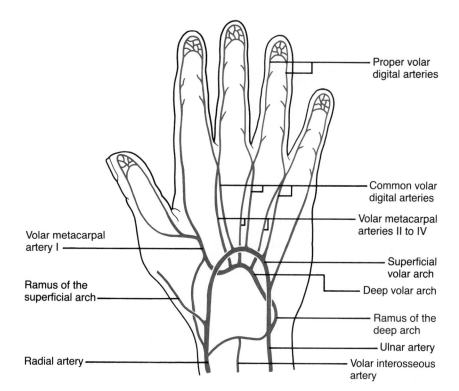

**FIGURE 6–32** ■ Blood supply to the hand.

*(labels on figure)*
Proper volar digital arteries
Common volar digital arteries
Volar metacarpal arteries II to IV
Superficial volar arch
Deep volar arch
Ramus of the deep arch
Ulnar artery
Volar interosseous artery
Volar metacarpal artery I
Ramus of the superficial arch
Radial artery

aggravate and relieve the pain, and impact of prior treatment should be noted.

A comprehensive history can be compiled by the patient before the first visit if forms are supplied. Previous medical records and test results should be secured. Additional information can be gathered from the patient during the initial interview or subjective evaluation.

## Visual Examination

After the history, a general inspection of the involved upper extremity should be performed. The posture in which the patient holds and carries the entire upper extremity should be noted. The resting posture of the hand itself

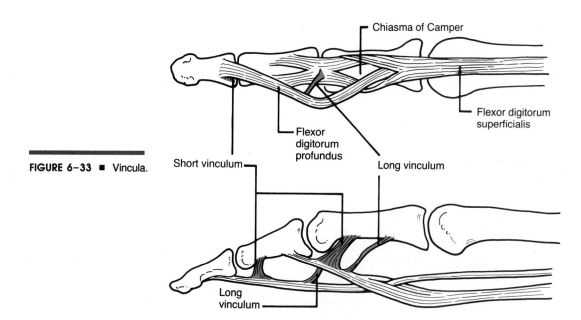

**FIGURE 6–33** ■ Vincula.

*(labels on figure)*
Chiasma of Camper
Flexor digitorum superficialis
Flexor digitorum profundus
Long vinculum
Short vinculum
Long vinculum

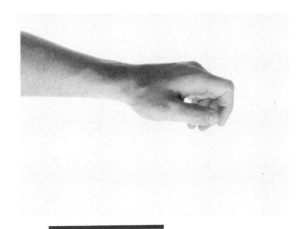

**FIGURE 6-34** ■ Resting posture of the hand.

should also be recorded, normal posture being increasing radial to ulnar flexion of the digits with the wrist in a neutral position (Fig. 6-34). Deviation from this usual flexed position of the digits may indicate tendon, joint, or peripheral nerve involvement. Any observed signs of pathology should be documented: muscle atrophy or hypertrophy; edema; wounds, scars, or skin discoloration; limited gross motion; and so forth.

Upon closer inspection, the practitioner should focus on the texture and color of the skin of the hand. Normally the palmar skin is moist, thick and irregularly textured, and tethered, allowing little motion of the skin over the deeper structures. The dorsal skin is thin and mobile. Creases of the hand and wrist are clearly defined (Fig. 6-35). Calluses are usually present, most commonly on the palmar surface of the hand at the level of the MP joints and at the pulps of the fingers. Changes in texture (skin atrophy) and altered sweating patterns may indicate vasomotor problems. The amount and distribution of sweat should be recorded and can be measured by using the ninhydrin test for sudomotor function.[26,27] Color changes (red, pale, or cyanotic) may indicate vascular problems and can be

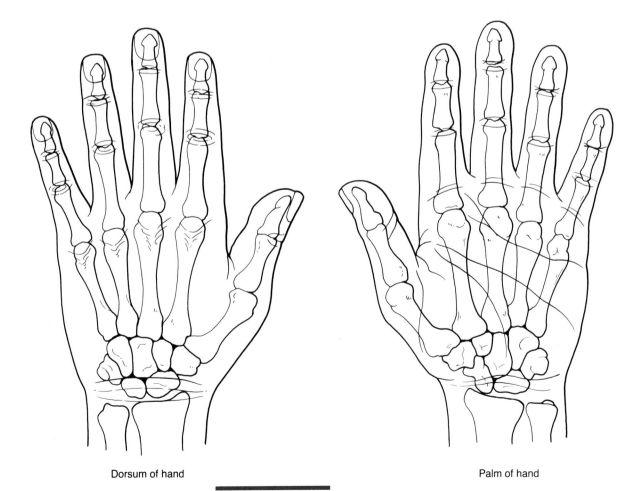

Dorsum of hand

Palm of hand

**FIGURE 6-35** ■ Creases of the hand and wrist.

recorded on a diagram or photograph. The nails should be examined for ridging, discoloration, or other deformities. Edema should be noted and measured volumetrically or, if that is not possible, by circumferential measurements of the digits, wrist, and forearm with a flexible tape measure. Characteristics of wounds and scars should be described. Lack of mobility of scar tissue can contribute to limited joint range of motion and tendon excursion and consequently function.

## Tactile Assessment

After visual assessment, palpation verifies observed symptoms in the hand and wrist and provides additional information. Palpation should be gentle and pressure modified in response to the patient's discomfort or pain. Areas of hypersensitivity or decreased sensation can be identified and specific changes in sensitivity evaluated later in the examination.

Palpation of the temperature of the skin is also important because it can be indicative of vascular problems. If objective measurement of temperature is desired, a thermistor or cutaneous temperature gauge can be utilized. Normal digital temperature ranges from 30 to 35°C. The radial and ulnar pulses can be taken as well. Patency of the arteries is determined by the Allen test.[24,28] In this test, both arteries are compressed and the patient is instructed to open and close the hand several times (Fig. 6–36). The hand appears blanched. Upon release of one of the arteries, the hand should fill and appear flush in the pattern

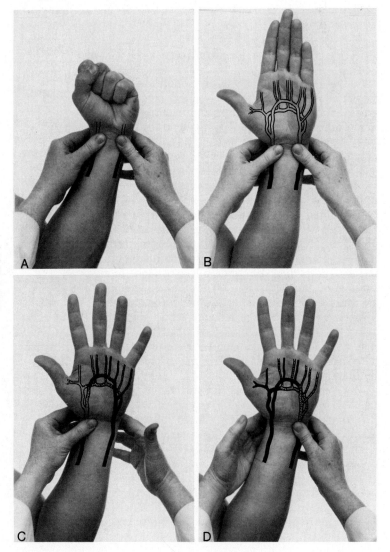

**FIGURE 6–36** ■ Allen test. (A) While the examiner compresses the radial and ulnar arteries, the patient should quickly open and close the fist. (B) As a result, the hand will blanch. (C) The examiner releases compression from the ulnar artery and observes the filling pattern. (D) The process is repeated to check the patency of the radial artery.

of circulation of that artery, indicating its patency. These steps are then repeated for the other artery. This procedure can also be performed with a single digit. The nails can also provide information about the circulation of the hand. Pressure over the nail bed causes blanching of the fingertip, but when pressure is removed the fingertip should flush with color if circulation is not impaired.

Deeper palpation of the hand and wrist assesses bones, joints, and areas overlying bursae and tendon sheaths. Palpation of joints and tendon sheaths reveals synovial effusion, swelling, or thickening, if present. Areas of tenderness or acute pain should be noted. Gentle mobilization (anterior, posterior, and lateral stresses provide joint play) of digital joints and the carpal bones can reveal ligamentous laxity. This last procedure should always be performed with care and may be contraindicated in some patients after trauma or surgery.

## Range-of-Motion Evaluation

Active and passive range of motion should be measured using objective tools and recorded in great detail. Crepitus, clinks, and clunks occurring during motion are also to be documented. The evaluation should focus not only on joint range of motion but also deficits in range resulting from other limiting factors such as extrinsic tendon tightness, intrinsic tightness, adherence, or a combination thereof. These limitations can be identified as the practitioner determines end feel on passive movement of the joints and compares the active and passive measurements of motion. Range-of-motion measurements should include both blocked and full-excursion measurements. Blocked range of motion is evaluated as the practitioner stabilizes the proximal segment of the joint in extension while the joint being measured is actively or passively flexed (Fig. 6–37). Full-excursion measurements are taken after the patient makes a fist or fully opens the hand (Fig. 6–38).

More specifically, to test for intrinsic tightness, the MP joint is held in full extension while the PIP joint is passively flexed (Fig. 6–39A and B). Then, with the MP joint held in flexion, the PIP joint is passively flexed again. If PIP joint flexion is greater with the MP joint in flexion than in extension, tightness of the intrinsic muscles is present and must be addressed in treatment.[24]

A similar procedure is followed when testing for oblique retinacular ligament tightness, except

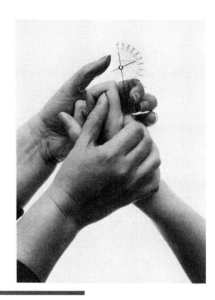

**FIGURE 6–37 ■** Blocked flexion range-of-motion measurement.

that the PIP and not the MP joint is held flexed and extended while the DIP joint is passively flexed (Fig. 6–40A and B). When tightness is present, DIP joint flexion is limited. If DIP joint flexion is greater when the PIP joint is held in a flexed position, tightness of the oblique retinacular ligament is present.[24]

When testing for either intrinsic muscle or oblique retinacular ligament tightness, if PIP and DIP joint motions are equal in both positions, it can be assumed that the functional ROM is limited by capsular dysfunction. Other limiting factors such as tendon adherence are usually influenced by position.

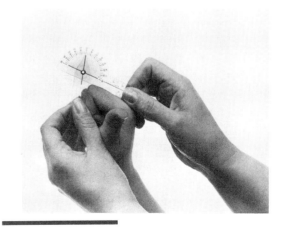

**FIGURE 6–38 ■** Full excursion flexion range-of-motion measurement.

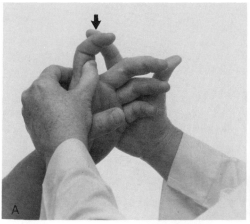
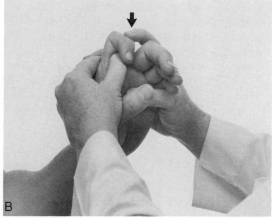

FIGURE 6-39  ■  (A and B) Intrinsic tightness test.

Other factors that can limit range of motion include tendon adherence. This is most easily assessed during examination of active range of motion. If joint motion is greater in the blocked position than in full excursion, it may be caused by limited excursion of the tendon(s). Altering wrist position can enhance the limitation of motion.

## Strength Assessment

Strength assessment is modified according to the diagnosis. Application of force, even for testing purposes, can disrupt damaged or surgically altered structures. Certainly, in a case involving a 4-week-old flexor tendon repair, a thorough evaluation of strength would be deferred.

Strength can be measured by manual and mechanical means. Manual muscle testing is used to assess the strength of the muscles of the hand and wrist. Muscle bellies and tendons are palpated to determine whether the muscle is being contracted when a manual force is applied. For details of proper test positions and testing technique, see Kendall and McCreary's *Muscles, Testing and Function.*[29] This text is an excellent reference for manual muscle testing.

Grip strength is measured using a grip dynamometer, and pinch strength by a pinch meter. Use of a grip dynamometer allows the practitioner to assess the strength of all the muscles contributing to grip in a functional manner.[30] The Jamar grip dynamometer (Asimov Engineering, Los Angeles, CA), by means of an adjustable handle, allows the assessment of grip in five positions (half-inch increments from 1 to 3 inches). To test grasp, the patient is asked to grip the

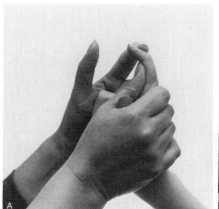
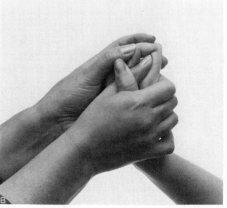

FIGURE 6-40  ■  (A and B) Oblique retinacular ligament tightness test.

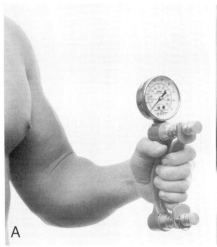
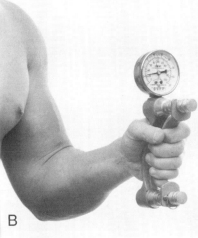

**FIGURE 6-41** ■ (A and B) Jamar test position.

dynamometer in each of the five positions, alternating between the uninvolved and the involved extremity. The elbow should be positioned at 90 degrees of flexion, the upper arm adducted by the patient's side, and the forearm maintained in neutral (Fig. 6–41). The patient should avoid a ballistic or jerking effort because this can result in falsely recording higher grip strength. The initial position is more indicative of intrinsic strength, the 3-inch position of extrinsic strength. Normally, grip strength is less at the extreme positions. If the strengths recorded at the five positions are plotted, a bell curve commonly results.[24,31] Limited range of motion, sensory deficits, pain, muscle development associated with occupation, and submaximal effort are factors that can cause a deviation from the bell curve.

A pinch meter is utilized to measure pinch strength. Three types of pinch strength are commonly measured: pulp to pulp, lateral or key pinch (Fig. 6–42A and B), and three-jaw chuck (not shown). The position described for grip testing is utilized for pinch testing. Assessment of these three pinch strengths can indicate dysfunction of the anterior interosseus and ulnar nerves and/or joint problems, particularly with the joints of the thumb.

To interpret the results of these strength tests, the patient's measurements can be compared to normative data.[32,33] However, because these norms may not be directly applicable to the specific patient, it is more effective to use the test results for the uninvolved extremity as the "norm" for that patient.

## Assessment of Sensibility

For optimal functioning, the hand requires intact sensation. Therefore, assessment of the

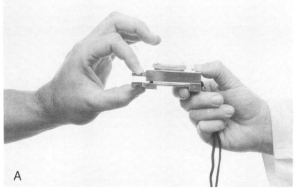
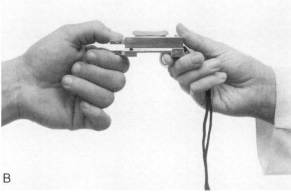

**FIGURE 6-42** ■ (A) Pulp to pulp (tip to tip) pinch measurement; (B) lateral or key pinch measurement.

hand's sensibility is an essential part of the evaluation process. Knowledge of the peripheral nerves, their patterns of innervation, and variations in innervation across individuals is required to interpret sensibility effectively. A variety of sensibility tests can be used, but the most commonly used tests include von Frey's filaments, Dellon's moving two-point discrimination test, Weber's two-point discrimination test, vibratory testing, and Moberg's pick-up test.

Adequate information can be obtained by performing a visual examination of the hand, Weber's static two-point discrimination test[34,35] (which evaluates the slowly adapting fiber-receptor system), and Dellon's moving two-point discrimination test[26,35] (which evaluates the quickly adapting fiber-receptor system). The results of these tests can indicate a need for further detailed assessment of the patient's sensibility. Visual examination was discussed earlier in the chapter. Static and moving two-point discrimination testing requires the use of a paper clip or an anesthiometer of some type—for example, the Disk-Criminator (Disk-Criminator, Baltimore, MD) or the Boley gauge (Research Designs, Houston, TX). If a paper clip is used, it must be bent so as to have two points that are level with one another. The space between the two points must be adjustable.

To perform static testing of a digit, the patient's hand (palm up) should be supported by the therapist's hand (Fig. 6–43) or by putty or a firm foam. Placing the points of the anesthiometer or paper clip longitudinally on the radial or ulnar aspect of the finger being tested, the therapist randomly alternates applying one and two points. The pressure applied should not exceed that which just causes blanching. The patient re-

**Table 6–1.** TWO-POINT DISCRIMINATION RATINGS

| Rating | Discrimination |
| --- | --- |
| Normal | Less than 6 mm |
| Fair | 6–10 mm |
| Poor | 11–15 mm |
| Protective | One point perceived |
| Anesthetic | No points perceived |

sponds to the number of points perceived (the patient's eyes are closed). The points are gradually brought closer together until the patient can no longer distinguish two points from one point.[26,35] Normal static two-point discrimination at the fingertip is less than 6 mm (see Table 6–1).[28]

Moving two-point discrimination testing is performed in a similar manner. The test procedure, as described by Dellon, begins with the points approximately 8 mm apart. The points are moved longitudinally from proximal to distal along the surface of the supported finger. Dellon states that "just sufficient pressure is utilized for the subject to appreciate the stimulus."[35] The stimulus is randomly alternated between one and two points with the patient responding with the number of points perceived (the patient's eyes are closed). The spacing between the two points should be decreased in 1- to 2-mm increments as the testing progresses; the final discrimination test is set at 2-mm spacing. Dellon suggests, "when the patient begins to answer slowly, and the moving two-point limit or threshold is being approached, [that] the patient be required to give seven of ten correct responses before proceeding to the next lower value."[35] Normal moving two-point discrimination is 2 mm at the fingertip.

## Functional Assessment

Further assessment of the functionality of the hand is necessary and can be accomplished by asking the patient to move and manipulate spheres, rods, and other objects of various sizes and by reviewing the patient's ability to perform activities of daily living, tasks that must be performed each day.

More specific assessment of the functional status of the hand includes the standardized manual dexterity and coordination tests described in the literature. These include the Purdue Peg-

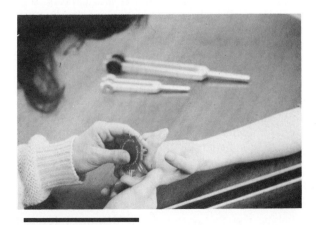

**FIGURE 6–43** ■ Two-point discrimination sensory testing.

board Test, in which the patient places small washers and collars on pegs placed in holes of a board (Fig. 6–44); the Minnesota Rate of Manipulation Test, in which the patient grasps and places blocks into spaces on a board; and the Jebson-Taylor Hand Function Test, in which the patient grasps and manipulates objects of various sizes and shapes. Some standardized tests require the use of tools as part of the test: the O'Connor Test, the Crawford Small Parts Dexterity Test, and the Bennett Hand-Tool Test.

General task and specific work simulations also provide information regarding the functional abilities of the hand and upper extremity as a whole. General task-oriented activities and work-stations can be utilized, with the therapist focusing on the patient's ability to perform the task, the manner in which it is performed, the length of time required to complete it, and the ability of the patient to repeat or maintain the task over time. Additional information can be gained through the use of a work simulator (Fig. 6–45) (BTE Work Simulator; BTE, Hanover, MD), a device that records torque, distance, and time measurements and calculates the amount of work performed and the power generated while simulating the task.

## Psychosocial Assessment

The psychologic and social aspects cannot be overlooked when dealing with patients with upper extremity dysfunction. In many cases, the lives of these patients are severely disrupted. They may be unable to work (either temporarily or permanently), incapable of caring for themselves independently at home, and no longer able to engage in their usual social and avocational activities. There can be loss of self-esteem and disruption of body image. Because the psychologic and social implications of these limitations can be staggering, it is essential that these aspects be evaluated and treated. In many cases, this extends beyond the capabilities of the therapist and the patient should be referred to a social worker, psychologist, or psychiatrist. If the psychologic and social dysfunctions are not dealt with, the treatment may be less effective and the patient's prognosis limited.

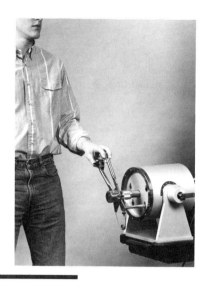

**FIGURE 6–45** ■ Functional tasks and work simulation (BTE Work Simulator).

## Basis of Rehabilitation

Management of hand injuries and conditions is based on the principles of wound healing. A thorough discussion of wound healing is beyond the scope of this chapter. Tables 6–2 and 6–3 provide a review of the phases of wound healing and typical healing times of the tissues of the hand. Although specific guidelines for treatment of injuries, diseases, and dysfunction are discussed later, it is important to recognize that general factors can influence healing; these include the patient's age, the patient's general health and nutrition, mechanism of injury, type of wound, and expertise of the surgeon. Therefore, a thorough knowledge of the principles of wound healing and prognosis for tissue recovery enables the therapist to alter treatment for the specific patient. Each case must be studied and

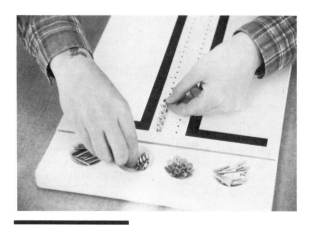

**FIGURE 6–44** ■ Standardized dexterity testing (Purdue Pegboard Test).

###### Table 6-2. PHASES OF WOUND HEALING

| Phase | Timetable | | | Pathophysiology | Wound Strength | Management |
|---|---|---|---|---|---|---|
| | Onset | Peak | Duration | | | |
| Traumatic inflammation | 0 | 12 hours | 24–48 hours | Vascular response: bleeding, edema<br>Cellular (phagocytosis) response: leukocytes, macrophages | Negligible | Rest<br>Elevation<br>Ice |
| Proliferation of fibroblasts | 12 hours | 2–5 days | 10 days | Fibroblasts proliferate, migrate, and bridge wound edges by 5 days | Some | Rest<br>Elevation |
| Collagen (fibroplasia) | 5 days | 3 months | 6 months | Collagen fibrils: initially weak random fibrils; later strong flexible fibers depending on the stress placed on them | Rapid rise | Splintage of the repaired tissue<br>Exercise |
| Remodeling | 1 month ────────→ 2 years plus | | | Collagenase removes excess collagen, fibroblasts contract, and there is vascular and wound shrinkage | Continued gradual rise | Exercise and return of function |

From Morrin JB, Davey V, Donolly WB: The Hand—Fundamentals of Therapy. London: Butterworth-Heinemann Ltd., 1985, p 3.

managed on an individual basis; one should not treat all patients with flexor tendon repair, carpal tunnel release, or Colles' fracture in the same way.

# TREATMENT

## Exercise

Range-of-motion exercises play a major role in the rehabilitation of the hand. Active, active assisted, passive, and resistive exercises are all used in hand rehabilitation. Active range-of-motion exercises promote tendon excursion and prevent tendon adherence, reduce or prevent ligament tightness, guide scar tissue formation, aid in reduction or prevention of edema, increase joint motion, and increase muscle strength and endurance. Passive exercises primarily increase joint motion and guide the formation of scar tissue. Resistive exercise is reserved for strengthening when indicated. The practitioner must apply his or her knowledge of the anatomy of the intrinsic muscle system, the extensor mechanism, and the influence of joint position on the ligaments of the joints when selecting exercises to be included in a specific treatment program.

In treatment of the hand, exercises should be performed slowly and should not cause pain; however, slight discomfort is acceptable. Treatment that is too aggressive may result in pain and edema, which can cause or increase stiffness

###### Table 6-3. HEALING TABLE[a]

| Tissue | Early Healing (Movement Without Stress) | Consolidated Healing (Can Take Full Stress) |
|---|---|---|
| Skin | 1 week | 3 weeks |
| Tendon to tendon | 3 weeks | 6–12 weeks |
| Tendon to bone | 3 weeks | 6–12 weeks |
| Ligament repair | As for tendon | As for tendon |
| Nerve | 3 weeks | 6 weeks |
| Bone to bone | 3 weeks | 6–12 weeks |

[a] These healing times vary according to the age, local blood supply, and general condition of the patient.
From Morrin JB, Davey V, Donolly WB: The Hand—Fundamentals of Therapy. London: Butterworth-Heinemann Ltd., 1985, p 4.

and dysfunction. Painful exercise causes fear and anxiety in patients and can influence their motivation and compliance with the program.

In addition to the exercises performed in the clinic, a home exercise program is a necessary part of the treatment. Even if the patient is seen on a daily basis in the clinic, this one-time daily exercise session is insufficient in treating the characteristic problems suffered by hand patients. Home exercises should be performed at least four to six times daily, with the number of repetitions determined by the practitioner. The program should be reviewed and updated at each clinic visit.

## Edema Management

Several methods for controlling edema are available to the clinician. Types of edema respond differently to the various treatment methods. For example, acute edema responds well to elevation and retrograde or fluid-flushing massage. Subacute edema is responsive to a more aggressive program of intermittent compression and pressure wrapping or pressure garments, in combination with elevation and massage. Brawny edema is difficult to manage. High-voltage galvanic stimulation can be added to the aforementioned treatment techniques.

The most commonly used method of edema management is elevation. The elevated position places the upper extremity above the horizontal position (commonly referred to as "the hand above the heart"). Venous return and lymphatic return are assisted by this position. Pillows or commercially available foam elevators can be used to achieve the optimal position. It is not advisable to ask the patient to maintain the elevated position actively for prolonged periods because muscle fatigue and soreness result.

Also used to assist venous and lymphatic return is retrograde or fluid-flushing massage. With the hand and upper extremity adequately lubricated and in the elevated position, the therapist applies pressure in a distal-to-proximal fashion. The amount of pressure utilized is based on the patient's tolerance; retrograde massage should not cause discomfort or pain. Contraindications for retrograde massage include infection, severe skeletal instability, and inability to maintain protective positioning while performing the massage. Patients and their families should be instructed in this technique when the therapist deems it appropriate.

Other options in edema management are constant and intermittent compression. Various materials are available that maintain light but constant pressure on the edematous area. On larger areas, an Ace wrap can be used. For the hand, elastic materials such as Coban, a self-adherent wrap (Medical Products Division/3M, St. Paul, MN), or Compressogrip bandage, an elasticized tubing, are appropriate substitutes because the area to be wrapped tends to be small (e.g., a single digit). Other materials that can be used to apply pressure include T-foam, cotton string, and elasticized gloves. With pressure wrapping, either the figure-of-8 or the angled circumferential wrapping technique can be used (Fig. 6–46). The wrap should be applied in a distal-to-proximal fashion. It is also recommended that the distal end of each digit remain exposed so that monitoring of skin color and temperature is possible. Coban wrap can be used almost constantly unless discomfort or vascular compromise is experienced. String should be applied for only 5-minute periods. Signs of excessive pressure include a change in skin color and a decrease in skin temperature. Air splints can also be used to apply constant or intermittent pressure. It is advisable to reserve string wrapping and air splints for the responsible, compliant patient with an uncomplicated diagnosis or condition because it is difficult to monitor signs of excessive pressure. Contraindications to pressure application include infection and vascular compromise or repair.

A commonly used modality for edema control is intermittent compression. Commercially available units include the Jobst compression pump (Jobst Institute, Toledo, OH). This method of treatment is most effective on large, edematous

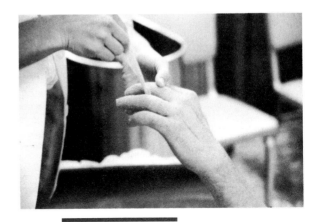

**FIGURE 6–46** ■ Coban wrapping of digits.

areas; it is not effective in treating edema in the fingers. An elevated position should be maintained while compression is being applied. On average, treatment duration is 30 to 45 minutes. Pressure delivered must exceed capillary pressure (25 mm Hg), if tolerated by the patient. It is important that the pressure delivered by the unit not exceed the patient's diastolic pressure minus 10 mm Hg.

Active range of motion is effective in reducing edema. Movement of the fingers tends to disperse fluids proximally, and muscle contractions serve to pump fluids from the edematous area. Active exercise must be monitored because aggressive exercise can increase edema resulting from inflammation. For patients who are unable to contract muscles effectively, electrical stimulation is an option. Electrode placement must be accurate in order to stimulate the motor point. A comfortable but fair grade of contraction should be elicited to be effective.

High-voltage galvanic stimulation is also utilized in edema management. Two methods can be used. One is to place the electrodes in the tank while using a whirlpool. The second is to apply wet gauze wrap circumferentially to the distal half of the upper extremity, with the electrodes encompassed within the wrap. Distribution of the edema determines electrode placement; the edematous area can be sandwiched by the electrodes, or the electrodes can be applied to the same surface over the edematous area.

## Pain Management

When treating the hand patient, it becomes obvious that there are many causal factors in pain. Joint stiffness, muscle spasm, edema, scar tissue adhesions, and nerve injury all contribute to pain. Effective treatment depends on identifying the cause(s) and then determining the most effective way to manage and/or alleviate the problem.

Various modalities are used for pain management. Heat is effective in relieving joint stiffness and muscle spasm. Popular choices of heat modalities include moist hot packs, paraffin, whirlpool, and Fluidotherapy (Henle Int., Sugar Land, TX). In deciding which to choose, consider whether moist or dry heat is preferable, what degree of elevation of the upper extremity is possible, and whether active motion is to be performed while the heat is being administered.

Decreasing edema in itself offers relief of pain or discomfort. Increased pressure within or surrounding structures causes pain, and decreasing edema results in a decrease in pressure. Edema management has been discussed previously.

Active use of the hand (range-of-motion exercises and functional activities) can alleviate pain or discomfort caused by joint stiffness and edema. In addition, when an exercise is performed slowly and deliberately, it stretches the joint capsule, thereby reducing joint stiffness. Motion also tends to disperse fluids from the fingers and, by way of muscle contraction, from the hand and forearm. It is important to monitor hand-forearm volume and complaints of pain or discomfort when using exercise and functional activities to reduce stiffness and swelling, because too much active motion may increase edema and pain of inflammation.

Massage is another treatment technique for alleviating pain and discomfort. The physiologic effects of massage help to reduce muscle spasm, joint stiffness, and edema. Deep friction massage is effective for scar tissue management. In the presence of pain caused by neuromas (sensitive, scarred nerve endings), massage serves to desensitize the painful area.

Other modalities that are useful in the management of pain are ultrasound, phonophoresis, electrical stimulation, and transcutaneous nerve stimulation (TENS). Pain resulting from muscle spasm, joint stiffness, and possibly scar tissue adherence can be influenced by ultrasound, phonophoresis, and electrical stimulation. TENS can be especially effective in cases of nerve pain. These include nerve compressions, nerve lacerations with repair, and amputations. Electrodes can be placed on or directly adjacent to the painful area, on acupuncture points, over dermatomes, or along the path of the nerve. When following the path of the nerve, electrodes can be placed proximal and distal to or only proximal to the painful area. Experimentation may be necessary to determine the optimal electrode placement as well as the optimal TENS settings (e.g., waveform, pulse rate, intensity).

## Management of Scar Tissue

Mobilization of scar tissue is accomplished by various methods. Deep friction massage can be performed manually or by using a device, such as a golf ball or others that are commercially available. Deep friction massage, when performed over adherent structures or tissues, promotes softening and increased mobility of the scar tissues. The combination of motion and pressure provides stretch to the collagen fibers. A lubricant should be used during manual massage to decrease shear forces over the skin and simultaneously provide skin care. Application of pressure to encourage softening and mobilization of scar tissue can also be achieved through the use of plaster of Paris, foam rubber, or elastomer, held in place by Coban or pressure gloves (Fig. 6–47). Elastomer (Dow Corning, Midland, MI) is a silicone rubber compound that conforms well to the scarred area. When used in conjunction with Coban or other compressive garment, it applies adequate pressure to the tissues, causing them to flatten and soften. Joint motion should not be inhibited by these various methods unless they are being used within a static splint.

Vibration and ultrasound are modalities that can be used in scar tissue management. Both are aimed at softening and/or altering the collagen fibers. The use of ultrasound for this purpose is controversial, but when it is used to disperse molecules of an applied topical medication (phonophoresis) it is more acceptable. Ultrasound should not be used during the first 4 to 8 weeks after tendon or nerve repairs. Additional research is needed to determine the effectiveness or ineffectiveness and guidelines for use of this modality in scar management.

Lastly, active and passive range-of-motion exercises are effective in managing scar tissue. The stresses applied to the collagen fibers during motion result in guiding or orientation of collagen formation and provide elongating forces across the fibers. The most effective technique is that of slow, active and/or passive stretch, lasting approximately 30 to 60 seconds. These stretches must be repetitious to be effective. Heat and massage can be used to prepare the tissues for this technique. It is important to note that scar tissue does not reach maturity for 6 to 12 months. Therefore, continued effort is worthwhile when dealing with resistant tissues.

The treatment techniques just discussed are utilized on a daily basis in the rehabilitation of hand and upper extremity problems. These problems include fractures, tendon and peripheral nerve repairs, joint arthroplasties, tendinitis, pain conditions, and a multitude of others. The following discussion concerns injuries, diseases, and conditions commonly seen by a physical therapist, particularly one who specializes in hand and upper extremity rehabilitation. The pathology, etiology, clinical signs, and treatment by physicians (nonsurgical and surgical) are discussed briefly. Physical therapy–related management is presented in more detail with the aim of providing sufficient information for the general clinician or novice hand therapist to feel comfortable in treating these problems.

## Common Fractures

Fractures of the wrist and hand can be simple to manage if they are stable and nondisplaced. These fractures are splinted or casted, immobilizing the joints just proximal and distal to the fracture to protect and permit healing of the bone. Frequently, this immobilization is discontinued after 2 to 3 weeks and minimal stiffness and compromise of function ensue. However, unstable, comminuted, and displaced fractures are more complex. Management of these fractures often requires surgical intervention, involving open reduction and internal fixation of the fracture with wire sutures, Kirschner wires (K-wires), screws, or plates. Splinting or casting is necessary in most cases after the surgical intervention to protect the fracture and external fixators. The duration of immobilization varies, but when stability has been achieved with internal or external fixation and the bone involved has good vascularity, mobilization is permitted. Intra-articular fractures and fractures involving severe comminution are not easily stabilized, and as much as 12 to 15 weeks of immobilization may be required in these cases. The disruption of the joint and the extended immobility complicate the course of rehabilitation with greater losses in range of motion, strength, and function.

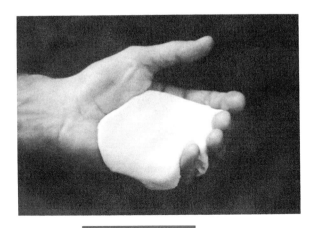

**FIGURE 6–47** ■ Elastomer mold.

## Extra-articular Fractures of the Wrist

### COLLES' FRACTURE

The most common fracture at the wrist is Colles' fracture. It is classified as an extra-articular fracture of the distal radius with dorsal displacement of the distal fragment and radial shift of the carpus and hand (Fig. 6–48). The fracture is usually incurred by falling on an outstretched arm with forces borne by the volar surface of the radius, the initial fracture site. The greater the angle of wrist extension at impact, the greater the forces placed on the distal radius. This results in more extensive injury, such as comminution of the dorsal portion of the radius.

Management of Colles' fractures ranges from closed reduction with casting or external fixation to surgical reduction with internal fixation.[36,37] Immobilization leads to joint stiffness, tendon tightness, and edema. Therefore, after application of the cast or fixator or after operation, it is important to initiate active and passive range-of-motion exercises of all uninvolved joints (the digits, elbow, as possible, and shoulder). These exercises maintain the integrity of joint capsules, help to reduce edema, and prevent tendon tightness and adherence of the uninvolved joints. The exercises should not cause pain. Aggressive management can slow healing and cause such complications as reflex sympathetic dystrophy (RSD).

Generally, consolidation of the fracture takes 5 to 8 weeks. This time frame may be lengthened by complications including injury to the distal radioulnar and radiocarpal joints. Loss of stability of these joints because of fracture or loss of ligamentous support complicates the management of these fractures and the treatment regimen.

Full functional recovery takes from 4 months to a year. Complications affecting the recovery process include median nerve compression and development of RSD. Unfortunately, some patients never recover fully from this injury. Limited range of motion of the wrist and/or forearm and decreased grip strength are among the residual symptoms of Colles' fracture. In cases involving RSD, the residual symptoms and resultant functional impairment are more significant.

### SMITH'S FRACTURE

This extra-articular fracture is the reverse of Colles' fracture. The distal portion of the radial fracture dislocates palmarly rather than dorsally and the hand and distal fragment displace radi-

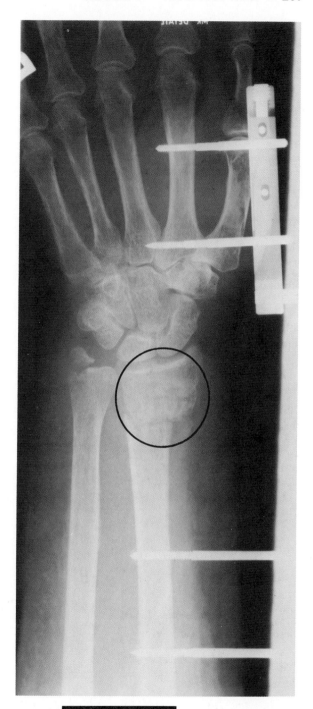

**FIGURE 6–48** ■ Colles' fracture (x-ray).

ally (Fig. 6–49). Like Colles' fracture, the most common cause of Smith's fracture is a fall. Often the fall is backward and the outstretched arm is supinated with the wrist dorsiflexed; therefore, the forces are borne across the volar surface of the radius.

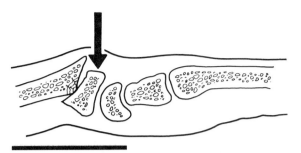

**FIGURE 6–49** ■ Smith's fracture. Arrow indicates palmar dislocation of the distal radius.

Surgical management is commonly required in cases of Smith's fractures.[36] If surgery is not performed, closed reduction with casting or external fixation is the method of treatment. The effects of immobilization, the use of exercise, and the effects of excessively aggressive treatment are similar to those in Colles' fracture.

On average, consolidation of the fracture takes 5 to 9 weeks. Recovery may be slower if the distal radioulnar and radiocarpal joints are injured. Loss of stability of these joints because of fracture or loss of ligamentous support complicates the management of these fractures.

In these cases, full functional recovery, if achieved, takes from 6 months to a year. Complications affecting the recovery process include median nerve compression and development of RSD. Some patients never recover fully from this injury. Limited range of motion of the wrist and/or forearm and decreased grip strength are among the residual symptoms after Smith's fracture.

## Carpal Fractures

### SCAPHOID FRACTURE

Fractures of the scaphoid (Fig. 6–50) constitute approximately 60% of all carpal fractures.[38] These fractures are most frequently caused by a fall on an outstretched hand and less commonly by a direct blow to the hand. In both cases,

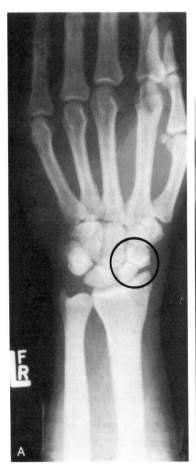

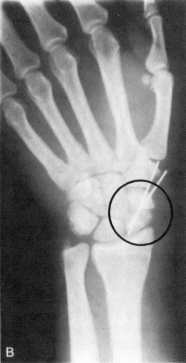

**FIGURE 6–50** ■ Scaphoid fracture. (A) Before treatment; (B) after reduction and fixation.

when the forces are borne by the bone rather than the supporting ligaments, fracture occurs. Fractures of the scaphoid occur at three levels: the distal pole, the midportion, and the proximal pole. Rate of healing and extent of complications depend on the location of the fracture because of the differentiated blood supply to the scaphoid. The middle and distal portions of the scaphoid are well vascularized and healing is faster than that of fractures involving the proximal portion. Poor vascular supply lengthens healing time and can lead to avascular necrosis of that portion of the scaphoid or nonunion of the fracture. The presence or absence of displacement of the fractured pieces also influences the rate of healing and frequency of complication. Capitate and lunate dislocations and fractures are often associated with scaphoid fracture.

Management of scaphoid fractures varies.[3,9,36,39] Nondisplaced fractures are easily managed by cast immobilization. Middle and distal portion fractures are placed in a cast for 4 to 8 weeks, proximal pole fractures for 12 to 24 weeks. Operative treatment is required for displaced scaphoid fractures. Open reduction with internal fixation using a K-wire, followed by application of a thumb spica cast, is common.

Rehabilitation should be initiated after application of the cast (with or without operative intervention). Active and passive range-of-motion exercises of the digital joints, elbow, and shoulder should be performed. These aid in reducing edema and prevent capsular and tendon tightness. Pain should not accompany exercise. Overly aggressive therapy can result in complications, including RSD. Instruction concerning elevation of the involved extremity should be given. On removal of the cast, active motions of the thumb and wrist are performed within a pain-free range. Support should be provided just proximal to the joint being moved, isolating the forces provided by the tendon(s) to move that joint efficiently.

Edema should be managed aggressively. Elevation, retrograde or fluid-flushing massage, and active range-of-motion exercises facilitate edema reduction. Other methods of edema control, such as Jobst compression, compression garments, and high-voltage galvanic stimulation, may be necessary.

## KIENBÖCK'S DISEASE

Kienböck's disease is a result of avascular necrosis of the lunate (Fig. 6–51); however, the specific cause of the avascular necrosis is not known. In a percentage of cases, a difference is noted in the articular surfaces of the radius and ulna. Normally the articular surfaces of these two bones are level with one another, resulting in even loading across the lunate. In many cases of Kienböck's disease, the articular surface of the ulna lies proximal to that of the radius, a condition termed ulnar minus or negative ulnar variant.[36,39-41] The lunate is then subjected to uneven loading because it receives no support from the ulna. With the wrist in the dorsiflexed position, the lunate is actually compressed between the ulnar border of the radius and the capitate.

Symptoms of Kienböck's disease include point tenderness over the dorsal aspect of the lunate, wrist pain, limited wrist dorsiflexion, and decreased grip strength. Treatment of the condition

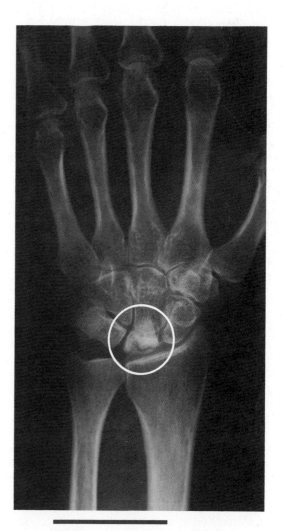

**FIGURE 6–51** ■ Kienböck's disease.

depends on the stage of the disease (I through IV), with stage I characterized by minimal destruction of the lunate and stage IV by collapse and fragmentation of the lunate with perilunate osteoarthritis.[36,40,41] Prolonged immobilization is the method of treatment employed early in the disease. Correction of the ulnar minus condition can also be a preferred treatment method.[42] In the late stage of the disease, several salvage procedures can be considered. One option consists of a lunate implant combined with arthrodesis of the scaphoid, trapezium, and trapezoid. Wrist implants are no longer a treatment of choice because silicone synovitis has become a notable complication. A more aggressive procedure would be a total wrist arthrodesis.

Rehabilitation of patients with Kienböck's disease depends on the treatment method selected. Therapy is focused on pain management and maintenance of digital, elbow, and shoulder range of motion while the wrist is immobilized. After removal of the cast, gentle active range-of-motion exercises of the wrist should be initiated (except in the case of the total arthrodesis) with the end goal of a functional range of motion, not normal range of motion. Addition of passive and resistive exercises to the rehabilitation program depends on the diagnosis. The clinician should be aware of the specifics of each case in order to select the appropriate treatment strategy. Range of motion and strength should not be gained at the expense of pain and instability.

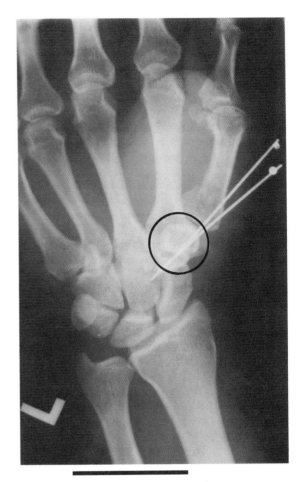

**FIGURE 6-52 ■** Bennett's fracture.

## Metacarpal and Phalangeal Fractures and Dislocations

### BENNETT'S FRACTURE

Bennett's fracture is a common fracture of the thumb. It involves fracture and displacement of the first metacarpal from its proximal end, the site of a strong ligamentous attachment (the anterior oblique carpometacarpal ligament). This ligamentous attachment site is the location of the oblique intra-articular fracture (Fig. 6–52). The pull of the abductor pollicis longus, which has its insertion at the base of the metacarpal, serves as a deforming force in this fracture.

Management of this dorsal fracture dislocation varies.[9] Closed reduction and immobilization are used, but in many cases it is difficult to maintain the reduction. When this is chosen, it is necessary to immobilize the thumb and wrist in a short arm cast for 6 to 8 weeks. A complication of this method is skin necrosis over the dorsum of the thumb because traction and pressure forces are applied by the cast to maintain the

reduction. Skeletal traction and open reduction with external fixation are also accepted methods of treatment.

During the period of immobilization, it is important to focus on edema control and maintenance of range of motion of the uncasted joints of the upper extremity. On removal of the cast, gradual mobilization of the thumb and wrist joints is necessary. Edema management must be continued and active blocked and full-excursion exercises initiated. Gentle passive motion is performed within a comfortable range.

### BOXER'S FRACTURE

A boxer's fracture is a fracture of the fifth metacarpal at the level of the neck (Fig. 6–53). It is called a boxer's fracture because in most instances the injury is sustained during a fight. Because of the forces borne by the metacarpals on impact, acute angulation of the head of the metacarpal into the palm occurs at the time of fracture. The proximal segment moves dorsally

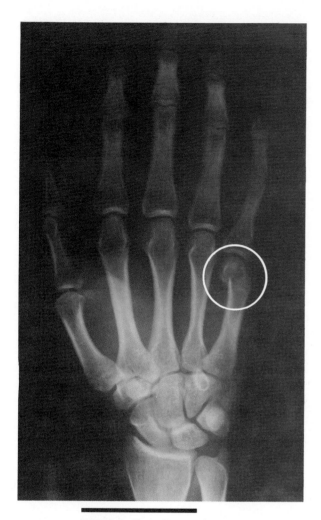

**FIGURE 6–53** ■ Boxer's fracture.

as a result of the impact forces and the pull of the interosseous muscles. The degree of angulation of the segments dictates the method of treatment.[43] For 20 to 30 degrees of angulation, closed reduction and casting are the preferred method of treatment. When greater angulation is present, closed reduction with K-wire fixation is required. When closed reduction is not possible or difficulty is encountered in maintaining the reduction, open reduction and plating of the metacarpal fracture are performed.

Closed reduction with a short arm cast or hand-based splint is the more common method of management. While the cast is in place, it is necessary to focus on maintaining motion of the uninvolved joints. Therefore, active and passive range-of-motion exercises of all uninvolved joints of the extremity are begun immediately. If the fifth metacarpophalangeal joint is not immobi-

lized, adequate stabilization of the metacarpal must be maintained during the exercise sessions. Measures to decrease or prevent edema should be used.

Splints and casts may be discontinued as early as 2 weeks after the injury, but in the majority of cases 4 weeks of protection are adequate. At this time, active and passive range-of-motion exercises are continued. Resistive exercises are usually initiated 2 weeks after removal of the cast or splint, and normal use of the hand is encouraged.

GAMEKEEPER'S THUMB

Stresses to the ulnar aspect of the thumb can result in rupture of the ulnar collateral ligament of the MP joint of the thumb (Fig. 6–54). The ligament itself can rupture or avulse from bone, most often at the proximal phalanx. This injury results in lateral instability of the thumb. Ulnar collateral ligament injuries are frequently sustained when skiing. During a fall, forces are frequently placed on the thumb via the ski pole.

These injuries are managed nonoperatively by reduction and casting or splinting. In cases of significant displacement of the bone fragment, the surgeon may perform an open reduction with internal fixation. After injury, range of motion of the uninvolved joints of the extremity is begun. The usual steps to control or prevent edema are taken. In either case, the thumb spica cast or splint (hand or forearm based) is usually removed at 6 weeks, when active and gentle passive range-of-motion exercises are initiated. In nonoperative cases, resistive exercises are given at the eighth week and normal use of the hand is encouraged. Where open reduction with internal fixation is required, the cast is removed at 6 weeks and the K-wire or wire pull-out suture at 8 weeks. Therefore, resistive exercises are not begun and normal use of the hand is not encouraged until the 10th week.

# Management of Flexor Tendon Repairs

## Primary Tendon Repairs

One area of challenge to clinicians who see hand patients is that of postoperative management of flexor tendon repairs. Tendon injuries can have varied appearances, from clean, tidy lacerations to untidy, mangled disruption compli-

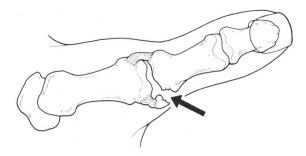

**FIGURE 6-54** ■ Gamekeeper's thumb (arrow).

cated by skeletal, vessel, and/or nerve damage. The mechanism of injury, status of the wound, and status of the patient all influence the immediate management of the tendon injury. The lacerated tendon may be repaired primarily, or repair may be delayed. In a primary repair, the tendon is sutured within 24 hours after injury; delayed primary repair is performed between 24 hours and 10 days after injury. Cash[10] also defines early secondary and late secondary repair. Delayed repairs often involve a staged procedure in which an artificial tendon is inserted for an average of 3 months, followed by a tendon graft. Surgical repair techniques are beyond the scope of this chapter, but the practitioner should be aware of common surgical techniques and their impact on the rehabilitation process.

A review of the literature yields various methods of postoperative management of flexor tendon repairs, ranging from complete immobilization for 3 weeks to early active mobilization. The most popular treatment programs, those which advocate immediate controlled mobilization, are described by Kleinert and colleagues[44-46] and Duran and Houser.[47,48] Other postoperative management programs are proposed by Young and Harmon[12,47,48,48a] and Chow et al.[49] Although these approaches vary, they are all based on the principles of wound healing. The ultimate goal of all is to manage the tissues through the appropriate wound-healing phases so that collagen is remodeled to allow tendon glide.

The phases of wound healing are summarized here, but it is recommended that further reading be done to supplement this information. The articles by Mason and Allen[50] and Peacock[51] are excellent. The three phases of healing are the exudative or inflammatory phase, the phase of fibroplasia, and the remodeling phase. The first two phases are typical of all healing wounds; the remodeling phase is specific to tendon healing.

The inflammatory phase of healing begins at the time of injury and lasts 4 to 6 days. During this phase there is a vascular and cellular response to injury. Reactions occur to fight infection, to rid the area of dead tissue, and to prepare the tissue for healing to begin. The second phase, proliferation, lasts 2 to 4 weeks depending on the site and size of the wound. Collagen formation and deposition occur in this stage. Toward the end of this phase, a counterbalancing of collagen synthesis and destruction must occur. Without this equilibrium, a tendon callus of great magnitude would develop and tendon glide could not occur. The third phase, maturation, lasts many months. Remodeling of the collagen network occurs through this period of time. The collagen fibers proceed from a disorganized, random arrangement to an oriented, organized structure. The effects of this remodeling can be seen both visually and functionally. Cross-linking of the collagen fibers at the tendon interface occurs, resulting in increasing tensile strength.

From a plot of tensile strength versus time (the phases of healing), it is apparent that during the initial 4 to 6 days after suture, the gross tensile strength drops below that found immediately after repair because of disintegration of the tendon ends. The sutures could be pulled from the tendon because of the softening that occurs at the tendon ends (loss of holding power). Around the fifth day, tensile strength begins to increase, and it returns to its baseline by approximately the ninth day. Holding power of the tendon ends returns to baseline by the 12th to 14th day. A plateau is noted around the 19th day, but another increase then occurs through the 21st day. A second plateau lasts approximately 14 days before further increase in tensile strength is noted. This period of increase (extending beyond the phase of fibroplasia) corresponds to the functional demands or stress placed on the tendon.[50-52]

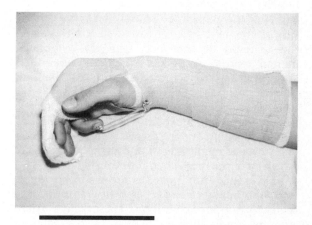

**FIGURE 6-55** ■ Protective splint for flexor repair.

With knowledge of the phases of healing and the vulnerability of the tendon repair during each phase, as well as the fact that tensile strength is directly related to the amount of stress placed on the tendon during the remodeling phase, postoperative management of tendon repairs has evolved. The goals of treatment after tendon repair are initially to protect the repair and then to mobilize the repair. As collagen is laid down, mobilization must begin to guide the collagen formation. As the collagen matures, it is necessary to continue to apply forces to prevent shortening or contracture of the tissues. Inappropriate management (improper splinting and mo-

bilization) can result in tendon lengthening because of stretching or gapping at the repair site, which can result in inadequate tendon excursion and therefore a poor functional result. Tendon rupture can also result from inappropriate management.

Immediately after a surgical repair, a plaster protective splint is usually applied. The splint maintains the digits and wrist in a flexed position that maintains slack on the repaired tendons. The protective splint (Fig. 6-55), which extends from the upper forearm to slightly beyond the fingertips, maintains the wrist in approximately 45 degrees of flexion and the MP and PIP joints in 20 degrees of flexion. In conjunction with the splint, rubber band traction is applied; that is, rubber bands are attached by a suture through the nail or a hook glued to the nail of the involved digits to a safety pin located at wrist level. The rubber bands maintain the IP joints in approximately 30 to 50 degrees of flexion but should be sufficiently light in tension to allow full IP extension within the bounds of the splint. The purpose of the rubber band traction is to flex the digit passively after active extension, decreasing tension on the repair site. Synergistic relaxation of the flexor muscles is achieved by the rubber band (Fig. 6-56). This splint is worn for 3 to 4 weeks and is then replaced by a less restrictive method of protection.

An Ace wrap or wide Velcro strap is worn around the wrist, and the safety pin is attached.

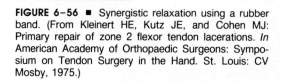

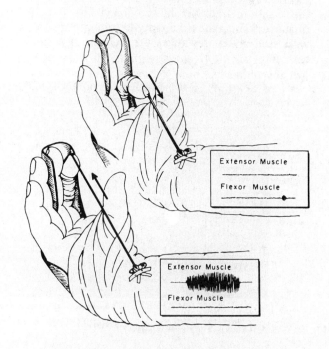

**FIGURE 6-56** ■ Synergistic relaxation using a rubber band. (From Kleinert HE, Kutz JE, and Cohen MJ: Primary repair of zone 2 flexor tendon lacerations. *In* American Academy of Orthopaedic Surgeons: Symposium on Tendon Surgery in the Hand. St. Louis: CV Mosby, 1975.)

The rubber band traction is utilized for an additional 1 to 2 weeks.

Generally, treatment is initiated 2 to 3 days postoperatively. Wound and skin care, edema management, and exercise are performed. Management of edema includes elevation and fluid flushing or retrograde massage. Fluid-flushing massage must be done cautiously, making sure that protective positioning is maintained.

Appropriate exercise consists of passive flexion and extension of the digits; digital extension is performed one joint at a time while the remaining digital and wrist joints remain flexed. The purpose of passive exercise is to prevent joint contractures of the digits, particularly the PIP joint, which is prone to flexion contracture with the use of rubber band traction. PIP joint contractures can occur if the tension provided by the rubber band is too great and does not allow the patient to reach full active extension of the IP joints within the bounds of the splint, or if the importance of achieving full extension is not stressed to the patient. If a contracture occurs, the clinician can extend the PIP joint passively by flexing the wrist and MP joint to slacken the repair tendon(s), extending the joint by moving the middle phalanx while stabilizing the proximal phalanx. Applying pressure to the middle phalanx does not stress an FDP repair as well, because the force is more effectively directed to the PIP joint. The same principles apply if a DIP joint contracture develops. To extend the joint passively, flex all proximal joints to slacken the repaired tendons and then apply force directly to the distal phalanx while stabilizing the middle phalanx. The patient should remain relaxed while the passive exercises are performed to en-sure that no tension is placed across the suture site of the involved tendons. All joint contractures should be managed aggressively because limited tendon excursion may result in adherence. Splinting for joint contractures can be initiated as early as 4 weeks if the digits and wrist can be positioned comfortably to avoid tension across the tendon repairs. This early splinting would apply only in cases of severe contractures. With proper management and compliance of the patient, contractures should not result.

Active extension exercises are also performed, with the rubber bands passively returning the digits to the flexed position. These active extension exercises allow excursion of the tendons through their sheaths to prevent adhesions. It is often helpful for the patient to flex the MP joint passively while extending the IP joints actively. Doing so more adequately directs the pull of the extensors to the IP joints. These active extension and passive flexion and extension exercises continue throughout the treatment program.

Passive extension of the wrist toward neutral while maintaining the digits in a fully flexed position is allowed in the second week. Prevention of joint stiffness is the purpose of this exercise.

At the end of the third week, gentle active flexion is initiated. The patient should be instructed in full-excursion flexion and in flexion of the IP joints only (hook fist position). These two types of flexion (Fig. 6–57A and B) allow differential gliding of the flexor digitorum profundus and superficialis tendons, which is especially important when both tendons have been repaired. Differential gliding prevents the repair sites from adhering to one another, which would limit active range of motion. Be cautious if

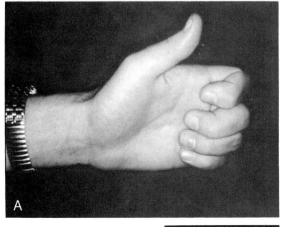
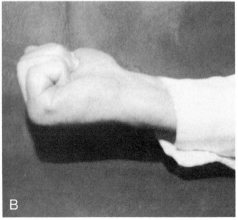

**FIGURE 6–57** ■ (A) Hook fist. (B) Full fist.

blocking is necessary when performing the hook fist exercise, because blocking can provide resistance to the proximal segment, resulting in resistance to the repaired flexor tendon. Another active exercise used to encourage tendon excursion is isometric fist exercise. The digits are passively placed in a fully flexed position and the patient is asked to hold that position (contract the flexors). This exercise is especially useful early in treatment, when few patients can achieve full flexion actively because of muscle weakness. Active and passive extension and passive flexion exercises continue. For these exercises, the wrist can be placed in the neutral position.

In the fourth week, splinting is discontinued unless circumstances of the injury or repair or the patient's compliance indicate otherwise. If continued protection is needed, an Ace wrap about the wrist to which the rubber band is anchored is an alternative to the splint (Fig. 6–58). Active and passive flexion and extension exercises are continued.

At 6 weeks, active flexion and extension exercises can be performed more aggressively and full passive extension of digits and wrist can begin simultaneously. Protective splinting is discontinued and dynamic splinting for joint contractures, if present, is indicated at this time. Flexor tendon tightness can be actively addressed at this time. Gentle active stretching can be performed by placing the wrist in a position in which full digital extension cannot be achieved. Gentle stretch can be applied actively at this position. Splinting for flexor tendon tightness is initiated during the seventh to eighth week. Light functional activities can be resumed at this time.

Resistive exercises can begin at the eighth

week. Initially, manual resistive exercise is most appropriate. As resistance is graduated, gentle resistance can be provided by a soft therapeutic putty or foam rubber ball, which allows dynamic motion, and hand exercisers, which provide a more isometric form of exercise. Both types should be employed. Hand boards composed of rubber bands can also be used for strengthening.

Over the next several weeks, more aggressive resistive exercises are performed to improve strength and endurance. Firmer putties and hand exercisers, along with weight cuffs and dumbbells, are utilized. By week 12, all restrictions on activities are eliminated. Return to work can be anticipated. Work hardening may be indicated to prepare the patient for return to work.

### Flexor Tendon Graft

When extensive damage has been sustained by the tendon(s), tendon sheath, and other digital structures, a primary repair may be contraindicated. Such injuries usually require surgical débridement and, if necessary, skeletal stabilization, vessel and nerve repair, and soft tissue coverage. Wound management, skeletal stability, and viability of the involved parts are the initial priorities of the surgeon. For the clinician, wound closure, scar management, and range of motion are the initial treatment priorities. Later, a tendon graft procedure can be performed. It must be decided whether a graft can be performed or a staged procedure is necessary. This decision depends on the extent of injury sustained initially and the current status. Soft, mobile scar tissue and normal to near-normal joint range of motion are necessary before the graft is surgically placed. Less extensive injury with minimal damage to the tendon sheath, pulley system, and other structures could indicate a primary graft, whereas more extensive injury would require placement of a tendon spacer first to allow for formation of a tendon sheath and bed. Several months later, a graft would be threaded through the newly formed sheath.

Management after a tendon graft is more conservative than that after a primary repair. The tendon graft is essentially a nonvascularized entity that is pulled through into the bed created by the tendon spacer and sutured to the proximal and distal ends of the remainder of the muscle-tendon unit. It takes approximately 3 weeks for the tendon graft to receive sufficient vascularization. Also, the graft has two suture sites, compared to the one site of the primary repair. Therefore, more caution is exercised when

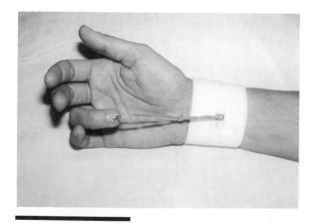

**FIGURE 6–58** ■ Dynamic traction using a rubber band anchored to an elastic wrap.

mobilizing a graft. The primary goal of tendon graft rehabilitation is well described by Wilson,[53] who states that "it is necessary to achieve both stability and balance in the digit and to have the graft act primarily to flex the more proximal joint. Less motion but more power is required at the distal joint."

Immediately after operation, a protective splint maintains the wrist in 30 to 40 degrees of flexion and the MP joints in 50 to 60 degrees of flexion. Rubber band traction is used as described in the section on primary flexor tendon repairs. The IP joints assume a semiflexed resting position, although the splint and tension offered by the rubber bands should permit full extension. Wound and skin care is provided and edema controlled (details have been given previously). Gentle passive joint flexion is performed by the clinician. Active and passive IP joint extension exercises are performed with the wrist and MP joints in flexion. Proper stabilization of proximal segments should be provided when performing active and passive extension exercises. This treatment program continues through the third week. With wound closure, aggressive scar management should be initiated.

During the fourth week, the dorsal protective splint can be discontinued and the rubber band attached to a wrist band. An exception is made in the case of a patient who has full or nearly full excursion flexion, because a free-moving tendon is considered more vulnerable to rupture at this time. Gentle active flexion of the IP joints while stabilizing the MP joint in increasing degrees of extension is added to the exercise program. Passive exercises should continue.

The pull-out wire or suture is removed at week 5. Active IP joint flexion and extension are increased and passive flexion and extension exercises continue. During the sixth week, hook fisting is initiated and more vigorous active PIP joint flexion is encouraged.

At the seventh week, gentle resistive flexion and extension are permitted. Splinting should be discontinued, if not already done, and the patient encouraged to utilize the hand in light activities. Extension exercises should become more aggressive in the eighth week. Joint contractures can be splinted at this time, being cautious not to place excessive tension across the graft. A gradually increasing resistive exercise program should be initiated, utilizing therapeutic putties, hand exercisers, and so forth.

In managing flexor tendon grafts, the clinician must be aware of complications of this procedure. With primary flexor tendon repairs, joint contracture and stiffness can develop and tendon rupture is possible. More specific to a flexor tendon graft are bowstringing and the tendency toward development of a swan-neck or lumbrical plus deformity. Bowstringing of the tendon is a result of an inadequate pulley system. In the absence of particularly the $A_2$ and $A_4$ pulleys, the tendon is not adequately restrained and a poor mechanical advantage exists for the tendon. Therefore, when the muscle contracts, the tendon is unable to transmit the force efficiently, resulting in decreased flexion and grip strength. Swan-neck deformity can develop if imbalances exist between the extrinsic flexors and the intrinsic system. If the tendon graft is too long, causing the profundus to retract proximally into the palm and resulting in increased tension on the lumbrical, a lumbrical plus deformity can develop. Lumbrical plus deformity can be seen as the patient actively flexes the fingers; increased MP joint flexion results in IP joint extension.

If damage to the pulley system and tendon sheath and bed is extensive, it is necessary to reconstruct the pulley system and create a bed and sheath into which a tendon graft can later be placed. Therefore, a two-stage tendon repair is indicated. This procedure involves insertion of a tendon spacer or implant, which is secured by a screw to the distal phalanx and untethered at its proximal end in the proximal palm or forearm. The spacer is flexible yet firm so that it does not buckle as the digit is flexed. As motion of the finger occurs, the spacer glides freely and, as a result, a new sheath begins to form around it. The tendon spacer remains in place approximately 12 to 16 weeks. During this time, the new sheath matures and fluid develops, which aids in the gliding of the graft once in place.

Use of active tendon implants has been described. Hunter et al[54] have inserted Dacron cords that are secured both distally to the distal phalanx and proximally to the proximal tendon motor, which allows the implant to impart active motion to the involved digit. This implant allows utilization of the graft motor through the 12th to 16th week and testing of reconstructed pulleys.

Treatment after insertion of the tendon spacer includes wound and skin care, scar management as indicated, edema control, pain management, and passive range of motion to minimize joint stiffness and prevent joint contracture. Complications that can accompany this procedure include excessive edema, excessive scar tissue, pain, joint contracture, digital deformity resulting from the imbalance associated with the unopposed pull of the extensor tendon(s), and tenosynovitis. The clinician should be aware of the earliest symptom and deal with each aggressively to avoid the consequences.

Postoperatively, a dorsal protective splint is applied, maintaining the wrist in approximately 30 degrees of flexion, the MP joints in 60 degrees of flexion, and the IP joints in full extension. Early range of motion consists of gentle active extension and passive flexion exercises. Passive flexion can be accomplished by the therapist and patient passively moving the involved finger and also by allowing the patient to trap the involved finger between adjacent uninvolved fingers. Buddy taping can be used to simulate active flexion as well. If pain develops during the early postoperative weeks, the use of TENS is suggested.

At 3 weeks, protective splinting is discontinued. Splints or web straps can be used to improve passive flexion if limited. Buddy taping or Velcro strapping can be used to encourage motion of the involved finger(s) during light activities.

By the sixth week, the patient can return to work if it is deemed safe. Aggressive management of joint stiffness and contracture and scar tissue is mandatory. The clinician and patient must remain focused on the goals of treatment because the success of the subsequent tendon graft depends on successful management of this initial stage.

## Tenolysis

If tendon adherence remains a problem despite aggressive efforts to encourage tendon excursion, the patient may be a candidate for a flexor tenolysis. This surgical procedure involves excision of scar tissue about the tendon that binds the tendon within the sheath. On average, at least 12 weeks must elapse from the date of primary tendon repair or tendon graft to when tenolysis is performed.[55,56] This time delay allows slowing of scar tissue formation or tissue equilibrium before introducing further surgical trauma. Other requirements for the procedure are normal or nearly normal passive range of motion, functional sensation, and adequate muscle strength.

Active motion should be initiated within 12 hours after surgery. Edema must be monitored carefully. Strickland[56] states that "the first several days after this procedure are critical, and it is rare to see a substantial improvement of range of motion that is actively achieved during the first week." Postoperatively, it is important to control edema and pain. Methods of edema con-

trol have been discussed previously. TENS may be used for pain management after tenolysis. Some authors advocate the use of local anesthesia during the first postoperative week.[55] Pain must be managed so that the patient can perform effectively the active exercises that are begun immediately after surgery. Isometric fist exercise is the key exercise because it is most effective in encouraging tendon excursion. The fingers are moved passively into a full fist and the patient is asked to hold them actively in that position. Gentle active blocked IP joint flexion and active extension are also permitted. Exercises are performed on an hourly basis, and it is important that the patient be instructed in proper exercise techniques. Electrical stimulation is indicated if muscles are weakened.

## Extensor Tendon Injuries

Rehabilitation of extensor tendon injuries is based on knowledge of wound healing, biomechanics, and anatomy of the extensor system. At various levels throughout the system, there are differences in nutrition and vascularity that affect healing and biomechanics because of the interrelationships of various structures. To become more familiar with specifics of the extensor system, it is necessary to present details of its structure.

The extrinsic extensor digitorum communis tendons traverse the distal forearm and carpus and then fan out over the metacarpals to enter each digit. As each tendon passes over the MP joint, it becomes entangled in an intricate system of ligaments, fascial bands, and other tendons, termed the extensor mechanism. Some structures of this mechanism function to transmit tension, resulting in active motion of the finger, and other structures contribute to stabilization of the mechanism.

Dorsally, over the distal end of the metacarpal and at the MP joint level, a fibrous dorsal hood composed of the extensor tendon, tendinous junctions, and sagittal bands is formed (Fig. 6–59). The latter two structures contribute to maintaining the central position of the common extensor tendon and stabilizing the tendon as it transmits forces. As the sagittal bands connect the extensor tendon to the volar plate and proximal phalanx (Fig. 6–60), they function to extend the MP joint. According to Rosenthal,[19] the sagittal bands also act as "functional slings that pass between the joint capsule and the intrinsic muscles. They hood the axis of joint motion during

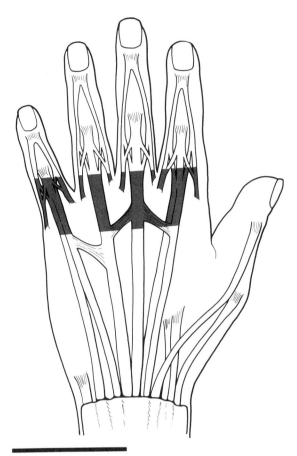

**FIGURE 6-59** ■ Common extensor tendons, tendinous junctions, and sagittal bands.

extension and pass distally to the axis of motion during flexion." The intrinsic muscles, both the lumbricals and interossei, contribute to the extensor mechanism via their connection to a wide fibrous dorsal hood (Fig. 6–61). This dorsal hood is divided into two sections, the oblique portion and the transverse portion. The interosseous muscles contribute to the transverse portion of the hood and, therefore, function to flex the MP joint when contracted. The lumbrical insertions converge into the oblique portion of the hood. This configuration permits them to function as IP joint extensors.

At the level of the middle phalanx, fibers from the oblique portions of the extensor hood blend into another structure, termed the lateral bands (Fig. 6–62). Also contributing to the lateral bands are fibers from the central tendon. Lateral bands from each side of the finger move dorsally and distally along the middle phalanx, where they join to form one tendon, the terminal extensor tendon. This terminal tendon inserts into the base of the distal phalanx and functions to extend the distal phalanx. The central extensor tendon inserts into the distal middle phalanx and, along with the oblique fibers of the dorsal hood, functions to extend the PIP joint.

The transverse retinacular, triangular, and oblique retinacular ligaments also contribute to the extensor mechanism. These ligaments are similar in function to the previously mentioned sagittal bands. The structures contributing to the

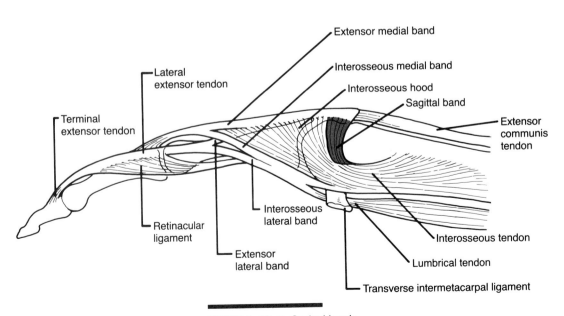

**FIGURE 6-60** ■ Sagittal bands.

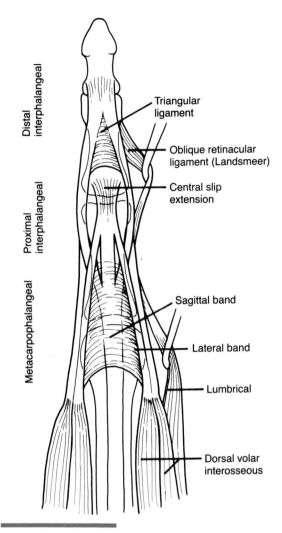

**FIGURE 6-61** ▪ Interossei and lumbricals to dorsal hood.

transverse retinacular ligament are the flexor sheath and the volar plate of the PIP joint. This ligament lies volar to the lateral bands and functions as a stabilizer of the PIP joint and the lateral bands. Fibrous extensions from the intrinsic and central extensor tendons and the lateral bands compose the triangular ligament and enable it to assist in extension of the middle phalanx. The oblique retinacular ligament also originates from the flexor sheath, at the level of the proximal phalanx. It inserts into the base of the distal phalanx along with the terminal tendon. As this ligament passes volar to the PIP joint axis, it functions to assist in the extension of the DIP joint.

The complexity of the extensor mechanism is obvious. A delicate balance is maintained within

this system and any disruption of a contributing structure can have dramatic effects. The clinician must have a thorough understanding of the system to manage injuries to the mechanism appropriately and to treat or prevent accompanying deformities.

Rehabilitation of extensor tendon injuries is different from that of flexor tendons. Structural and nutritional differences make a more conservative treatment approach necessary. Extensor tendons are injured five times more frequently than flexor tendons, in part because of their subcutaneous location. Extensor injuries are generally considered less complicated to treat than flexor tendon injuries; however, if they are treated improperly a simple extensor or complicated extensor injury can be as compromising to the integrity of hand function as a flexor tendon injury.

The extensor tendons are flat, ribbon-like structures composed of longitudinally oriented fibers that do not easily retain sutures. In the case of the extensor tendons, healing occurs despite the large separation between the two ends. This separation appears to be progressive; it is greater at 6 weeks than at 3 weeks or 3 days. Extensor tendons' ability to hold sutures diminishes more rapidly and to a greater extent than flexor tendons'. Suture pull-out may occur even at 21 days. In the case of wound healing, the curve for the extensor tendons is similar in appearance to that for the flexors, but it progresses at a slower pace. The extensor tendons have less excursion than the flexors, which makes preservation of tendon length critical during repair.

Like the flexor tendon anatomy, the extensor anatomy has zones that are defined by anatomic relationships.[17,18] There are seven extensor tendon zones (Fig. 6–63):

**Zones 1 and 2** are defined distally by the insertion of the terminal extensor tendon into the distal phalanx and terminate just distal to the attachment of the central slip to the proximal end of the middle phalanx. Also included is the area of insertion of the oblique retinacular ligament into the terminal tendon.

**Zones 3 and 4** encompass the attachment of the central slip to the middle phalanx, PIP joint, transverse retinacular ligament, transverse portion of the extensor hood, and insertion of the lateral bands.

**Zone 5** extends from the proximal end of the proximal phalanx to the metacarpal neck.

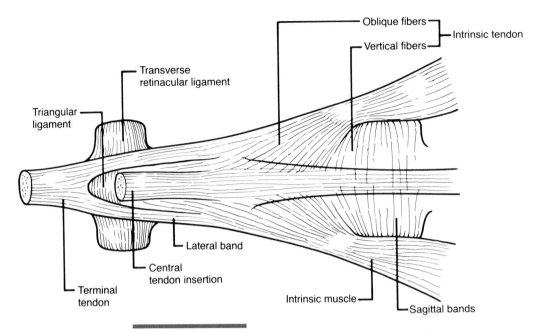

**FIGURE 6-62** ■ The extensor mechanism at the PIP joint level.

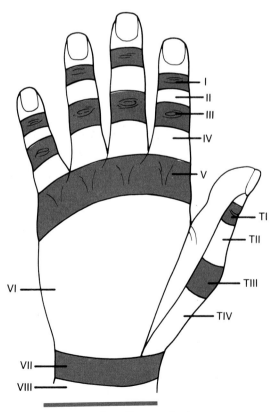

**FIGURE 6-63** ■ Extensor tendon zones.

Structures included in this zone are the sagittal bands located at the MP joint level.

Zone 6 is defined distally by the metacarpal neck and proximally by the carpometacarpal joints.

Zone 7 corresponds to the area overlying the carpus.

The rehabilitation of extensor tendon injuries is designed by zones. Having the necessary knowledge of extensor anatomy, biomechanics, and healing, the appropriate management should easily be understood.

**Injuries in Zones 1 and 2.** In zones 1 and 2, the most frequently treated injury is rupture of the terminal tendon. This injury occurs when a direct blow is sustained by the distal end of the finger, forcing the distal phalanx into an extremely flexed position. As a result, the tendon ruptures or a fragment of bone is pulled from the distal phalanx where the tendon inserts. The loss of the support offered by this tendon results in a "mallet" deformity (Fig. 6-64).

In the absence of other associated injuries, such as open injury to the tendon and fracture dislocation, conservative treatment is appropriate in cases of acute injury. This consists of continuous immobilization of the DIP joint in 0 degrees

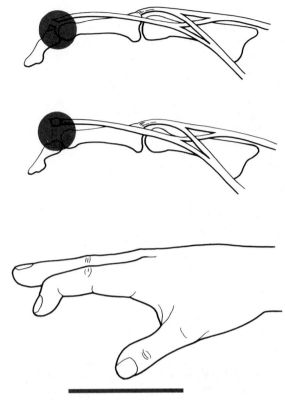

**FIGURE 6-64** ■ Mallet deformity.

of extension to approximately 10 degrees of hyperextension for 6 to 8 weeks. Maintenance of the joint in this position allows healing of the tendon through scar tissue formation or healing of the bone by callus formation. A splint fabricated from a thermoplastic material can be used to immobilize the joint, or foam-covered aluminum splints or the commercially available Stack splint (Link America, Inc., East Hanover, NJ) can be substituted. It is recommended that the splint be applied to the dorsal aspect of the distal and middle phalanx so as not to interfere with sensory function and full flexion ability of the PIP joint. Doing so eliminates the option to use a Stack splint. Caution must be exercised to avoid vascular compromise and skin breakdown caused by the splint. Hyperextension of the DIP joint can compromise circulation to the dorsum of the distal phalanx and lead to skin necrosis. Also, because splinting is continuous, moisture from perspiration can accumulate and lead to maceration of the skin. To avoid this complication, the splint can be lined with an absorbent material such as moleskin and an alternate splint made available to replace one that becomes wet. Pa-

tients and their families must be instructed in splint replacement. It is critical that the DIP joint remain fully extended while the splint is being replaced to avoid interfering with or interrupting the healing process. A family member can support the joint in the extended position during the change, or the patient can use the edge of a table to support the distal phalanx while alternating splints.

In the presence of associated injuries, surgical repair of the tendon and reduction of a dislocated fracture may be necessary. In these cases, immobilization of the joint is accomplished using a K-wire.

During the 6- to 8-week period of immobilization, the patient should be seen weekly for wound and skin care and splint adjustments necessitated by changes in dressing volume and edema. Range of motion of all uninvolved joints must be monitored to ensure that normal motion is maintained. During this time, the clinician must look for any tendency toward development of a swan neck deformity. Should this tendency develop, the PIP joint must be splinted in 35 to 45 degrees of flexion, which removes tension from the extensor mechanism. The DIP joint should continue to be splinted in full extension to slight hyperextension. In many cases, only 2 to 3 weeks of PIP joint splinting is required to overcome the tendency toward the swan neck deformity.

At the sixth week, gentle active flexion exercises are begun, with the patient instructed in proper stabilization techniques (support of the proximal and middle phalanges in extension). Only 20 degrees of flexion should be allowed to avoid the potential for overstretching or rupture of the tendon. If an extension lag develops at this time, active exercise should be stopped and the DIP joint continuously splinted for an additional 2 to 3 weeks. If the healing tendon tolerates the active flexion exercises, the arc of motion can be increased in week 7 to 30 to 35 degrees of flexion.

By the eighth week and in the absence of extension lag, daytime splinting can be discontinued and active flexion increased. Splinting at night should continue for an additional 3 to 4 weeks. The patient should be encouraged to use the hand in light activities, although resistive exercises are avoided until the 12th week.

**Injuries in Zones 3 and 4.** Postoperative management of injuries in zones 3 and 4 is similar to that described for zones 1 and 2 except that the

PIP joint becomes the area treated. Damage to the central extensor tendon and the triangular ligament is sustained when injury occurs within this area, and therefore a boutonnière deformity is commonly observed. Acute, closed injuries can be managed conservatively by 6 weeks of immobilization. The PIP joint is splinted in full extension, while the DIP joint remains mobile. DIP joint flexion is encouraged to stretch the oblique retinacular ligaments and lateral bands. Associated injuries, such as involvement of the lateral bands, may necessitate surgical repair and immobilization of both IP joints.

The patient should be seen weekly to monitor wound and skin conditions, edema, splint fit, and range of motion of all uninvolved joints. Edema is a common complication of this injury. It must be managed aggressively using Coban wrap, circumferential splinting or casting, and retrograde massage.

With repair of the lateral bands, immobilization of the DIP joint is maintained for 4 to 6 weeks. Therefore, gentle active DIP joint flexion exercises may begin at 4 weeks. Active PIP joint motion is deferred for an additional 2 weeks. PIP joint exercises include gentle active flexion and aggressive active extension. Proper stabilization of the proximal segments is critical when performing these exercises. During active flexion, the proximal phalanx should be stabilized in the extended position. For active extension exercises to be effective, the proximal phalanx must be stabilized in the flexed position to achieve maximum intrinsic extension.

Extension splinting continues for a total of 8 to 10 weeks, but the splint is removed for exercise beginning at the sixth week. If PIP joint flexion is difficult and minimal extension lag is present, dynamic flexion splinting can begin at the eighth week. Appropriate splinting schedules require careful monitoring of the patient's range of motion. When daytime splinting is no longer necessary, functional use of the hand is encouraged. Resistive exercises are added to the program at approximately the 9th to 10th week.

**Injuries in Zones 5 and 6.** Opinion varies regarding the timing of mobilization of extensor tendon repairs in zones 5 and 6. Timing is critical. As tensile strength permits, increased tension is applied to elongate the scar. The goal is to manage the tissues appropriately as dictated by the various phases of wound healing so that collagen is remodeled to allow tendon glide. To obtain optimal results, the clinician must consider the anatomic characteristics of the area, the

correct position for immobilization, and the proper timing of mobilization. Improper splinting and timing of mobilization can result in an increase in tendon length through stretch or gapping at the repair site, resulting in an extension lag that cannot be overcome.

A supportive and protective splint is applied immediately after surgery. The splint spans from the upper forearm to slightly beyond the fingertips. If only one or two digits are involved, adjacent fingers should be included in the splint because of the action of the juncturae tendinum. To support the joints properly, the wrist is positioned in approximately 40 degrees of extension while all digital joints are maintained in full extension. This protective position must be maintained when the hand is out of the splint, to avoid placing tension across the repair site.

Wound and skin care, edema management, and exercise are initiated 3 to 5 days after surgery. Wound and skin care can be accomplished by using a sterile whirlpool bath (with hand and wrist adequately supported). This cleans and débrides the wound and softens the skin. Edema control may be necessary. Elevation, retrograde massage, and Coban wrapping are methods used to control acute edema. Later in the treatment program, intermittent compression and/or compression gloves may be added. Exercises include active blocked flexion and passive extension of each digital joint individually. Passive MP flexion between the ranges of slight hyperextension through 10 degrees for the index and long fingers and 15 degrees for the ring and small fingers should be performed. This allows approximately 2 mm of excursion of the tendons to discourage tendon adherence.[57] The clinician can also appreciate possible joint problems while doing this maneuver.

After 2 weeks, the splint is cut back to free the DIP joints but continue to support all other proximal joints. Upon closure of wounds, scar management is essential. Mobilization of scar tissue is accomplished by various methods. Manual massage or massage using a device, such as a golf ball or others now available on the market, promotes softening and increased mobility of the scar tissues. Application of pressure to encourage softening and mobilization can also be achieved through the use of foam rubber or elastomer, held in place by Coban wrap or gloves. Vibration and ultrasound are other options for scar management. Active DIP and PIP joint flexion exercises with the MP and wrist joints held in extension are performed during each therapy session.

At 3 weeks, the static splint can be cut back to free the PIP joints, allowing active PIP joint flexion exercises to be added to the home program. To avoid excessive tension across the extensor repairs resulting in extension lag, a hand-based support that can be affixed to the static splint is fabricated. When the patient is not exercising, this extension support should be utilized. In place of the static splint, a dynamic MP extension splint can be fitted. This option should be reserved for the cooperative patient and those in whom MP joint stiffness is a problem.

Four weeks after surgery, gentle active and active assistive extension exercises are permitted. In order to isolate the EDC tendons, the patient should be instructed in "clawing." The IP joints are semiflexed while the MP joints are extended (Fig. 6–65), resulting in tendon glide. To work on MP joint flexion, the intrinsic plus position should be utilized. The patient should actively extend the IP joints, then flex the MP joints (Fig. 6–66). This maneuver protects the repair site during the exercise. Wrist mobilization can begin within a limited range. With the digital joints extended, the patient can actively flex the wrist to neutral.

At 5 weeks, the static splint is cut back to the level of the distal palmar crease; doing so permits MP flexion. In addition to the foregoing exercises, gentle full-excursion flexion may begin. When performing this exercise, it is important to limit the amount of tension across the repair site; therefore, the wrist should be positioned in extension.

Splinting is discontinued at the sixth week. Full-excursion flexion exercises are performed more aggressively, and simultaneous finger and

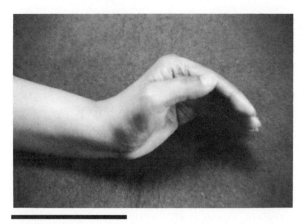

FIGURE 6–66  ■ Intrinsic plus position for exercise used to improve MP joint flexion.

wrist flexion exercises are initiated. The patient should be encouraged to use the hand in light daily activities. In cases of extension contracture, dynamic flexion splinting is appropriate.

Gentle resistive exercise is initiated in the 8th week and becomes more aggressive in the 10th week. Work hardening may be indicated at this time. Return to unrestricted activity occurs at the 12th to 14th week.

**Injuries in Zone 7.** Injuries in zone 7 require immobilization of the wrist and MP joints only. A static splint should be fabricated to position the wrist in 30 to 40 degrees of extension and the MP joints in full extension. Early treatment is geared toward preserving full IP joint motion. By the third week, exercises are selected that encourage differential gliding. In cases in which multiple EDC tendons are repaired, the tendons heal together en masse unless measures are taken to allow them to move independently. This can be accomplished by moving one finger individually while maintaining all other fingers in full extension. During the third week, about 30 degrees of flexion is tolerated. Each subsequent week, an additional 15 to 20 degrees of flexion should be added. Full flexion should be achieved by the sixth week. In addition to the finger exercises described, active wrist flexion and extension and radial and ulnar deviation can begin in the fourth week. In the flexion-extension plane, a gradual progression to the neutral position takes place during weeks 4 and 5. With regard to radial and ulnar deviation, approximately 15 degrees in each direction is permitted.

At the sixth week, the static splint is cut back to the level of the distal palmar crease. Splinting of the wrist continues to the eighth week and

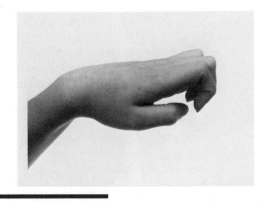

FIGURE 6–65  ■ Intrinsic minus or clawing exercise used to encourage EDC tendon excursion. (From Evans RB, Burkhalter WE: A study of the dynamic anatomy of extensor tendons and implications for treatment. J Hand Surg 11(5):774–779, © 1986, Churchill Livingstone, New York.)

full flexion and radial and ulnar deviation should not be attempted before that time. Gentle resistive exercises begin at approximately the 10th week and become more aggressive by the 12th to 14th week. Referral to work hardening may be appropriate at the 12th week.

### Extensor Tendon Injuries to the Thumb

**Injuries in Zone 1.** Treatment of extensor tendon injuries in zone 1 is similar to that outlined for the fingers. Without associated injuries, conservative management consisting of 8 weeks of continuous splinting is appropriate. The IP joint should be positioned in full extension to slight hyperextension to allow the tendon to "scar in." After this period of continuous immobilization, gentle active flexion and extension exercises are begun. An additional 2 to 3 weeks of splinting is indicated.

When surgical intervention is necessary, continuous immobilization of the DIP joint for 6 weeks is appropriate. At that time, gentle active flexion and extension exercises are initiated. Splinting should continue through the eighth to ninth week.

**Injuries in Zone 2.** Extensor tendon injury in zone 2 requires immobilization of both the MP and IP joints of the thumb. The IP joint should be positioned in full extension and the MP in radial extension. After 4 to 5 weeks of continuous splinting, gentle active range-of-motion exercises are begun. Interrupted immobilization continues an additional 2 to 3 weeks.

**Injuries in Zones 3 and 4.** Treatment is similar for injuries sustained in zones 3 and 4. Because of the tendon anatomy in this region, immobilization of the thumb MP and wrist joints is required. The MP joint should be supported in full extension, with the first metacarpal held in a slightly abducted position. The wrist is immobilized in about 30 degrees of extension. The IP joint remains free to flex and extend. After 4 weeks of continuous immobilization, gentle active MP joint flexion and extension and carpometacarpal joint abduction exercises are begun. Splinting for a total of 5 to 6 weeks is appropriate.

**Injuries in Zone 5.** Management of zone 5 injuries is challenging to the therapist. The area where the extensor pollicis longus passes under the extensor retinaculum is prone to adhesion formation and, therefore, a balance between im-

mobilization and motion must be identified. Thumb-index web space contracture is another likely complication. Initially, static splinting is used to protect the tendon repair. Positioning requirements include the MP joint in full extension, the first metacarpal in slight abduction, and the wrist in approximately 30 degrees of extension. After 3 to 4 weeks of static splinting, dynamic splinting utilizing the same joint positions becomes appropriate. Gentle active exercises are begun at week 4. Corrective dynamic splints can be applied during the sixth week, focusing on any contractures that remain at this time.

## Commonly Treated Tenosynovitis and Tendinitis

### De Quervain's Disease

De Quervain's disease is tenosynovitis of the first dorsal compartment. The tendons of the extensor pollicis brevis and the abductor pollicis longus are housed within this compartment (Fig. 6–67). This condition is related to excessive mechanical stresses, often attributable to a work-re-

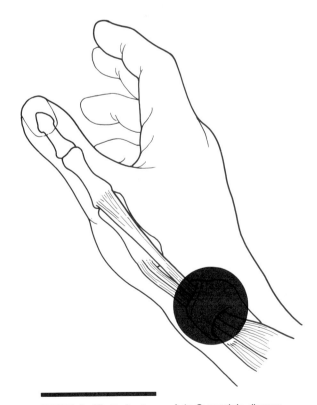

**FIGURE 6–67** ■ Anatomy of de Quervain's disease.

lated or avocational-related task. It is included in the list of cumulative trauma disorders.

Pain, swelling, and decreased range of motion of the thumb are characteristic of this disease. Patients complain of pain in the thumb and wrist, sometimes radiating into the forearm. Weakness of grip and pinch and pain on motion of the thumb, wrist, and forearm are also complaints. Clinical signs include swelling localized in the area of the radial styloid, decreased grip and pinch strength, and pain or tenderness on palpation of the first compartment. Finkelstein's test may be useful in diagnosing the disease.[28,58] When performing this test, the patient is asked to flex the thumb into the palm, enclosing it in a fist (Fig. 6–68). Then either active or passive ulnar deviation of the wrist is executed. This motion results in moderate to severe pain.

Treatment of de Quervain's disease can be conservative or surgical in nature.[58] In most cases, conservative treatment is recommended. Immobilization of the thumb and wrist (excluding the IP joint) and nonsteroidal anti-inflammatory agents are initially prescribed. If the symptoms persist after 3 to 4 weeks, a local steroid injection is usually given. Immobilization should continue for an additional 2 to 4 weeks. A second injection may be given should the symptoms persist for an additional 4 to 6 weeks. A third injection is not highly recommended because of the effects of steroids on tendons and tendon sheaths. Surgical intervention is indicated in these cases of persistent symptoms. During surgery, the compartment is opened and decompressed and a tenosynovectomy performed. When there is significant involvement of the tendon sheath, the sheath may be excised.

Postoperative treatment includes immobilization of the thumb and wrist for 3 to 5 days. Active range-of-motion exercises are then initiated. Scar management is important because adherence can be a postoperative complication. Desensitization is also begun after wound closure because neuromas and sensitivity of the dorsal radial sensory nerve may be caused by adherence. Gentle resistive exercise can begin during the fourth to fifth week. A gradual return to unrestricted activity supplements the strengthening program.

## Management of Rheumatoid Arthritis

Management of the rheumatoid hand can be of an early, conservative nature or of a postoperative nature. Early, conservative management is geared toward prevention or reduction of deformity by way of splinting, exercise, and education of the patient in the area of joint protection. Postoperative management includes splinting, exercise, and education of the patient after various surgical procedures and is geared toward obtaining a pain-free, functional hand.

Conservative management of the disease includes drug therapy and physical and occupational therapy or hand therapy. Goals of treatment include pain management, particularly during a flare-up. Modalities such as hot packs, paraffin, whirlpool, and TENS provide some relief. Massage is also beneficial. Exercise is used to maintain motion, not necessarily to improve range or strengthen the hand. Splints are utilized to prevent or reduce deformity and offer protection to and support of the joints. Evaluation of activities of daily living is important in order to recognize activities to be adapted or instances in which assistive devices may be useful. Education must be provided in the areas of joint protection and work simplification. Activities that place deforming stresses on the joints should be identi-

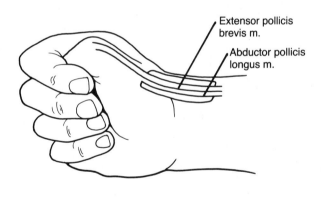

Extensor pollicis brevis m.

Abductor pollicis longus m.

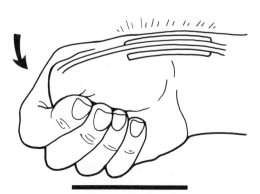

**FIGURE 6–68** ■ Finkelstein's test.

fied and alternative methods taught. Unfortunately, in many cases, these conservative measures are ineffective in preventing further joint destruction and deformity and surgical intervention becomes necessary. Surgical management can include synovectomy, arthrodesis (joint fusion), soft tissue reconstruction, or arthroplasty (joint replacement). When wrist deformities are also present, correction of the wrist deformities is necessary before surgery on the digits can be attempted.

Frequently, the initial involvement at the wrist is synovitis of the distal radioulnar joint and ECU. As the disease progresses, destruction of the triangular fibrocartilage complex and subluxation of the ECU tendon occur. Rupture of the ECU is commonly seen. With loss of the stabilizing power of the ECU and destruction of the triangular fibrocartilage complex, the ulnar carpal bones tend to shift volarly, the scapholunate relationship is altered, and a radial rotation or supination of the carpus results. In the presence of synovitis of the digital joints, particularly the MP joints, the abnormal forces transmitted through the unstable wrist contribute to the development of digital ulnar drift.[59,60]

Surgical correction of wrist problems can include relocation of the ECU, excision of the distal ulna (termed a Darrach procedure), synovectomy of the flexors and extensors, restoration of a normal scapholunate relationship through ligamentous reconstruction, reconstruction of the triangular fibrocartilage complex, ECRL tendon transfer to the ulnar side of the hand to control volar shift of the carpus and radial metacarpal shift, carpal and radiocarpal wrist joint arthroplasties (joint replacements), soft tissue spacers, and wrist arthrodesis.[59-61]

Postoperative management of the various arthroplasty procedures is similar with the exception of the length of immobilization after surgery. Moderate lengths of immobilization are necessary for formation of a stable joint capsule and protection of the tendon weaves or relocations that accompany the joint replacement.

**Trapezium**—immobilized in a short arm thumb spica for 6 weeks. K-wires used for fixation are removed at 3 to 4 weeks.
**Lunate**—immobilized in a short arm cast for 6 weeks. K-wires are removed at 3 to 4 weeks.
**Ulnar head**—in short arm cast or splint for 3 to 4 weeks. If fabricating a splint, the wrist should be positioned in slight dorsiflexion.
**Radiocarpal wrist**—in short arm cast for 2 to 4 weeks (wrist is positioned in neutral).

After removal of the cast, active range of motion of the wrist should be initiated. Modalities are used as indicated. Progression of activities continues with the patient returning to full activity by the 12th to 14th week. The key to wrist rehabilitation is a pain-free, stable wrist, sacrificing near-normal range of motion for this goal.

The ultimate stabilizing procedure for the wrist is arthrodesis. Here, the wrist is immobilized in a short arm cast for 6 to 8 weeks before hand function is allowed without support.

When wrist problems have been corrected, deformities of the digits can be addressed. The deforming forces or contributing factors that accompany the pathologic changes of rheumatoid arthritis are many. Normal anatomic and dynamic characteristics of the hand and wrist that act as or contribute to deforming factors[59,62,63] include the following:

■ Asymmetry of the metacarpal heads and the metacarpophalangeal ligaments
■ Location of synovial recesses and bursae
■ Insertion of the intrinsic muscles on both sides of each finger
■ Ulnar bias of the flexor tendons and the tendency of the proximal finger joints to deviate ulnarly during flexion
■ Force of gravity
■ Continual excessive pressures on the radial side of the index finger

The pathologic changes and changes occurring secondary to the disease process include the following:

■ Loss of bone and joint stability
■ Tissue laxity
■ Subluxation of the flexor and extensor tendons
■ Contracture of the intrinsic muscles
■ Increased intra-articular pressures

Coupling the normal anatomic and dynamic characteristics of the hand and wrist that act as or contribute to deforming factors with these pathologic changes, the common deformities of MP joint flexion—ulnar drift, swan-neck, and boutonnière—result. To further detail the MP joint flexion deformity, the interosseous muscles normally exert a volar displacement force that increases as MP joint flexion progresses. This deforming action is greater when contractures develop in the muscles and hold the joint in flexion and volar displacement.

Another deforming force involves the ulnar bias of the pull of the extrinsic digital flexors. The metacarpophalangeal and metacarpoglenoid portions of the collateral ligaments and the pal-

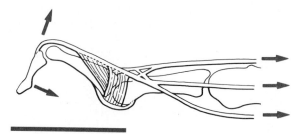

**FIGURE 6–69 ■** Swan-neck deformity. Overpull of forces contributes to PIP joint deformity.

mar plate serve as the anchor pulley that balances the normal ulnar pull of the flexors. Stretching or tearing of these structures results in displacement of the entrance of the pulley to a ulnar and palmar direction and, hence, an increase in the ulnar pull by the flexors.

Intrinsic contracture and extensor problems can result in the swan-neck and boutonnière deformities of the digits.[59,63–66] In general, swan-neck deformities involve dorsal subluxation of the lateral tendons causing hyperextension of the PIP joint and flexion of the DIP joint (Fig. 6–69). In the rheumatoid hand, because of flexor synovitis, pull of the flexor tendons is concentrated on the MP joints. This facilitates the pull of the intrinsic muscles to the central tendon across the PIP joint. Over time, imbalance of forces increases and stretching out of the transverse retinacular ligaments allows subluxation of the lateral tendons, which increases the extensor pull over the PIP joint. The oblique retinacular ligaments at the DIP joint become stretched, resulting in lengthening of the lateral tendons and overpull of the FDP tendon.

The boutonnière deformity is caused by the distended capsule of the PIP joint weakening the central tendon and transverse fibers, resulting in lengthening of the tendon and ligaments (Fig.

6–70). This results in volar subluxation of the lateral tendons and increased extensor pull over the distal phalanx, giving the PIP joint flexion and the DIP joint hyperextension characteristic of the deformity.

## Management of Metacarpophalangeal Arthroplasties

Surgical management of these digital deformities involves soft tissue reconstruction and joint replacement. MP joint arthroplasties are the most frequently performed arthroplasties in the rheumatoid hand. The surgical procedure involves removal of the residual joint surfaces of both the metacarpal and proximal phalanx bones. The implant is a single piece of silicone that is placed centrally in both bones (Fig. 6–71). After placement of the implant in the bones, the joint capsule is repaired and surgical steps are taken to eliminate the various deforming forces on the joints. The implant serves as a dynamic spacer around which a new capsuloligamentous system forms (a process termed encapsulation). This system serves to hold the implant in position but must be adequately flexible to allow motion of the joint. Therefore, the primary goal of the rehabilitation program is to create a joint capsule that is tight laterally and elastic volarly and dorsally. The ultimate result is a pain-free, stable joint that moves through a functional range of motion. This is accomplished through treatment methods that are geared toward guiding the formation of the capsular scar tissue through controlled application of stress.

The postoperative management program includes static and dynamic splinting, heat modalities such as hot packs and/or paraffin or whirlpool (with measures taken to support the hand while in the tank), and massage for scar mobili-

**FIGURE 6–70 ■** Boutonnière deformity.

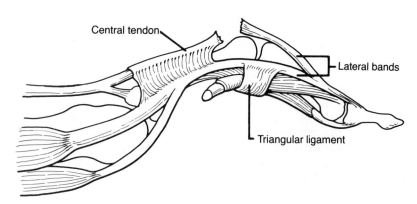

Central tendon

Lateral bands

Triangular ligament

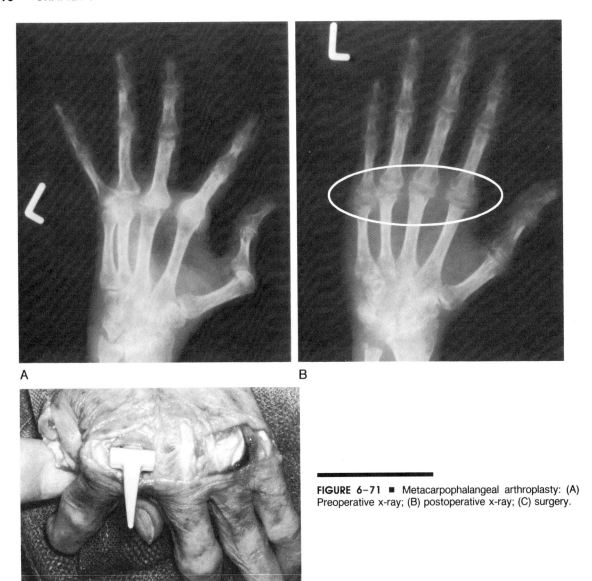

**FIGURE 6-71** ■ Metacarpophalangeal arthroplasty: (A) Preoperative x-ray; (B) postoperative x-ray; (C) surgery.

zation and edema reduction. In addition, exercise and joint protection and work simplification programs are formulated.

Various authors have described postoperative management programs for MP joint arthroplasties, with those of Swanson et al[67] and Madden et al[68] being the best known. Madden's program is a more conservative approach to mobilization. Many clinicians combine aspects of each in order to deliver the most effective postoperative program for individual cases.

Within 24 to 48 hours of surgery, splints are applied to maintain the MP joints in full extension. Dynamic splinting is favored for daytime

and static splinting for night use. The dynamic splint positions the wrist in approximately 20 to 30 degrees of extension and the MP joints are supported by finger cuffs in full extension (Fig. 6-72). A radial pull is applied to the finger cuffs so that the radial aspect of the capsule becomes somewhat shortened and tight, because many daily tasks result in radial forces across the MP joints. Neither IP joint is incorporated in the splint. A static splint is preferred for night use because of its streamline construction (no outrigger). The splint maintains the wrist in 20 to 30 degrees of extension and all digital joints in full extension (Fig. 6-73A). Proper alignment of the

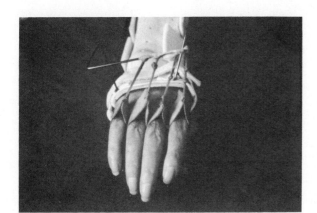

**FIGURE 6–72** ■ Dynamic extension splint. Note the radial pull component.

fingers is guaranteed by placing spacers or gutters in the splint (Fig. 6–73B), not allowing the digits to shift to the ulnar direction.

From the second day to the third week, treatment includes wound and skin care, edema management, moist heat, and exercise. Each MP joint should be moved passively through a complete pain-free range approximately 10 times. Proper alignment of the digits must be maintained at all times when they are unsplinted. Axial alignment must be controlled and no radial or ulnar deviation permitted. A goal of postoperative management is to maintain 70 degrees of passive flexion.

Active range-of-motion exercises begin within the dynamic splint on the third to sixth day after

surgery, depending on the patient's pain and edema status. Simultaneous PIP-DIP joint flexion is performed while supporting the MP joint in full extension (Fig. 6–74). This blocked (or hook) flexion provides stretch to the intrinsics. Another important exercise is MP joint flexion while maintaining both IP joints in extension. For patients who have difficulty with this exercise, static finger splints should be fabricated (or tongue depressors used), allowing them to then isolate flexor pull to the MP joints directly (Fig. 6–75). Patients must also be taught to activate the extrinsic extensor tendons by extending the MP joints and flexing the IP joints (the claw or intrinsic minus position). This position allows the extensor tendons and extensor hoods to glide maximally and eliminates intrinsic overactivity, which is frequently seen. These active exercises should be performed five times each hour.

At 3 weeks, any residual flexor weakness should be treated aggressively. As mentioned previously, 70 degrees of flexion is desired. If difficulty is encountered in reaching this goal, flexion splinting can be initiated at 4 weeks. If the IP joints are stable, rubber bands attached to Velcro hooks or hooks glued to the nails can be affixed to a wrist cuff, maintaining a flexed position. If IP joint instability is a problem, a dynamic splint can be fabricated, utilizing finger cuffs over the proximal phalanx to provide passive flexion. The therapist must be willing to sacrifice a few degrees of extension to achieve functional flexion. Flexion splinting can be alternated with extension splinting.

Active exercise out of the splint can begin at

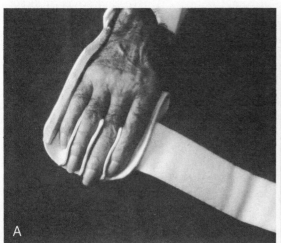

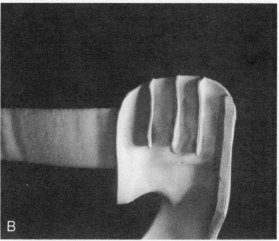

**FIGURE 6–73** ■ Static extension splint, dorsal views. (A) Hand in splint; (B) splint without hand. Spacers maintain proper alignment of the digits.

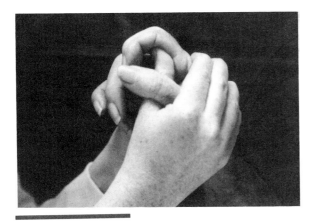

FIGURE 6-74 ■ Active blocked PIP flexion exercise with adequate proximal stabilization.

the third to fourth week. Exercises to be emphasized include active blocked (hook) flexion, full-excursion flexion (making a fist) and extension, pure EDC extension, and passive intrinsic stretching. In addition, radial strengthening exercises are begun. This can be accomplished by radial "finger walking"; with the fingers resting in the extended position on a flat surface, the patient should slide each finger individually in the radial direction, contracting the radial deviating muscles of the finger. Again, if the patient has difficulty maintaining IP joint extension, finger gutters or splints can be used.

Daytime splinting is discontinued at the sixth to eighth week. The patient should be encouraged to utilize the hand in light activities. At eight weeks, all restraints are eliminated. A strengthening program can be initiated but should not be aggressive. Thought must be given

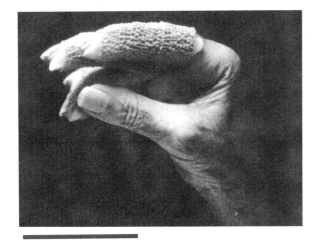

FIGURE 6-75 ■ Gutter splints used for MP joint exercises.

to the fact that the original deforming forces would be strengthened. A gradual return to functional activities along with isometric exercises can serve as the strengthening program. The full program of exercise and stretching should be carried out for 3 months. Night splinting is continued to the 12th to 14th week and longer if necessary (if extension lag persists).

## Management of Proximal Interphalangeal Joint Arthroplasties

Postoperative management for PIP arthroplasties differs from that of the MP joint because of the differences in joint shape, supporting structures, and biomechanics. The PIP joint may be replaced for reconstruction of a stiff joint or reconstruction of a swan-neck deformity or a boutonnière deformity, and postoperative management differs for each procedure.[62,64,65,67] The differences result from the varying soft tissue reconstructive procedures that accompany the joint replacement. Having already described these deformities, we present postoperative treatment of each procedure. These programs are based on the fact that reconstructed joints begin tightening during the second postoperative week and are quite tight by the end of the third week. Therefore, if the desired range of motion has not been achieved by the third week, it is difficult to gain further improvement in motion.

After surgical correction of the stiff PIP joint, mobilization begins within 3 to 5 days. While supporting the proximal phalanx, active flexion and extension are performed. Support of the proximal phalanx is necessary so as to direct the flexor forces to the PIP joint. A small thermoplastic or foam-covered aluminum splint is used to maintain the PIP joint in extension when it is not being exercised. The splint can be applied slightly to the radial or ulnar side of the digit to correct any angular deformity. It is worn mainly at night for 3 to 6 weeks, depending on the severity of extension lag. In most cases, a few degrees of extension lag remain after this type of surgery. Should inadequate flexion be a problem, dynamic flexion splinting can begin at 3 to 4 weeks. Ideal range of motion is 0 through 70 degrees.

Management of reconstruction of a swan-neck deformity involves immobilization of the PIP joint in 10 to 20 degrees of flexion and the DIP joint in neutral for 10 days. Active range of motion is then initiated with proper support provided to obtain maximum flexion. Passive range of motion is not indicated until the second to third week because surgical correction involves stepcutting and suturing the central tendon. It is important to obtain a 10- to 15-degree flexion contracture of the PIP joint to prevent recurrent hyperextension tendencies.

In the postoperative management program of the boutonnière deformity, it is important to maintain the extension of the PIP joint and allow flexion of the DIP joint. Because of the reconstruction of the extensor mechanism, the finger should be immobilized for about 10 days. A thermoplastic splint should support the PIP joint in extension; the DIP joint should not be immobilized but should flex freely. Ten to 14 days after surgery, active flexion and extension exercises are usually begun, alternating with use of the extension splint. Splinting should continue at night until the joint position is stable and the degree of extension lag acceptable. This may require up to 10 weeks.

## Peripheral Nerve Injuries

Peripheral nerve injuries range from compression neuropathies to complete laceration of a nerve. A thorough understanding of the anatomy, physiology, and healing process of the nervous system is necessary for delivery of appropriate treatment. Knowledge of anatomy and motor and sensory innervation patterns allows the clinician to determine which nerve is involved, the level of involvement, and the appro-

priate splinting configurations to protect the nerve and prevent deformities resulting from muscle weakness or paralysis. Wound healing dictates the timing of the rehabilitation process. General anatomy (the course of the nerves) was discussed earlier but is reviewed in this section. Anatomy of nerves is presented here.

The basic unit of a peripheral nerve is the axon, which is composed of nerve cells (Fig. 6–76). Surrounding the axon is the myelin layer across which impulses travel. The cells composing this myelin layer are called Schwann cells. The outer layer of the axon is the endoneurium. This entire structure constitutes the nerve fiber. Nerve fibers are grouped together in bundles or fasciculi. A sheath, the perineurium, encases each fasciculus. Fasciculi are then grouped together and enclosed by epineurium. A nerve sheath, or the epineural sheath, is the outermost layer of the nerve.

When a peripheral nerve is injured, the myelin sheath and axon suffer the greatest damage. Degeneration of the myelin (wallerian degeneration) and axon begins within the first week after injury and continues for varied lengths of time. Then the process of regeneration begins.

Injuries to nerves can be classified according to severity. Two popular classification systems are a three-class system proposed by Seddon and a five-degree system described by Sunderland.[22,69] The first level of injury according to Seddon is neurapraxia. This class corresponds to Sunderland's first-degree lesion. The myelin layer is damaged but no other structures are compro-

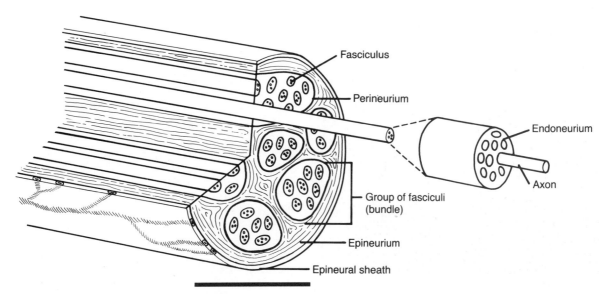

**FIGURE 6–76 ■** Anatomy of a peripheral nerve.

mised. Compression neuropathies fall into this category. The condition is reversible and the prognosis excellent.

Axonotmesis is the second level of Seddon's classification system and is equivalent to Sunderland's second-degree and mild third-degree lesions. Compression damages the myelin layer and axon, and degeneration occurs distal to the lesion. Severe nerve compressions and crush injuries are included in these categories. This condition is also reversible and the prognosis is good.

Neurotmesis is the third level of Seddon's system and corresponds to Sunderland's moderate to severe third-degree and fourth-degree lesions. Significant damage is sustained by the fasciculi and perineurium. Because of the severity of injury, prognosis for motor recovery is poor. The prognosis for sensory recovery is fair to good. Complete laceration of the nerve corresponds to Sunderland's fifth-degree lesion. The entire nerve is damaged.

## Compression Neuropathies

Various compression-entrapment neuropathies of the peripheral nerves of the upper extremity have been documented in the literature.[22,23,25,69]

Levels of compression or entrapment presented in this chapter include those of the forearm and wrist. Specific to the median nerve, pronator syndrome, anterior interosseous nerve syndrome, and carpal tunnel syndrome are discussed; to the ulnar nerve, entrapment at the elbow and in Guyon's canal; and to the radial nerve, compressions of the posterior interosseous nerve and superficial radial nerve. In discussing each of these syndromes, the anatomy is reviewed, followed by a description of clinical signs, diagnostic tests, and appropriate management programs (both conservative and postoperative).

### MEDIAN NERVE COMPRESSION SYNDROMES

#### Carpal Tunnel Syndrome

Carpal tunnel syndrome, the most commonly treated compression neuropathy, involves compression of the median nerve at the level of the wrist.[23,70-73] As they approach the hand, the median nerve and nine flexor tendons pass through a confined space, the carpal tunnel. This tunnel is formed by the carpus and the transverse carpal ligament (Fig. 6–77). Problems evolve when there are conditions that result in alteration of

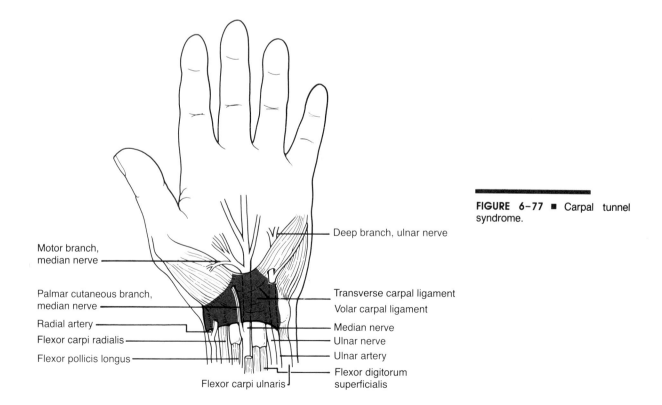

**FIGURE 6–77** ■ Carpal tunnel syndrome.

Deep branch, ulnar nerve

Motor branch, median nerve

Palmar cutaneous branch, median nerve

Radial artery

Flexor carpi radialis

Flexor pollicis longus

Flexor carpi ulnaris

Transverse carpal ligament
Volar carpal ligament
Median nerve
Ulnar nerve
Ulnar artery
Flexor digitorum superficialis

any of the structures forming or contained within the tunnel. Radioulnar, radiocarpal, and carpal fractures; swelling of the median nerve; swelling of the flexor tendon sheath; anatomic variants or abnormalities; and tumors are among these conditions. Swelling of the nerve and/or flexor tendons frequently results from repetitive wrist motions and static or dynamic grip and pinch. Other causes of carpal tunnel syndrome include systemic diseases such as rheumatoid arthritis and osteoarthritis, diabetes, and thyroid disorders and hormonal changes of pregnancy and menopause.[22,73] Appropriate treatment depends on the cause of the compression, the severity of the symptoms, the extent of nerve degeneration, and the duration of the compression. Conservative treatment is indicated in many cases, whereas in others surgical intervention is the only appropriate treatment.

Symptoms of carpal tunnel syndrome include numbness and tingling (initially at night), pain, clumsiness, and weakness. As the syndrome progresses, night symptoms become more severe and remain throughout the day, and radiating or referred pain at the shoulder may be experienced. Clinical signs include diminished sensation of the median nerve distribution (palmar surface of the thumb, index finger, middle finger, and radial half of the ring finger), pseudomotor changes of the skin, atrophy of the thenar muscles, and positive Phalen's, Tinel's, and pinch tests. Phalen's test[73] involves constricting the space within the carpal tunnel by positioning the patient's wrist in full flexion for 1 minute (Fig. 6–78). The fingers should remain relaxed during the test. For patients with even mild carpal tun-

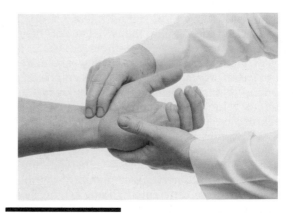

**FIGURE 6–79 ■** Tinel's test (percussion over the median nerve).

nel syndrome, this induced compression results in numbness throughout the median nerve distribution (a positive test).

Tinel's test[22,23] is also used to indicate the presence of carpal tunnel syndrome. Percussion of a compressed median nerve at the level of the tunnel elicits tingling through the palm to the fingertips, resulting in a positive test (Fig. 6–79). Many patients describe the tingling sensation as "electric shocks."

The pinch test[71] is used to determine the involvement of the lumbrical muscles in the syndrome. The patient is asked to pinch a piece of paper with a three-jaw chuck pinch (pinching the thumb against the tips of the index and middle fingers). The patient attempts to hold onto the paper as the examiner pulls it away. A positive result is noted when the patient experiences numbness of the median innervated fingertips and/or cramping in the midpalm region within 1 minute.

Electrodiagnostic studies can confirm the diagnosis of carpal tunnel syndrome. Studies of median nerve conduction may reveal slowing of conduction velocities. Electromyographic studies of the median nerve–innervated thenar muscles may show abnormal patterns.

Frequently, conservative treatment is an effective management method. Thompson and Koppell[74] and Ditmars and Houin[71] found that in 60% of patients with mild carpal tunnel syndrome, conservative treatment was sufficient. Splints are used to rest or support the wrist in 0 to 20 degrees of extension; the patient's comfort should be considered. Activities that contribute to the symptoms must be avoided. Therefore, education of the patient is a priority. In conjunction with splinting, oral nonsteroidal anti-inflam-

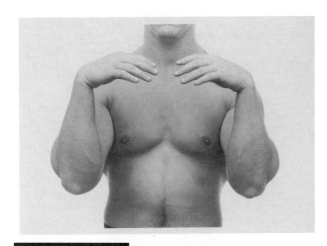

**FIGURE 6–78 ■** Phalen's test (constriction of the median nerve).

matory drugs and local steroid injections can be beneficial in decreasing the swelling of tissues about the nerve. Several authors advocate the use of vitamin B$_6$.[69] After several weeks of rest, an exercise program can begin with emphasis on motions that promote gliding of the nerve and tendons.[74] Included in the program are making a hook fist, isolated DIP and PIP joint flexion with the MP joints in flexion, full-excursion flexion (fist exercise), and simultaneous wrist and finger extension exercises. Scar tissue adherence about the tendons and nerve is minimized by these motions because differential gliding of the flexor digitorum profundus and superficialis and the median nerve is accomplished. After 4 to 5 weeks of continuous splinting followed by 4 to 5 weeks of exercise and gradual weaning from the splint, the carpal tunnel syndrome should be resolved.

Surgical release of the carpal tunnel is indicated when conservative treatment is ineffective, acute compression is caused by injury, and diagnostic tests and physical examination reveal a more chronic condition with moderate nerve involvement. The surgical procedure involves cutting the transverse carpal ligament with or without reattachment before closure. Removal of scar tissue about the nerve (external neurolysis) and within the nerve (internal neurolysis) and tenosynovectomy may be necessary. A newer development in carpal tunnel surgery involves the use of an endoscope through which a fiberoptic lens and microsurgical scalpel are passed. The carpal ligament is located using a television monitor and then cut. The procedure requires only two small incisions, so postoperative recovery is shortened. This is not yet a widely accepted method of treatment by hand surgeons.

Postoperative management of the standard carpal tunnel release consists primarily of home program instruction and weekly to biweekly monitoring. Many physicians do not refer these patients for rehabilitation except in cases in which significant deficits existed preoperatively and complications arise postoperatively. Three to seven days of immobilization is recommended, followed by instruction in scar management, desensitization techniques, and range-of-motion exercises that promote differential tendon gliding. Strengthening of the hand and wrist is frequently incorporated in the gradual return to unrestricted activity. Complications that can develop include pain and sensitivity of the scar, restrictive scar tissue formation, and weak and/or painful grip. With periodic monitoring, these complications may be avoided or effectively

managed. Return to work is dependent on the patient's job demands. When a job task contributed to the onset of the syndrome, work hardening and ergonomic analysis are indicated. Ultimately, it may be necessary to impose job restrictions or require a job change. The reported success rate of this surgery varies. Ditmars and Houin[71] report a 60% success rate.

### Pronator Syndrome

Just distal to the elbow, the median nerve passes between the two heads of the pronator teres muscle before providing innervation to that muscle. Compression of the nerve can occur at this level with contribution from the lacertus fibrosis (Fig. 6–80). Symptoms of pronator syndrome include pain, tenderness, and cramping of the proximal anterior forearm; paresthesias that radiate distally to the hand; weakness of pinch; and occasionally numbness of the median nerve distribution of the thumb and index and middle fingers. Clinical signs are increased pain upon resisted pronation, tenderness on palpation of the pronator teres muscle, and weakness of the flexor pollicis longus, flexor digitorum profundus

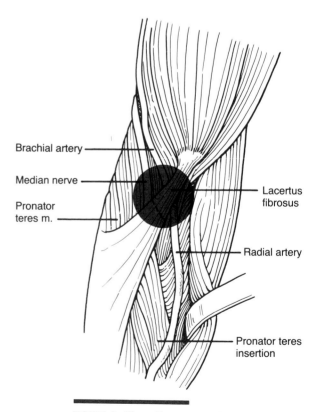

**FIGURE 6–80** ■ Pronator syndrome.

of the index and middle fingers, and pronator quadratus. Electromyographic studies may confirm the diagnosis.

Conservative management may be effective in treating this condition. Rest and immobilization are the primary treatment. Support of the wrist, thumb, and index and middle fingers eliminates contraction of the flexor muscle mass and tension across the nerve. The wrist is placed in the neutral position and the digits in functional position (thumb abducted and extended and fingers with the MP joints in flexion and the IP joints in extension). After 4 to 6 weeks of continuous splinting, an additional 4 to 6 weeks are allowed for gradual splint removal. Active range-of-motion exercises can begin during the weaning process. The patient must also be educated to avoid any provocative motions, such as repetitive elbow flexion-extension and forearm supination-pronation and static forearm pronation. Should the condition persist after 8 to 12 weeks of conservative treatment, surgical intervention is indicated.

During surgery, the lacertus fibrosus and any other constricting fibrous structures are cut. To relieve pronator muscle compression, the nerve can be moved to a subcutaneous position above the muscle mass and the pronator lengthened.[22] Neurolysis may also be indicated. Postoperative management is similar to that described for conservative treatment. Four to six weeks of immobilization is recommended. Then active range-of-motion exercises are begun. Scar management and desensitization are included in the postoperative program. In cases of subcutaneous translocation, tenderness over the area of the nerve may persist.

### Anterior Interosseous Nerve Syndrome

The anterior interosseous nerve, a branch of the median nerve, originates in the forearm at the level of the cubital fossa. It innervates the flexor pollicis longus, flexor digitorum profundus (FDP) of the index and middle fingers, and pronator quadratus. Compression occurs at the point of division from the median nerve, near the tendinous insertion of the pronator teres muscle (Fig. 6–81). The patient's chief complaint is that of weakness of pinch. Pain is not usually associated with this condition. The primary clinical sign is weakness of the flexor pollicis longus and FDP of the index and middle fingers. Aside from manual muscle testing, the patient can be asked to maintain a thumb-to-index/middle fingertip pinch against resistance. Because of muscle

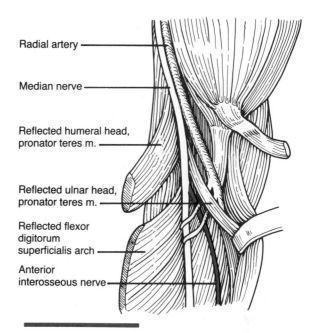

Radial artery
Median nerve
Reflected humeral head, pronator teres m.
Reflected ulnar head, pronator teres m.
Reflected flexor digitorum superficialis arch
Anterior interosseous nerve

**FIGURE 6-81** ■ Anterior interosseous nerve compression.

weakness, the patient cannot hold the position. Electromyography may reveal some abnormalities.

Conservative management consists of rest and immobilization. Support of the wrist, thumb, and index and middle fingers eliminates contraction of the flexor muscle mass and tension across the nerve. The wrist is placed in the neutral position and the digits in the functional position (thumb abducted and extended and the fingers with the MP joints in flexion and the IP joints in extension). After 4 to 6 weeks of continuous splinting, an additional 4 to 6 weeks are allowed for gradual splint removal. Active range-of-motion exercises can begin during the weaning process. Should the condition persist after 8 to 12 weeks of conservative treatment, surgical intervention is indicated. Postoperative management is similar to that described for conservative treatment.

### ULNAR NERVE COMPRESSIONS

### Entrapment at the Elbow

Another common neuropathy is entrapment of the ulnar nerve at the elbow. The sites of compression or trauma are at the arcade of Struthers, the groove of the humeral medial epicondyle (the cubital tunnel), and the level of the flexor carpi ulnaris (FCU) (Fig. 6–82A and B). Subluxation of the nerve at the condylar groove, repeti-

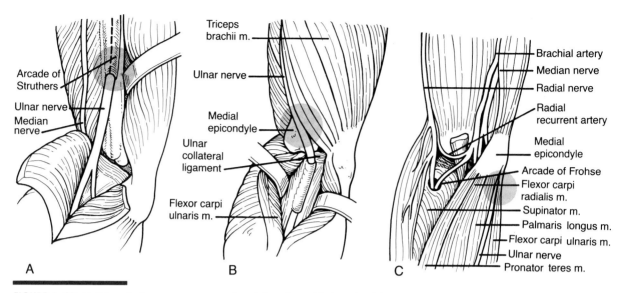

**FIGURE 6-82** ■ Sites of ulnar nerve compression at the elbow. (A) Arcade of Struthers; (B) medial epicondyle; (C) compression from the flexor carpi radialis muscle.

tive stretching of the nerve, and external pressure of long duration to the nerve around the condyle result in repeated trauma to the nerve. Compression of the nerve by the FCU also provides insult to the nerve. Appropriate treatment depends on the cause of the trauma, the severity of the symptoms, the extent of nerve degeneration, and the duration of the compression. Conservative treatment is recommended whenever possible. In cases of unsuccessful conservative management and long-standing cases in which muscle atrophy and joint deformities are present, surgical intervention becomes necessary.

Symptoms of cubital tunnel syndrome include numbness and tingling (paresthesias) distal to the elbow through the ulnar nerve sensory distribution, most often of the small finger and ulnar side of the ring finger; pain and tenderness about the medial aspect of the elbow; and weakness of grip and pinch. Numbness, tingling, and pain are frequently aggravated by resting the flexed elbow on a firm surface. As the syndrome progresses, referred pain in the scapular region can be experienced. Clinical signs include diminished sensation of the ulnar nerve distribution (the small finger and the palmar and dorsal surfaces of the ulnar half of the ring finger and the ulnar border of the hand), pseudomotor changes of the skin, a positive Tinel's sign, and a positive Froment's sign.[22,28] This test assesses weakness of the ulnar nerve–innervated muscles used for pinching. Normally, in holding a piece of paper between the thumb and lateral aspect of the index finger (lateral or key pinch) against resist-

ance, the adductor pollicis, along with other muscles, is activated. If weakness of the adductor pollicis exists, the patient recruits the flexor pollicis longus to substitute in an attempt to hold the paper. Flexion of the thumb IP joint results, giving a positive Froment's sign. Weakness of the FCU, FDP of the ring and small fingers, lateral half of the flexor pollicis brevis, interossei, ulnar two lumbricals, and hypothenar muscles and muscle atrophy are also observed. Electrodiagnostic studies can confirm the diagnosis. Studies of ulnar nerve conduction frequently reveal slowing of conduction velocities. Electromyographic studies of the ulnar nerve–innervated muscles may show changes.

Conservative treatment consists primarily of rest, immobilization, and elimination of the external cause, if present. Splinting of the elbow and wrist is advised, but caution must be used in the fabrication process so that pressure is not placed on the nerve by the splint. Flaring or bubbling the area at the medial epicondyle prevents this pressure. In addition, foam padding may be placed within the bubbled area. Positioning of the elbow is also critical when fabricating the splint. The splint must maintain the elbow in a position that does not place tension across the nerve. Thirty to 45 degrees of flexion is a good position. The wrist should be held in neutral. Nonsteroidal anti-inflammatory drugs are sometimes prescribed.

Surgical management offers several options, depending on the etiology.[22] Constriction by the aponeurosis of the FCU is managed surgically by cutting the structure to relieve the compression. Alternatively, a medial epicondylectomy can be performed. With removal of the medial epicondyle and the adjacent supracondylar ridge and reattachment of the flexor pronator muscle origin to adjacent soft tissues, decompression can be accomplished with minimal trauma to the nerve. In cases in which the ulnar nerve is subjected to subluxation, stretching, and external pressure, several surgical options exist. The nerve can be removed from the groove and transposed anteriorly (an anterior transposition). More involved procedures include subcutaneous, intramuscular, and submuscular transpositions. In other words, the ulnar nerve can be moved superficially to the flexor pronator muscles, or it can be placed inside (intramuscular transposition) or under (submuscular transposition) the flexor pronator muscle mass. The intramuscular and submuscular transpositions are preferred for the padding or coverage provided to the nerve. When the transposition is complete, suspected areas of compression must be released before closure.

After surgery, a period of immobilization is required. The splinting requirements described in conservative treatment are appropriate, although a greater degree of elbow flexion is desired. Particularly after the submuscular and intramuscular transpositions, approximately 90 degrees of flexion should be maintained. Scar and pain management are important in the postoperative treatment program. Deep and cross friction massages are performed as tolerated by the patient. Elastomer molds, foam, and so forth are used to provide pressure in the scar region. Desensitization must be initiated on wound closure. Active exercise is beneficial in scar management. Gentle active range-of-motion exercises are begun during the third week after surgery. Motion should be performed within a range that does not elicit paresthesias or increased pain or discomfort because of tension across the nerve. In cases involving reattachment of the flexor pronator muscles, motion should be within a range that protects this soft tissue procedure. Complications of this surgery (any of the foregoing procedures) include scar tissue adhesions, neuromas, and chronic pain.

Compression at the Wrist (Guyon's Canal)

Compression of the ulnar nerve at the level of the wrist and palm occurs in Guyon's canal (Fig. 6–83). Guyon's canal is formed by the pisiform and the volar carpal and transverse carpal ligaments. At this level, the ulnar nerve divides, giving rise to the superficial, deep motor, and dorsal radial sensory branches. Sensation to the palmar surface of the small and ulnar side of the ring fingers is provided by the superficial branch, dorsal sensation by the dorsal sensory branch. The deep motor branch innervates the ulnar two lumbrical, interosseus, hypothenar, and adductor pollicis muscles. Because the division of the dorsal sensory branch from the main nerve occurs just proximal to the wrist, distal pathology does not compromise dorsal sensation. The superficial and deep motor branches divide distal to the wrist. Compression of the ulnar nerve at the level of Guyon's canal affects palmar sensation and motor abilities. Causes of this compression include repeated or chronic trauma to the area (often attributed to tool usage or use of hand in accomplishing a job task), bone or soft tissue injury, and ganglia.

Clinical signs of ulnar nerve compression at the wrist include diminished palmar sensation, paresthesias of the palmar distribution, and intrinsic muscle weakness. Identification of the clinical signs and knowledge of the anatomy allow the clinician to determine which branch is affected. At the level of or proximal to Guyon's canal, both motor and sensory deficits are noted. Distal compression of only the deep motor branch results in only motor deficits, whereas compression of the superficial branch yields only sensory deficits. Electrodiagnostic studies provide useful information in confirming the diagnosis.

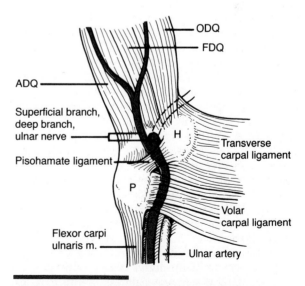

**FIGURE 6–83** ■ Ulnar nerve compression at Guyon's canal. ODQ, opponens digiti quinti (minimi); FDQ, flexor digiti quinti (minimi); H, hamate; P, pisiform; ADQ, abductor digiti quinti (minimi).

Abnormalities in conduction velocities and electromyography can be measured.

Conservative management and postoperative management are similar. The wrist should be splinted in order to remove tension across the nerve. The ulnar two digits may be included in the splint. Immobilizing the wrist in neutral and the fingers in semiflexion prevents this stretch from occurring. Full IP extension must be allowed within the splint to discourage development of flexion contractures. Mobilization occurs in approximately 4 weeks if the condition is managed conservatively. In cases of surgical management, motion can be initiated after 2 weeks of splinting. Elimination of the cause must also be addressed. Education of the patient is essential. Patients must avoid pressure and repeated trauma to the nerve. Job modifications, restrictions, or change may be necessary.

## RADIAL NERVE COMPRESSION NEUROPATHIES

### Posterior Interosseous Nerve Syndrome

The radial nerve gives rise to the posterior interosseous nerve (PIN) just proximal to the head of the radius. The PIN innervates the extensor carpi radialis brevis, then courses distally to pass between the two heads of the supinator muscle, the arcade of Frohse (Fig. 6–84). The nerve innervates the supinator, the extensor digitorum communis, extensor digiti minimi, extensor carpi ulnaris, abductor pollicis longus, extensor pollicis longus and brevis, and extensor indicis proprius, in that order. The PIN terminates at the wrist and provides innervation to that joint. No sensory innervation is provided by the nerve. The primary source of compression of the PIN is the arcade of Frohse. Other causes of PIN syndrome include fractures or dislocations of the radial head and needle injections.

Symptoms of the syndrome include pain in the area of the lateral epicondyle, aching of the posterior aspect of the forearm, and weakness of finger extension. Symptoms can lead to a misdiagnosis of lateral epicondylitis. To test specifically for PIN syndrome, ask the patient to extend the elbow and, while maintaining this position, resist extension of the middle finger. A positive result is pain at the EDC origin.[22] Direct pressure over the course of the nerve also produces pain. Another clinical sign is weakness of the PIN-innervated muscles, particularly the EDC. Electrodiagnostic studies may reveal abnormalities.

Conservative treatment focuses on immobiliza-

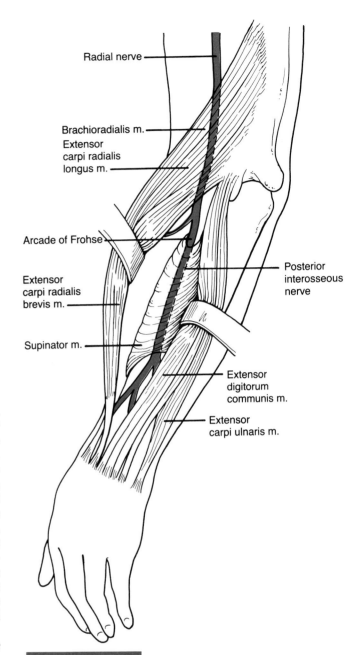

**FIGURE 6–84** ■ Common site of posterior interosseous nerve syndrome.

tion. The wrist should be splinted in approximately 20 degrees of extension and MP joints of the digits in 0 degrees of extension. Dynamic splinting may also be considered for daytime use. Again, the wrist should be maintained in 20 to 30 degrees of extension, while the finger cuffs support the proximal phalanges in full extension. Active flexion against the tension provided by rubber bands should be possible. Four to 6 weeks of continuous splinting followed by an additional 4 to 6 weeks of gradual weaning from the splint is suggested. Active range-of-motion exercises can begin at that time. Should symptoms persist after 8 to 12 weeks of conservative treatment, surgical intervention is necessary. During surgery, compressing fibrous structures including the arcade of Frohse are cut and neurolysis is performed if necessary. Postoperative treatment is similar to the conservative methods already described.

### Superficial Radial Nerve Entrapment

The superficial radial nerve courses the forearm to provide sensation to the hand. The various branches of the superficial radial nerve (Fig. 6–85) supply the radial two thirds of the dorsum of the hand, the entire dorsum of the thumb, and the dorsum of the index finger, long finger, and radial half of the ring finger from MP to PIP joint level. Most often, compression of this nerve is due to direct trauma to the forearm or dorsum of the hand by a direct blow, a tight cast or watchband, or handcuffs. Patients' complaints include local tenderness, pain in the forearm, and numbness and painful paresthesias of the dorsum of the hand. Diagnosis must be made primarily from these complaints. The condition may sometimes be confused with de Quervain's disease.

Conservative management consists of rest and immobilization, anti-inflammatory medication, and desensitization. A wrist splint, positioning the wrist in neutral, can remove tension from the nerve as well as protect the sensitive area from the external environment. Treatment can continue for at least 4 to 6 months.

Surgical treatment involves decompression, dissection from adhesions, and management of neuromas if present. In this case, the nerve may be divided and the ends embedded in muscle. Postoperatively, the wrist should be splinted in mild flexion and ulnar deviation. Gentle active range-of-motion exercises can begin after 7 to 10 days of immobilization. Scar massage is important and should be initiated as soon as the wound can tolerate tension. Surgical management is not highly successful.

## Peripheral Nerve Lacerations

Complete laceration of a peripheral nerve must be repaired surgically. The goal of nerve repair is to approximate the nerve ends to align the fascicular groups without producing tension across

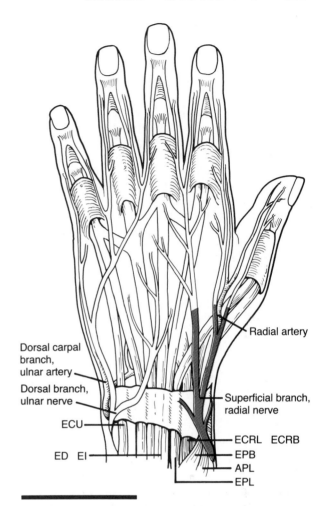

**FIGURE 6–85** ■ Entrapment of superficial branch of the radial nerve. APL, abductor pollicis longus; EPB, extensor pollicis brevis; ECRB, extensor carpi radialis brevis; ECRL, extensor carpi radialis longus; ED, extensor digitorum; EI, extensor indicis; ECU, extensor carpi ulnaris.

the repair. Postoperative management must maintain these goals. Appropriate treatment protects the integrity of the repair and avoids tension across the nerve.

After surgery, a protective splint must be fabricated to immobilize the joints above and below the nerve repair. Deformities must also be corrected by the splint. Deformities result from muscle imbalance that is created by the muscle weakness or paralysis that accompanies nerve injury. Scar management and desensitization should be included in treatment. Active range-of-motion exercises can begin during the third to fourth week. Initially, paresthesias should be avoided during exercise because they can be indicative of tension across the nerve.

During the fourth to fifth week, protection of the nerve repair no longer requires immobilization of the adjacent joints and the protective splint can be discontinued. The current splint can be modified or a new one fabricated. The purposes served by the replacement splint are correction of deformities to protect joints and muscles and to improve functionality of the hand. This is necessary because motor recovery may take many months. The splint can be dynamic or static depending on the nature of the muscle deficits. For example, a static hand-based dorsal splint is most functional in correcting the "claw" deformity (the intrinsic minus hand). The splint blocks the MP joints in flexion in order to isolate the pull of the EDC to the IP joints, thereby improving the function of the hand. Conversely, a dynamic splint is more appropriate in posterior interosseous nerve injuries, because the dynamic component allows functional use of the hand (the hand-forearm component stabilizes the wrist and the dynamic outrigger supports the MP joints in extension but allows active flexion against the rubber bands).

At the seventh to eighth week, resistive exercises are added to the treatment program. Treatment frequency can be decreased at this time, when only periodic monitoring of signs of motor and sensory recovery is required. Long-term treatment goals include strengthening of recovering muscles and sensory re-education.

## Other Common Hand Conditions and Disorders

### Reflex Sympathetic Dystrophy

Reflex sympathetic dystrophy (RSD) is one of the most difficult, challenging problems for the clinician to treat. It is defined as a vasomotor dysfunction.[75] Pain is the primary symptom and is the reason for this difficulty. Patients who suffer from RSD are not tolerant of many of the modalities and techniques that therapists use in treatment. Several treatment options are discussed here, and the clinician must be prepared to make changes in the treatment program at any time.

The cause of this condition appears to be abnormal sympathetic reflex. Lankford[75] states that the following three conditions must be present for the development of the syndrome: (1) a persistent painful lesion (traumatic or acquired), (2) diathesis (predisposition, body characteristic, sus-

ceptibility), and (3) an abnormal sympathetic reflex. Pain and edema can develop after trauma to the upper extremity. The susceptible patient guards the painful extremity, and limited mobility or total immobilization ensues. An increase in edema and joint stiffness develop because of the immobilization and results in increased pain. Ultimately, the extremity is painful, swollen, and stiff (Fig. 6–86). The goal of treatment is to break the cycle. Elimination of one or more of the contributing factors can lead to resolution of the syndrome.

Three stages are used to describe the course of RSD. The first stage corresponds to the acute phase of injury. The duration of this stage is approximately 3 months. Pain and edema are characteristic symptoms. Discoloration of the hand develops, with redness being especially obvious around the MP and PIP joints. Hyperhidrosis (excessive sweating) results from increased sudomotor activity. Despite its appearance, the hand tends to be cool in temperature. Radiologic examination would reveal osteoporosis as the acute phase progresses.

The subacute phase or second stage extends from the 3rd through the 10th to 12th month. Pain and edema remain as the primary symptoms and, in fact, tend to be worse during this phase, resulting in increased joint stiffness. As time passes, the red discoloration dissipates and is replaced by a pale cyanosis. Hyperhidrosis changes to dryness. Skin and subcutaneous tissue atrophy becomes obvious and the bones become more osteoporotic.

The last stage of the syndrome is characterized by marked joint stiffness and deformity. Thickening of the palmar fascia contributes to joint deformity. Severe osteoporosis is seen on x-ray films. Skin and subcutaneous atrophy is more severe. The skin is pale, dry, and shiny; skin creases cannot be seen. Pain may continue to be severe or may have diminished by this time. Edema begins to subside.

The key to treatment of RSD is early detection and appropriate aggressive management. Obviously, pain and edema control are critical components of the treatment program. Nerve blocks can be utilized in an attempt to interrupt the abnormal sympathetic reflex, including stellate ganglion blocks, somatic nerve blocks, and perineural infusion. Anesthetic drugs (lidocaine [Xylocaine] and bupivacaine hydrochloride [Marcaine]), reserpine, and guanethidine are delivered by injection or by indwelling catheter.[75] In conjunction with the nerve blocks, adjunctive treat-

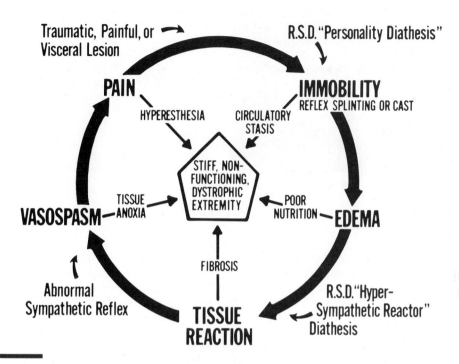

**FIGURE 6-86** ■ Reflex sympathetic dystrophy cycle. (From Lankford LL: Reflex sympathetic dystrophy. *In* Green DP: Operative Hand Surgery, Vol 1. New York: Churchill Livingstone, 1982, p. 549.)

ment is necessary. This includes psychologic, physical, and occupational therapy.

For the physical and occupational therapists, management of pain and edema is critical. Splinting, heat, massage, TENS, electrical stimulation of acupuncture points, and stress loading (weight bearing)[76] are viable methods of controlling pain. Edema management includes elevation, retrograde massage, compression wrapping or garments, intermittent compression, high-voltage galvanic stimulation, and gentle, controlled active motion. If pain begins to get out of control, patients cannot tolerate many of these treatment methods. When the therapist realizes that the current method of treatment is ineffective, a change must be made quickly. In addition, gentle dynamic splinting and controlled range-of-motion exercises are included in the treatment pro-

gram to discourage joint stiffness and deformity. The clinician must exercise caution in determining the amount of force to be applied by the splint and the appropriate number of repetitions and frequency of exercise sessions. Aggressive treatment aggravates and perpetuates the syndrome. When splinting the hand, functional positioning is critical. The wrist should be maintained in 35 to 45 degrees of extension, the MP joints in approximately 70 degrees of flexion, and the PIP joints in 20 to 30 degrees of flexion. This is a position of balance. All joint structures and muscles are placed in an optimal position to discourage muscle imbalance and joint contracture.

Treatment is dictated by the course of the syndrome, but common goals can be identified that are not altered by the syndrome. These include

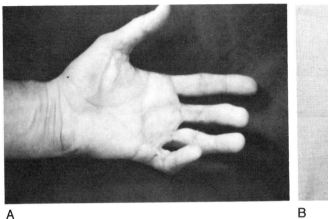
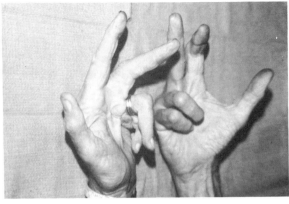

A                                          B

FIGURE 6-87 ■ Hand with Dupuytren's disease. Note the palmar nodules and cords (A) and resultant deformity (B).

pain and edema control, maintenance of functional range of motion, and prevention of joint deformities.

### Dupuytren's Disease

Dupuytren's disease is a common condition affecting the palmar fascia lying between the skin and flexor tendons in the distal palm and fingers. The pathologic event that initiates the disease is unknown, but the course after that change is well documented.[77,78] Fibroblastic proliferation and collagen formation are characteristic. Beginning as a nodule in the palm or finger, the condition progresses to the formation of fibrous bands and joint contractures (Fig. 6-87). The MP joint is most frequently involved, followed by the PIP joint. The DIP joint is only occasionally affected.

Other characteristics of the disease include its genetic origin. It frequently occurs in people of northern European descent. It is most often seen in older men, although it can appear in females. An association exists between this disease and others such as diabetes, epilepsy, and alcoholism.[78] The condition is usually not painful.

The most frequent and successful treatment of Dupuytren's disease is surgery. Conservative management by steroid injection, vitamin E, splinting, and exercise is seldom effective. Generally, hand surgeons permit the disease to take its course (the rate of progression of the disease is variable) and intervene when joint contractures result in functional limitation. Surgical techniques that have been successful for treatment of the disease include fasciotomy and fasciectomy.[77,78] Currently, excision of the palmar fascia or fas-

ciectomy is the surgical treatment of choice (Fig. 6-88). Wound closure techniques are also varied. Traditionally, after excision of the diseased tissue, the surgical wounds were closed by sutures and pressure dressings were applied. Closure of the wounds in this manner resulted in closure under tension, which frequently led to complications in healing such hematoma, tissue necrosis, and infection. If skin coverage was not adequate, skin grafts were used. Similar postoperative complications resulted. These complications encourage increased scar tissue formation, which compromises the ultimate postoperative result. Scar tissue contracture and subsequent joint contractures and tendon adherence provide a less than desirable functional outcome. In 1964, McCash introduced a technique that involved leaving the surgical wounds open after excision, allowing them to heal by secondary intention.[77] This pro-

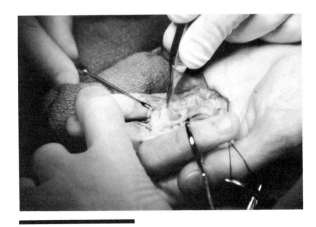

FIGURE 6-88 ■ Surgical procedure for Dupuytren's disease.

cedure is widely practiced today and results in a more favorable long-term result; fewer postoperative complications occur. The McCash procedure does have disadvantages. Because the wounds are left open, infection can result and healing time is prolonged. Therefore, postoperative management must focus on prevention of infection and other factors that inhibit healing, including hypergranulation, wound tension, and edema.

Other surgical procedures may be involved in the management of Dupuytren's disease because the involvement of the disease can be so extensive. If the disease is long-standing, joint contraction can occur and fasciectomy may not be sufficient to improve joint motion. Surgical release of the involved joints (capsulectomy or capsulotomy) may be indicated. The practitioner may also encounter cases in which nerve and/or artery repairs are associated with the normal surgical management of the disease. The digital nerves and arteries are frequently surrounded by diseased fascia, so damaged or severed nerves and vessels can result despite meticulous surgical technique. The practitioner must be aware of these associated procedures in order to provide the most appropriate and effective postoperative treatment.

Early physical therapy intervention focuses on wound and skin care, dressing changes, edema control, active and gentle passive range of motion, and splinting. On the day after surgery, the patient should be seen for fabrication of a resting splint (Fig. 6–89). The hand-based splint should not place tension across the wounds but should maintain the joint extension gained during surgery. It should also provide mild pressure to the palmar surface of the hand, which is helpful in

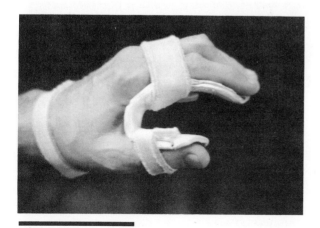

FIGURE 6–89 ■ Static resting splint with thumb component.

managing scar tissue formation. Factors to be considered when fabricating the splint include neurovascular status of the involved digits, presence of infection, and whether surgical release of any joints was performed. These factors can influence the degree of extension in which the joints are maintained.

On day 3, use of a sterile whirlpool (water temperature ranging from 98 to 100°F) is initiated for cleansing the wounds. Povidone-iodine (Betadine; Purdue Frederick, Norwalk, CT) can be added to the water for its antibacterial properties. Avoid positioning the hand in a dependent position in the whirlpool because this encourages edema. Ask the patient to maintain the elbow in at least 90 degrees of flexion and to flex and extend the digits and wrist periodically while in the water. After the whirlpool, the hand should be rinsed with clear water or saline solution to remove remaining bacteria from the wounds. The extremity should then be elevated on a pillow for the remainder of the treatment session.

Skin care can include application of a lubricant such as lanolin, avoiding the wounds. A dry, sterile dressing is then applied. Measures should be taken to control edema, aside from elevation and active range of motion. Retrograde massage may be difficult at this time because of the extensiveness of the wounds, but intermittent compression can be used. Initially, a pressure of 30 to 40 mm Hg for 30 minutes is appropriate. Because retrograde massage is an effective method of removing fluid from the hand, it should be initiated as soon as possible. When limited dressing is required, Coban wrapping of the digits may be added to edema control measures. Coban can hold smaller gauze pads in place, and it is not necessary to wait for complete wound closure. Starting at the fingertip, the Coban should be wrapped in the proximal direction with minimal tension applied because circulation is frequently compromised in the involved digits. The fingertip may be left uncovered to monitor the color of the finger, which would indicate any circulatory distress. Another option in the control of edema is use of an Isotoner glove (Aris Isotoner, New York, NY).

Range-of-motion exercises should include active and gentle passive flexion and extension of the digital joints. Use of both blocked and full-excursion exercises ensures that both joint motion and tendon excursion are addressed. Opposition of the thumb to each finger and abduction and adduction of all fingers should also be performed. Do not neglect the other joints of the upper extremity in the exercise program. Initially, 10 repetitions of each exercise are appropriate for the treatment session and the home program. Generally, the exercise program should be performed four to six times daily. As motion improves and time since the operation increases, the exercise program should be modified. Gentle manual resistive exercise or the use of soft putty may be initiated at 4 weeks. Unrestricted use of the hand generally occurs in 6 to 8 weeks.

Because of changes in the volume of the hand, range of motion of the joints, and amount of dressing required, continued monitoring of the splint is necessary. During each visit, the therapist should carefully mold the splint, allowing each joint to be held gently in extension. As healing progresses, a more aggressive approach must be taken to optimize the gains made surgically in joint motion. An effective alternative to the palmar hand-based splint is the dorsal splint, illustrated in Figure 6–90. Although considered a static splint, it is somewhat dynamic in nature because tension can be increased or decreased with the Velcro closures. This can prove to be of greater benefit in promoting extension than the palmar splint when precautions no longer need to be considered. In either case, a static extension splint is used continuously for the first 3 to 4 weeks and removed only for exercise. After that time, static splints are worn at night and as deemed necessary during the day. Another option to day splinting is dynamic extension splinting (see Fig. 6–47). Dynamic splinting can be more effective in managing more severe and stubborn cases of joint contracture, and it allows active flexion of the joints and functional use of the hand. Day splinting is reduced as indicated

by joint status, but night splinting continues for at least 4 to 6 months. When considering elimination of night splinting, it may be beneficial to wean the patient from the splint slowly rather than to discontinue its use abruptly. This allows the patient and therapist to observe any tendency of a joint to return to flexion.

Crucial to the postoperative treatment of Dupuytren's disease is the management of scar tissue. Considering the nature of the disease and the surgical procedures used to treat it, the difficulty encountered in attempting to manage it is great. Compounding factors include inappropriate splinting and exercise and uncontrolled edema. Therefore, the therapist must execute all aspects of treatment appropriately but be aggressive in dealing with the scar tissue; otherwise, a poor functional outcome will result. As wounds close, massage should be initiated to soften scar tissue and promote its mobility. Lanolin or other lubricants are used during massage. Scar massage consists of small, circular motions incorporating as much pressure as tolerated by the patient. It is beneficial to do scar massage before exercise, because the increase in local circulation and softening of the tissue are conducive to exercise. At least six 10-minute sessions should be performed daily. Another technique used to soften and flatten scar tissue is the application of elastomer. This material is prepared and spread over all scar areas, allowing it to conform to the surfaces to which it is applied. After several minutes, the material becomes firm and can be held in place by Coban (Fig. 6–91). Elastomer can be used before wounds are completely closed; small open areas can be covered by a nonadhering gauze. The molds can be used under splints as long as

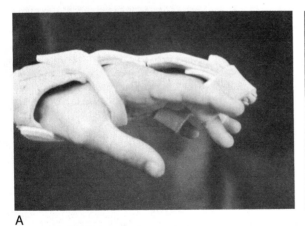

A

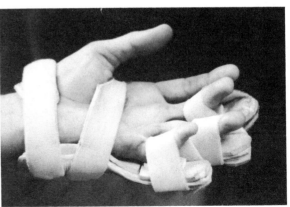

B

**FIGURE 6–90** ■ Dorsal dynamic splint or rack splint, lateral (A) and palmar (B) views.

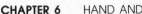

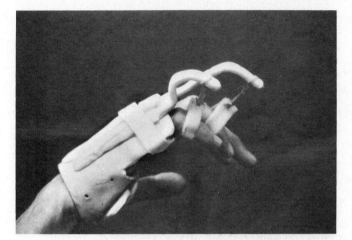

**FIGURE 6-91** ■ Dynamic PIP extension splint.

modifications are made to the splints. Continued monitoring of scar areas is necessary to determine when new molds are required or elastomer can be discontinued. Raised scars may require fabrication of new molds as remodeling occurs, in order to maintain effective pressure on the scar. When scars are flat and no longer reactive, elastomer molds can be discontinued.

## SUMMARY

This chapter has presented the basics in the areas of anatomy, wound biology, biomechanics, pathology, and therapeutic assessment and treatment. In addition, it has discussed various medical conditions, injuries, and diseases commonly seen by many therapists. The goal has not been to provide a cookbook approach to treatment of patients with hand and upper extremity problems; the postoperative management programs presented here should serve only as guidelines when treating the specific condition or injury. Many other factors must be considered when treatment plans are made: the patient's age, the mechanism and severity of injury, preoperative delay, suture material and technique, operative handling of the tissues, tension of repairs, the patient's ability to modify scar tissue biochemically, and the patient's cooperation and compliance during the rehabilitation process and how these factors determine the timing involved and techniques chosen. Tailoring the treatment program for each individual yields a better result.

Treament guidelines are helpful but cannot replace the fundamentals. A good grasp of the basics allows the practitioner to successfully manage not only the common diagnoses but also the uncommon. A sound foundation in anatomy, wound biology, biomechanics, physiology, physical agents, and therapeutic exercise enables the therapist to identify undiagnosed problems and conditions, design appropriate, flexible treatment programs, and successfully manage problems not seen on a daily basis. This chapter has attempted to provide a thorough review of these basics and insight into the management of various hand and wrist problems.

## CASE STUDY 1

### ▼HISTORY

The patient is a 53-year-old male, right-hand dominant electrician who was referred to therapy with the chief complaint of proximal forearm pain. He relates a 3-month history of dull aching pain on the lateral aspect of his right forearm and elbow. The onset of the pain was gradual, but at this time he describes it as a constant pain that is aggravated by certain motions and is frequently worse at night. After 6 weeks of increasing pain, the patient sought medical attention form his family physician. The patient received a cortisone injection at the elbow and instructions to rest his arm. The injection produced no response. Five weeks later, he returned to his family doctor, who prescribed anti-inflammatory medicine and physical therapy. The patient has continued to work since the onset of the pain. No significant past medical history exists. Currently, he is taking no other medications.

### PHYSICAL EXAMINATION

On physical examination, the girth of the right proximal forearm was comparable to that of the left. No postural abnormalities were noted in the cervical and thoracic spinal regions or the shoulder girdle. Range of motion of all joints of the right upper extremity (RUE) was within normal limits. Focusing on the area of pain, palpation about the lateral epicondyle and radial head elicited no response from the patient. Distal palpation at the level of the neck of the radius, in the area of the extensor muscle bellies (the mobile wad), elicited pain. Specifically, the area between the brachioradialis and the extensor carpi radialis brevis was tender. No other areas of tenderness were defined. Gross manual muscle testing revealed no weakness, although resisted supination with the elbow in a flexed position elicited pain. Based on these findings (areas of tenderness and painful resisted supination), the middle finger test was performed. With the elbow extended, the wrist in neutral and the digital joints in extension, the patient was asked to maintain extension of the middle finger against resistance. This maneuver caused pain in the area of the mobile wad. These positions and maneuvers did not elicit the same response when done on the LUE. A radial nerve compression syndrome was suspected, and a thorough evaluation of the sensory distribution of the radial nerve was performed but revealed no disturbances or deficits.

## TREATMENT

The initial treatment session focused on patient education. Conservative treatment emphasizes rest, splinting, avoidance of provocative motions, and task modification. What constitutes provocative motions (repetitive supination and pronation, static pronation, and repetitive wrist flexion) was explained to the patient as was the rationale of why to avoid these motions. Assessment of home and work tasks that require these motions were identified, and modifications to the working position, the work station, or work tasks were detailed. The importance of rest was emphasized.

A static wrist splint was fabricated to maintain the wrist in approximately 10 to 15 degrees of extension. Proper positioning of the splint was outlined and a wearing schedule defined. The patient should wear the splint at night and as possible throughout the day. He was told to wear the splint at work whenever possible.

A 1-week follow-up visit allowed for a check of the splint; whether it fit properly, were there any areas of pinch, and was it being used (was it dirty). A review of the information given during the first session was also conducted.

Conservative treatment can continue for 3 to 6 months. Therefore, the patient should be monitored by monthly visits. If symptoms persist, surgical decompression is indicated.

## CASE STUDY 2

### ▼HISTORY

The patient is a 44-year-old, right-hand dominant accountant who was referred to therapy 6 weeks after surgical repair of the left index finger flexor digitorum profundus and superficialis, the extensor digitorum communis (the extensor indicis proprius was lacerated but not repaired), and the radial digital nerve and artery. There was also a fracture of the second metacarpal at the level of the head. The injury was sustained when the patient's hand was caught between his boat and the dock. He reported being hospitalized for 4 days, followed by weekly visits to his physician. The patient presented with a plaster static extension splint that had been fabricated by the physician. The splint maintained the wrist in neutral and the MP joint in full extension and the PIP and DIP joints unsupported. Referral to therapy was for active range of motion. No significant past medical history existed. He was taking Tylenol for pain management; no other medications were being taken.

### PHYSICAL EXAMINATION

On examination, the left index finger was moderately edematous and red. Extensive scarring was noted over the dorsal surface and lateral aspect of the proximal phalanx, extending into the thumb/index web space and palm Fig. 6–92. The scar tissue was hypertrophic in areas and extremely adherent to the underlying structures. The resting position of the index

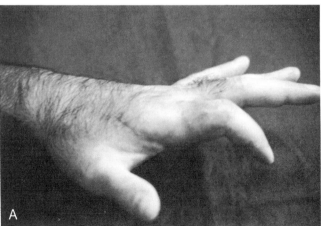
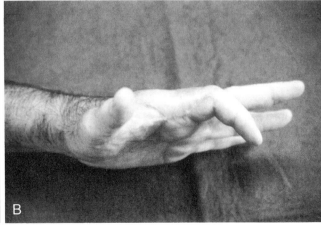

**FIGURE 6–92.** ■ Scarring over the dorsal and lateral aspect of the proximal phalanx (A) and extending into the thumb/index web space and palm (B).

finger was with the MP joint in full extension, the PIP joint in 65 degrees of flexion, and the DIP joint in 10 degrees of flexion. Active blocked and full-excursion range-of-motion measurements of the index finger were the same as those noted in the resting position. Passive blocked range of motion was slightly greater: MP = 0/20 degrees, PIP = 55/75 degrees, and DIP = 5/30 degrees. Limiting factors included joint contracture, absent tendon gliding (or pullthrough), and scar tissue adherence. The EDC, FDP, and FDS tendons were palpable on active extension and flexion. Range of motion of all other digital joints of the left hand, wrist, elbow, and shoulder was within normal limits both actively and passively. A thorough evaluation of strength was deferred, although cursory manual muscle testing revealed near-normal strength of the uninvolved digits. Assessment of sensation revealed a deficit in the radial aspect of the index finger; two-point discrimination was > 10 mm.

## TREATMENT

Initially, priorities of treatment included scar tissue management, edema control, and increasing joint motion. The typical treatment session during the first several weeks in physical therapy consisted of heat (whirlpool), retrograde massage and elevation for edema management, deep friction massage for scar mobilization, and active and passive blocked and full-excursion range-of-motion exercises. Protection of tendon repairs was not of great concern because tendon gliding was so compromised by adherence. A hand-based (not across the wrist) dynamic PIP extension splint was fabricated (Fig. 6–93) and the patient was instructed to wear it 20 minutes every hour. Approval for an MP flexion splint could not be obtained from the physician. An elastomer mold was made at the same time so that the splint was fitted over the mold.

A home program included Coban wrapping of the digit (worn except when exercising), elevation, retrograde (fluid flushing) and deep friction massages, ac-

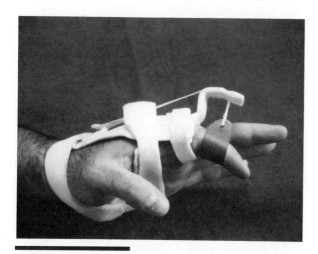

**FIGURE 6–93. ■** A hand-based dynamic PIP extension splint.

tive and passive blocked and full-excursion range-of-motion exercises of all digital joints, passive stretching of the thumb/index web space, and active range of motion of the wrist, elbow, and shoulder. Massage was to be done as often as possible (at least six times per day) and exercises were to be done on an hourly basis (repetitions as tolerated). The patient was encouraged to use the hand, including the index finger, in his daily activities, and not to get in the habit of isolating the digit from the remainder of his hand.

As time after surgery increased, treatment became more aggressive. Ultrasound was added to soften scar tissue. It became obvious that certain compromises would have to be made in treatment. For example, dynamic MP flexion splinting was added at 12 weeks postoperatively, despite an active extension lag at the MP and PIP joints. It became apparent that additional surgery was going to be necessary if a functional digit was desired. Therefore, increasing passive joint motion and managing scar tissue became the primary goals of treatment.

Sensibility was frequently reassessed so that sensory re-education could be initiated when indicated. Monitoring advancement of Tinel's sign showed no change; there was no advancement of the level of regenerating axons. Owing to the amount and density of the scar tissue, the nerve repair was more than likely "caught up" in scar tissue. The regenerating axons could not cross or bridge the gap between the proximal segment of the nerve and its distal nerve stump.

Over the course of treatment, passive range of motion of the index finger improved, but minimal change occurred in active range of motion. Passive range of motion was as follows: MP = 0/30 degrees, PIP = 20/90 degrees, and DIP = 0/60 degrees. Extensibility, mobility, and softness of the scar tissue also improved, although it remained the primary limiting factor to active range of motion. Tendon gliding did not improve, nor did sensation.

Because the scar tissue remained "active," reconstructive surgery was delayed until 11 months following injury. Plans for surgery included an MP joint capsulectomy, neurolysis of the radial digital nerve, and tenolysis of the flexor tendons. Extensor tendon surgery was to be performed at a later date.

## *References*

1. Brown DE, Lichtman DM: Midcarpal instability. Hand Clin 3(1):135–140, 1987.
2. Green DP: Carpal dislocations. *In* Operative Hand Surgery (Green DP, ed). New York: Churchill-Livingstone, 1982, pp 703–742.
3. Kleinman WB: Management of chronic rotary subluxation of the scaphoid by scapho-trapezio-trapezoid arthrodesis. Rationale for the treatment, postoperative changes in biomechanics, and results. Hand Clin 3(1):113–133, 1987.
4. Weber ER: Concepts governing the rotational shift of the intercalated segment of the carpus. Orthop Clin North Am 15(2):193–208, 1984.

5. Palmer AK: The distal radioulnar joint. Anatomy, biomechanics, and triangular fibrocartilage complex abnormalities. Hand Clin 3(1):31–40, 1987.
6. Mayfield JK: Wrist ligamentous anatomy and pathogenesis of carpal instability. Orthop Clin North Am 15(2):209–216, 1984.
7. Taleisnek J: Ligaments of the wrist. J Hand Surg 1:110–118, 1976.
8. Tubiana R: Examination of the Hand and Upper Limb. Philadelphia: WB Saunders, 1984.
9. Weeks PM: Acute Bone and Joint Injuries of the Hand and Wrist—A Clinical Guide to Management. St. Louis: CV Mosby, 1981.
10. Cash SL: Primary care of flexor tendon injuries. In Rehabilitation of the Hand: Surgery and Therapy, 3rd ed (Hunter JM, Schneider LH, Mackin EJ, et al, eds). St. Louis: CV Mosby, 1990, pp 379–389.
11. Chase RA: Anatomy and kinesiology of the hand. In Rehabilitation of the Hand: Surgery and Therapy, 3rd ed (Hunter JM, Schneider LH, Mackin EJ, et al, eds). St. Louis: CV Mosby, 1990, pp 13–28.
12. van Strien G: Postoperative management of flexor tendon injuries. In Rehabilitation of the Hand: Surgery and Therapy, 3rd ed (Hunter JM, Schneider LH, Mackin EJ, et al, eds). St. Louis: CV Mosby, 1990, pp 390–409.
13. Cambridge CA: Range-of-motion measurements of the hand. In Rehabilitation of the Hand: Surgery and Therapy, 3rd ed (Hunter JM, Schneider LH, Machin EJ, et al, eds). St. Louis: CV Mosby, 1990, pp 82–92.
14. Kauer JMG, de Lange A: The carpal joint. Anatomy and function. Hand Clin 3(1):23–29, 1987.
15. Ruby LK, Cooney WP, An KN, et al: Relative motion of selected carpal bones. A kinematic analysis of the normal wrist. J Hand Surg [Am] 13:1–10, 1988.
16. Doyle JR: Extensor tendons—acute injuries. Operative Hand Surgery (Green DP, ed). New York: Churchill-Livingstone, 1982, pp 1441–1464.
17. Evans RB: Therapeutic management of extensor tendon injuries. In Rehabilitation of the Hand: Surgery and Therapy, 3rd ed (Hunter JM, Schneider LH, Mackin EJ, et al, eds). St. Louis: CV Mosby, 1990, pp 492–511.
18. Evans RB: Therapeutic management of extensor tendon injuries. Hand Clin 2(1):157–168, 1986.
19. Rosenthal EA: The extensor tendons. In Rehabilitation of the Hand: Surgery and Therapy, 3rd ed (Hunter JM, Schneider LH, Mackin EJ, et al, eds). St. Louis: CV Mosby, 1990, pp 458–491.
20. Gray H: Gray's Anatomy. Philadelphia: Running Press, 1974.
21. Warfel JH: The Extremities, 4th ed. Philadelphia: Lea & Febiger, 1974.
22. Eversmann WW: Entrapment and compression neuropathies. In Operative Hand Surgery (Green DP, ed). New York: Churchill-Livingstone, 1982, pp 957–1009.
23. Spinner M: Injuries to the Major Branches of the Peripheral Nerves in the Forearm, 2nd ed. Philadelphia: WB Saunders, 1978.
24. Aulicino PL, DuPuy TE: Clinical examination of the hand. In Rehabilitation of the Hand: Surgery and Therapy, 3rd ed. (Hunter JM, Schneider LH, Mackin EJ, et al, eds). St. Louis: CV Mosby, 1990, pp 31–52.
25. Howard FM: Compression neuropathies in the anterior forearm. Hand Clin 2(4):737–745, 1986.
26. Callahan AD: Sensibility testing: clinical methods. In Rehabilitation of the Hand: Surgery and Therapy, 3rd ed (Hunter JM, Schneider LH, Mackin EJ, et al, eds). St. Louis: CV Mosby, 1990, pp 594–610.
27. Swanson AB, de Groot Swanson G, Goran-Hagert C: Evaluation of impairment of hand function. In Rehabilitation of the Hand: Surgery and Therapy, 3rd ed (Hunter JM, Schneider LH, Mackin EJ, et al, eds). St. Louis: CV Mosby, 1990, pp 109–138.
28. American Society of Surgery of the Hand: The Hand—Examination and Diagnosis, 3rd ed. New York: Churchill-Livingstone, 1990.
29. Kendall, FP, McCreary EK: Muscles, Testing and Function, 3rd ed. Baltimore: Williams & Wilkins, 1983.
30. Bechtol CD: Grip test: use of a dynamometer with adjustable handle spacing. J Bone Joint Surg [Am] 36:820, 1954.
31. Fess EE: Documentation: essential elements of an upper extremity assessment battery. In Rehabilitation of the Hand: Surgery and Therapy, 3rd ed (Hunter JM, Schneider LH, Mackin EJ, et al, eds). St. Louis: CV Mosby, 1990, pp 53–81.
32. Kellor M, Frost J, Silberberg N, et al: Hand strength and dexterity: norms for clinical use. Am J Occup Ther 25:77–83, 1971.
33. Mathiowetz V, Kashman N, Volland G, et al: Grip and pinch strength: normative data for adults. Arch Phys Med Rehabil 66(1):69–74, 1985.
34. Bell-Krotoski JA: Sensibility testing: state of the art. In Rehabilitation of the Hand: Surgery and Therapy, 3rd ed (Hunter JM, Schneider LH, Mackin EJ, et al, eds). St. Louis: CV Mosby, 1990, pp 575–584.
35. Dellon AL: Evaluation of Sensibility and Re-education of Sensation in the Hand. Baltimore: Williams & Wilkins, 1981.
36. Frykman GK, Nelson EF: Fractures and traumatic conditions of the wrist. In Rehabilitation of the Hand: Surgery and Therapy, 3rd ed (Hunter JM, Schneider LH, Mackin EJ, et al, eds). St. Louis: CV Mosby, 1990, pp 267–283.
37. Weber ER: A rational approach for the recognition and treatment of Colles' fracture. Hand Clin 3(1):13–21, 1987.
38. Gelberman RH, Manske PR: Factors influencing flexor tendon adhesions. Hand Clin 1(1):35, 1985.
39. Taleisnek J: Fractures of the carpal bones. In Operative Hand Surgery (Green DP, ed). New York: Churchill-Livingstone, 1982, pp 669–702.
40. Almquist EE: Kienböck's disease. Hand Clin 3(1):141–148, 1987.
41. Gelberman RH, Szabo RM: Kienböck's disease. Orthop Clin North Am 15(2):355–367, 1984.
42. Linscheid RL: Ulnar lengthening and shortening. Hand Clin 3(1):69–79, 1987.
43. Wilson RL, Carter MS: Management of hand fractures. In Rehabilitation of the Hand: Surgery and Therapy, 3rd ed (Hunter JM, Schneider LH, Mackin EJ, et al, eds). St. Louis: CV Mosby, 1990, pp 284–294.
44. Kleinert HE, Cash SL: Current guidelines for flexor tendon repair within the fibro-osseous tunnel: indications, timing, and techniques. In Tendon Surgery in the Hand (Hunter JM, Schneider LH, Mackin EJ, eds). St. Louis: CV Mosby, 1987.
45. Kleinert HE, Kutz JE, Ashbell TS, Martinez E: Primary repair of lacerated flexor tendons in no-man's land. J Bone Joint Surg [Am] 49:577, 1967.
46. Kleinert HE, Kutz JE, Cohen MJ: Primary repair of zone 2 flexor tendon lacerations. In AAOS Symposium on Tendon Surgery in the Hand. St. Louis: CV Mosby, 1975, pp 91–104.
47. Stewart KM: Review and comparisons of current trends in the post-operative management of tendon repair. Hand Clin 7(3):447–460, 1991.
48. Duran RJ, Houser RG: Controlled passive motion follow-

ing flexor tendon repair in zones II and II. *In* AAOS: Symposium on Tendon Surgery in the Hand. St. Louis: CV Mosby, 1975, pp 105–114.

48a. Young RES, Harmon JM: Repair of tendon injuries of the hand. Ann Surg 151:562–566, 1960.

49. Chow JA, Thomes LJ, Dovelle S, et al: A combined regimen of controlled motion following flexor tendon repair in "no man's land." Plast Reconstr Surg 79(3):447–455, 1987.

50. Mason ML, Allen HS: The rate of healing of tendons: an experimental study of tensile strength. Ann Surg 113:424, 1941.

51. Peacock EE: Biological principles in the healing of long tendons. Surg Clin North Am 45:461–476, 1965.

52. Evans RB: An update on wound management. Hand Clin 7(3):409–432, 1991.

53. Wilson RL: Flexor tendon grafting. Hand Clin 1(1):103, 1985.

54. Hunter JM, Singer DI, Mackin EJ: Staged flexor tendon reconstruction using passive and active tendon implants. *In* Rehabilitation of the Hand: Surgery and Therapy, 3rd ed (Hunter JM, Schneider LH, Mackin EJ, et al, eds). St. Louis: CV Mosby, 1990, pp 427–457.

55. Schneider LH, Mackin EJ: Tenolysis: dynamic approach to surgery and therapy. *In* Rehabilitation of the Hand: Surgery and Therapy, 3rd ed (Hunter JM, Schneider LH, Mackin EJ, et al, eds). St. Louis: CV Mosby, 1990, pp 417–426.

56. Strickland JW: Flexor tenolysis. Hand Clin 1(1):130, 1985.

57. Evans RB, Burkhalter WE: A study of the dynamic anatomy of extensor tendons and implications for treatment. J Hand Surg [Am] 11:774, 1986.

58. Kirkpatrick WH: De Quervain's disease. *In* Rehabilitation of the Hand: Surgery and Therapy, 3rd ed (Hunter JM, Schneider LH, Mackin EJ, et al, eds). St. Louis: CV Mosby, 1990, pp 304–307.

59. Swanson AB: Pathomechanics of deformities in hand and wrist. *In* Rehabilitation of the Hand: Surgery and Therapy, 3rd ed (Hunter JM, Schneider LH, Mackin EJ, et al, eds). St. Louis: CV Mosby, 1990, pp 891–902.

60. Taleisnek J: Rheumatoid arthritis of the wrist. Hand Clin 5(2):257–278, 1989.

61. Ferlic DC: Implant arthroplasty of the rheumatoid wrist. Hand Clin 3(1):169–179, 1987.

62. Flatt AE: The Care of the Rheumatoid Hand, 3rd ed. St. Louis: CV Mosby, 1974.

63. Swanson AB: Pathogenesis of arthritic lesions. *In* Rehabilitation of the Hand: Surgery and Therapy, 3rd ed (Hunter JM, Schneider LH, Mackin EJ, et al, eds). St. Louis: CV Mosby, 1990, pp 885–890.

64. Ferlic DC: Boutonnière deformities in rheumatoid arthritis. Hand Clin 5(2):215–222, 1989.

65. Nalebuff EA: The rheumatoid swan-neck deformity. Hand Clin 5(2):203–214, 1989.

66. Smith RJ: Intrinsic contracture. *In* Operative Hand Surgery (Green DP, ed). New York: Churchill-Livingstone, 1982, pp 515–537.

67. Swanson AB, de Groot Swanson G, Leonard J, et al: Postoperative rehabilitation programs in flexible implant arthroplasty of the digits. *In* Rehabilitation of the Hand: Surgery and Therapy, 3rd ed (Hunter JM, Schneider LH, Mackin EJ, et al, eds). St. Louis: CV Mosby, 1990, pp 912–928.

68. Madden JW, Arem A, DeVore G: A rational postoperative management program for metacarpophalangeal joint implant arthroplasty. J Hand Surg 12:358–366, 1977.

69. Spinner M: Nerve lesions in continuity. *In* Rehabilitation of the Hand: Surgery and Therapy, 3rd ed (Hunter JM, Schneider LH, Mackin EJ, et al, eds). St. Louis: CV Mosby, 1990, pp 523–529.

70. Chaplin E, Kasden ML, Corwin HM: Occupational neurology and the hand. Differential diagnosis. Hand Clin 2(3):513–524, 1986.

71. Ditmars DM, Houin HP: Carpal tunnel syndrome. Hand Clin 2(3):525–532, 1986.

72. Heckler FR, Jabaley ME: Evolving concepts of median nerve decompression in the carpal tunnel. Hand Clin 2(4):723–736, 1986.

73. Phalen GS: The carpal tunnel syndrome. Clinical evaluation of 598 hands. Clin Orthop 83:29, 1972.

74. Thompson WAL, Koppell HP: Peripheral entrapment neuropathies of the upper extremity. N Engl J Med 260:1261, 1959.

75. Lankford LL: Reflex sympathetic dystrophy. *In* Rehabilitation of the Hand: Surgery and Therapy, 3rd ed (Hunter JM, Schneider LH, Mackin EJ, et al, eds). St. Louis: CV Mosby, 1990, pp 763–786.

76. Waylett-Rendall J: Therapist's management of reflex sympathetic dystrophy. *In* Rehabilitation of the Hand: Surgery and Therapy, 3rd ed (Hunter JM, Schneider LH, Mackin EJ, et al, eds). St. Louis: CV Mosby, 1990, pp 787–792.

77. McCash CR: The open palm technique in Dupuytren's contracture. Br J Plast Surg 17:271, 1964.

78. McFarlane RM: Dupuytren's contracture. *In* Operative Hand Surgery (Green DP, ed). New York: Churchill-Livingstone, 1982, pp 463–498.

## Bibliography

Amadio PS, Jaeger SH, Hunter JM: Nutritional aspects of tendon healing. *In* Rehabilitation of the Hand: Surgery and Therapy, 3rd ed (Hunter JM, Schneider LH, Mackin EJ, et al, eds). St. Louis: CV Mosby, 1990, pp 373–378.

Beckenbaugh RD, Linscheid RL: Arthroplasty in the hand and wrist. *In* Operative Hand Surgery (Green DP, ed). New York: Churchill-Livingstone, 1982, pp 141–184.

Bell-Krotoski J: Advances in sensibility evaluation. Hand Clin 7(3):527–546, 1991.

Botte MJ, Gelberman RH: Fractures of the carpus, excluding the scaphoid. Hand Clin 3(1):149–161, 1987.

Cannon NM, Strickland JW: Therapy following flexor tendon surgery. Hand Clin 1(1):147–165, 1985.

Caplan HS, Hunter JM, Merklin RJ: Intrinsic vascularization of flexor tendons. *In* AAOS: Symposium on Tendon Surgery in the Hand. St. Louis: CV Mosby, 1975, pp 48–58.

Dovelle S, Heeter P: Early controlled mobilization following extensor tendon repair in zones V–VI of the hand: preliminary report. Contemp Orthop 4(11):41–44, 1985.

Doyle RF, Blythe W: The finger flexor tendon sheath and pulleys: anatomy and reconstruction. *In* AAOS: Symposium on Tendon Surgery in the Hand. St. Louis: CV Mosby, 1975, pp 81–87.

Eaton RG: Joint Injuries of the Hand. Springfield, IL: Charles C Thomas, 1971.

Froimson AI: Tenosynovitis and tennis elbow. *In* Operative Hand Surgery (Green DP, ed). New York: Churchill-Livingstone, 1982, pp 1507–1514.

Gelberman RH, Woo S: The physiological basis for application of controlled stress in the rehabilitation of flexor tendon injuries. J Hand Ther 2(2):66–70, 1989.

Green DP: Carpal dislocations. *In* Operative Hand Surgery (Green DP, ed). New York: Churchill-Livingstone, 1982, pp 703–742.

Hunter JM: Recurrent carpal tunnel syndrome, epineural fibrous fixation, and traction neuropathy. Hand Clin 7(3):491–504, 1991.

Jaeger SH, Singer DI, Whitenack SH: Nerve injury complications: management of neurogenic pain syndromes. Hand Clin 2(1):217–224, 1986.

Ketchum LD: Primary tendon healing: a review. J Hand Surg 2(6):428, 1977.

Lane C: Therapy for the occupationally injured hand. Hand Clin 2(3):593–602, 1986.

Leddy JP: Flexor tendons—acute injuries. *In* Operative Hand Surgery (Green DP, ed). New York: Churchill-Livingstone, 1982, pp 1347–1373.

Leslie BM: Rheumatoid extensor tendon ruptures. Hand Clin 5(2):191–202, 1989.

Lister GD, Kleinert HE, Kutz JE, et al: Primary flexor repair followed by immediate controlled mobilization. J Hand Surg 2(6):441–455, 1977.

Lundborg G, Rank F: Experimental intrinsic healing of flexor tendons based upon synovial fluid nutrition. J Hand Surg 3(1):21, 1978.

Manske PR, Whiteside LA, Lesker PA: Nutrient pathways to flexor tendons. J Hand Surg 3:32, 1978.

Miller-Breslow A, Millender LH, Feldon PG: Treatment considerations in the complicated rheumatoid hand. Hand Clin 5(2):279–289, 1989.

Morrin J, Davey V, Conolly WB: The Hand—Fundamentals of Therapy. London: Butterworth-Heinemann, 1985.

Mullins PAT: Use of therapeutic modalities in upper extremity rehabilitation. *In* Rehabilitation of the Hand: Surgery and Therapy, 3rd ed (Hunter JM, Schneider LH, Mackin EJ, et al, eds). St. Louis: CV Mosby, 1990, pp 195–220.

O'Brien ET: Fractures of the metacarpals and phalanges. *In* Operative Hand Surgery (Green DP, ed). New York: Churchill-Livingstone, 1982, pp 583–588.

O'Donovan TM, Ruby LK: The distal radioulnar joint in rheumatoid arthritis. Hand Clin 5(2):249–256, 1989.

Omer GE: Nerve response to injury and repair. *In* Rehabilitation of the Hand: Surgery and Therapy, 3rd ed (Hunter JM, Schneider LH, Mackin EJ, et al, eds). St. Louis: CV Mosby, 1990, pp 515–522.

Peacock EE, Van Winkle W: Surgery and Biology of Wound Repair. Philadelphia: WB Saunders, 1970.

Philips CA: Management of the patient with rheumatoid arthritis. Hand Clin 5(2):291–309, 1989.

Potenza AD: Prevention of adhesions to healing digital flexor tendons. JAMA 187:187, 1964.

Strickland JW: Biologic rationale, clinical application and results of early motion following flexor tendon repair. J Hand Ther 2(2):71–83, 1989.

Totten PA, Hunter JM: Therapeutic techniques to enhance nerve gliding in thoracic outlet syndrome and carpal tunnel syndrome. Hand Clin 7(3):505–520, 1991.

Tubiana R, ed: The Hand, Vol 3. Philadelphia: WB Saunders, 1987.

Watson HK, Black DM: Instabilities of the wrist. Hand Clin 3(1):103–111, 1987.

Williams HB, Jabaley ME: The importance of internal anatomy of the peripheral nerves to nerve repair in the forearm and hand. Hand Clin 2(4):689–707, 1986.

Wilson RL, Carlblom ER: The rheumatoid metacarpophalangeal joint. Hand Clin 5(2):223–237, 1989.

Wray RC: Repair of sensory nerves distal to the wrist. Hand Clin 2(4):767–772, 1986.

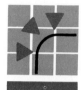

# Hip

## BARNEY LeVEAU

## INTRODUCTION

The major functions of the hip joint are to provide support for the transmission of superincumbent forces to the lower limb and to allow ease of motion for ambulation. These functional demands require the hip joint to have great stability along with a wide range of motion. The hip joint is constructed so that the bones and soft tissue ensure stability while they permit freedom of motion. Because the hip joint is located so deeply in the body, it presents numer-

ous problems in evaluation and diagnosis of disorders.

A review of the anatomy of the hip enables the therapist to identify normal structural relationships of the region. Based on this information, an effective objective evaluation of child and adult patients can be discussed. These findings from the initial evaluations determine the differential diagnosis. Rehabilitation programs are individualized to the diagnosis and the patient's age, general physical status, social support system, and so forth. Home exercise programs reinforce clinical therapeutic exercise programs and make the patient an active participant in the recovery.

The superincumbent weight and the muscular loading of the hip cause mechanical disorders of the hip. These include dislocations, subluxations, fractures, and degeneration of the cartilage and bone. Treatment of these disorders is often related to restoration or approximation of the normal joint mechanics along with relief of pain and correction of structural deformities and gait abnormalities.

## ANATOMY

### Bone

The hip joint is composed of a globular projection on the proximal end of the femur that fits deeply into a socket formed by the pelvic bone (Fig. 7–1).

#### *Proximal End of Femur*

The proximal end of the femur includes the head, the neck, and the trochanters (Fig. 7–2). The femoral head is approximately two thirds of a sphere. The shape of this projection is nearly, but not completely, spheric.[1-3] The surface is smooth and covered almost entirely with cartilage. At one point on the head, just below the center of the head, lies a depression or fovea for attachment of the ligament of the head of the femur. The head and neck join at an area called the subcapital sulcus. The subcapital sulcus is more evident at the superior and inferior aspects of the neck. The neck is mainly pyramidal in shape and is about three fourths the diameter of the head. This size differential allows a wide range of motion. The neck is covered with periosteum to which a fold of joint synovium is attached.

The angle of the neck with the femoral shaft, the angle of inclination (Fig. 7–3), varies from birth to adulthood. The angle between the neck and shaft at infancy is approximately 175 degrees. As the neck lengthens it also descends, decreasing the angle to about 125 degrees in adulthood.

The neck also causes the head to be projected forward (Fig. 7–4). The angle of torsion is about 40 degrees at birth, creating anteversion. With age, this angle decreases to approximately 12 to 15 degrees. If the torsion of the neck is projected backward it is called retroversion.

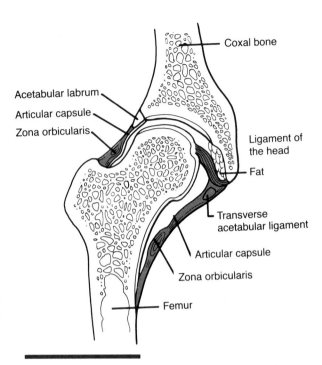

**FIGURE 7–1** ■ Frontal section through the hip joint. Synovial membrane is shown lining the articular capsule and reflected around the neck of the femur and the ligament of the head to the articular cartilage. The zona orbicularis consists of circular fibers in the fibrous capsule.

The superior aspect of the neck is shorter than the inferior aspect. The superior aspect terminates distally at the greater trochanter, and the inferior aspect terminates at the lesser trochanter. These trochanters are prominent processes that provide increased leverage for some of the muscles that cross the hip.

The greater trochanter is a large, irregular quadrilateral projection located at the lateral junction of the femoral neck and shaft. It is directed outward and slightly backward as it provides an attachment for several muscles (gluteus minimus, gluteus medius, piriformis). It is located approximately 2 cm below the head of the femur. On the medial aspect of the greater trochanter is a deep depression called the trochanteric fossa. This depression allows greater range of motion of the hip joint.

The lesser trochanter is a small conical prominence projecting medially and slightly posteriorly from the medial junction of the neck and shaft on which the iliopsoas muscle attaches. Its triangular base is connected to three easily discerned borders: the lower border of the femoral neck, the posterior intertrochanteric line, and the pectineal line.

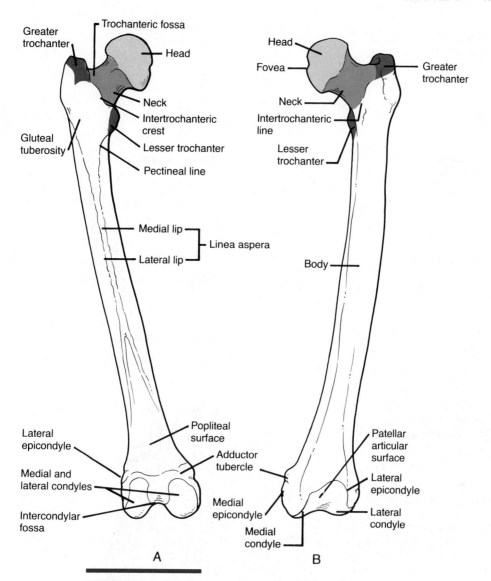

FIGURE 7–2 ■ Anterior (A) and posterior (B) views of the femur.

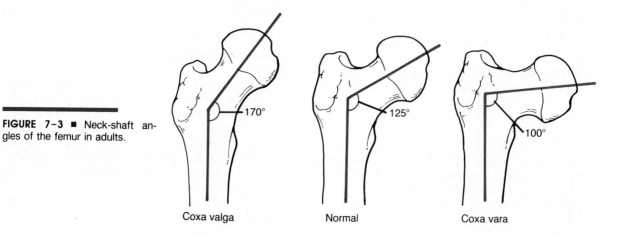

FIGURE 7–3 ■ Neck-shaft angles of the femur in adults.

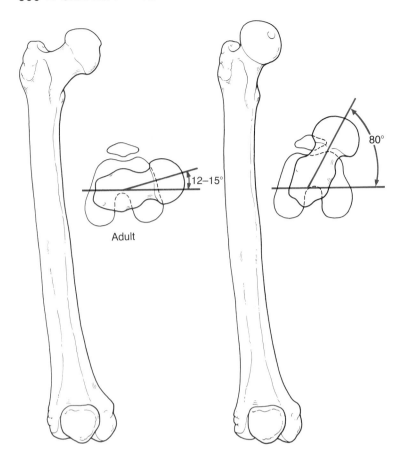

Adult

**FIGURE 7-4** ■ The femoral anteversion angle: the angle formed by the intersection of the femoral condyle's coronal plane with a line drawn through the femoral neck and femoral head center (head-neck axis).

Several other important landmarks are located near the junction of the neck and shaft of the femur (see Fig. 7-2). On the posterior aspect, the posterior intertrochanteric line (intertrochanteric crest) extends from the greater trochanter to the lesser trochanter. From the anterior aspect of the femur, the intertrochanteric line, along which the articular capsule attaches, spirals below the lesser trochanter and continues posteriorly as the pectineal line on which the pectineus muscle attaches. The pectineal line continues distally as the medial edge of the linea aspera. The medial and lateral edges of the linea aspera provide attachment for several muscles of the thigh, as described later in the section concerning muscles.

### Pelvis

The adult pelvis is composed of four bones: a pair of coxal bones, the sacrum, and the coccyx (Fig. 7-5). The ilium, ischium, and pubis, which fuse during late adolescence, make up each coxal bone. In the infant these are three separate bones.

The ilium is a large wing-like bone that is the most superior of the three components of the coxal bone (Figs. 7-6 and 7-7). It has smooth lateral and medial surfaces. Notable landmarks along the border of the ilium are the anterior inferior iliac spine, the anterior superior iliac spine (ASIS), the iliac crest, the posterior superior iliac spine (PSIS) the posterior interior iliac spine, and the greater sciatic notch. The medial surface landmarks are the iliac fossa and the iliac tuberosity. The fossa on the lateral surface of the ilium is traversed by the inferior gluteal line, the anterior gluteal line, and the posterior gluteal line.

The ischium is an irregular-shaped bone that is inferior to the ilium and posterior to the pubis. The notable landmarks on the ischium, the most posterior coxal component, are the ischial spine, the lesser sciatic notch, the ischial tuberosity, and the ramus of the ischium. This ramus forms the posterior and part of the interior walls of the obturator foramen.

The component anterior to the ischium is the pubis. It has a superior ramus and an inferior

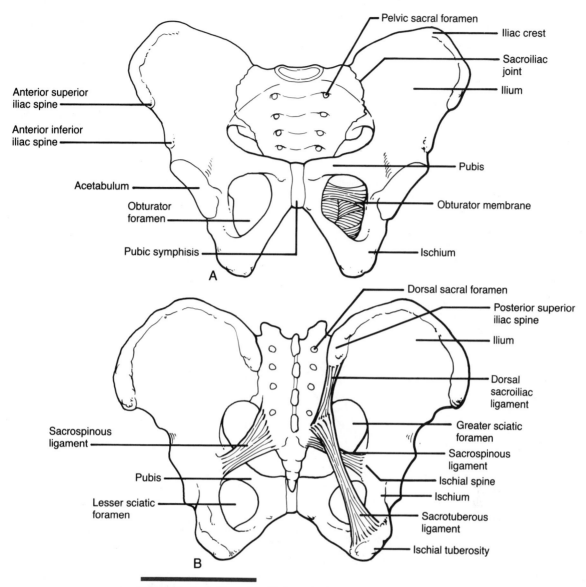

**FIGURE 7–5** ■ The pelvis (A) from the front and (B) from behind.

ramus, which complete the obturator foramen. Anteriorly are the pubic crest and the pubic tubercle.

The acetabulum is a cup-shaped concavity on the lateral side of the pelvis that faces laterally, anteriorly, and inferiorly (Fig. 7–8). The horizontal obliquity of the acetabulum as measured in x-rays studies is approximately 30 degrees at birth and decreases to its adult value of about 20 degrees by the age of 3 years.[4] The horizontal obliquity remains at this orientation throughout adulthood.

The acetabulum is formed by the joining of the ilium superiorly, the ischium inferolaterally, and the pubis medially (Fig. 7–9). The triradiate cartilage forms the area of contact between these bones and allows endochondral growth of the acetabular cup. The acetabulum is not a full circle but resembles a horseshoe or inverted U with an indentation, called the acetabular notch, at its inferior aspect (see Fig. 7–8). The inferior aspect of the circumference of the acetabulum is completed by the transverse ligament, which crosses the distal aspect of the notch. The deep area within the U is called the acetabular fossa. A raised rim (acetabular labrum) outlines the ace-

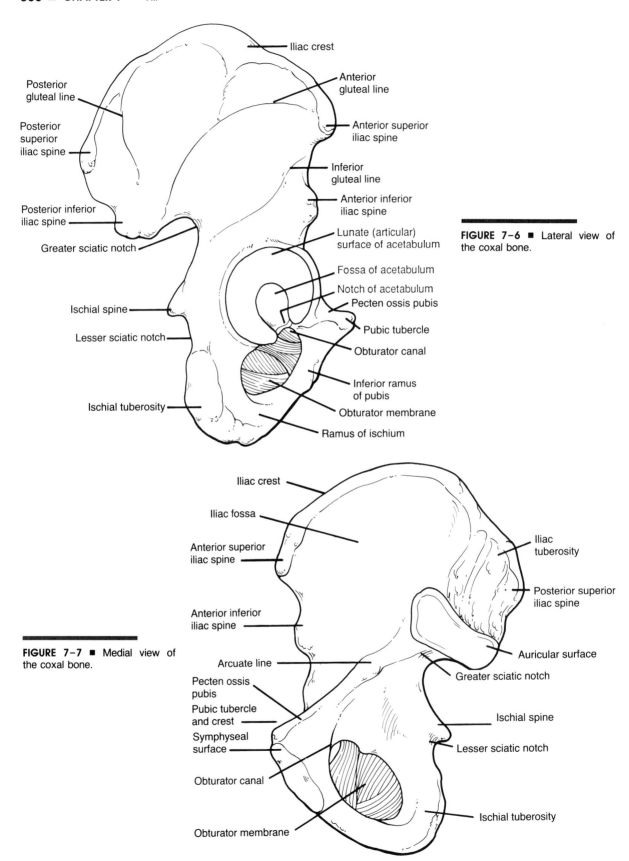

Iliac crest

Posterior gluteal line

Anterior gluteal line

Posterior superior iliac spine

Anterior superior iliac spine

Inferior gluteal line

Anterior inferior iliac spine

Posterior inferior iliac spine

Lunate (articular) surface of acetabulum

Greater sciatic notch

Fossa of acetabulum

Notch of acetabulum

Pecten ossis pubis

Ischial spine

Pubic tubercle

Lesser sciatic notch

Obturator canal

Inferior ramus of pubis

Ischial tuberosity

Obturator membrane

Ramus of ischium

**FIGURE 7–6** ■ Lateral view of the coxal bone.

Iliac crest

Iliac fossa

Iliac tuberosity

Anterior superior iliac spine

Posterior superior iliac spine

Anterior inferior iliac spine

Auricular surface

Arcuate line

Greater sciatic notch

Pecten ossis pubis

Pubic tubercle and crest

Ischial spine

Symphyseal surface

Lesser sciatic notch

Obturator canal

Ischial tuberosity

Obturator membrane

**FIGURE 7–7** ■ Medial view of the coxal bone.

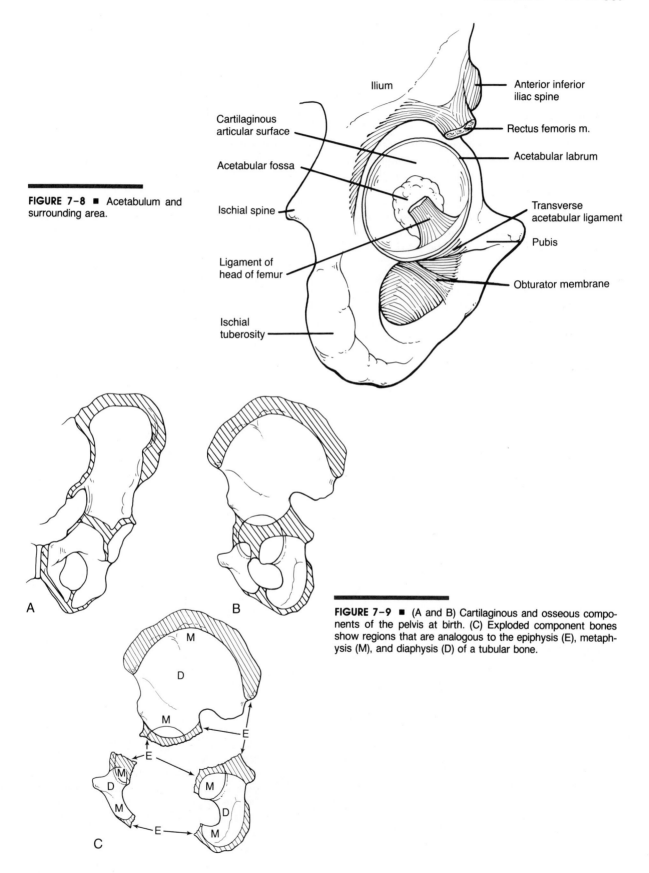

**FIGURE 7–8** ■ Acetabulum and surrounding area.

Ilium

Anterior inferior iliac spine

Cartilaginous articular surface

Rectus femoris m.

Acetabular fossa

Acetabular labrum

Ischial spine

Transverse acetabular ligament

Pubis

Ligament of head of femur

Obturator membrane

Ischial tuberosity

A

B

**FIGURE 7–9** ■ (A and B) Cartilaginous and osseous components of the pelvis at birth. (C) Exploded component bones show regions that are analogous to the epiphysis (E), metaphysis (M), and diaphysis (D) of a tubular bone.

M

D

M

E

E

M

D

M

E

M

D

M

C

tabulum. This rim is highest superiorly at its apex, where body weight is accommodated, and lower inferiorly, where no body weight is carried.

## Cartilage

Four types of cartilage occur in the acetabular area (Fig. 7–10): physeal cartilage (triradiate cartilage), fibrocartilage of the labrum, articular cartilage, and undifferentiated hyaline cartilage.

The triradiate cartilage is located in the physeal regions of the ischium, ilium, and pubis. These regions grow in the same manner as the epiphyseal plates of long bones. The endochondral growth process allows the acetabular cavity to expand progressively as the femoral head grows.[5]

The fibrocartilaginous labrum of the acetabulum is a tough, mobile annulus that attaches to the bony acetabular rim but does not extend over the acetabular notch. The labrum increases the depth of the acetabulum and thus stabilizes the hip joint. It extends beyond the greatest circumference of the head of the femur, thus preventing femoral head dislocation from the acetabulum. The labrum holds the femoral head so effectively that the head can be removed from the acetabulum only if the labrum is stretched or ruptured, as in a total hip replacement.[2] The superior margin of the labrum is quite mobile and may fold into the hip joint cavity of a congenitally dislocated hip, blocking reduction of the dislocated femoral head.[3]

The articular cartilage covers a portion of the acetabulum forming a broad horseshoe-shaped area that opens downward. The upper portion of the acetabulum is the major weight-bearing site of the articulation. The articular cartilage is thickest at this upper area and around the outer periphery of the horseshoe shape as it carries the body weight. Thinning of the cartilage occurs toward the center and lower portion of the acetabulum. The nonarticular portion of the acetabulum or acetabular fossa and a fat pad covered with synovial fluid are found within the horseshoe. The subchondral bone and synovial fluid provide nutrition for the articular cartilage. Repair of damaged articular cartilage in the hip joint is limited because the cartilage is not supplied directly from blood vessels.

Articular cartilage covers the entire surface of the femoral head except at the fovea. The cartilage is thicker at the center of the femoral head, where it makes contact with the acetabulum, and thinner at the circumference of the joint. The articular cartilage of the femoral head terminates at the junction of the femoral head and neck, the subcapital sulcus.

## Capsule

A strong fibrous capsule encloses the articulating surfaces of the hip joint and a large portion of the femoral neck. The capsule attaches to the edge of the acetabulum, the acetabular labrum, and the transverse ligament, forming a closely fitting cuff around the neck of the femur. The capsule attaches anteriorly on the femur along the intertrochanteric line and posteriorly on the neck about 1.5 cm above the intertrochanteric crest. This capsular design places the lateral half of the neck in an extracapsular position posteriorly and the anterior surface and the medial half of the posterior surface of the femoral neck in an intracapsular position. The capsule is thick and strong over the upper and anterior portion of the joint and thinner and weaker over the lower and posterior joint area.

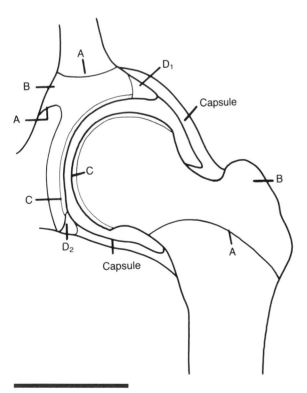

**FIGURE 7–10** ■ Four basic types of cartilage found in the region of the hip: (A) physeal (growth); (B) hyaline (epiphyseal); (C) articular; (D$_1$) fibrocartilage of the labrum; and (D$_2$) fibrocartilage of the transverse acetabular ligament.

## Ligaments

The capsule is reinforced by three strong fibrous longitudinal ligaments that originate on the pelvis and terminate on the femur (Fig. 7–11). These ligaments are named according to the bone areas that they connect (the iliofemoral, pubofemoral, and ischiofemoral ligaments).

The iliofemoral ligament, the ligament of Bigelow, is the strongest of the three. It extends from the anterior inferior iliac spine of the pelvis, crosses in front of the joint, splits into two bands forming an inverted Y, and attaches along the intertrochanteric line of the femur. It is considered the strongest ligament in the body[6] and is rarely ruptured; however, it acts as a point of pivot during hip dislocation. The iliofemoral ligament is loose in flexion and becomes taut during full hip extension. In extension it resists the movement of the pelvis posteriorly on the femoral head and pulls the femoral head more firmly into the acetabulum.

The pubofemoral ligament originates on the pubic portion of the acetabular rim and partly on the superior pubic ramus of the pelvis. It passes obliquely to the underside of the femoral neck. The ligament is relatively weak, but it limits hip abduction and becomes tight in hip extension.

The ischiofemoral ligament is a weaker ligament that arises from the ischial portion of the acetabular rim. It spirals around the femoral neck and attaches to the greater trochanter just posterior to the attachment of the iliofemoral ligament and therefore also becomes tense during hip extension.

A fourth ligament connecting the acetabulum and the femoral head is the ligament of the head of the femur, which originates from both sides of the acetabular notch and the floor of the acetabular fossa deep to the transverse ligament, runs to the head of the femur, and inserts loosely onto the upper part of the fovea of the femoral head. It is surrounded by synovial membrane. This ligament serves to conduct blood vessels to the femoral head. If this ligament is ruptured, loss of blood supply can lead to aseptic necrosis of the femoral head.

## Muscles

The bone configuration and the ligaments and joint capsule provide a considerable amount of stability to the hip joint while allowing extensive hip movement. These movements about the hip consist of flexion, extension, abduction, adduction, outward rotation, inward rotation, horizontal flexion, horizontal abduction, and circumduction. As they cross the hip, the muscles provide hip movement and additional joint stability (Figs. 7–12 to 7–15). The function of each muscle depends on its anatomic relationship to the axis of the hip joint, positional relationship to the force of gravity on the body part to which it attaches, simultaneous activity of other muscles, and inertia of the body part to which it attaches (Table 7–1). Therefore, knowledge of a muscle's attachments allows an individual to determine the muscle's function. The size and shape of the muscle also contribute to the muscle's function, the force of contraction, and the distance it travels.

The iliacus, a flat triangular muscle, attaches proximally to the upper two thirds of the iliac

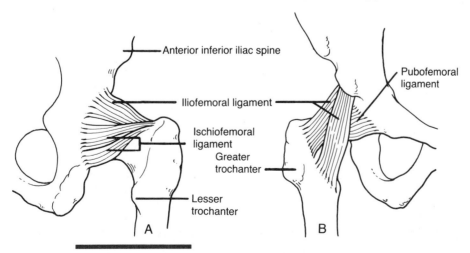

**FIGURE 7–11** ■ Left hip joint (A) from the front and (B) from behind.

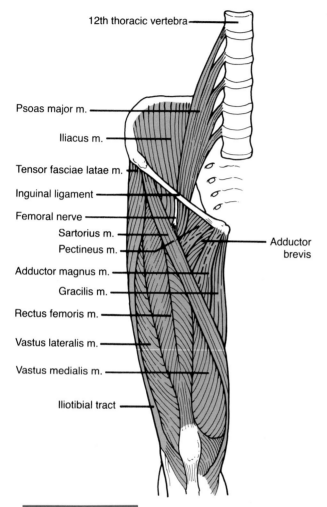

12th thoracic vertebra

Psoas major m.

Iliacus m.

Tensor fasciae latae m.

Inguinal ligament

Femoral nerve

Sartorius m.

Pectineus m.

Adductor
brevis

Adductor magnus m.

Gracilis m.

Rectus femoris m.

Vastus lateralis m.

Vastus medialis m.

Iliotibial tract

**FIGURE 7–12** ■ More superficial muscles of the anterior aspect of the thigh. The space between the pectineus and the adductor longus is exaggerated so that the position of the adductor brevis can be shown.

and extends over two joints, the hip and the knee. It arises from the ASIS and the upper half of the notch below it. The muscle passes across the anterior and medial aspects of the thigh. Its tendon attaches distally in front of the gracilis and semitendinosus muscles on the upper part of the tibia below the tibial tuberosity. It provides flexion, external rotation and minimal abduction of the thigh, and flexion of the leg.

The rectus femoris is the part of the quadriceps that crosses two joints (the hip and the knee). It arises from the ASIS and a small tendinous part from the ilium just above the acetabulum. It joins the other quadriceps muscles as it attaches on the tibial tuberosity. It flexes the thigh and extends the leg.

The adductor longus arises from the pubis tubercle and attaches on the linea aspera between the attachments of the vastus medialis and the

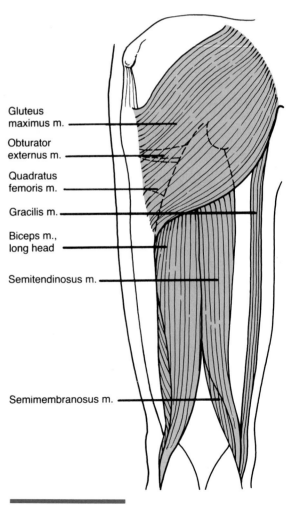

Gluteus
maximus m.

Obturator
externus m.

Quadratus
femoris m.

Gracilis m.

Biceps m.,
long head

Semitendinosus m.

Semimembranosus m.

**FIGURE 7–13** ■ Posteriorly placed adductors of the thigh.

fossa and the inner margin of the iliac crest, the base of the sacrum, the iliolumbar ligament, the anterior superior and inferior iliac spines and notch between them, and the capsule of the hip joint. The psoas, a long fusiform muscle, arises from the front of the bases and lower borders of the transverse recesses of the five lumbar vertebrae and the sides of the bodies of the last dorsal and all five lumbar vertebrae. Both the iliacus and psoas muscles have a common distal attachment onto and below the lesser trochanter of the femur. These two muscles combine to flex, externally rotate, and minimally adduct the thigh of a free limb.

The sartorius is the longest muscle in the body

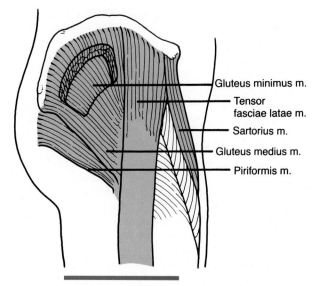

**FIGURE 7–14** ■ Abductors of the thigh.

| Motion | Primary | Secondary |
|---|---|---|
| Abduction | Gluteus medius<br>Gluteus minimus<br>Tensor fasciae latae | Piriformis<br>Sartorius<br>Obturator internus<br>Gluteus maximus<br>  (upper) |
| Adduction | Adductor magnus<br>Adductor longus<br>Pectineus<br>Adductor brevis<br>Gluteus maximus<br>Obturator externus<br>Quadratus femoris | Gracilis<br>Semitendinosus<br>Biceps (long head) |
| Flexion | Iliopsoas<br>Tensor fasciae latae<br>Sartorius<br>Rectus femoris | Pectineus<br>Adductor longus<br>Adductor brevis<br>Adductor magnus |
| Extension | Gluteus maximus<br>Hamstrings<br>Adductor magnus | Piriformis<br>Obturator internus<br>Gluteus medius |
| Internal rotation | Gluteus medius<br>  (anterior fibers)<br>Tensor fasciae latae<br>Pectineus | Gracilis<br>Adductor magnus<br>Adductor longus<br>Adductor brevis<br>Medial hamstrings |
| External rotation | Gluteus maximus<br>Iliopsoas<br>  (in infants)<br>Obturator internus<br>Obturator externus<br>Piriformis | Sartorius<br>Biceps |

adductor magnus. It assists with adduction, flexion, and internal rotation of the thigh.

The gracilis is also a two-joint muscle. It arises from the interior ramus of the pubis and from the ramus of the ischium. It attaches distally on the medial surface of the upper end of the tibia close to the attachments of the sartorius and semitendinosus. It adducts, flexes, and medially rotates the thigh and flexes the leg.

The adductor brevis comes from the body and inferior ramus of the pubis. It attaches on the lower part of the line between the lesser tro-

**FIGURE 7–15** ■ Posteriorly placed external rotators of the thigh. The gluteus minimus has long been regarded as aiding external rotation, but its participation has not been shown electromyographically.

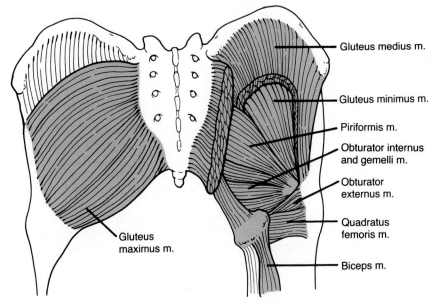

chanter and the linea aspera and into the upper portion of the linea aspera. It flexes, adducts, and medially rotates the thigh.

The adductor magnus arises from the inferior ramus of the pubis, the ramus of the ischium, and, the ischial tuberosity. It attaches along the linea aspera distal to the adductor tubercle. Its major function is to adduct the thigh, with anterior fibers flexing the thigh and posterior fibers extending the thigh.

The pectineus comes from the superior ramus of the pubis. It attaches to the femur just below the lesser trochanter. It flexes, adducts, and medially rotates the thigh.

The semitendinosus, which crosses two joints, arises from the ischial tuberosity and passes down the medial side of the posterior thigh. It attaches medial and distal to the tibial tuberosity. It extends the thigh and flexes and medially rotates the leg.

The semimembranosus crosses two joints arising from the ischial tuberosity and crosses under the semitendinosus and long head of the biceps. It attaches on the posteromedial side of the medial tibial condyle. It extends the thigh and flexes and medially rotates the leg.

The biceps femoris has two heads. The long head arises from the ischial tuberosity and crosses two joints. The short head arises from the linea aspera on the posterior surface of the femur. The heads of the muscle join and attach to the head of the fibula. The muscle extends the thigh and flexes and laterally rotates the leg.

The gluteus maximus is a large superficial posterior hip muscle. A small part of the crest of the ilium is in the region of the PSIS. It arises from a small part of the crest of the ilium in the region of the PSIS, the posterior surface of the lower part of the sacrum, the side of the coccyx, and the aponeurosis of the erector spinae muscle, the sacrosciatic ligament, and fascia covering the gluteus medius. About three fourths of the muscle attaches distally to the iliotibial band, which continues across the knee and attaches anterolaterally on the lateral tibial condyle. The remainder inserts on a rough line on the femur extending from the greater trochanter to the linea aspera. It extends and laterally rotates the thigh, with the upper fibers abducting and the lower fibers adducting the thigh.

The gluteus medius is a broad triangular muscle on the lateral side of the pelvis. The posterior third is covered by the gluteus maximus and the anterior two thirds by the fasciae latae. It arises on the surface of the ilium between the superior and middle gluteal lines and from gluteal apo-

neurosis. It is divided into three parts whose distal tendons unite and attach to the outer surface of the greater trochanter. It abducts the thigh, with the anterior fibers flexing and medially rotating the thigh and the posterior fibers minimally extending and laterally rotating the thigh.

The gluteus minimus lies immediately below the gluteus medius. It is a fan-shaped muscle that arises from the outer surface of the ilium between the middle and inferior gluteal lines and from the margin of the greater sciatic notch. Its distal tendon attaches to the anterior border of the greater trochanter. It is an abductor of the thigh.

The tensor fasciae latae arises from the anterior portion of the outer lip of the crest of the ilium and from the outer surface of the ASIS and part of the outer border of the notch below the ASIS. It attaches distally to the iliotibial band, which continues distally to the tuberosity of the tibia. It flexes and medially rotates the thigh and may assist in abduction of the thigh.

The piriformis is a flat muscle that lies parallel to the posterior border of the gluteus medius. It arises from the front of the sacrum between S-1 to S-4, the sacrosciatic foramen and the anterior surface of the great sacrosciatic ligament, passes through the sacrosciatic foramen, and attaches to the upper border of the greater trochanter. It rotates the thigh laterally when the thigh is extended and abducts the thigh when the thigh is flexed.

Inferior to the piriformis are the obturator internus and two associated muscles, the gemelli. The obturator internus arises from the inner surface of the anterior and external walls of the pelvis, the obturator membrane, and the edges of the obturator foramen. It fills the lesser sciatic foramen and attaches just above the trochanteric fossa. These muscles rotate the thigh laterally when the thigh is extended and abduct the thigh when the thigh is flexed.

The superior and inferior gemelli serve as accessory muscles to the obturator internus. The superior gemellus arises from the ischial spine and inserts on the upper border of the obturator internus tendon. The inferior gemellus arises from the ischial tuberosity and inserts on the lower border of the obturator internus tendon.

The obturator externus lies behind the adductor muscles. It arises from the outer surface of the pelvis from the obturator membrane and around the obturator foramen, passes behind the hip joint, and attaches to the trochanteric fossa. It rotates the thigh laterally.

The quadratus femoris is a small rectangular

muscle. It arises from the ischial tuberosity and attaches to the femur midway between the lesser and greater trochanters. It laterally rotates and adducts the thigh.

## Bursae

Several bursae are related to the muscles that cross the hip joint (Fig. 7–16). The most commonly inflamed bursae are the iliopectineal bursa, the trochanteric bursa, and the ischiogluteal bursa.

The iliopectineal bursa, the largest of the three bursae identified, lies between the deep surface of the iliopsoas muscle and the anterior aspect of the hip joint, between the iliofemoral and pubofemoral ligaments. In approximately 15% of normal hips, this bursa communicates with the hip joint. Because it is in close proximity to the femoral nerve, pain may radiate down the front of the thigh. The trochanteric bursa lies between the gluteus maximus muscle and the posterolateral surface of the greater trochanter, and pain may occur during flexion and internal rotation of the thigh because of compression by the gluteus maximus. The ischiogluteal bursa is located over the ischial tuberosity and covers the sciatic nerve and the posterior femoral cutaneous nerve. This bursa often becomes inflamed during prolonged sitting, and irritation may occur down the sciatic nerve distribution.

## Blood Supply

Branches from the obturator, gluteal, and femoral arteries nourish the acetabulum and the head, neck, and trochanteric areas of the femur (Figs. 7–17 and 7–18). Because the femoral head suffers more vascular disorders than any other skeletal element,[3] the patency of the blood supply to this region is clinically important.

The acetabular branch of the obturator artery supplies blood to the medial aspects of the acetabular rim, the surface of the acetabulum, and the transverse acetabular ligament.[1] A small branch of this artery traverses from the acetabulum to the fovea with the ligament of the head of the femur and therefore nourishes a limited portion of the femoral head. The amount of capital area supplied by this artery is highly variable. The extent of the supply of blood to the head of the femur determines remodeling and healing after femoral neck fracture or hip dislocation.

The superior gluteal artery supplies the upper portion of the acetabulum, and the inferior gluteal artery furnishes blood to the inferior and posterior portions of the acetabular rim. The medial and lateral femoral circumflex arteries supply the proximal end of the femur. Branches from these arteries surround the femoral neck and ascend along the neck to form a ring around the upper regions of the neck at the subcapital sulcus. At this location small branches are sent into the head and travel parallel to the epiphyseal plate or scar. The lateral epiphyseal, superior metaphyseal, and inferior metaphyseal arteries all come from the medial circumflex artery. The lateral epiphyseal arteries are important to the health of the hip joint because they supply about two thirds of the femoral head.[7] The blood vessels divide at the zones of provisional calcification. The circumflex arteries serve the proximal area; the metaphyseal vessels supply the distal area. Several anastomoses occur in the femoral neck area and provide good alternative blood supply to the femoral neck,[3] but no intraosseous anastomotic flow occurs between the head and neck,[8] limiting nutrition to the head after injury. Joint fluid supplies nutrients to the cartilage and zone of cell proliferation, which limits nutrition to these areas.

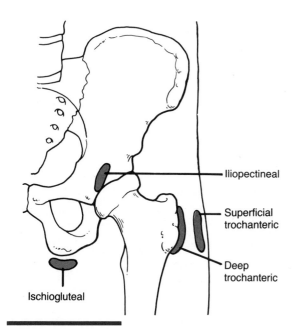

Iliopectineal

Superficial trochanteric

Deep trochanteric

Ischiogluteal

**FIGURE 7–16** ■ Most commonly affected bursae about the hip.

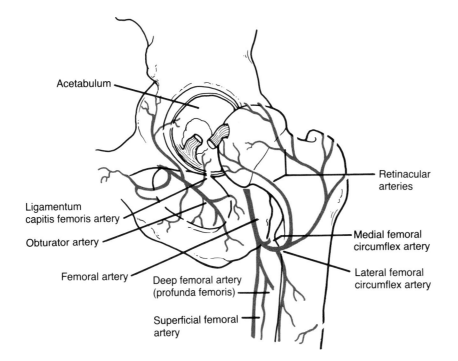

**FIGURE 7–17** ■ Arterial supply to the femoral head and neck (anterior view).

Acetabulum

Retinacular arteries

Ligamentum capitis femoris artery

Obturator artery

Medial femoral circumflex artery

Femoral artery

Lateral femoral circumflex artery

Deep femoral artery (profunda femoris)

Superficial femoral artery

## Nerves

The pattern of hip joint innervation is an important factor in hip joint function because pain is often associated with hip disorders. The hip joint is densely innervated by primary and accessory articular nerves. These nerves are formed from direct articular branches of adjacent nerve trunks and from articular twigs from nerves that innervate muscles around the joint (Fig. 7–19).

Three articular nerves branch directly to the hip joint: the posterior articular nerve, the medial articular nerve, and the nerve to the ligamentum capitis femoris.[9] The posterior articular nerve branch to the quadratus femoris muscle is the

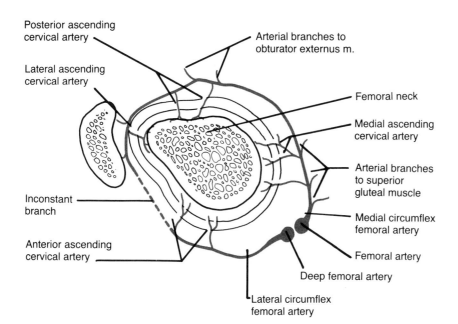

Posterior ascending cervical artery

Arterial branches to obturator externus m.

Lateral ascending cervical artery

Femoral neck

Medial ascending cervical artery

Arterial branches to superior gluteal muscle

Inconstant branch

Medial circumflex femoral artery

Anterior ascending cervical artery

Femoral artery

Deep femoral artery

Lateral circumflex femoral artery

**FIGURE 7–18** ■ Proximal left femur cross section at the neck base shows the extracapsular arterial ring and arteries traversing the capsule. Broken lines indicate inconstant connections between anterior and lateral ascending cervical arteries. Note that the lateral ascending cervical artery branches after traversing the capsule. In young children, this artery can be compressed in the narrow space between the femoral neck and greater trochanter as the artery passes through the capsule.

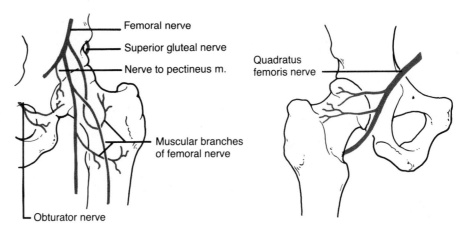

**FIGURE 7-19** ■ Usual pattern of nerve supply to the hip joint.

most extensive nerve supply of the hip joint. The anterior branches of this nerve arise at intervals from the lateral aspect of the main nerve trunk proximal to its termination in the quadratus femoris. These branches pass laterally on the surface of the ischium, beneath the obturator internus tendon and gemelli muscles, and enter the posterior capsule of the joint. The middle and superior branches curve upward along the acetabular rim to supply the posterior joint capsule and continue to the inferior border of the gluteus medius muscle. The inferior branch travels along the border of the obturator externus muscle and is distributed to the posterior and inferior regions of the joint capsule and to the ischiofemoral ligament.[9]

The medial articular nerve arises from the anterior division of the obturator nerve and divides into medial and lateral branches as it passes through the obturator canal. The lateral branch gives off a medial articular twig before terminating in the pectineus and adductor muscles. This medial articular twig divides into filaments that supply the anteromedial and inferior aspects of the joint capsule and the medial plane of the iliopsoas muscle.[9]

The nerve to the ligamentum capitis femoris arises from the muscular branch of the posterior division of the obturator nerve. It enters the acetabular notch with blood vessels and breaks into filaments along the ligamentum capitis femoris, supplying this ligament and the acetabular fat pad in the cotyloid notch.[9]

A small portion of the hip joint is supplied by accessory articular nerves. Muscular branches from the femoral nerve provide most of the accessory articular innervation. Most commonly, the anterior medial and inferior joint capsules are supplied from the nerve to the pectineus muscle.[7,9]

Three common types of nerve endings are located in the hip joint.[9] One type profuses the inferior capsular regions, anterior and posterior to the joint. These nerve endings are low-threshold, slowly adapting mechanoreceptors and affect muscle tone reflexively at rest and during movement. They are the principal contributors to perceptual awareness. A second type are high-threshold, slowly adapting nerve endings, confined to the joint ligaments. Unencapsulated nerve endings (pain receptors) are arranged in a plexus in the joint capsule. They are most dense posteriorly and inferiorly. No nerve endings of this type are found in the synovial tissue. Denervation of the joint eliminates the joint's sensitivity to stretch, motion, and compressive forces. Thus, the protective mechanism of the joint is destroyed, resulting in trauma and degenerative changes.[10]

## EVALUATION

A patient comes to the clinic to seek help with a problem often related to pain, loss of joint function, a deformity, or a limp. Each of these problems can be related to a failure of or damage to the normal anatomy of the hip joint.

The practitioner's task is to determine the cause and extent of the presenting problem. Although some problems may be readily evident, a consistent evaluation procedure should be conducted. This procedure should consist of a history; a physical examination including observation, palpation, functional testing, and special tests; a radiographic examination; and laboratory examinations.

## History

An accurate and complete history should be obtained from the patient. However, a history from a very young patient with hip problems is usually obtained from one or both parents. Preliminary data on age, sex, race, economic status, occupation, past and present activity levels, and family responsibilities are important in reference to hip problems. Several disorders of the hip are related to the patient's age, gender, race, or activity level. The patient or patient's parent is asked about prior medical problems such as previous illnesses, injuries, and operations. Information should also be obtained about previous and present treatments and medications. If trauma occurred, the mechanism of injury, immediate effect of the trauma, and immediate treatment of the trauma should be ascertained.

Additional information must be collected for the infant patient. The history of the infant should include the genetic history if known; pregnancy, labor, and delivery details; and perinatal and neonatal events. For example, is there a family history of congenital disorders? What was the mother's state of health during the pregnancy? Did the mother have any illness or trauma or take medications during pregnancy? Was the labor spontaneous or induced? Was the labor prolonged? Was the delivery traumatic? Was the delivery vertex or breech? What are the color, appearance, and activity of the newborn? What was the child's gestational age? What was the child's birth weight? Does the child cry when the hip is touched or moved? Is the child irritable? Does the child have a poor appetite? Do you have difficulty changing diapers? What motor milestones has the infant achieved and when? After the preliminary data are considered, the chief reason for the patient's visit should be noted.

Pain is the most common complaint of the patient with hip disease.[11] Accurate information concerning the patient's pain is essential. The therapist should attempt to determine whether the pain is localized or general. The therapist can ask the patient to point to the point or area of pain and outline the area if the pain radiates or spreads. The patient should be able to state the time of occurrence, the suddenness of onset, and the duration of pain. The patient should also be able to identify activities or positions that cause, aggravate, or ease the pain. The patient should also discuss activities that are limited because of the pain. The location of pain is also important. It may occur first in the midinguinal region and later, as it progresses, in the anterior thigh and knee.[12] Hip problems refer pain to the knee without the patient perceiving hip pain. Posterior area hip pain may be referred from the lower lumbar vertebrae or sacrum, but upper lumber vertebrae may refer pain to the anterior thigh. Vascular disorders can cause buttock or anterior thigh pain. Referred pain can be related to the obturator, sciatic, or femoral nerve patterns. In addition, hip pain may originate from lumbosacral or visceral disorders.

Altered physical appearance may bring the patient in to see the practitioner for assistance. Deformity of the hip, knee, ankle, or foot can be related to a hip problem. The patient should be asked the following questions. What is your concept of the deformity? When and by whom was the deformity first noted? Was the onset of the deformity associated with an injury or disease process? Is the deformity progressing? What disability do you have related to the deformity?

The patient may arrive at the clinic because of diminished function. The patient's concept of the dysfunction should be determined. The patient should be questioned concerning the time of onset, degree and extent of dysfunction, and progress of dysfunction.

## Physical Examination

### Observation

With the patient adequately exposed, the practitioner should observe the alignment of the body parts and skin color and texture and should look for swelling, scars from previous surgery, deformity, and muscle atrophy. The infant should be observed while in the supine and prone positions. Children and adults should be observed while standing. In the newborn the practitioner should note the position of the lower limbs, observe spontaneous limb movement, check the level of the gluteal folds to obtain information concerning deformity, and note any lack of desire of the infant to move. As the older patient is standing, the practitioner should observe whether the patient is standing with equal weight on both limbs, whether the pelvis is level, whether there is an increase in lumbar lordosis, and whether the lower limbs are aligned normally. Such observations may provide clues related to pain, limb length, muscle contractures, or hip deformity.

If the patient is able to walk, the practitioner should observe the patient's walking habits. Abnormal gait patterns may reveal pain, deformity, muscle weakness, muscle tightness, or joint stiffness. A few characteristic gait types are as follows.

The antalgic gait occurs as the patient attempts to avoid pain. The hip may be held in slight flexion, abduction, and external rotation. The patient takes quick steps on the involved side to reduce the time spent on the painful hip. Slipped capital femoral epiphysis may be suspected if an obese adolescent walks with an antalgic gait.

The gluteus medius (Trendelenburg) gait occurs if the patient has weakness of the hip abductor muscles. If the pelvis on the opposite side of the hip with muscle weakness drops during the stance phase of the involved side, the gait is termed uncompensated gluteus medius gait. A compensated gluteus medius gait occurs as the patient moves the upper body laterally toward the hip with muscle weakness. Such movement reduces the abductor muscle force necessary to keep the pelvis level. If the patient's hip abductor muscles are weak on both sides, the patient thrusts the trunk laterally from side to side. This gait pattern is often referred to as a waddling gait.

If the patient has weakness of the gluteus maximum muscle, the knee on the weak side is held in extension and the trunk is thrust backward (gluteus maximus lurch). Such action reduces the opportunity for the patient's trunk to fall forward. This gait pattern may be bilateral if weakness exists in both gluteus maximus muscles. In such cases the patient keeps the pelvis forward and the trunk back at all times.

A short leg gait is present if one limb is longer than the other. During the stance phase of the short limb, the pelvis on the short limb side drops and the trunk bends laterally toward the short limb side. Patients with unilateral hip dislocations exhibit this pattern of gait.

## Palpation

The practitioner should palpate the joint to find evidence of swelling, abnormal mass, local heat, deformity, or local tenderness. The practitioner should palpate in the groin area of the newborn to check the position and motion of the femoral head. Local tenderness should be determined anterior and posterior to the hip joint and over the greater trochanter. Such tenderness may be isolated over a specific bursa or other particular structure. Strained muscles may be tender to palpation. The crests of the ilium, the anterior superior iliac spines, the posterior superior iliac spines, and the greater trochanters should be palpated to determine the position of the pelvis and related problems such as a short limb.

## Functional Testing

Functional testing includes evaluation of the range of motion of the joint and muscle strength. A major component of function is the range of motion of the hip joint (Fig. 7–20). Tables 7–2 and 7–3 show the normal ranges for hip movements. During the range-of-motion evaluation, the patient should lie on a firm treatment table to reduce substitutions for motion. Pain in the painful arc should be noted as the joint is moved. For objective evaluation a goniometric device should be used. The following motions should be measured.

For the newborn and young infant the practi-

■■■■ **Table 7–2.** HIP MOTION IN FEMALES (IN DEGREES)

| Motion | 4 years n = 52 | 6 years n = 52 | 8 years n = 52 | 11 years n = 69 | 15 years n = 57 | Adults n = 104 |
|---|---|---|---|---|---|---|
| Flexion | 151, 140–162[a] | 149, 135–162 | 146, 136–157 | 139, 126–153 | 141, 129–153 | 141, 127–155 |
| Extension | 29, 24–35 | 26, 15–38 | 27, 21–34 | 25, 10–40 | 26, 19–33 | 26, 16–35 |
| Abduction | 55, 46–64 | 53, 43–62 | 50, 41–58 | 46, 35–56 | 46, 36–57 | 42, 35–50 |
| Adduction | 30, 24–35 | 30, 25–36 | 28, 22–34 | 29, 21–35 | 28, 21–35 | 30, 24–37 |
| Internal rotation | 60, 40–80 | 58, 41–75 | 57, 40–73 | 50, 33–68 | 48, 31–66 | 52, 34–71 |
| External rotation | 44, 25–63 | 44, 29–59 | 43, 27–58 | 42, 27–57 | 42, 28–56 | 41, 25–56 |
| Total rotation | 104, 89–119 | 102, 86–119 | 99, 84–115 | 92, 77–108 | 90, 75–105 | 92, 73–112 |

[a] Mean, 2 SD.

From Svenningsen S, Terjesen T, Auflem M, et al: Hip motion related to age and sex. Acta Orthop Scand 60:97–100, 1989. © 1989, Munksgaard International Publishers Ltd., Copenhagen, Denmark.

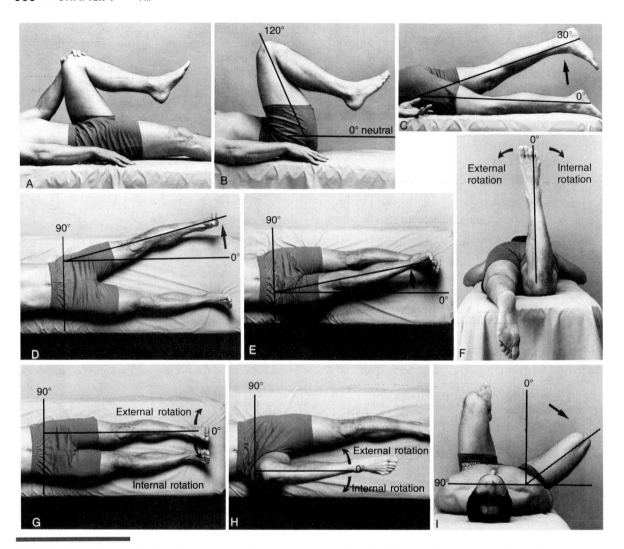

**FIGURE 7–20** ■ Standard method for measuring hip motion. Measure all motion from a defined zero starting position. Compare the motion to the opposite side and describe motion as active or passive. (A) Flexion. Zero starting position, right hip. The patient holds the opposite hip in full flexion. This action flattens the lumbar spine and reveals any hip flexion contracture. (B) Record flexion. Place one hand on the iliac crest to note the point at which the pelvis begins to rotate. (C) Extension. Record the upward hip motion from the zero starting position with the knee straight or flexed. (D) Abduction. Zero starting position: the patient lies supine with the legs extended at right angles to a transverse line across the anterior superior pelvic spines. Measure the outward motion. (E) Adduction. Elevate the opposite extremity to allow the leg to pass under it. (F) Rotation in extension. Zero starting position: The patient lies prone. Flex the knee to 90 degrees, perpendicular to the transverse line. Measure external rotation by rotating the leg upward. (G) Measure rotation in extension supine as indicated. (H) Measure rotation in flexion or extension. Zero starting position in flexion: flex the hip and knee 90 degrees with the thigh perpendicular to a transverse line. Internal rotation: measure by rotating the leg away from the midline with the thigh as the rotation axis. External rotation: measure by rotating the leg toward the trunk midline with the thigh as the rotation axis. (I) Abduction in flexion is usually measured in 90 degrees of flexion.

tioner gently grasps the leg and carefully moves the hip through the various ranges of motion estimating the values. In the newborn the hips are in the flexed and externally rotated position. The movement of flexion is limited by the protuberance of the abdomen, and extension is limited by a flexion contracture of approximately 28 degrees.[1] Abduction with the hips flexed is nearly 90 degrees.[13] Any limitation or asymmetry is abnormal and may indicate dislocation of the hip. External rotation may reach approximately 90 degrees at birth but decreases to approximately 48 degrees by 6 weeks of age.[1] Internal rotation is less than external rotation until about the age

■■■■■ **Table 7–3.** HIP MOTION IN MALES (IN DEGREES)

| Motion | 4 years n = 51 | 6 years n = 50 | 8 years n = 52 | 11 years n = 65 | 15 years n = 57 | Adults n = 102 |
|---|---|---|---|---|---|---|
| Flexion | 149, 137–161[a] | 147, 138–157 | 146, 134–158 | 137, 121–152 | 138, 124–152 | 137, 125–148 |
| Extension | 28, 21–34 | 25, 12–38 | 27, 22–33 | 25, 12–38 | 25, 18–32 | 23, 16–30 |
| Abduction | 53, 45–61 | 50, 41–60 | 47, 41–53 | 44, 33–55 | 42, 33–50 | 40, 33–47 |
| Adduction | 30, 26–36 | 30, 26–34 | 28, 23–35 | 29, 23–34 | 29, 23–34 | 29, 23–35 |
| Internal rotation | 51, 36–67 | 51, 33–69 | 51, 33–70 | 46, 32–61 | 41, 26–56 | 38, 23–53 |
| External rotation | 48, 33–62 | 47, 29–65 | 42, 23–62 | 42, 27–58 | 43, 29–57 | 43, 29–56 |
| Total rotation | 99, 81–117 | 98, 83–113 | 94, 83–113 | 88, 72–105 | 84, 68–100 | 81, 67–96 |

[a] Mean, 2 SD.

From Svenningsen S, Terjesen T, Auflem M, et al: Hip motion related to age and sex. Acta Orthop Scand 60:97–100, 1989. © 1989, Munksgaard International Publishers Ltd., Copenhagen, Denmark.

of 3 years, after which it may become slightly greater than external rotation.[13] Range of motion in internal rotation is less if measured with the hip in extension than with the hip flexed.[1] Adduction is not tested in the newborn or infant.

The range of motion of the child and adult is evaluated in the following manner.

**Flexion.** With the patient supine the practitioner pulls the patient's opposite limb to the patient's abdomen. With the knee flexed, the practitioner moves the involved hip through the available range.

**Abduction-adduction.** With the patient supine the practitioner keeps the pelvis level. The pelvis is stabilized by placing the patient's opposite limb over the side of the treatment table[14] or by the practitioner placing a hand on the iliac crest.[15] The practitioner moves the hip in abduction and adduction. The practitioner should not allow pelvic motion during this measurement.

**Inward-outward rotation.** This motion may be tested with the patient supine or prone. With the patient supine, place both the hip and knee at 90 degrees of flexion. The practitioner rotates the leg inward and outward. With the patient prone and knees together, the practitioner flexes the knee to 90 degrees. The practitioner rotates the leg outward and then inward by crossing the legs. Knee laxity would alter the results by causing increased rotational values.

**Extension.** With the patient prone the practitioner raises the thigh upward without increasing the lumbar lordosis. The patient can flex the opposite hip over the edge of the treatment table to reduce the chance of increased lordosis. The angle of the thigh with the horizontal is measured.

A second component of function is muscle strength. Strength of the hip flexor, extensor, abductor, adductor, and rotator muscle groups along with the knee flexor and extensor muscles should be evaluated bilaterally. Testing muscle strength of neonates and infants is impossible, but observation of their spontaneous movement provides evidence of this muscular function. Lack of spontaneous motion may indicate a septic hip or fracture.

For a general screening of the muscle strength the patient can be in the supine position. The practitioner then provides manual force to the limb, asking the patient to resist the manual force. If the patient cannot provide resistance, the practitioner should ask the patient to move the limb against gravity. In case of weakness, typical manual muscle testing procedures should be applied. If the patient can provide resistance to the practitioner, a hand-held dynamometer is useful for obtaining strength values for future comparisons. The muscle strength should be tested bilaterally and compared. Painful or weak contractions should be noted. The most painful actions should be tested last.

## Special Tests ← Infants

**Piston test or Dupuytren's sign** (Fig. 7–21). This is a telescope test. The infant is supine. The hip is flexed to 90 degrees and abducted and the knee is flexed. The practitioner grasps the thigh with one hand and holds the pelvis firmly with the other. The thigh is pressed downward and then lifted upward. The stability or movement of the thigh should be noted. A normal hip feels stable with little movement occurring, whereas a dislocated hip has piston mobility.

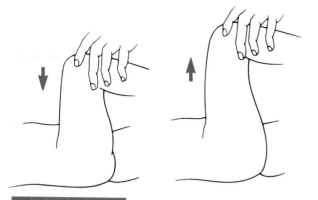

**FIGURE 7-21** ■ Telescoping of the hip. (From Magee DJ. Orthopedic Physical Assessment, 2nd ed. Philadelphia: WB Saunders, 1992, p 349.)

**Allis' test** (Fig. 7–22). This is a leg length comparison test. The infant is supine, the hips and knees are both at 90 degrees, and the shins are held parallel with the heels aligned. Note any difference in thigh length. If one knee is lower than the other, the infant may have a hip dislocation, a short thigh, or a short tibia.

**Ortolani's test** (Fig. 7–23). The patient is supine. The practitioner places one hand on the opposite side of the infant's pelvis for stabilization. The practitioner's other hand is applied to the infant's involved limb to flex the knee maximally and flex the hip to 90 degrees. Then the practitioner abducts the hip gently and raises the thigh with the fingers. The practitioner should note the

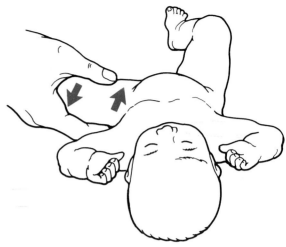

**FIGURE 7-23** ■ The Ortolani maneuver. In this technique, the hip is abducted gently and the thigh is raised with the fingers to reduce the hip gently. When performing the test, one hand should always be used to stabilize the pelvis; therefore, only one hip at a time can be examined.

feeling of the femoral head sliding into the acetabulum, often with a click. Such a result indicates a dislocated hip.

**Barlow's test** (Fig. 7–24). The patient is supine with the pelvis stabilized by the practitioner's hand. The practitioner's other hand

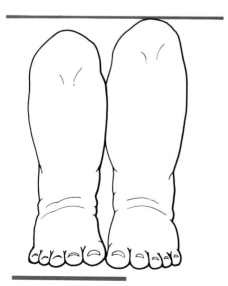

**FIGURE 7-22** ■ Galeazzi's sign (Allis' test).

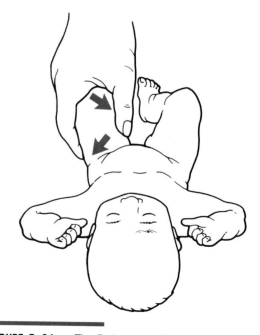

**FIGURE 7-24** ■ The Barlow test. The thumb is placed on the inner aspect of the thigh and the hip is adducted, with longitudinal pressure exerted on the thigh, pushing it toward the table. The examiner again uses one hand to stabilize the pelvis, testing one hip at a time.

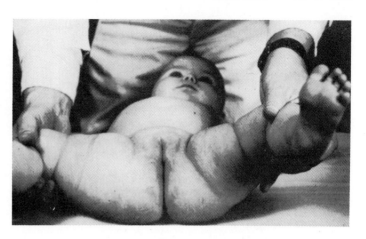

**FIGURE 7–25** ■ Abduction test for unilateral dysplasia of the hip in an infant 8 months of age who has subluxation on the left side. When the test is positive, the thigh on the dysplastic side cannot be abducted as far as the thigh on the side with a normal hip. Note deepening of the proximal fold in the left thigh, which also suggests dysplasia. (From MacEwen GD, Bunnell WP, Ramsey P: The hip. *In* Pediatric Orthopedics, Vol 2. [Lovell WW, Winter RB, eds]. Philadelphia: JB Lippincott, 1986, p. 711.)

is applied to the involved limb to flex the knee maximally and flex the hip to 90 degrees. The practitioner adducts the hip slightly beyond midline with slight downward and lateral pressure on the inner thigh with the thumb. The practitioner should note possible dislocation of the hip. If dislocation occurs as a result of this movement, it should reduce with abduction.[16] An unstable hip is dislocated with this maneuver.

**Abduction test (Hart's sign)** (Fig. 7–25). The hips of the supine infant are abducted passively. The practitioner should note any limitation or asymmetry of the movement. Limited abduction may indicate hip dislocation. In this position, asymmetric gluteal folds may be observed in infants with a dislocated hip.

**Ely's test** (Fig. 7–26). This is a test for a contracture of the rectus femoris. The infant is placed prone with the knee flexed. The practitioner notes the position of the hip. If

the hip flexes, the rectus femoris is classified as tight.

**Ludloff's sign.** While flexing and abducting the hip, the practitioner attempts to extend the knee. The knee should not extend. If knee extension does occur and no systemic flaccidity is present, the hip is probably unstable. This test may be useful up to 6 months of age.[13]

## Special Tests — Adults

**Thomas' test** (Fig. 7–27). This is a test for hip flexor muscle tightness or contracture. The patient is positioned supine and is asked to bring both knees to the chest. The patient holds the nontested knee tightly to the chest and slowly lowers the limb being tested into extension. The final hip position of the tested side is measured with a goniometer to

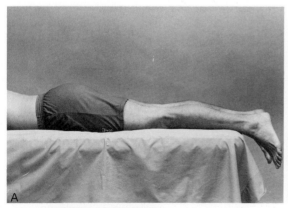
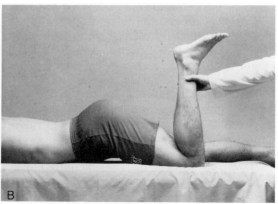

**FIGURE 7–26** ■ Ely's test for tight rectus femoral. Hips and knees are extended while in prone position.

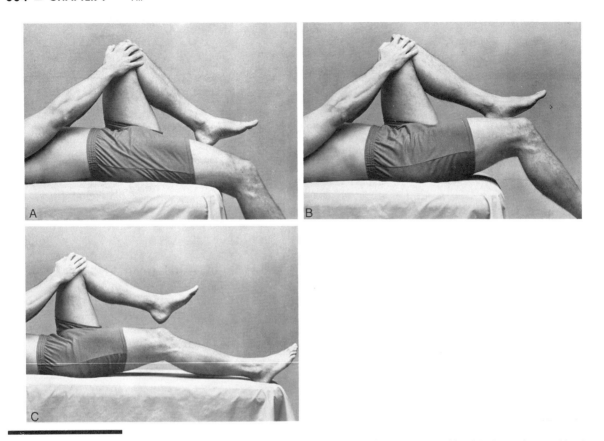

**FIGURE 7-27** ■ Thomas' test. (A) Negative test. (B) Positive test. (C) False-positive test caused by tight hamstrings and heel on plinth.

determine the degree of hip flexion tightness.

**Ober's test** (Fig. 7-28). This is a test for iliotibial band tightness. The patient is positioned lying on the side, and the hip and knee of the bottom limb are flexed. The hip of the limb to be tested (upper) is abducted and extended and the knee flexed to 90 degrees. The patient lowers the tested (upper) limb to the treatment table. If the limb does not drop to the table the test is positive, indicating a tight iliotibial band.

**Ely's test** (see Fig. 7-26). This is a test for rectus femoris muscle tightness as previously described in special tests for infants.

**Craig's test** (Fig. 7-29). This is a test for the angle of anteversion of the femoral neck. The patient is positioned prone and the knee is flexed to 90 degrees. The patient's hip is rotated internally until the therapist can tell by palpation that the greater trochanter is parallel to the table top. From this position the hip is rotated so that the tibia is vertical.

The therapist measures the angle between the two positions of the tibia with a goniometer and notes the degree of hip anteversion.

**Trendelenburg's test** (Fig. 7-30). This is a test for hip abductor muscle abnormality on one side. An abnormality is common to many hip disorders involving deformity and abductor muscle weakness. The patient stands on one leg with the opposite limb raised from the ground. The therapist notes whether the pelvis on the side of the raised limb rises or drops. If that side of the pelvis does not rise but falls, the test is considered positive for gluteus medius weakness or dysfunction of the hip such as dislocation, coxa vara, or femoral neck fracture. of the standing

**Leg length** (Figs. 7-31 and 7-32). The patient should be in the supine position with the malleoli together. For true leg length the practitioner should measure with a tape from the most distal edge of the ASIS to the tip of the malleoli. For apparent leg length

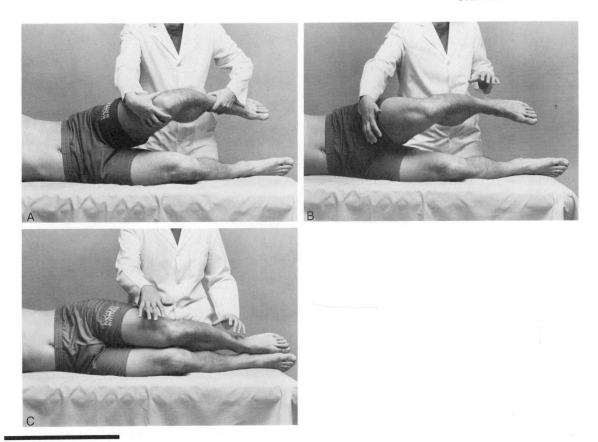

**FIGURE 7–28** ■ Ober's test. (A) Starting position. The hip is passively extended by the examiner to ensure that the tensor fasciae latae runs over the greater trochanter. (B) A positive test is indicated when the leg remains abducted while the patient's muscles are relaxed. (C) A negative test is indicated when the hip adducts.

**FIGURE 7–29** ■ Craig's test for femoral anteversion. (Modified from Magee DJ: Orthopedic Physical Assessment, 2nd ed. Philadelphia: WB Saunders, 1992, p. 344.)

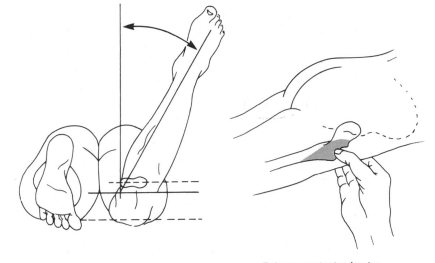

Degree of anteversion

Palpate greater trochanter
parallel to table

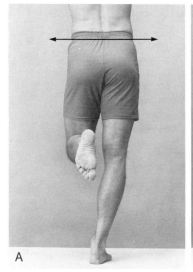
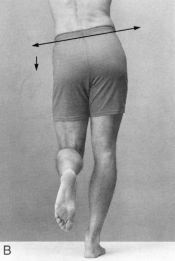

FIGURE 7-30 ■ Trendelenburg's sign. The patient stands with the back toward the examiner and flexes one hip and knee, raising the foot off the ground. The examiner places one hand on each iliac crest. Normally, the iliac crests are level or, on the side on which the leg is lifted, the pelvis is higher (A). If the sign is positive, the iliac crest drops on the side on which the leg is lifted (B). This indicates gluteus medius and minimus weakness on the side on which the patient is standing.

the practitioner measures from the umbilicus to each malleolus. Differences in the actual and apparent leg lengths can indicate abductor or adductor muscle contractures or pelvis obliquity.[13]

**Thigh girth.** With the patient supine, the practitioner should use a tape to measure the girth of the thigh. The thighs should be measured individually at precisely the same level, 2 inches above the patella, with the tape around the thigh and perpendicular to the thigh. A difference in circumference measurement indicates muscle atrophy.

## Radiographic and Other Diagnostic Tests

A comprehensive evaluation of disorders affecting the hip joint cannot be complete without the findings of general medical diagnostic tests. These tests include x-ray, scintigraphy (bone scan), tomography, magnetic resonance imaging, arthrography, ultrasound, and aspiration. Characteristics of radiography, computed tomography (CT), ultrasound, and magnetic resonance imaging are shown in Tables 7-4 to 7-7.

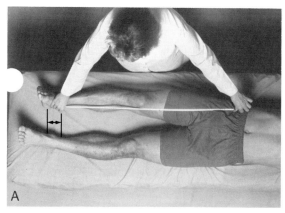
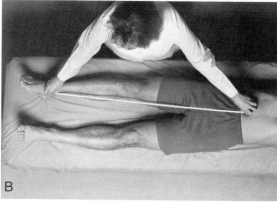

FIGURE 7-31 ■ Measurement of true leg length. (A) Measuring as is to the medial malleolus. (B) Measuring from the umbilicus to the lateral malleolus.

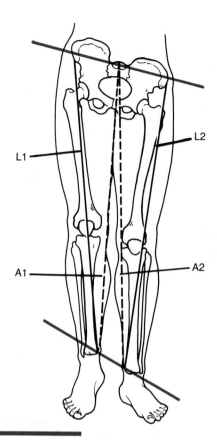

**FIGURE 7-32** ■ Points of reference in measuring true and apparent leg lengths. In the case illustrated, the right leg appears shorter because of pelvic tilt and A1 < A2, but true leg lengths are equal (L1 = L2).

**Table 7-5.** CHARACTERISTICS OF COMPUTED TOMOGRAPHY

Provides sectional images; three-dimensional information
Provides information based on tissue absorption of x-ray photons
Uses ionizing radiation
Provides good spatial resolution
Provides good contrast resolution
Commonly requires contrast agents
Allows image processing
Cannot be adapted for real-time imaging
Is not portable
Has fair throughput
Is expensive

From Merritt CRB, Bluth EI: Techniques for diagnostic imaging. Postgrad Med 77(6):56–73, 1985.

## X-ray Studies

Initial x-ray studies should include an anterior-posterior view of the pelvis and both hips and a lateral view of each hip (Fig. 7–33); other views may include "frog-leg" and oblique positions. Several important features should be observed by inspection of x-ray films:

*The angle of inclination* (neck-shaft angle), which is the angle formed by the neck and shaft of the femur, can easily be determined to reveal coxa vara or coxa valga (Fig. 7–34).

*Shenton's line* is a line that curves upward along the medial border of femur and continues as a smooth arc along the inferior edge of the pubis (Fig. 7–35).

**Table 7-4.** CHARACTERISTICS OF CONVENTIONAL RADIOGRAPHY

Provides two-dimensonal summation image
Allows limited sectional imaging (tomography)
Provides information based on tissue absorption of x-ray photons
Uses ionizing radiation
Provides high spatial resolution
Provides poor contrast resolution
Requires contrast agents for many examinations
Cannot readily provide processed images
Can be adapted for real-time imaging (fluoroscopy)
May use portable equipment
Is rapid (excellent throughput)
Is relatively inexpensive

From Merritt CRB, Bluth EI: Techniques for diagnostic imaging. Postgrad Med 77(6):56–73, 1985.

**Table 7-6.** CHARACTERISTICS OF ULTRASOUND

Provides sectional images in any plane; three-dimensional information
Provides information based on acoustic (elastic) properties of tissues
Uses no ionizing radiation; safe
Provides excellent spatial resolution
Provides good to excellent contrast resolution
Requires no contrast agents
Allows image processing
Allows real-time imaging
Uses portable equipment
Has good throughput
Is relatively inexpensive
Is limited by bone and gas
Is operator dependent

From Merritt CRB, Bluth EI: Techniques for diagnostic imaging. Postgrad Med 77(6):56–73, 1985.

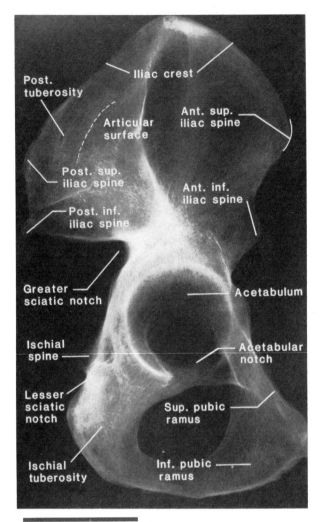

FIGURE 7-33 ■ Lateral specimen radiograph of the innominate bone with anatomic labels. (From Berquist TH, Coventry MB: The pelvis and hips. *In* Imaging of Orthopedic Trauma and Surgery [Berquist TH, ed]. Philadelphia: WB Saunders, 1986, p 183.)

*Hilgenreiner's line* is a horizontal line from the most inferior part of the ilium on one side of the pelvis to the lowest part of the ilium on the other side (see Fig. 7-35). The level of the upper femoral epiphysis should be noted.

*Perkins' line* is a vertical line drawn through the outermost point of the acetabulum (see Fig. 7-35).

The *acetabular index* represents the slope of the acetabulum (roof of acetabulum). It is the angle formed by the line drawn from the lateral edge through the medial edge with Hilgenreiner's line (see Fig. 7-35).

The *symphysis-os ischium angle* is determined by two lines drawn from the most prominent

**Table 7-7.** CHARACTERISTICS OF MAGNETIC RESONANCE IMAGING

Provides sectional images in any plane; three-dimensional information
Provides images based on tissue proton density, T1 and T2 relaxation times, and flow characteristics
Uses no ionizing radiation; safe
Provides good spatial resolution
Provides excellent contrast resolution
May require paramagnetic contrast agents to increase specificity
Allows image processing
Cannot be adapted for real-time imaging
Has limited throughput
Is not portable
Is expensive
Is investigational for many applications
Requires gating for cardiac and abdominal applications

From Merritt CRB, Bluth EI: Techniques for diagnostic imaging. Postgrad Med 77(6):56-73, 1985.

point of the symphysis to the inside of the pelvis to the highest inside of the os ischium (Fig. 7-36).

*Wiberg's (center edge) angle* is the angle formed by the vertical line through the center of the femoral head with the line through the center of the femoral head and the lateral rim of the acetabulum (Fig. 7-37).

*Nélaton's line* is the line drawn from the ante-

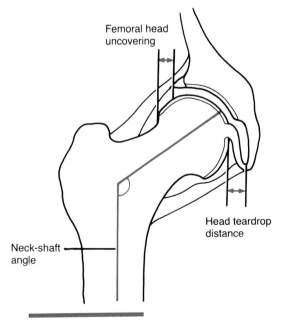

FIGURE 7-34 ■ Three radiologic measurements.

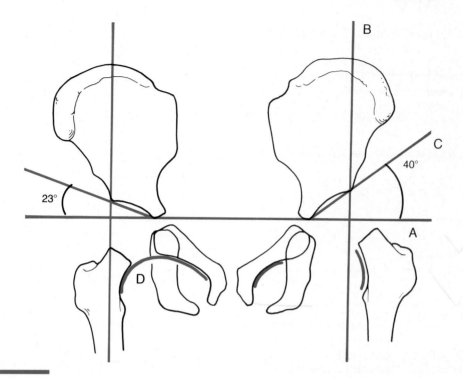

**FIGURE 7-35** ■ Radiologic signs of congenital hip dislocation. A horizontal line (A) is drawn through the junctions of the iliac, ischial, and pubic bones at the center of the acetabulum (Hilgenreiner's line). A perpendicular line (B) is drawn through the outer border of the acetabulum (Perkins' line). The secondary ossification center of the femoral head (or, in its absence, the medial metaphyseal beak of the proximal femur) should lie within the inner lower quadrant formed by the intersection of these lines. The acetabular index, a measure of acetabular depth, can be estimated by inscribing a line (C) joining the inner and outer edges of the acetabulum. The angle formed by this line and line A is normally less than 30 degrees. Increased angles indicate acetabular hypoplasia. Shenton's line (D) is inscribed along the inferior border of the femoral neck and inferior border of the superior pubic ramus. It is ordinarily smooth and unbroken. Proximal displacement of the femoral head in congenital hip dislocation results in interruption of line D.

rior superior iliac spine to the ischial tuberosity (Fig. 7–38).

*Bryant's triangle* is a triangle formed by a line from the ASIS to the top of the greater tro-

chanter and two intersecting perpendicular lines, one drawn posteriorly from the ASIS and one drawn superiorly from the tip of the greater trochanter (Fig. 7–39).

**FIGURE 7-36** ■ Inclination of the pelvis is determined by an angle between the highest medial points of the os ischium and the symphysis. (From Tonnis D: Normal values of the hip joint for the evaluation of x-rays in children and adults. Clin Orthop 119:39–47, 1976.)

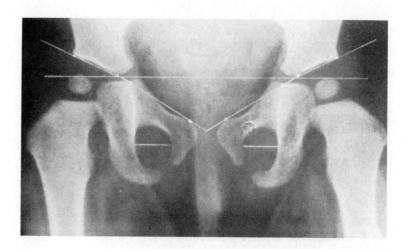

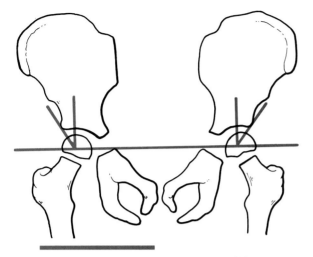

**FIGURE 7-37** ■ The center-edge angle of Wiberg.

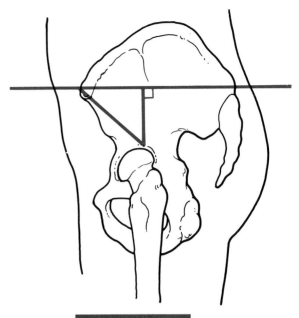

**FIGURE 7-39** ■ Bryant's triangle.

## Scintigraphy

In nuclear imaging (bone scans), bone-seeking radionuclides are used to detect a wide variety of lesions in bone. The bone scans show changes of local blood flow in bone and the degree of metabolic activity in the bone. Areas of increased radionuclide uptake or "hot spots" and areas of decreased radionuclide uptake or "cold spots" are readily seen (Figs. 7-40 and 7-41) and these findings are used to formulate the clinical diagnosis.

## Computed Tomography

CT provides accurate images of thin "slices" or sections of the body in coronal, sagittal, and oblique planes. This method differentiates clearly between radiographic densities of various tissues,[17] and CT scans (Fig. 7-42) provide more information about the bone and soft tissue than conventional tomography and x-rays.[18] These scans can easily show the structures through materials such as the plaster of an abduction splint.

## Magnetic Resonance Imaging

Magnetic resonance imaging allows visualization of soft tissue (Fig. 7-43), especially articular

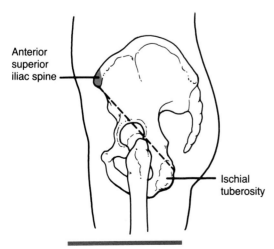

Anterior superior iliac spine

Ischial tuberosity

**FIGURE 7-38** ■ Nélaton's line.

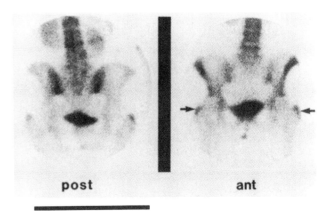

post        ant

**FIGURE 7-40** ■ Anterior and posterior spot views showing linear uptake in the lateral aspects of both greater trochanters (arrows) indicating bilateral disease. (From Allwright SJ, Cooper RA, Nash P: Trochanteric bursitis: bone scan appearance. Clin Nucl Med 13:561-564, 1988.)

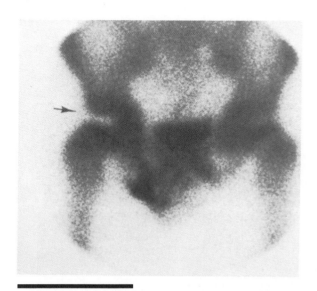

**FIGURE 7–41** ■ Technetium-99m methylene diphosonate scan of a 7-year-old male with a limp and hip pain shows a well-defined photon-deficient area in the right femoral head (arrow). Radiographic findings were consistent with Legg-Calvé-Perthes disease. (From Berquist TH, Coventry MB: The pelvis and hips. *In* Imaging of Orthopedic Trauma and Surgery [Berquist TH, ed]. Philadelphia: WB Saunders, 1986, Fig. 1–28.)

cartilage.[19] It is an excellent noninvasive technique for viewing the hip. With this method the shape and containment of the femoral head may be discerned without injection of a contrast agent.

### Arthrography

Arthrography reveals the true shape of the joint as represented by the articular cartilage (Fig. 7–44). The procedure uses iodinated organic compounds injected into the joint. An x-ray film is obtained within about 10 minutes of the injection. Arthrography is generally not used for diagnosis but may be used to assess development of the acetabulum and femoral head and remodeling of the hip after reduction.

### Ultrasonography

Some authors consider ultrasound an excellent method for screening hip dysplasia in newborn babies[20] and a reliable technique for determining hip joint morphology up to the age of 1 year,[21] but others have questioned its use.[22,23] The technique appears to be more sensitive than plain x-ray films in detecting hip effusion. It is recom-

mended as a complementary examination when inflammation is suspected.[24,25] Ultrasonography is a noninvasive method used to differentiate between solid lesions and fluid-filled areas (Fig. 7–45).

## Laboratory Examinations

Examination of synovial fluid, obtained by aspiration (Fig. 7–46), may help differentiate among disorders of trauma, infections, and so forth. The fluid color, clarity, and viscosity are classified. In addition, the extracted sample of the synovial fluid may be examined under a microscope or by cultural analysis.

## DIFFERENTIAL DIAGNOSIS

An accurate diagnosis of disability of the hip joint area depends on a thorough history (Table 7–8), a complete physical examination, and proper selection and interpretation of radiologic techniques. Some of these techniques are summarized in Table 7–9. Analysis of the patient's pain and demographic characteristics complements the findings of the patient's physical examination and radiologic studies.

## Age

The age of the patient is one of the major determinants in the differential diagnosis of a hip problem. Several disorders of the hip are commonly associated with a specific age range (see Table 7–9). Septic arthritis and congenital problems are commonly seen at birth to 2 years of age. Transient synovitis, Legg-Calvé-Perthes disease, and coxa vara are most often seen between 2 and 12 years. Slipping of the epiphysis occurs between 8 and 17 years. Older children and young adults may have osteochondritis desiccans. During adulthood, rheumatoid arthritis may begin between the ages of 20 and 40 years, idiopathic avascular necrosis between 30 and 50 years, and degenerative joint disease after 30 years. Hip fractures may occur at any age but are most common after 50 years. Fractures in children are rare but if they occur are considered very serious. Soft tissue injury such as muscle strains may occur in active individuals at any age because of trauma or overuse activities.

A screening program for all newborns and infants helps differentiate among the common hip

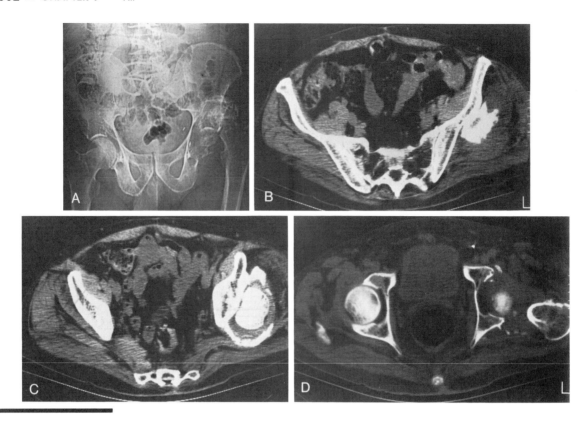

**FIGURE 7–42** ■ (A) Digital radiograph of pelvis demonstrating dislocation of femoral head with fragmentation about the acetabulum. (B) CT scan at the level of the iliac crest, showing a displaced femoral head with a large soft tissue hematoma. (C) CT scan with soft tissue technique at the supra-acetabular level, showing the displaced femur and ectopic ossification surrounding it. (D) CT scan through the acetabulum demonstrating small bony fragments anteriorly and posteriorly. A portion of the femoral head is still within the acetabulum. Shortening of the femur is identified, as the lesser trochanter is at the level of the acetabulum. (From Dalinka MK, Neustadter LM: Radiology of the hip. *In* The Hip and Its Disorders [Steinberg ME, ed]. Philadelphia: WB Saunders, 1991, Fig. 4–10.)

problems at this age. A breech position at birth may make one suspect congenital dislocation of the hip (CDH). If the neonate or infant has a deformation such as torticollis, CDH may also be present. Positive results of the Ortolani, piston, and Barlow tests indicate the presence of CDH. If the neonate or infant has the hip in a flexed, abducted, and externally rotated position, holds the limb still, and is irritable to palpation and passive movement, septic arthritis of the hip should be highly suspected. If the patient with hip pain has a history of infection, antibiotic treatment, steroid treatment, or venipuncture, septic arthritis is highly suspected. Near the age of 2 years, the Ortolani and Barlow signs are less valuable in determining CDH, but limited hip abduction, adductor muscle contracture, pistoning, short limb, and asymmetric gluteal folds may indicate CDH.

If a child has a limp with a painless hip and a short leg, CDH or coxa vara may be suspected.

Congenital dislocation of the hip or hip subluxation may be missed in the first 2 years. It may become more noticeable as the child holds the hip in external rotation, and the thigh may be swollen. A radiogram or arthrogram may clarify the diagnosis of CDH and rule out coxa vara.

Septic arthritis rarely occurs at this age but must be ruled out as a potential diagnosis because of its serious consequences. Children with septic arthritis, transient synovitis, and slipped capital femoral epiphysis have decreased hip motion and often hold the hip in flexion, abduction, and external rotation. Pain may be referred to the knee in all three disorders. Children with septic arthritis and transient synovitis usually refuse to walk. The child with transient synovitis who does walk may walk with an antalgic gait if an acute slip is present; however, a child with a chronic slip may have a Trendelenburg gait. The child with Legg-Calvé-Perthes disease usually has an antalgic gait after activity. Usually, pres-

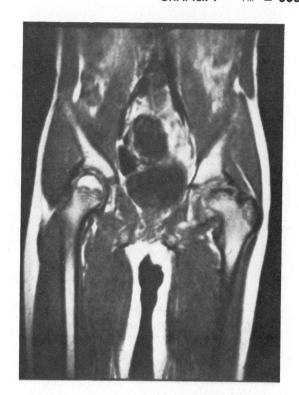

**FIGURE 7-43** ■ Magnetic resonance imaging in Legg-Calvé-Perthes disease of the left hip. (From Tachdjian MO: Pediatric Orthopedics, 2nd ed. Philadelphia: WB Saunders, 1990, Fig. 3-140.)

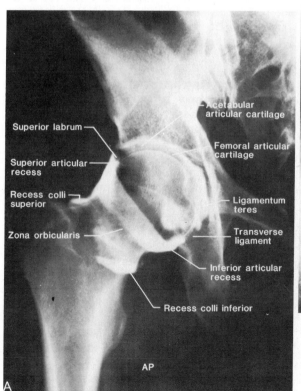

Superior labrum

Superior articular recess

Recess colli superior

Zona orbicularis

Acetabular articular cartilage

Femoral articular cartilage

Ligamentum teres

Transverse ligament

Inferior articular recess

Recess colli inferior

AP

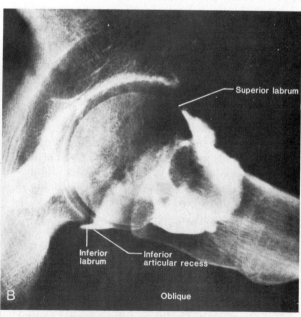

Superior labrum

Inferior labrum

Inferior articular recess

Oblique

B

**FIGURE 7-44** ■ Normal hip arthrogram with anatomy labeled. (A) Anteroposterior view. (B) Oblique view. (From Berquist TH, Coventry MB: The pelvis and hips. *In* Imaging of Orthopedic Trauma and Surgery [Berquist TH, ed]. Philadelphia: WB Saunders, 1986, Fig. 4-99.)

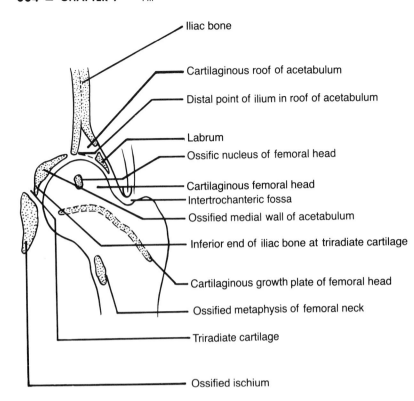

Iliac bone

Cartilaginous roof of acetabulum

Distal point of ilium in roof of acetabulum

Labrum

Ossific nucleus of femoral head

Cartilaginous femoral head

Intertrochanteric fossa

Ossified medial wall of acetabulum

Inferior end of iliac bone at triradiate cartilage

Cartilaginous growth plate of femoral head

Ossified metaphysis of femoral neck

Triradiate cartilage

Ossified ischium

**FIGURE 7–45** ■ Ultrasonography of the hip in congenital hip dislocation. (Redrawn from Tachdjian MO: Pediatric Orthopedics, 2nd ed, Vol 1. Philadelphia: WB Saunders, 1990, Fig. 2–113B.)

ence of fever, abnormal radiograms, and an abnormal CT scan indicate septic arthritis. Joint aspiration revealing an increased white blood cell count and polymorphonuclear leukocytes verifies septic arthritis.

Children with transient synovitis usually have relief of symptoms after about 10 days. If they do not, they may have early Legg-Calvé-Perthes disease.

One of the main differences between Legg-Calvé-Perthes disease and slipped capital femoral epiphysis is the age of onset. Legg-Calvé-Perthes disease occurs about 6 to 8 years earlier. Radiograms should confirm slipping, especially those taken with the patient in the frog-leg position.

## Pain

A patient often comes to the clinic because of pain that is causing functional impairment or gait disturbances. Pain in the hip area may be related to hip disorders but may often be referred to that area from a dysfunction in the lumbar or the sacroiliac region. This referred pain is often perceived in the gluteal area and posterior thigh.

Roberts and Williams described a systematic approach to hip disorder diagnosis in relation to pain.[26] They based their differential diagnosis on the history of pain (such as its onset, timing, and relationship to previous injury or disorder), the location of the pain, and physical examination of the patient.

**Onset and Intensity of Pain.** Knowing the onset of pain may be useful in determining a differential diagnosis. Acute, severe pain often results from trauma such as hip fracture, muscle strain, tendinitis, or bursitis. Septic arthritis also has a rapid onset of severe pain, whereas transient synovitis and avascular necrosis may have sudden severe onset of pain or may develop with insidious pain. Only a few children with slipping of the epiphysis have sudden, severe onset. Disorders such as degenerative joint disease, Legg-Calvé-Perthes disease, slipped capital femoral epiphysis, avascular necrosis, and transient synovitis begin with low-level pain that slowly progresses to become more intense. The pain in Legg-Calvé-Perthes disease tends to be a dull ache. Patients with a slipped capital femoral epiphysis generally have minimal, vague pain with an increase in intensity at the extremes of motion.

In some disorders there is an increase in intensity of pain with use. These include degenerative

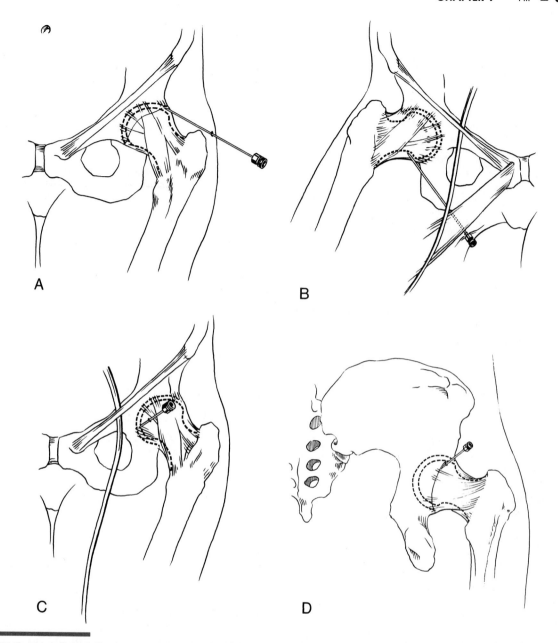

**FIGURE 7–46** ■ Routes for hip aspiration: (A) lateral; (B) medial; (C) anterior; (D) posterior. (From Collins DN, Nelson CL: Infections of the hip. *In* The Hip and Its Disorders [Steinberg ME, ed]. Philadelphia: WB Saunders, 1991, Fig. 31–6.)

joint disease (DJD), muscle strain, tendinitis, and Legg-Calvé-Perthes disease. The pain may be made more intense by weight bearing or repetitive activities. Tumors cause constant pain, and neurogenic pain is worse at rest. Pain caused by tumors and chronic infections is often perceived as greater at night.

**Location of Pain.** The location of the pain may also assist the practitioner in making a dif-

ferential diagnosis (Table 7–10). As mentioned earlier, pain located in the buttock and the lateral and posterior thigh may originate from a lower spinal problem. Posterior hip and thigh pain may also be related to ischial bursitis or muscle strain. If the posterior pain is enhanced with active and resisted movement, it is probably muscle strain; if the pain occurs during passive hip movement, it is more likely to originate in the joint. Posterior hip pain associated with backward or forward

■■■■■■ **Table 7–8.** RADIOLOGIC STAGING OF AVASCULAR NECROSIS OF THE FEMORAL HEAD

| Stage | Criteria |
|---|---|
| 0 | Normal x-ray film, normal bone scan, and MRI |
| I | Normal x-ray film, abnormal bone scan, or MRI |
| | A. Mild (<15%) |
| | B. Moderate (15–30%) |
| | C. Severe (>30%) |
| II | Sclerosis and/or cyst formation in femoral head |
| | A. Mild (<15%) |
| | B. Moderate (15–30%) |
| | C. Severe (>30%) |
| III | Subchondral collapse (crescent sign) without flattening |
| | A. Mild (<15%) |
| | B. Moderate (15–30%) |
| | C. Severe (>30%) |
| IV | Flattening of head *without* joint narrowing or acetabular involvement |
| | A. Mild (<15% of surface and <2 mm depression) |
| | B. Moderate (15–30% of surface *or* 2–4 mm depression) |
| | C. Severe (>30% of surface or >4 mm depression) |
| V | Flattening of head *with* joint narrowing and/or acetabular involvement |
| | A. Mild |
| | B. Moderate  } (determined as above plus estimate of acetabular involvement) |
| | C. Severe |
| VI | Advanced degenerative changes |

From Steinberg ME (ed): The Hip and Its Disorders. Philadelphia: WB Saunders, 1991, p. 634.

bending while sitting and while coughing generally radiates from the back.

Almost any hip pathology can cause pain in the trochanteric area, but more often the pain results from trochanteric bursitis or a tight fascia lata. Local tenderness over the greater trochanter usually indicates trochanteric bursitis.

Many of the disorders of the hip produce pain in the anterior groin area. If anterior hip pain is present in a patient over the age of 50 years, the diagnosis is most likely DJD of the hip. Muscle strain and tendinitis are also common in this area, as is iliopectineal bursitis. Other possible causes in the anterior groin area are hip fracture, septic arthritis, and avascular necrosis. Further information is needed to differentiate these causes of pain.

**Type of Pain.** Interarticular disorders often cause pain during passive internal and external rotation and hip flexion. Interarticular pain also may occur at the extremes of any passive range of motion. However, if the pain is worse at the limit of extension, early degenerative joint disease is suggested.

## Radiologic Signs

Radiologic measurements assist in differentiating disorders of the hip, following the progress of the disease, and evaluating the effect of treatment. They are ordered by physicians and interpreted by radiologists but should be read by the physical therapist to reinforce the other practitioner's impressions.

In the newborn the cartilaginous structures of the proximal end of the femur are difficult to evaluate. Some radiographic measurements, however, may indicate specific disorders. In a patient with a dislocated or subluxated hip, Shenton's line is discontinuous, the shaft of the femur may be lateral to Perkins' line, von Rosen's line passes through the anterosuperior iliac spine, the acetabular index may be greater than 30 degrees, and a false acetabulum may be apparent. At this early age a patient with septic arthritis may have normal radiographs, but a few months later the radiographs may show increased separation of the secondary ossification center of the femoral head from the lateral pelvic teardrop margin and an osteoporotic acetabulum and proximal femur. Coxa vara is indicated by a decreased angle of inclination on the anterior-posterior radiograph and a triangular fragment on the inferomedial aspect of the femoral neck.

The first radiologic changes (Fig. 7–47) seen in Legg-Calvé-Perthes disease may be the small ossified center of the involved femoral head and the increase in distance between the ossified head and the teardrop margin of the acetabulum (or the bony crescent sign). As the disorder progresses through its stages, widening of the epiphyseal line occurs, the epiphysis becomes more dense, the head appears to become fragmented, and the head flattens and is displaced laterally. Later the head and metaphysis reossify with some possible deformities such as a wide flat head and lateral displacement of the head.

In the preslip phase of slipped capital femoral epiphysis, the femoral growth plate widens and a demineralized area between the growth plate and metaphysis may appear. The clearest picture (Fig. 7–48) of slipping is seen in the frog-leg view.[8,27] This view may help differentiate between Legg-Calvé-Perthes disease and slipping of the epiphysis. In this view the crescent sign may be seen in Legg-Calvé-Perthes disease and the actual slipping may be seen in slipped epiphysis.

In the adult, radiographs can help differentiate among fractures, idiopathic avascular necrosis,

*— mostly held in flexion, ABduction & ext. rot.*

**Table 7–9.** CLINICAL DIFFERENTIATION

| Factor | Disorder | | | | | | | | | | |
|---|---|---|---|---|---|---|---|---|---|---|---|
| | Congenital Hip Dislocation | Septic Arthritis | Coxa Vara | Legg-Calvé-Perthes | Transient Synovitis | Slipped Femoral Capital Epiphysis | Bursitis | Osteochondritis Deseccans | Avascular Necrosis | Degenerative Joint Disease | Fracture |
| Age (most common average age) | Birth | Less than two years; rare in adults | Childhood | 2–13 years X = 6 years | 2–12 years | Males 10–17 years X = 13 years Females 8–15 years X = 11 years | | Older children Young adults | 30–50 years | Greater than 40 years | Older adults |
| Incidence Male:Female | 1:8 F Left > right Blacks < whites 20% bilateral | | 1:1 | M 4:1 Rare in blacks 15% bilateral | M 2:1 Unilateral | M 2:1 Blacks > whites | | Males greater than females | M 7:3 | Women greater than men | Women greater than men |
| Observation | Short limb; associated with torticollis | Irritable child; motionless hip; prominent greater trochanter, mild illness | Short limb | Short limb; high greater trochanter; quad atrophy; adductor spasm | Decreased flexion; abduction; external rotation; thigh atrophy; muscle spasm | Short limb; obese; quadricep atrophy; adductor spasm | | Thigh atrophy | | Frequently obese, joint crepitus, atrophy of gluteal muscles | Ecchymosis, may be swelling, short limb |
| Position | Flexed and abducted | Flexed; abducted; externally rotated | Mild hip flexion contracture; may be excessive lordosis | | | Flexion, abduction, external rotation | Abduction, external rotation | | | | External rotation |
| Pain | Mild pain with palpation and passive motion; often referred to knee | | | Gradual onset; aching in hip, thigh and knee; tenderness | Acute: severe pain in knee, Moderate: pain in thigh and knee; tenderness over hip | Vague pain in knee, suprapatellar area, thigh and hip; also in extreme motion | Severe over bursa area | Intermittent mild pain | 50% sharp pain 50% insidious and intermittent pain in extreme ends of range | Insidious onset, pain with fall in barometric pressure | Severe pain in groin area |

Table continued on following page

367

**Table 7-9.** CLINICAL DIFFERENTIATION *Continued*

| Factor | Disorder | | | | | | | | | | |
|---|---|---|---|---|---|---|---|---|---|---|---|
| | Congenital Hip Dislocation | Septic Arthritis | Coxa Vara | Legg-Calvé-Perthes | Transient Synovitis | Slipped Femoral Capital Epiphysis | Bursitis | Osteochondritis Deseccans | Avascular Necrosis | Degenerative Joint Disease | Fracture |
| History | May be breech birth | Steroid therapy Fever | | 20–25% familial; low birth weight; growth delay | Low grade fever | May be trauma | May be associated with rheumatoid arthritis, overuse | | | May be prolonged trauma, faulty body mechanics | May be trauma, fall |
| Range of motion | Limited abduction | Decreased | Limited abduction, extension | Limited abduction, extension | Decreased flexion; limited extension, internal rotation | Limited internal rotation, abduction, flexion, increased external adductor spasm | | Stiffness in internal rotation, abduction, and flexion | Decreased range of motion | Decreased motion external, internal rotation, and extreme flexion | Limited |
| Special tests | Galeazzi's sign Ortolani's sign Barlow's sign Piston's sign | Joint aspiration | | | | | | | | | |
| Gait | | Refused to walk | Painless limp Trendelenburg | Antalgic gait after activity | Refused to walk; antalgic limp | Acute: antalgic Chronic: Trendelenburg External rotation | Acute: antalgic Chronic: Trendelenburg | Trendelenburg; Gluteus medius gait | Coxalgic limp | Limp | |
| Radiologic findings | Upward and lateral displacement, delayed development of acetabulum | CT scan: localized abscess; increased separation of ossification center from the lateral pelvic teardrop margin | Defect in ossification; increased angle of inclination | In stages: increased density, fragmentation, flattening of epiphysis | Normal at first, widened medial joint space | Displacement of upper femoral epiphysis; especially in frog position | | Localized necrosis; head slightly flattened or deformed; fragments | Flattening followed by collapse of femoral head | Increased bone density, osteophytes, subarticular cysts; degenerated articular cartilage | Fracture line, possible displacement; short femoral neck |

**Table 7–10.** DIFFERENTIAL DIAGNOSIS BY REGION[a]

| Anterior Groin | Lateral | Buttock |
|---|---|---|
| Osteoarthritis—primary or secondary | Trochanteric bursitis | Muscular pain owing to strain or posture, tight hip flexors |
| Rider's (adductor) strain | Osteoarthritis | |
| Iliopsoas tendinitis | Tight fasciae latae | "Fibrositis nodules," tender points, trigger points |
| Iliopectineal bursitis | Radiating pain from lumbar disc or facet disease | |
| Hip fracture | | Radiation from lumbar disc or facet disease |
| Septic joint | Hip fracture | |
| Inflammatory synovitis (e.g., rheumatoid arthritis, ankylosing spondylitis, systemic lupus) | Radiating pain from the knee | Sciatic nerve irritation from trauma or sitting |
| | Meralgia paresthetica (lateral femoral cutaneous nerve entrapment) | Sacroiliitis from spondyloarthropathy |
| Aseptic necrosis of the femoral head | Bone tumor | |
| Loose body (e.g., from severe osteoarthritis, osteochondromatosis) | | |
| Bone tumor | | |
| Crystal-induced synovitis (gout) | | |
| Ureteral stone | | |
| Hernia | | |

[a] The diagnoses are listed in rough order of decreasing prevalence.
From Roberts WN, Williams RB: Hip pain. Primary Care 15(4):783–793, 1988.

and degenerative joint disease. The fracture line and displacement may easily be identified on the radiograph. Idiopathic avascular necrosis probably appears normal in the early stages but later follows the typical changes of the progressive stages. Degenerative joint disease is characterized by unequal cartilage loss and osteophytes.

Bone scans help differentiate several hip disorders. This procedure shows the extent of the involvement in avascular necrosis, tumors, and fractures. It can show the position of the femoral head in the acetabulum even while the patient is in a splint. A bone scan is often used to differentiate Legg-Calvé-Perthes disease from transient synovitis. It may also show local abnormality in septic arthritis.

Ultrasound and arthrography may be used to visualize the hip joint more clearly and completely than radiographs if the diagnosis is still unclear.[28–31] Ultrasound provides sectional images in any plane and excellent spatial resolution.[28] The arthrogram gives a clear picture of the joint and shows femoral head contours revealing surface irregularities and loose bodies.[1]

## TREATMENT

### Congenital Dislocation of the Hip

CDH is one of the most common and challenging congenital abnormalities of the musculoskeletal system (Fig. 7–49). Often it is not readily obvious at birth and may not be recognized until after the child has started to walk. It can progress to a painful degenerative arthritis in later years if not appropriately treated early.[17] Early diagnosis and treatment may allow the hip joint to develop a normal or nearly normal configuration.

The cause of CDH may be genetic, hormonal, or mechanical. A genetic cause may be indicated if more than one member of the family has CDH. The genetic influence is often related to acetabular dysplasia or joint laxity.[30] A hormonal cause is thought to be related to the ligament-relaxing hormone (relaxin) and estrogen reaching the fetal circulation.[30,32] Common mechanical causes are related to malposition in the mother's uterus; the breech position is a common (about 20% of the cases) cause of the disorder.[17]

Specific terminology is used to describe CDH. A hip is *dislocated* when the femoral head is completely displaced from the acetabulum but remains in the stretched joint capsule. In these cases the femoral head must be actively reduced. A hip is considered *dislocatable* when the head is in the acetabulum but can be completely displaced by a provocative maneuver such as Barlow's test. A hip is *subluxated* when the femoral head is significantly but not completely out of the acetabulum. The head of the femur rests on the edge of the acetabulum. If the hip joint is flexed and abducted, the joint can be reduced and stabilized. However, if the hip joint is extended and adducted it becomes subluxated. The

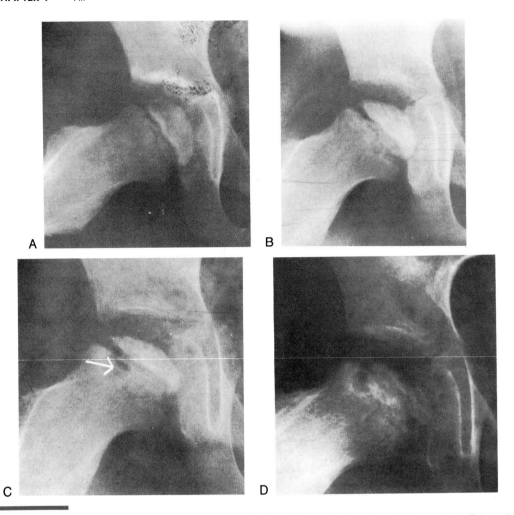

**FIGURE 7–47** ■ (A) Six-year-old male child with symptoms of pain and limp affecting the right lower limb. This radiograph, taken 6 weeks after onset, was reported to be negative. (B) Four months later, this radiograph was interpreted as showing early involvement with Legg-Calvé-Perthes disease. (C) Seven months after the initial radiograph, the alterations suggested more extensive involvement including the appearance of a metaphyseal "cyst" (arrow). (D) Eleven months after the initial radiograph, the femoral epiphysis was almost totally fragmented. (From Katz JF: Legg-Calvé-Perthes disease. *In* Management of Hip Disorders in Children [Katz JF, Siffert RS, eds]. Philadelphia: JB Lippincott, 1983, Fig. 9–9.)

normal bone development of the acetabulum or femoral head is disrupted if the hip joint is dislocated or subluxated. This disruption of forces directed through the joint causes abnormal development of the hip joint or *dysplasia*. The term *unstable* can mean any situation ranging from minimal displacement to complete dislocation of the femoral head; it is a confusing term and should not be used.

The incidence of CDH has been reported to be about 1.5 per 1000 live births.[17] MacEwen and Ramsey have divided the incidence as follows:[16]

| | |
|---|---|
| Dislocated | 1.3/1000 |
| Dislocatable | 1.2/1000 |
| Subluxatable | 9.2/1000 |
| Total | 11.7/1000 |

The disorder is unilateral in about 50 to 80% of cases[16,17] and involvement of the left side is about three times that of the right side. Girls are affected up to eight times more than boys and whites are affected more than blacks.[17] The diagnosis of CDH should be made as soon as possible after birth. The prognosis for CDH depends greatly on the age at which the disorder is diagnosed.[33] Unfortunately, neonatal screening does not detect all cases of a congenitally dislocated hip. There is growing evidence that some hips, normal at birth, dislocate after the neonatal period,[1,33] so continued inspection of the hip joint is necessary. Tachdjian recommends that the hip of the infant be evaluated at birth, 3 weeks, 6 weeks, 3 months, and 6 months.[30]

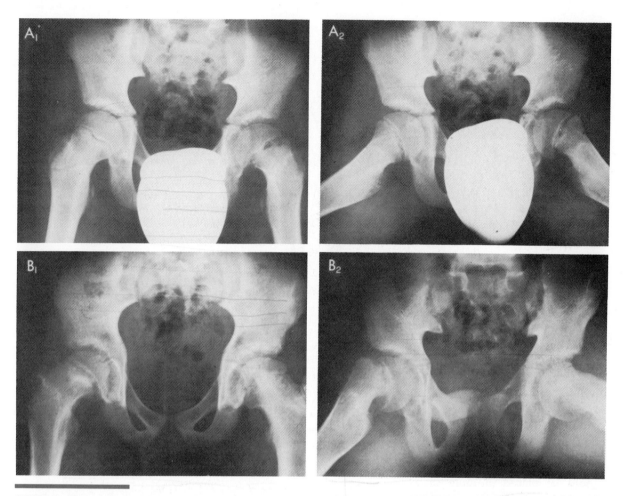

**FIGURE 7-48** ■ Acutely slipped capital femoral epiphysis in a 10-year-old boy with acute left hip and thigh pain. (A) Anteroposterior views of both hips. A line drawn along the superior surface of the femoral head, as seen on the right side, should intersect a corner of the femoral head. The left femoral head has slipped inferiorly. (B) "Frog leg" lateral roentgenograms of both hips demonstrate the mild displacement of the left femoral head more clearly. There is no evidence of remodeling in this acute slip. (From Scoles PV: Pediatric Orthopedics in Clinical Practice, 2nd ed. Chicago: Year Book Medical Publishers, 1988, Fig. 6-4.)

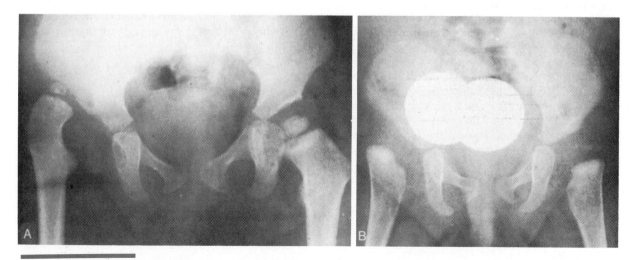

**FIGURE 7-49** ■ (A) High dislocation of the right hip. (B) Intermediate dislocation of the right hip. (From Sherlock DA, Gibson PH, Benson MKD: Congenital subluxation of the hip. J Bone Joint Surg [Br] 67:390-398, 1985.)

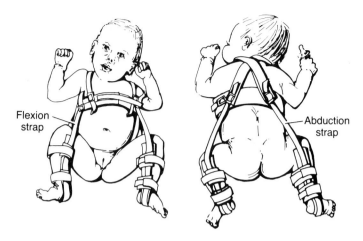

Flexion strap

Abduction strap

FIGURE 7-50 ■ The Pavlik harness. The shoulder and chest straps hold the harness in place. The flexion strap is adjusted to hold the leg flexed between 90 and 100 degrees. The strap must be lengthened with growth. The abduction strap should never be tight. It is a checkrein to limit adduction and is not to force abduction. (From Morrissy RT: Congenital dislocation of the hip. *In* The Hip and Its Disorders [Steinberg ME, ed]. Philadelphia: WB Saunders, 1991, Fig. 18-5.)

Treatment of CDH should begin as soon as possible after diagnosis. The treatment goal is to maintain a joint position that is favorable to reduction. Early treatment includes reduction of the hip joint and maintenance of this reduction until the acetabulum and femoral head develop sufficiently to reduce the chance of further dislocation or subluxation. If diagnosed early in infancy (0 to 6 months), congenital hip dysplasia can be managed effectively with the Pavlik harness (Fig. 7-50) in 90% of cases.[34] The hip should be placed in more than 90 degrees of flexion and moderate abduction. The harness should be worn for 22 to 24 hours per day[29] for at least 4 months. Controlled activity should be encouraged. The Frejka and von Rosen splints (Figs. 7-51 and 7-52) are recommended by some clinicians.[1,35] These positioners place the hip in flexion and abduction using growth principles to shape the femoral head and the acetabulum. After the age of 3 months care must be taken to avoid too much abduction, which places force on adduction contractures. Too much pressure on the femoral head may result in avascular necrosis. Devices such as double and triple diapers should not be used because the hips are not placed in flexion. The conservative treatment of splinting works best when the femoral head is not firmly dislocated and can easily slide in and out of the acetabulum, when soft tissue contractures are mild, and when the child is less than 6 months of age.[1]

After the age of 6 months a commonly recommended treatment for CDH is skin traction followed by closed reduction and a spica cast (Figs. 7-53 and 7-54). The skin traction is used for up to 4 weeks to pull the femoral head below the acetabulum. The maximum weight used is

2.4 kg. Pin traction may be used if skin traction is not effective. The closed reduction is done with the patient under general anesthesia. An alternative treatment for the patient over 6 months of age is surgery.[1] Surgical options include adductor tenotomy, inverted labrum re-

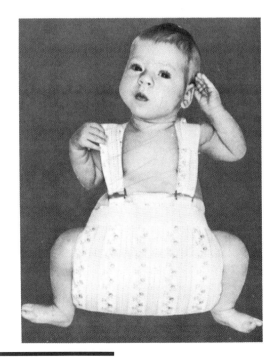

FIGURE 7-51 ■ Frejka pillow splint. This 2-month-old girl had a congenitally unstable left hip joint with a positive Ortolani test. The pillow splint keeps the hips in the stable position of flexion and abduction while allowing some active movement of the hips. (From Salter RB: Textbook of Disorders and Injuries of the Musculoskeletal System, 2nd ed. Baltimore: Williams & Wilkins, 1983, Fig. 8-21.)

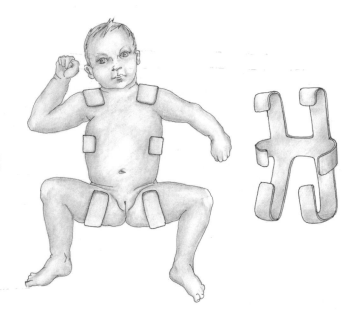

FIGURE 7-52 ■ Von Rosen's splint. (From Tachdjian MO: Pediatric Orthopedics, 2nd ed. Philadelphia: WB Saunders, 1990, Fig. 2-133.)

moval, acetabular osteotomy, and intertrochanteric osteotomy. In both treatment approaches, care should be taken to avoid avascular necrosis, joint stiffness, redislocation, and femoral fracture after immobilization. Sherlock et al. present a diagram for treatment of congenital hip dislocation[36] (Fig. 7-55).

A night splint should be used after removal of the case. A Pavlick harness is used for infants under 6 months of age and a Denis Browne abduction splint for older children. This splint should be used from 3 to 12 months depending on the development of the hip joint.[30] Full weight bearing can begin 4 to 6 weeks after removal of the cast.

Range-of-motion exercises are needed by children who have had surgery or immobilization. Emphasis should be placed on hip flexion, abduction, and internal rotation. Hip external rotation and adduction should be avoided. Motion of the knees may also be restricted by hip immobilization, and range-of-motion exercises for the knees may be required. Active and resistive exercises for both hips and both knees may be needed to strengthen the gluteus maximus, gluteus medius, quadriceps, and hamstrings. For the child who is of walking age, gait training should follow the therapeutic exercise program. Because children may not be motivated to follow a precise exercise protocol, the clinician must be cre-

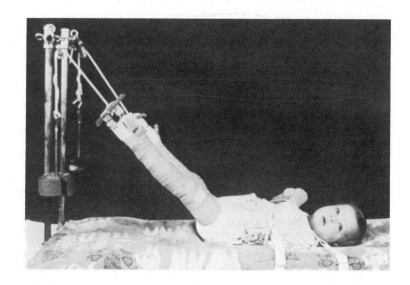

FIGURE 7-53 ■ Continuous skin traction via adhesive tape on the lower limb for congenital dislocation of the hip in a 1-year-old girl. The traction, which is maintained for a few weeks, gradually stretches the shortened muscles about the hip in preparation for a safe and gentle closed reduction. (From MacEwen GD, Bunnell WP, Ramsey P: The hip. In Pediatric Orthopedics, Vol 2. [Lovell WW, Winter RB, eds]. Philadelphia: JB Lippincott, 1986, p 716.)

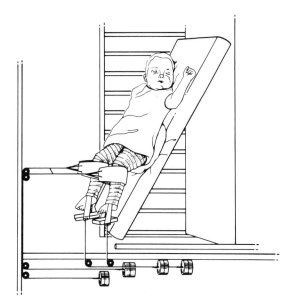

FIGURE 7-54 ■ Traction for congenital dislocation of the hip. The patient is placed on a Bradford frame with the feet elevated about 30 degrees. The patient serves as the counter traction. Skin traction from ankle to groin is used, and hips are kept flexed about 45 degrees. (From Morrissy RT: Congenital dislocation of the hip. *In* The Hip and Its Disorders [Steinberg ME, ed]. Philadelphia: WB Saunders, 1991, Fig. 18-6.)

ative in designing a program that will be adhered to by the child. Exercises in water may give the child incentive to perform. Cryotherapy can be used to control hip pain.

For children of walking age, open reduction or osteotomy may be needed. After the reduction, a spica cast (Fig. 7-56) is applied with the hip positioned in 90 degrees of flexion and abduction between the maximum abduction and unstable adduction positions.[16]

## Septic Arthritis

Septic arthritis of the hip is an acute, rapidly progressive infection of the hip joint (Fig. 7-57). Severe destruction of the joint may occur if effective treatment is not initiated early in the disease process.[1,17,37]

The most common cause of the disorder is spread of pyogenic bacteria from hematogenous osteomyelitis in the proximal metaphyseal region of the femur directly into the hip joint.[17,37] Subcutaneous abscesses, otitis media, pneumonia, umbilical infections, gluteal infections, transfusions through umbilical catheters, and femoral venipuncture[1] may also cause spread of microorganisms into the joint.

The disease is not common, but it is serious. It is most common in children less than 2 years old, less common in older children, and rare in adults. However, children or adults receiving prolonged adrenocorticosteroid therapy have a higher than average incidence.[1,17]

The disorder is difficult to recognize in the neonate and infant because its clinical picture is similar to that of other diseases. The most common sign and possibly the only initial sign is irritability of the infant. The disease causes severe pain in the joint that intensifies with movement. The neonate and infant hold the hip joint still in the position of flexion, abduction, and external rotation and respond adversely to palpation and passive motion. The older child may appear to be very ill with systemic symptoms of fever, sweating, chills, tachycardia, dehydration, and anorexia. The child often refuses to stand and the pain may be referred to the knee. The child may have a short leg, flexion-adduction contracture about the hip, decreased range of motion of the hip, hip subluxation, a prominent greater trochanter, and swelling of the thigh.[1,17,37]

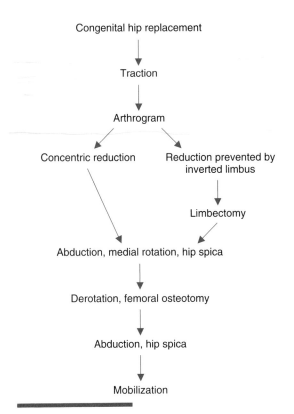

FIGURE 7-55 ■ The Somerville and Scott program of treatment for dislocated hips. (Redrawn from Sherlock DA, Gibson PH, Benson MKD: Congenital subluxation of the hip. J Bone Joint Surg [Br] 67:390-398, 1985.)

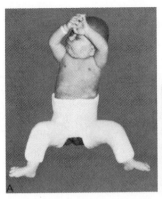
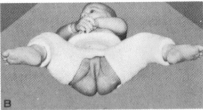

**FIGURE 7-56** ■ Bilateral hip spica plaster cast for congenital dislocation of the hip in a 1-year-old girl. This type of cast is applied after adductor tenotomy and gentle closed reduction and maintains the reduced hip in the stable position of marked flexion and moderate abduction (the "human" position). This child required a total period of 12 months in a cast, during which time the hip responded well. Earlier diagnosis and treatment would have shortened the period of immobilization. (From Salter RB: Textbook of Disorders and Injuries of the Musculoskeletal System, 2nd ed. Baltimore: Williams & Wilkins, 1983.)

If the diagnosis of septic arthritis of the hip is not made within a few days of onset, necrosis of the femoral head and irreparable damage to the hip joint often occur. Residual deformities may occur, even with early treatment, including shortened limb, coxa vara, coxa valga, hip subluxation, hip dislocation, or decreased size or absence of the femoral head.

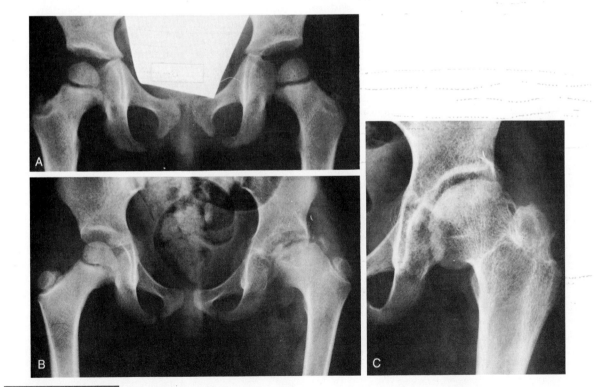

**FIGURE 7-57** ■ (A) Widening of the left joint space in a patient with septic hip caused by *Staphylococcus aureus*. (B) Seven months later, loss of capital femoral ossification and flattening similar to that in Legg-Calvé-Perthes disease are seen. (C) At 10 years of age, the capital femoral physis has closed spontaneously because of premature growth arrest. The greater trochanteric physis was closed surgically. (From Grogan DP, Sackett JR, Ogden JA: Infection of the hip. *In* The Hip and Its Disorders [Steinberg ME, ed]. Philadelphia: WB Saunders, 1991, p 359.)

Septic arthritis should be considered an emergency situation, and immediate treatment is essential. The treatment goals are to eliminate the infection and preserve the joint's integrity and function. When the problem is diagnosed, the joint should be aspirated; after a day or two, surgical drainage combined with intravenous antibiotics is instituted.[1,17,37] The intravenous antibiotics are generally used for 3 weeks, followed by oral antibiotics for the next 3 to 8 weeks. After surgical drainage, bilateral split Russell's traction (Fig. 7–58) or a splint or spica cast may be used to position the hip in slight abduction, flexion, and neutral or slight external rotation until healing is complete.[1,37,38] If the disorder is not treated quickly, residual deformities and joint destruction may occur, including hip subluxation, hip dislocation, or dissolution of the femoral head. A shoe lift may be used if the subluxation is mild and results in a leg length discrepancy. If the problem is more serious, surgery is necessary. For a dislocated hip, a capsular arthroplasty is performed to remove the scar tissue and deepen the acetabulum. Long periods of heavy traction follow this surgical procedure to overcome the capsular adhesions and shortened muscles and to reduce the head of the femur into the acetabulum. For a dissolved femoral head, a trochanteric arthroplasty can be used. After the surgery, the patient is placed in a hip spica cast. Upon removal of the cast, range-of-motion and muscle-strengthening exercises are initiated and partial weight-bearing on crutches is begun. The specific protocol used depends on the recommendations of the surgeon.[1,39] If an arthroplasty is not advisable, an arthrodesis that sacrifices joint motion may be performed.

## Coxa Vara

Coxa vara is a progressive disorder of the proximal end of the femur (Fig. 7–59). At birth the femoral neck forms an angle of approximately 175 degrees with the femoral shaft, and as the child ages this angle decreases to about 125 degrees. If the neck-shaft an angle is less than 120 degrees, it is classified as coxa vara.

The cause of coxa vara is unknown, but it is thought to be primarily an endochondral ossification defect in the femoral neck. Insufficient ossification of the medial portion of the capital femoral epiphysis may result from an embryonic vascular disturbance in the area or imperfect formation of the growth cartilage because of a defect in the cartilaginous anlage of the femur.[16]

The incidence of coxa vara is low[39] and appears to be equally distributed between the sexes. The disorder is usually not recognized until the child begins to walk. A painless limp and appearance of a short limb often become obvious. Excessive lordosis, limited abduction, mild hip flexion contracture, and limited hip extension may occur concomitantly. Coxa vara tends to be progressive unless surgically treated and may recur after treatment.

The goals for treatment of coxa vara are to increase the angle of inclination, promote ossifi-

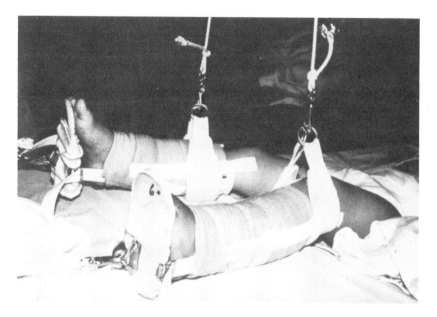

**FIGURE 7–58** ■ Bilateral split Russell's traction. Vertical force on strap around proximal tibia prevents hyperextension of knee, relieves resistance from weight of leg on bed, and controls amount of flexion of hip. (From Griffin PP: Acute septic arthritis of the hip in childhood. *In* The Hip: Proceedings of the Seventh Open Scientific Meeting of the Hip Society, 1979 [Sledge CB, ed]. St. Louis: CV Mosby, 1979.)

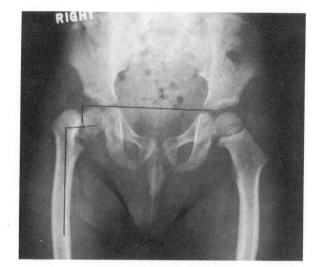

**FIGURE 7-59** ■ Anteroposterior view of pelvis demonstrating coxa vara. Note the vertical orientation of the growth plate and the triangle of bone on the inferomedial side of the neck. (From Peckham R, Dvonch VM: Coxa vara. Orthopedics 12:891–892, 1989.)

cation of the cartilaginous femoral defect, and reorient the growth plate to a more horizontal position.[16] If the angle of inclination is greater than 110 degrees, the condition is not treated but it is carefully observed; however, a lift in the shoe and stretching of the hip adductor and lateral rotator muscles may be needed. If the condition is progressive and falls below 110 degrees, surgery is usually the treatment of choice.[1,16] To obtain a more valgus position, a subtrochanteric or intertrochanteric osteotomy with a screw and plate or a bifurcated blade plate is used.[1] A more conservative alternative treatment recommended by some is abduction bracing to prevent adductor shortening or an adductor myotomy followed by abduction bracing.[1] However, some authors question the effectiveness of this alternative treatment.[30]

Various osteotomy procedures may be used depending on the surgeon's choice. After surgery in a child 6 years of age or younger, a one-and-one-half hip spica cast is applied for approximately 6 to 8 weeks. After the cast is removed, active, gentle range-of-motion exercise for the hips and knee is begun. Active side-lying hip abduction exercises and standing hip hiking (Trendelenburg's) exercises can be started. When full range of motion is obtained, partial weight bearing, three-point crutch walking is allowed. When the Trendelenburg sign is negative, gait may be progressed to full weight bearing. A spica cast is not necessary for older children if a bifurcated blade plate is used with the osteotomy. This plate is stable and partial weight bearing with crutches can begin 4 to 5 days after surgery. Active range-of-motion and strengthening exercises can begin at the discretion of the surgeon. This procedure heals in approximately 8 weeks.[30]

## Legg-Calvé-Perthes Disease

Legg-Calvé-Perthes disease begins as a vascular necrosis of the secondary epiphysis of the head of the femur (Fig. 7-60). It is generally a self-limiting disorder that may heal spontaneously with or without treatment. Its complications often cause musculoskeletal and functional problems. These complications include subchondral fracture in the epiphysis, hip subluxation, or flattening of the femoral head. If flattening of the femoral head occurs, the condition is often called coxa plana. The femoral head flattening makes the hip joint incongruous and degenerative joint disease develops later in life. Legg-Calvé-Perthes disease is one of the most important causes of painful limp in childhood.

The avascular necrosis is often initiated by a subchondral fracture,[40,41] by compression of the lateral epiphyseal artery by the external rotator muscles,[42,43] or by intraepiphysial compression of the blood supply to the secondary ossification center.[42,44] Scoles lists possible causes as metabolic bone disease, thrombotic vascular insults, trauma, infection, and transient synovitis.[8]

The disorder usually occurs in children between the ages of 2 and 12 years, most commonly around the age of 6 years. Most researchers have found the disorder to be more common in boys than girls, a ratio of about 4:1.[1,16,42] The disorder is rare in black children,

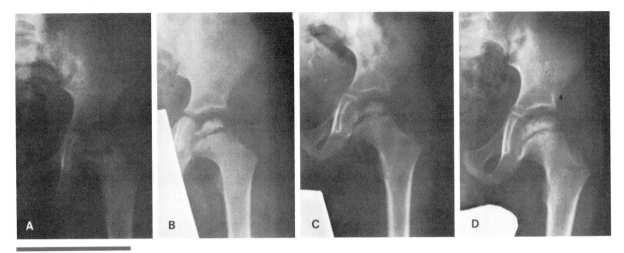

**FIGURE 7-60** ■ The four stages of Legg-Calvé-Perthes disease. The first changes are capsular swelling, increased joint space, and demineralization at the metaphyseal junction (A). This is followed by increase in density of the head (B), which flows into stage 3, in which radiolucent areas are present (C). Ultimately, the patient has an enlarged deformed femoral head, with widening of the neck of the femur (D). (From D'Ambrosia RD: The hip. *In* Musculoskeletal Disorders [D'Ambrosia RD, ed]. Philadelphia: JB Lippincott, 1986, Fig. 11–29.)

but Oriental and white children have a similar incidence. In about 15% of cases the disorder occurs bilaterally. There is a correlation between the presence of the disorder and low birth weight and growth delay.[1] The disorder appears to be familial in one fifth to one fourth of cases.[1]

Pain develops with a gradual insidious onset and fluctuates in severity depending on the stress placed on the hip joint. Usually the pain is an aching sensation rather than a sharp pain and is located in the hip, thigh, or knee. The anterior and posterior hip joint capsule may be tender on palpation. The child often has an antalgic gait, especially after activity. The hip joint may become stiff with a limited range of motion, especially in internal rotation and abduction. The adductor muscles may exhibit spasm, and atrophy may develop in the quadriceps muscles. The length of the involved limb may decrease by 1 to 2 cm. The greater trochanter becomes elevated and more prominent.

Generally, Legg-Calvé-Perthes runs its course and heals. The goals of treatment are containment of the femoral head in the acetabulum, maintenance of this reduction, restoration of motion, and relief of stress through the hip joint. Many patients with mild involvement may not need treatment; these individuals should be carefully observed for 2 to 4 months to follow the course of the disease.[16] The purpose of treatment is to provide protection against development of a deformity that will cause problems later in life. To allow the acute symptoms to subside, bed rest

and skin traction in balanced suspension for about 1 to 4 weeks are effective.[45] Rest removes the mechanical loading, which can cause pain, and traction helps relieve muscle spasm and tenderness around the joint.[8,16] Traction should not be done with the hip in extension. Full range of motion should be maintained, especially in abduction and internal rotation.

For children about 4 years of age with signs of joint problems, braces should be worn at night with the involved hip in 70 to 80 degrees of abduction and some internal rotation. The normal hip should be placed in 30 degrees of abduction. For children between the ages of 5 and 10 years, an abduction device should be worn both day and night (Figs. 7–61 to 7–63). Depending on the progression and severity of the disorder, the device may be worn for up to 18 months.[45] An active motion program with partial or full weight bearing should be conducted during this time.[16,46,47]

A typical protocol for conservative treatment includes traction, casting, bracing, and exercise. Traction, which can be done in the hospital or at home for several days, is used to rest the painful hip and help restore motion in abduction. When adequate abduction is achieved, a plaster cast is applied with the hips in abduction (10 degrees short of full) and slight internal rotation. The limbs of the cast are connected by a bar that is adjusted weekly to increase abduction. The child can be taught balance and gait activities while in the cast. The cast is removed after 6 to 8 weeks.

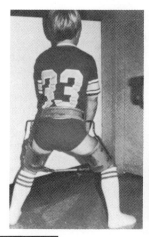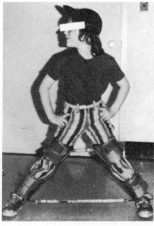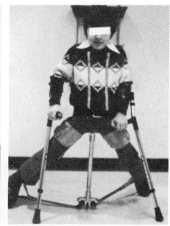

**FIGURE 7-61** ■ (A) Example of a child with Legg-Calvé-Perthes disease wearing an abduction brace developed at the Scottish Rite Children's Hospital in Atlanta. (B) Example of an abduction brace developed at the Blythedale Children's Hospital in Valhalla, NY. (C) Example of an abduction brace developed in Toronto and described by Bobetchko. (From Katz JF: Legg-Calvé-Perthes disease. *In* Management of Hip Disorders in Children [Katz JF, Siffert RS, eds]. Philadelphia: JB Lippincott, 1983, Fig. 9-10.)

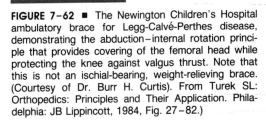

**FIGURE 7-62** ■ The Newington Children's Hospital ambulatory brace for Legg-Calvé-Perthes disease, demonstrating the abduction–internal rotation principle that provides covering of the femoral head while protecting the knee against valgus thrust. Note that this is not an ischial-bearing, weight-relieving brace. (Courtesy of Dr. Burr H. Curtis). From Turek SL: Orthopedics: Principles and Their Application. Philadelphia: JB Lippincott, 1984, Fig. 27-82.)

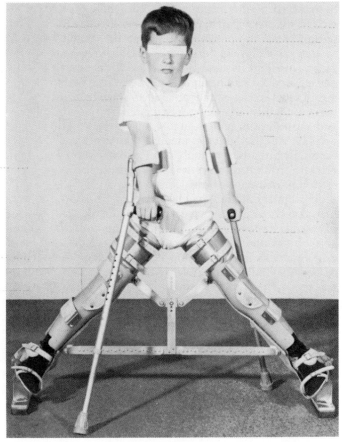

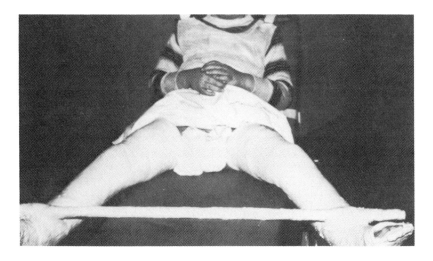

FIGURE 7–63 ■ Child in plaster casts held in abduction with a broomstick. This is a technique for centering subluxated femoral heads. The abduction is gradually increased by removing the broomstick and widening the abduction span. (From Katz JF: Legg-Calvé-Perthes disease. *In* Management of Hip Disorders in Children. [Katz JF, Siffert RS, eds]. Philadelphia: JB Lippincott, 1983, Fig. 8–8.)

While the cast is off for 2 to 3 days, the patient is restricted to bed rest but given range-of-motion exercises, preferably in the whirlpool or therapeutic pool. At this time the patient can be measured for an abduction orthosis, or the cast may be continued for another 6 to 8 weeks. If an orthosis is to be used, the cast is reapplied until the orthosis is ready. The cast is then removed to be replaced by the orthosis. Range-of-motion exercises are again performed. When in the abduction orthosis, the patient can pursue full activity as long as no weight is borne on the foot and limb. The splint is usually worn 24 hours a day and removed only for brief exercises and bathing. The exercises should include range of motion, especially hip abduction; internal rotation and knee flexion; and strengthening exercises especially for the gluteus medius, gluteus maximum, and quadriceps muscles. The hips should be held in abduction even during bathing. This total conservative treatment protocol may last for approximately 24 months.[42,48–53]

If these conservative measures are unsuccessful, surgery is necessary. The most common surgical procedure is a varus osteotomy or Chirari osteotomy[1,8,16] and abduction brace (see Figs. 7–61 and 7–62). About 12 weeks after the surgery, the patient may begin weight bearing. Another surgical procedure is an adductor tenotomy followed with a broomstick cast (see Fig. 7–63). Early surgery is done to prevent deformity, later surgery to improve existing deformity. Scoles reports that if significant femoral head deformity is present the results of surgical treatment are less predictable.[45] Evans and associates compared ambulation-abduction bracing with varus derotation osteotomy for patients over 6 years of age with severe Legg-Calvé-Perthes disease.[48] They found no difference in the results of the two treatment procedures; however, the bracing procedure may be more prolonged.

After the surgery, the patient's hip is immobilized in a spica cast using a non-weight-bearing crutch gait for approximately 6 weeks. After the cast is removed, exercises including active and passive hip, knee, and ankle range of motion and lower limb strengthening are begun. Gait progresses from partial weight bearing to full weight bearing when the patient has gained full range of motion and has a negative Trendelenburg sign.

## Transient Synovitis

Transient synovitis of the hip is the most common hip disorder causing a limp in children.[1,42] It is a self-limiting nonspecific inflammation of the synovium that occurs without apparent cause. Trauma, infection, and allergy[1] have been cited as possible causes of transient synovitis, but other researchers reject the causal relationship.[42] The disorder usually occurs in children between the ages of 2 and 12 years. Males are affected more frequently than females at approximately a 2 : 1 ratio.[54] Only one joint is commonly involved.

The synovitis may have either an acute or insidious onset of pain. If the disorder is severe, the pain is usually located in the hip, the child refuses to walk, and active and passive motion of the hip is limited. However, if the disorder is moderate, pain may be located in the thigh and knee as well as the hip, the child has an antalgic limp, and hip extension and internal rotation are limited.[1] The common posture of the hip is flexion, abduction, and external rotation. The patient may have a low-grade fever. The disorder seems to disappear after a few weeks or months without treatment.

The best treatment for transient synovitis is resting with the limb in a non-weight-bearing position. Buck's traction may be used if pain is severe. Local heat, massage, and aspirin may also help in relieving the pain. Partial weight bearing with crutches can be used when pain is decreased. The course of the disorder may last from 2 to 7 days.[1,16,45] If the symptoms are prolonged, the patient should be evaluated for Legg-Calvé-Perthes disease.

## Slipped Capital Femoral Epiphysis

The slipped capital femoral epiphysis is the most common hip disorder occurring during the adolescent period.[16] The epiphysis slips (Fig. 7–64) from its normal position on the femur. The lesion is found in the epiphyseal plate in the zone in which ossification occurs in adolescence.[55] The growth plate becomes disorganized as fibrous tissue increases and endochondral ossification becomes random.[8] Shearing weakens the growth plate. Trauma or weight bearing displaces the femoral head posteriorly and inferiorly.

The cause of the disorder is unknown. The problem may be related to the growth hormone that decreases the shear strength of the growth plate,[16] or it may be related to defective matrix production or endocrine abnormalities.[8]

Slipping of the epiphysis occurs during the latter part of adolescence in the final phase of growth after a rapid growth spurt. The age range is generally 10 to 17 years for boys with the mode about 13 to 14 years and 8 to 15 years for girls with the mode about 11 years. The disorder occurs at least twice as often in boys than in girls and about twice as often in black children than white children. About 75% of the cases occur in obese children with delayed maturation. Bilateral involvement occurs about 15% of the time.

Usually the onset of pain is minimal and vague. The pain is often felt in the knee, the suprapatellar area, the thigh, or the hip at extremes of motion. Tenderness may be felt in the anterior and lateral aspects of the hip. About 20% of those experiencing epiphyseal slipping have no pain. Approximately 14% of patients with the disorder have an acute onset.[16] In such cases pain is usually immediate and adductor spasm may occur.

Range of motion becomes limited in internal rotation, abduction, and sometimes flexion; conversely, extension may be increased. The position of most comfort appears to be flexion, abduction, and external rotation. Quadriceps atrophy often occurs and the limb length may shorten as much as 1 inch.[16] In the acute stages of the disorder the adolescent exhibits an antalgic gait, but during the chronic phase a Trendelenburg gait is usually present.

If treatment is administered early in the course of the disorder, the prognosis is good. If the disorder is recognized late in its course, permanent disability usually occurs.

Treatment of slipped capital femoral epiphysis

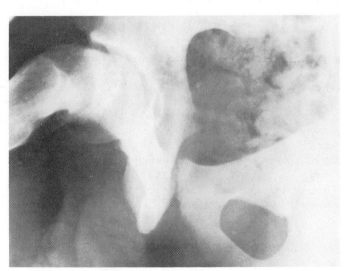

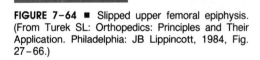
**FIGURE 7–64** ■ Slipped upper femoral epiphysis. (From Turek SL: Orthopedics: Principles and Their Application. Philadelphia: JB Lippincott, 1984, Fig. 27–66.)

should start immediately after its diagnosis. The slipping is considered an emergency condition[30] because minor trauma may cause further displacement. Once slipping of the head has begun, it continues until the epiphyseal plate is stabilized by skeletal maturation or by surgical procedures. The treatment should prevent further slipping. A conservative approach to treatment is to use a short leg cast with a cross bar or a spica cast. The hip is placed in abduction and internal rotation and the device should be worn for at least 12 to 14 weeks.[1] This treatment, however, is not recommended because conservative treatment has been shown to be successful. The treatment of choice is surgery.[1,8] As soon as the

slip is diagnosed, the patient should be admitted to the hospital and placed in split Russell's traction (see Fig. 7–58) to relieve muscle spasms and with medial straps to correct any lateral rotation contracture. After the muscle spasm is relieved, the condition should be re-evaluated[30] and the type of surgical procedure determined. If the slip is mild or moderate, pinning of the head in situ (Fig. 7–65), bone grafting across the physis, and use of a plate and pins are all typical surgical procedures.[45] The surgery should be followed by traction for 2 to 4 days and/or bilateral hip spica cast for immobilization. The patient should walk on crutches without weight bearing until pain-free range of motion is present. Weight bearing is

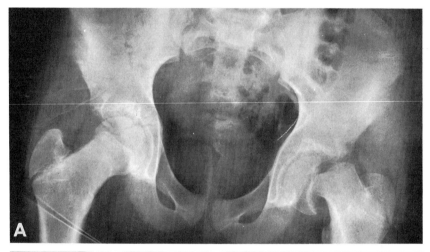

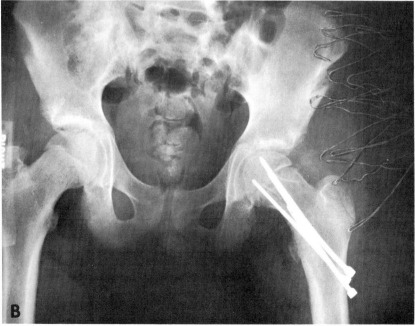

FIGURE 7–65 ■ (A) Complete slip of capital femoral epiphysis of left hip. (B) Same patient after operative replacement of the epiphysis, bone pegging of the growth line, and fixation with metallic pins. (Courtesy Dr. John Dowling, Lankenau Hospital, Philadelphia, PA. From Gartland JJ: Fundamentals of Orthopedics, 4th ed. Philadelphia: WB Saunders, 1987, Fig. 14–5.)

then gradually increased to full weight bearing in about 3 to 4 months[30,56] as the patient also performs range-of-motion and strengthening exercises. If the slip is severe, realignment of the head and neck should be accomplished in an osteotomy at the neck, intertrochanteric, or subtrochanteric regions.[45] Rehabilitation should proceed as previously discussed for an increase in range of motion and muscle strength.

## Bursitis

Bursitis is an inflammatory reaction in response to overuse or excessive pressure. The most common bursitis of the hip involves the deep trochanteric bursa. It may be caused by injury to the bursa from a direct blow, irritation of the iliotibial band, or rheumatoid arthritis. The iliopectineal and ischiogluteal bursae may also be injured by prolonged pressure.

Deep trochanteric bursitis is found in about 15% of rheumatoid arthritis patients, more commonly in women than in men. Therefore, all patients with rheumatoid arthritis with hip pain should be examined for bursitis.[57]

Bursitis is often accompanied by severe pain and tenderness over the bursa area and superior and posterior to the trochanter. Any motion may cause pain, which radiates down the posterior aspect of the thigh. Lateral thigh pain may be exacerbated by lying on the involved side. In deep trochanteric bursitis the limb is often positioned in abduction and external rotation. The patient may have an antalgic gait during acute bursitis and a Trendelenburg gait in the chronic stage. The disorder subsides with proper treatment and rest.

Active motion increases pain in patients with bursitis, and the treatment goals are relief of pain and resolution of the inflammatory process. After the pain is relieved, the goals should be return to normal function and prevention of recurrence. The patient should be educated to correct faulty postural and movement mechanics and to eliminate the cause of the irritation.

The patient should avoid activities and positions that irritate the bursa, such as rolling on the side, climbing stairs, and long walks.[12] In the early acute phase of the problem, cryotherapy (ice or cold pack) can reduce pain; during later stages, moist heat, ultrasound, and nonsteroidal anti-inflammatory drugs may be used to reduce the sharper pain.[26,58] Ultrasound to the site of the lesion is dramatically effective in about 3 to 6 minutes.[12] Raman and Haslock found that corticosteroid injected at the point of maximum tenderness of rheumatoid arthritic patients was an effective treatment for trochanteric bursitis.[57] As the pain subsides in cases of trochanteric bursitis, the tensor should be stretched to restore its full mobility. In cases of iliopectineal bursitis, the iliopsoas muscle should be stretched, the hip joint range of motion should be increased to normal, and the muscles surrounding the joint should be strengthened.

## Avascular Necrosis

Avascular necrosis is not a specific disease; it is the terminal phase of conditions that lead to impairment of the blood supply to the femoral head (Fig. 7–66). The lesion is most often located in the superior lateral area of the femoral head. Tissue death begins within 12 hours after the onset of circulatory impairment. A fracture of the proximal end of the femur (especially a transcervical fracture), slipped capital femoral epiphysis, hip dislocation, and hip manipulation may all impair circulation. The cause of avascular necrosis in adults is often unknown, but it may be related to alcoholism, sickle cell anemia, decompression sickness, major steroid therapy, and renal transplantation.[59]

Avascular necrosis may occur after hip fracture in about 65 to 85% of the patients. The factors leading to the avascular necrosis in these cases include severity of the fracture, quality of the reduction, delay in the reduction, and intracapsular pressure resulting from excessive body weight.[60] The incidence in nondisplaced fractures is approximately 14 to 44%; in displaced fractures it is significantly higher at 40 to 84%.[61] Avascular necrosis occurs less frequently in children than in adults because reossification occurs in children after a fracture, whereas in adults revascularization does not occur and the bone is not reossified.

Idiopathic avascular necrosis of the femoral head occurs more often in males (70%) and most commonly between the ages of 30 and 50 years. The disorder is often bilateral.[59] The course of the destruction of the femoral head depends on the cause of the necrosis and the age of the patient (Table 7–11). The healing potential is greater in children than in adults because the blood supply to the femoral head is less easily disturbed and more adaptable.[60]

Avascular necrosis that is secondary to another physical problem is evident at the time of the primary problem in only 15% of the cases; more

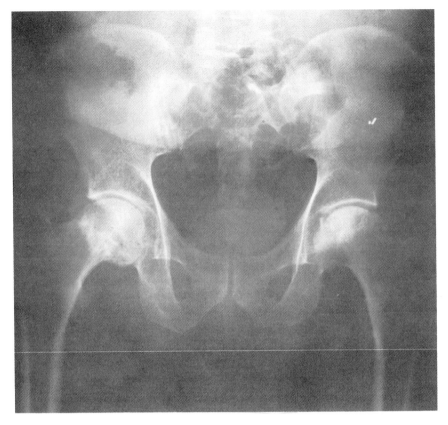

**FIGURE 7–66** ■ Avascular necrosis in a kidney transplant patient. Note the increased density (sclerosis) of the superior position of the femoral head, particularly on the left. (From D'Ambrosia RD: The hip. *In* Musculoskeletal Disorders [D'Ambrosia RD, ed]. Philadelphia: JB Lippincott, 1986, Fig. 11–10.)

commonly it may not be noticed for more than a year after treatment of the primary problem. The patient may have insidious pain in the hip or knee and a decreased range of motion.

Revascularization and reossification of the femoral head occur as it heals gradually over a period of 3 to 4 years in idiopathic avascular necrosis. The process takes many years and healing is never spontaneous. In the early stage of the disease process the patient is asymptomatic

and has no complaint of pain, hip range of motion is normal, and gait is normal. After a few months or even years of progression, intermittent pain in the groin radiates to the inner aspect of the thigh in about 50% of the patients. This mild intermittent pain is followed later by a sudden increase in pain. In about 50% of patients the earliest symptom of the problem is not the intermittent pain but the sudden severe pain as the femoral head fractures.[62] The joint slowly stiff-

---

**Table 7–11.** HISTORICAL CLUES TO DIAGNOSIS OF HIP PAIN

| History | Condition |
| --- | --- |
| Recent fall, old age, osteoporosis | Hip fractures; impacted femoral neck fracture may still allow walking |
| Abrupt onset, fever, immunosuppression | Septic joint |
| Subacute onset, oral corticosteroids, systemic lupus erythematosus | Avascular necrosis |
| History of inflammation in hand or foot joint | Inflammatory synovitis (e.g., gout, spondyloarthropathy, long-standing rheumatoid arthritis) |
| History of cancer | Bone metastasis |
| Horseback riding, straddling posture, accidental stepping into a hole | "Rider's" strain of adductors |

From Roberts WN, Williams RB: Hip pain. Primary Care 15(4):783–793, 1988.

ens, muscle spasms may occur, and motion, especially in abduction and internal rotation, becomes limited. Pain develops in forced extremes of motion and the patient walks with a coxalgic limp.[27]

In children, the femoral head affected by avascular necrosis reossifies. In this process the femoral head returns to normal or is slightly flattened. In adults, flattening and collapse of the femoral head are more common. Because the progress of the disease in adults is often irreversible, reconstructive surgery may be recommended for pain relief.

Avascular necrosis may run its course without surgical intervention. The goals of treatment are focused on preservation of the structure, preservation of function, and relief of pain. In the younger patient a nonsurgical approach would be to prohibit weight bearing for about 2 to 3 years to allow the femoral head to revascularize and heal without placing a weight-bearing load on the joint. In older patients, surgery should be done as soon as possible. Several stages are involved, and the treatment of choice varies depending on the stage of the disease process. Even in the earliest stage avoiding weight bearing for 6 to 9 months is rarely effective. Instead, drilling and grafting are more successful (Fig. 7–67). Holes are drilled along the axis of the femoral neck into the necrotic area of the head, and bone grafts from the tibia or fibula are inserted through these holes into the subchondral cortex of the head. The drilling hastens revascularization of the head, and the grafts assist in the repair process and provide support for the necrotic bone. If the case has progressed to necrosis but the head of the femur has not collapsed, the surgical procedure of choice is a varus derotation osteotomy of the femur. The osteotomy changes the position of the femoral head to place viable tissue in the weight-bearing region. This surgical procedure also stimulates revascularization. If the necrosis is extensive and the destruction is great, the surgical procedure is replacement of the head by an arthroplasty or total hip replacement[42] (Fig. 7–68). Depending on the extent of joint destruction, the type of surgical procedure, and the surgeon's beliefs, the rehabilitation of the postsurgical patient may vary. The goals of postsurgical rehabilitation are pain-free motion of the operated limb, independent ambulation, and independence in functional daily activities. The patient should be instructed in the rehabilitation procedures before the surgery in order to know what to expect after the operation.

The surgical procedure used may require cast-

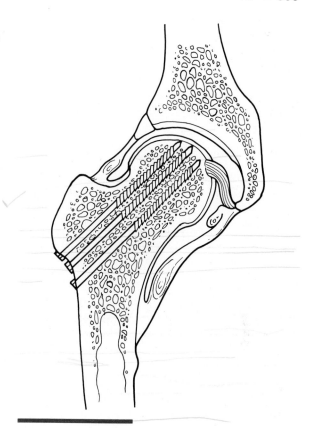

**FIGURE 7–67** ■ Avascular necrosis of femoral head, drilling and pegging operation. Ingrowths of vascular cellular tissue along the grafts from the vascular metaphysis repair the dead bone. The cortical transplants provide fixation, as does the threaded pin placed adjacent to the calcar. (From Turek SL: Orthopedics: Principles and Their Application. Philadelphia: JB Lippincott, 1984, p 1198. Modified from Phemister DB: Treatment of the necrotic head of the femur in adults. J Bone Joint Surg 31A:55, 1949.)

ing, which would be maintained for approximately 6 to 8 weeks. During this time the patient can be instructed in upper limb strengthening exercises, balance activities, and gait. Upon removal of the cast, exercises are begun for range of motion of the hips, knees, and ankles and strengthening of the lower limb muscles, especially the gluteus medius, gluteus maximus, and quadriceps. Gait is progressed from non–weight bearing with crutches to full weight bearing when the range of motion is nearly normal and the strength is sufficient to give a negative Trendelenburg sign.

If a device is used in the surgical procedure that gives sufficient stability to the joint without casting, range-of-motion and strengthening exercises and gait training are begun a few days after the surgery. The timing and vigor of the exercises depend on the wishes of the surgeon.

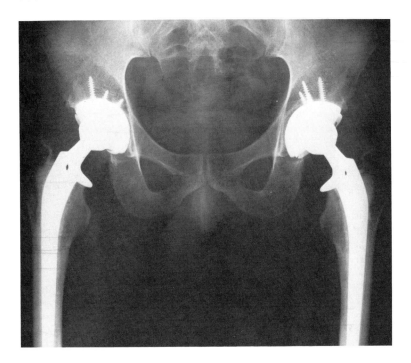

**FIGURE 7-68** ■ Bilateral "hybrid" total hip replacement in a young male with avascular necrosis after steroid administration. The clinical course is excellent. (From Steinberg ME, Steinberg DR: Avascular necrosis of the femoral head. *In* The Hip and Its Disorders [Steinberg ME, ed]. Philadelphia: WB Saunders, 1991, Fig. 30-27.)

## Degenerative Joint Disease

DJD is the most common disease affecting the hip.[12] DJD or osteoarthritis of the hip is a progressive deterioration of articular cartilage and overgrowth of periarticular bone (Figs. 7-69 and 7-70). As the articular cartilage degenerates, subchondral vascularity increases, the subchondral cortex thickens, marginal and central subchondral bone remodels, osteophytic outgrowths form peripherally, and subarticular bone cysts develop. Aging changes in the components of the articular cartilage gradually reduce its ability to withstand loading. Osteophytes generally occur throughout the joint except in the area of loading. In the area of greatest loading the old bone and newly formed bone are compressed, eroded, and develop minute fractures. This bone increases in density and changes to a hard, ivory-like mass, and the capsule becomes fibrous and hyperemic.[42]

The etiology of DJD is divided into two types: primary and secondary. The primary type develops spontaneously in middle age with no known predisposing cause; it appears to be idiopathic. The secondary type of DJD occurs in response to a known injury, deformity, or disease. A single trauma or several occasions of microtrauma may cause DJD. Repetitive loading of the joint can lead to degeneration of cartilage and changes in subchondral bone. Degenerative joint disease often develops as a secondary result of hip deformity and disease. The disorder may result from incongruity of the articular surfaces after such problems as a congenital dislocated hip, Legg-Calvé-Perthes disease, hip subluxation, hip fracture, septic arthritis, hip anteversion, coxa vara, coxa valga, and dysplasia of the acetabulum or femoral head. In most cases mechanical forces seem to be major determinants of DJD. Problems related to the development of DJD include obesity, hypothyroidism, pituitary dysfunction, and menopause. The disorder may develop more readily in some individuals than others be-

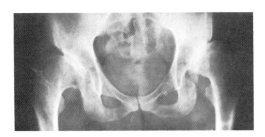

**FIGURE 7-69** ■ Degenerative joint disease of both hips in a 38-year-old woman secondary to residual subluxation after inadequate treatment of congenital dislocation of the hips in childhood. The patient walked with a marked limp and suffered pain in both hips. This serious and disabling condition could have been prevented by diagnosis and adequate treatment at birth. (From Salter RB: Textbook of Disorders and Injuries of the Musculoskeletal System, 2nd ed. Baltimore: Williams & Wilkins, 1983, Fig. 8-15.)

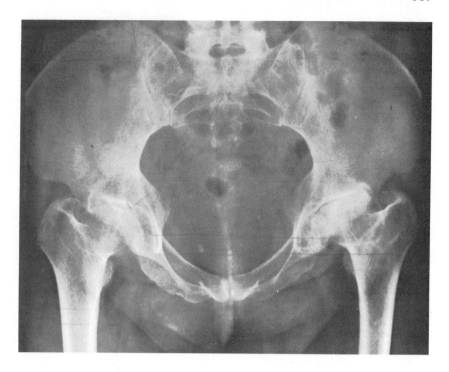

**FIGURE 7–70** ■ Osteoarthritis of the left hip, which has developed in a mechanically imperfect joint. The patient had Legg-Calvé-Perthes disease in both hips as a child. (From Gartland JJ: Fundamentals of Orthopedics, 4th ed. Philadelphia: WB Saunders, 1987, Fig. 89.)

cause of an inherent weakness of the articular cartilage.

Although DJD may occur in an infant or child, it is found most commonly in middle-aged and older adults. After age 60 approximately 25% of females and 15% of males have symptoms of DJD.[17]

The individual may first have an insidious onset of groin or trochanteric pain, especially after long periods of weight bearing. The pain may later be referred to the anterior thigh or knee. As the condition progresses, pain may be felt in the lateral and posterior thigh as well. Tenderness may occur over the site of capsular inflammation. In a few cases the pain may begin in the knee, although the degeneration is in the hip. In time the hip pain may become quite severe, especially after motion. As the course of the disorder progresses, pain may even be felt at rest. The severity of pain is not related to radiologic change, but the pain appears to become worse with a fall in barometric pressure. The individual generally comes to the clinic because of pain and disability.

The patient develops hip joint stiffness after rest, and a decrease of range of motion in extension, internal rotation, and extreme flexion occurs. Spasm of the adductor, flexor, and external rotator muscles can lead to contractures and joint deformity. The muscles surrounding the hip may atrophy, especially the abductor muscles and the gluteus maximus. Within the joint a moderate effusion may develop but with little accompanying synovial thickening. Joint crepitus including squeaking, creaking, and grating occurs.

The degree of physical dysfunction corresponds to the individual's degree of joint degeneration and pain. The individual may have difficulty performing strenuous exercise, bending at the hip, sitting, and rising from bed. The patient may also have an antalgic limp because of pain and limitation of motion. Everyone who reaches old age develops some degree of DJD. The hip joint has the worse prognosis of any joint because the disorder is permanent and progressive.

Degenerative joint disease cannot be cured but may be controlled with appropriate treatment.[17,58] The goals of treatment are to relieve the symptoms and to manage the effects of progression of the pathologic process. The symptoms involved are pain, inflammatory reaction in the synovial membrane, and decreased range of motion. The pathologic process may cause limb deformity, reduce function, and increase pain.

Bed rest may be necessary to reduce compression and shearing on the joint and to allow inflammation to subside. Ice packs over the joint may be needed to reduce pain and inflammation in acute cases. Traction may also be of value at this time to stretch the capsule and to separate the joint surfaces.[42] In the chronic situation heat, such as that provided by ultrasound, may be used to decrease pain and inflammation. This treatment should be followed by gentle, active assistive range-of-motion exercises and mobilization to restore and maintain normal capsular mobility. The joint should be moved through the full range of motion several times during the day to prevent capsular contraction. Extensibility of the iliotibial band and hamstrings, quadriceps, adductor, and hip flexor muscles should be increased. Excessive joint use and excessive motion in the extreme ranges should be avoided. A muscle-strengthening program for the hip abductor and hip and knee extensor muscles should be developed and isometric exercises may be best to avoid excessive joint motion.[42] Ambulatory devices such as a cane, crutches, or a walker may be needed to reduce the weight-bearing load on the joint. A raised heel may reduce pain by preventing full hip extension during gait. A long ischial weight-bearing caliper brace with a leather cuff may be used to reduce the load on the hip joint.[42] The patient should be provided with an educational program that addresses any need to decrease body weight, change adverse body mechanics, and avoid exercises and activities that place too much stress on the joint.

Therapeutic drugs such as salicylates in the form of aspirin or sodium salicylate may be used to decrease pain and inhibit cartilage deterioration.[17,42] More powerful drugs may be effective for relieving pain but may also produce unwanted side effects. Local interarticular injection of corticosteroids to relieve pain should be used sparingly if at all because of their potential serious side effects.[17]

Several types of surgical intervention may be used to relieve the pain and correct the deformity. These include an osteotomy, total or hemiarthroplasty, or arthrodesis.[17,63] An osteotomy (Fig. 7–71) is used to change the alignment of the bone architecture and improve the biomechanics of the joint. The hemiarthroplasty (Fig. 7–72) may be used for a patient who has de-

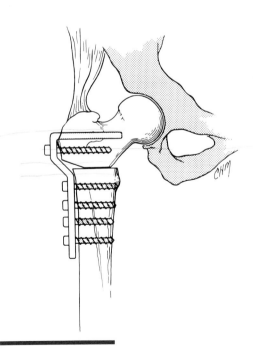

FIGURE 7–71 ■ Final appearance of the varus osteotomy after partial wedge resection and interfragmentary compression. (From Santore RF: Intertrochanteric osteotomy. *In* The Hip and Its Disorders. [Steinberg ME, ed]. Philadelphia: WB Saunders, 1991, Fig. 35–11.)

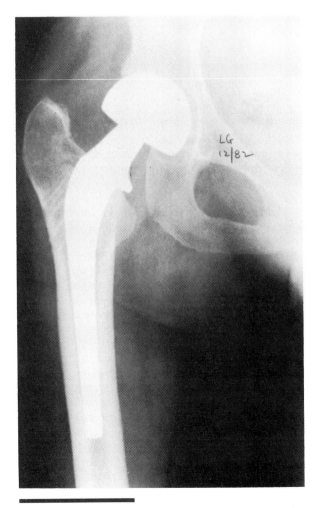

FIGURE 7–72 ■ Vitallium cap arthroplasty performed for painful degenerative arthritis after Legg-Calvé-Perthes disease. (From Stillwell WT: The Art of Total Hip Arthroplasty. Orlando: Grune & Stratton, 1987, p 171.)

generation of the femoral head but a nearly normal acetabulum in cases of significant joint degeneration. The total hip arthroplasty (Fig. 7–73) involves replacement of both the femoral head and neck and the acetabulum. A hip arthrodesis is a fusion of the joint that relieves the pain, but all joint motion is lost. Because the longevity of the total hip replacement is limited, this surgical procedure is usually reserved for the older, less active patient.

Rehabilitation of the patient after surgery is important. Such rehabilitation, however, begins with preoperative evaluation and instruction. The presurgical patient should have the affected hip range of motion and strength evaluated. Any contractures and deformities should be noted. Leg lengths should be measured. The presence of other joint problems should be recorded. The strength of the other limbs and gait pattern should also be evaluated.

Before surgery the patient should be instructed in use and protection of the affected hip in respect to the specific surgical procedure. The patient should be instructed in all postoperative exercises to be performed. These may include coughing and breathing exercises, ankle range-of-motion exercises, bed mobility exercises, and lower limb strengthening and range-of-motion activities. Proper positioning of the hip should be stressed. After the surgery, the exercises and activities learned preoperatively should be performed in a progressive manner in accordance with the patient's tolerance, the surgical procedure performed, and the surgeon's wishes. A general plan of postoperative treatment progression for a patient who has received a total hip replacement follows. Physical therapy should be given twice a day.[64]

Day 1
1. At all times use a device such as pillow or wedge to prevent adduction.

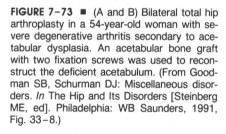

**FIGURE 7–73** ■ (A and B) Bilateral total hip arthroplasty in a 54-year-old woman with severe degenerative arthritis secondary to acetabular dysplasia. An acetabular bone graft with two fixation screws was used to reconstruct the deficient acetabulum. (From Goodman SB, Schurman DJ: Miscellaneous disorders. *In* The Hip and Its Disorders [Steinberg ME, ed]. Philadelphia: WB Saunders, 1991, Fig. 33–8.)

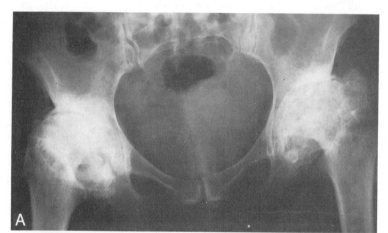

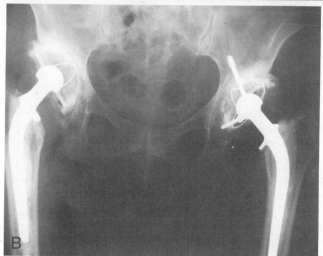

2. Perform active foot and ankle range-of-motion exercises.
3. Perform strengthening exercises for upper limbs and nonoperated limb.
4. Perform isometric exercises of major muscle groups on operated side.
5. Perform breathing exercises.
6. Review proper methods of moving in bed.
7. Transfer to built-up chair cautiously.
8. Avoid any position of instability.
9. Move toward nonoperated side during bed activities and transfers.
10. Avoid painful movements.
11. Avoid internal rotation.

Day 2
1. Initiate partial weight bearing as tolerated.
2. Begin active range of motion:
   Avoid adduction.
   Limited flexion to 30 degrees.
   Avoid extension if anterior surgical approach was used.
   Avoid resisted abduction for 3 weeks if trochanteric osteotomy was done.

Day 3
1. Continue all previous exercises.
2. Begin resisted range of motion noting previous precautions.
3. Begin home instructions related to commode transfers, automobile transfers, and so forth.

Day 4
1. Continue previous activities.
2. Progress hip flexion to 60 degrees on day 6 and to 90 degrees on day 10.

*Do not exceed 90 degrees of flexion.*

Upon return to home, the patient should be instructed to avoid specific activities and positions. These include:

*Do not* sit in low chairs.
*Do not* sleep on your side.
*Do not* cross your legs.
*Do not* flex your hips more than 90 degrees.
*Do not* force your hips to bend.
*Do not* drive.
*Do not* climb into bath tub.
*Do not* squat.
*Do not* do exercises not given by the physical therapist.

The patient should be told that after the first 6 weeks some of these prohibitions may be changed. The patient should be instructed to watch for infection and to avoid too much vigorous activity, such as running and jumping.

# Acute Injuries

## Fracture

Acute injuries to the hip present a major problem. This is especially true if the injury involves a fracture. Fractures of the femur in the hip joint area include extracapsular fractures involving the area of the trochanters and intracapsular fractures, which are fractures of the femoral neck (Fig. 7–74). The complications of hip fractures are the most troublesome of all fractures in the body.

The femoral neck of the child is strong; therefore, unless the trauma is severe, fracture in the femoral neck region is rare in children. However, those that do occur are serious. In the adult, femoral fractures are much more frequent. They are especially common in women above the age of 60 years because the bone is weakened by osteoporosis. Falls are a major cause of hip fractures in older individuals.[65]

The most common clinical feature of fracture of the proximal end of the femur is immediate and often severe pain in the groin area. Attempted movements of the hip are painful and tenderness occurs in the area anterior to the femoral neck. The fractured limb assumes a position of external rotation and appears to be shortened by 2 to 3 cm. The limb with an extracapsular fracture appears more shortened than one with an intracapsular fracture. No swelling is obvious in the intracapsular fracture, but the extracapsular fracture is swollen. Ecchymosis develops in a few days after the trauma in both cases.

Complications of a fracture in the hip joint area include avascular necrosis, nonunion or delayed union of the fracture, and degenerative joint disease, as well as the other major complications of fracture. Approximately 50% of patients have unsatisfactory results, including the previously listed complications. Intracapsular fractures have a much worse prognosis than extracapsular fractures. The disorder often changes the lifestyle of an ambulatory person to one who becomes bedridden. Physical and mental deterioration may follow and in some instances the patient may die within 6 months after the traumatic incident.[66]

In the elderly patient death may occur after a fracture. Therefore one of the goals in the treatment of the elderly patient who has suffered a hip fracture is early mobilization to avoid complications of bed rest. A second goal, especially

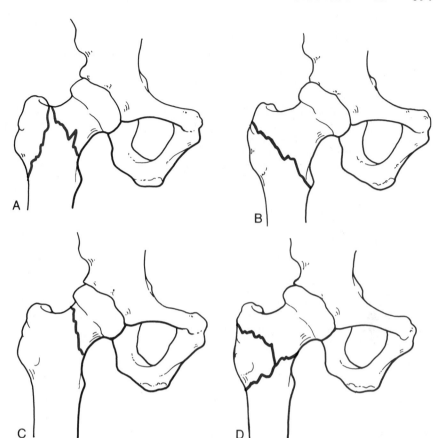

**FIGURE 7–74** ■ Classification of femoral neck fractures. (A) basal, pertrochanteric; (B) intertrochanteric; (C) subcapital, transcervical; (D) comminuted, subtrochanteric.

in adults, is to reduce the chance of avascular necrosis occurring. Other goals are reduction and stabilization of the fracture and restoration of normal hip function. In children the latter two goals are important. The key to successful surgery is adequate reduction of the fracture in response to the forces that caused it.[17] For displaced fractures, reduction and pinning of the fracture should be done as soon as possible. Reduction in many fractures is obtained by flexing, adducting, and then internally rotating and extending the hip.[17] Calandruccio reported that all nondisplaced and 94% of displaced fractures healed after treatment with multiple pin fixation[61] (Fig. 7–75). Impacted fractures are usually stable, and the younger patient is treated without surgery.[17] In the elderly, however, Laros recommends that pin fixation be used in both impacted and nondisplaced fractures.[67]

After the fracture is pinned, the patient can be permitted out of bed within a few days, and Salter states that partial weight bearing may be allowed within a few weeks.[17] Gartland and Laros recommend non–weight bearing until the fracture is healed, up to 6 months.[15,67] Patients with extracapsular fractures or with osteoporosis should be treated with nails or screws and a plate along the shaft of the femur.[15,61] If the head cannot be reduced satisfactorily or is avascular, a prosthesis should be used.[15,17] The goals of rehabilitation are to improve ambulation, reduce pain, improve hip motion, and increase muscle strength. The entire body, especially the ipsilateral lower limb joint, should be treated. Partial weight bearing should gradually progress to full weight bearing when the fracture is healed and the abductor muscles are sufficiently strong. Functional activities may begin about 2 weeks postoperatively. If a total hip replacement is used, the previous total hip replacement protocol should be followed.

Internal fixation of the hip fracture is often performed in the young adult. This procedure allows the patient to become ambulatory within a week; however, weight bearing on the involved limb must be restricted until the fracture

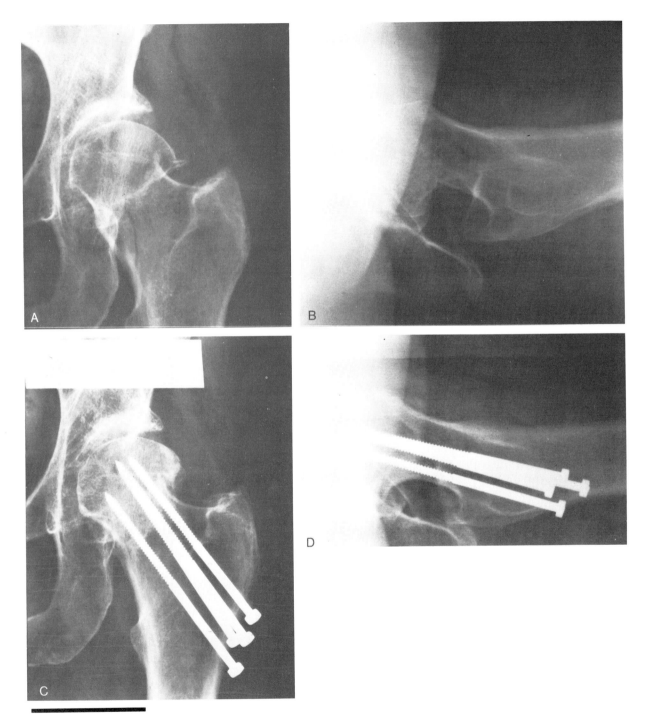

**FIGURE 7-75** ■ Radiographs of a 62-year-old female who fell at home. (A) Anteroposterior appearance after fracture, subcapital and comminuted. (B) Lateral appearance. (C) Anteroposterior appearance 9 months after closed reduction and internal fixation with four Knowles' pins. The fracture has healed in excellent position. (D) Lateral view. (From Berquist TH, Coventry MB: The pelvis and hips. *In* Imaging of Orthopedic Trauma and Surgery [Berquist TH, ed]. Philadelphia: WB Saunders, 1986, Fig. 4–79.) © Mayo Foundation, Rochester, Minnesota.

site is stable. Within the first week after surgery the patient should perform isometric exercises for the gluteus minimum, gluteus maximum, and quadriceps, and the feet and ankles should perform active range-of-motion exercises. A trapeze above the patient can help the patient exercise the upper limbs as well as get on the bed pan more easily. Active assistive hip range-of-motion exercises should be started approximately 3 days after surgery. The patient should be provided with home instructions to perform the exercises and functional activities such as using a raised toilet seat.

## Soft Tissue Injuries

Muscle strains are common traumatic injuries. The hip adductor muscles are the most injured muscle group, but the iliopsoas and hamstring muscles are also commonly injured. The injury may be caused by too much elongation of the muscle, by strong muscle contraction, or by a combination of a strong contraction opposed by an elongating force. The area of muscle tearing becomes very painful. Bleeding and swelling along the muscle may occur. Immediate treat-

**Table 7–12.** TREATMENT OF MUSCLE-TENDON INJURIES OF THE HIP AND PELVIS

| Treatment | Stage I—acute injury (first 24 to 72 hours) | Stage II—subsidence of acute symptoms | Stage III—able to do isometric exercises pain free | Stage IV—range of motion 95% of normal, strength 75% of normal leg | Stage V—strength 90% of unaffected leg |
|---|---|---|---|---|---|
| Rest | X | | | | |
| Ice | X | | | | |
| Compression | X | | | | |
| Elevation | X | | | | |
| Nonsteroidal anti-inflammatory medication | X | | | | |
| Contrast treatments | | X | X | | |
| Hydrotherapy | | X | X | | |
| Active range of motion | | X | X | | |
| Ultrasound | | X | X | | |
| Muscle stimulation | | X | X | | |
| Isometric exercise | | X | X | | |
| Well leg and upper extremity exercise | | X | X | X | |
| Isotonic and isokinetic exercises | | | X | X | |
| Stretching | | | X | X | |
| Aerobic activity | | | X | X | |
| Balance and coordination drill | | | | X | |
| Agility training | | | | X | |
| Sport-specific exercises | | | | X | |
| Jogging | | | | X | |
| Straight-ahead sprinting | | | | X | |
| Return to sports | | | | | X |
| Maintenance flexibility and strength program | | | | | X |

From Nichols JA, Hershman EB: The Lower Extremity and Spine in Sports Medicine, Vol. 2. St. Louis: CV Mosby, 1986, p 1142.

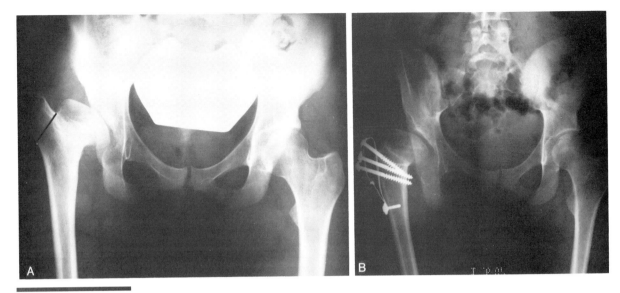

FIGURE 7-76 ■ Radiographs of a 26-year-old woman with dysplasia of the right hip. (A) Preoperative figure. Note differences in the acetabulum and proximal end of femur between the right and left sides. (B) View of trochanteric displacement osteotomy. (Courtesy of Frank Gottschalk, M.D.)

ment of a muscle strain should include ice, elevation, and compression. Anti-inflammatory agents reduce the pain and help limit inflammation.[12] Cryotherapy and compression treatment should be given daily. Crutch walking with reduced stress on the specific muscle may be necessary. Heat treatment in the form of hot packs, ultrasound, or hydrotherapy should not begin before the third day after the injury. Some therapists continue with cryotherapy for a much longer time. As the pain subsides, mild pain-free range-of-motion activities can be started. Strengthening exercises and gait activities can begin when the range of motion is pain free. Immediately after active exercises, cryotherapy should be used. When the injured muscle is approximately equal to the opposite uninjured muscle, the rehabilitation is complete; however, stretching and strengthening exercises should continue to prevent reinjury. Several common treatment modalities are presented in Table 7–12.

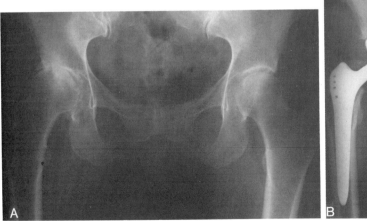

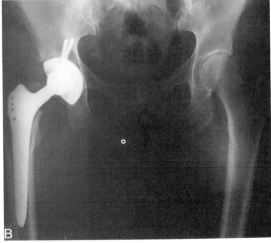

FIGURE 7-77 ■ Radiographs of a 64-year-old woman with degenerative arthrosis of the right hip. (A) Preoperative view. (B) View showing the uncemented total hip in place. (Courtesy of Frank Gottschalk, M.D.)

## CASE STUDY 1

▼The patient is a 26-year-old female with developmental dysplasia of the right hip. She had been treated for this problem as an infant. The patient had pain in the right hip area, deformity of the femoral head, and marked dysplasia of the acetabulum on the right side (Fig. 7-76A). A high-riding trochanter was also noted. The patient had a marked Trendelenburg gait.

A trochanteric displacement osteotomy was performed to improve the biomechanics of the hip abductor mechanism (Fig. 7-76B). Postoperatively, the patient's pain and gait improved. In the long term, the patient will require additional surgery because of the deformity of the hip. For 6 weeks after the surgical procedure, the patient was not allowed to flex the hip more than 45 degrees.

## CASE STUDY 2

▼The patient is a 64-year-old female with degenerative arthrosis of the right hip (Fig. 7-77A). She had difficulty functioning and was specifically limited in walking as well as dressing and other activities of daily living. Because her pain was no longer controlled with anti-inflammatory medicine and other nonoperative measures, she received an uncemented total hip replacement (Fig. 7-77B).

The patient's function improved satisfactorily with the postoperative physical therapy. The therapy program consisted of full weight bearing the day after surgery and specifically strengthening of the quadricep and hip abductor muscles. Later the patient progressed to riding an exercise bicycle and pool therapy.

## SUMMARY

This chapter reviewed the anatomy of the hip joint region, presented a variety of disorders found in the area, discussed differential diagnosis of the disorders, and provided methods for evaluation and treatment of these disorders. Although this chapter does not include all disorders related to the hip joint, it addresses a majority of the common problems. The causes, progression, and treatment of most of the disorders of the hip involve mechanical loading of the region. A thorough knowledge of biomechanics of the hip is essential for understanding care of the hip.

## References

1. Chung SMK: Hip Disorders in Infants and Children. Philadelphia, Lea & Febiger, 1981.
2. Singleton MC, LeVeau BF: The hip joint—structure, stability, and stress: a review. Phys Ther 55:957–973, 1975.
3. Harty M: The anatomy of the hip joint. In Surgery of the Hip Joint, 2nd ed (Tronzo RG, ed), Vol I. New York, Springer-Verlag, 1984, pp 45–74.
4. Harris NH: Acetabular growth potential in congenital dislocation of the hip and some factors upon which it may depend. Clin Orthop 119:99–106, 1976.
5. Ogden JA: Hip development and vascularity: relationship to chondro-osseous trauma in the growing child. In The Hip: Proceedings of the Ninth Open Scientific Meeting of The Hip Society, 1981 (Salvati EA, ed). St. Louis: CV Mosby, 1981, pp 139–187.
6. Moseley HF: Disorders of the hip. Clin Symp 5:35–60, 1983.
7. Muckle DS, Bentley G, Deane G, et al: Basic sciences of the hip. In Femoral Neck Fractures and Hip Joint Injuries (Muckle DS, ed). New York: John Wiley & Sons, 1977, pp 1–54.
8. Scoles PV: Pediatric Orthopedics in Clinical Practice, 2nd ed. Chicago: Year Book Medical, 1982, pp 141–157.
9. Dee R: Structure and function of hip joint innervation. Ann Coll Surg Engl 45:357–374, 1969.
10. Harty M: Anatomy. In The Hip and Its Disorders (Steinberg ME, ed). Philadelphia: WB Saunders, 1991, pp 27–46.
11. Caldwell DS, Rice JR: Evaluation of the patient with hip pain. In Common Disorders of the Hip (Singleton MC, Branch EF, eds). New York: Haworth, 1986, pp 35–47.
12. Kessler FM, Hertling D: The hip. In Management of Common Musculoskeletal Disorders, 2nd ed (Hertling D, Kessler RM, eds). Philadelphia: JB Lippincott, 1990, pp 272–297.
13. McGann WA: History and physical examination. In The Hip and Its Disorders (Steinberg ME, ed). Philadelphia: WB Saunders, 1991, pp 72–87.
14. Heath RD: Physical diagnosis of the hip. In Surgery of the Hip Joint, 2nd ed (Tronzo RG, ed), Vol I. New York: Springer-Verlag, 1984, pp 27–43.
15. Gartland JJ: Fundamentals of Orthopedics, 4th ed. Philadelphia: WB Saunders, 1987.
16. MacEwen GD, Ramsey PL: The hip. In Pediatric Orthopedics (Lovell WW, Winter RB, eds), Vol 2. Philadelphia: JB Lippincott, 1986, pp 703–780.
17. Salter RB: Textbook of Disorders and Injuries of the Musculoskeletal System, 2nd ed. Baltimore: Williams & Wilkins, 1983.
18. Helms CA, Hoagland FT, Murray W, et al: Computed tomography of the hip. In The Hip: Proceedings of the Thirteenth Open Scientific Meeting of The Hip Society, 1985 (Fitzgerald RH Jr, ed). St. Louis: CV Mosby, 1985, pp 143–149.
19. Genant HK, Jergenson HE, Heller M, et al: Magnetic resonance imaging of the hip. In The Hip: Proceedings of the Thirteenth Open Scientific Meeting of The Hip Society, 1985 (Fitzgerald RH Jr, ed). St. Louis: CV Mosby, 1985, pp 150–156.
20. Exner GU: Ultrasound screening for hip dysplasia in neonates. J Pediatr Orthop 8:656–660, 1988.
21. Castelein RM, Souter AJM: Ultrasound screening for congenital dysplasia of the hip in newborns: its value. J Pediat Orthop 8:666–670, 1988.
22. Bialik V, Reuveni A, Pery M, et al: Ultrasonography in developmental displacement of the hip: a critical analysis of our results. J Pediar Orthop 9:154–156, 1989.
23. Clarke NMP, Clegg J, Al-Chalabi AN: Ultrasound screening of hips at risk for CDH. J Bone Joint Surg [Br] 71:9–12, 1989.
24. Miralles M, Gonzales G, Pulpeiro JR, et al: Sonography of the painful hip in children: 500 consecutive cases. AJR 152:579–582, 1989.
25. Koski JM, Anttila PH, Isomäki HA: Ultrasonography of

the adult hip joint. Scand J Rheumatol 18:113–117, 1989.

26. Roberts WN, Williams RB: Hip pain. Prim Care 15(4):783–793, 1988.

27. McBeath AA: Some common causes of hip pain. Postgrad Med 77:189–195, 198, 1985.

28. Merritt CRB, Bluth EI: Techniques for diagnostic imaging. Postgrad Med 77:56–63, 67, 1985.

29. MacEwen GD, Mason B: Evaluation and treatment of congenital dislocation of the hip in infants. Orthop Clin North Am 19:815–820, 1988.

30. Tachdjian MO: Pediatric Orthopedics, 2nd ed, Vols 1 and 2. Philadelphia: WB Saunders, 1990.

31. Tonnis D, Storch K, Ulbrich H: Results of newborn screening for CDH with and without sonography and correlation of risk factors. J Pediatr Orthop 10:145–152, 1990.

32. Adams JC, Hamblen DL: Outline of Orthopedics, 11th ed. New York: Churchill-Livingstone, 1990.

33. Hazel JR, Beals RK: Diagnosing dislocation of the hip in infancy. West J Med 151:39–41, 1989.

34. Staheli LT: Management of congenital hip dysplasia. Pediatr Ann 18:25–32, 1989.

35. Miranda L, Palomo JM, Monzonis J, et al: Prevention of congenital dislocation of the hip in the newborn. J Pediatr Orthop 8:671–675, 1988.

36. Sherlock DA, Gibson PH, Benson MKD: Congenital subluxation of the hip. J Bone Joint Surg [Br] 67:390–398, 1985.

37. Jolley MN, Salvati EA, Wilson PD Jr: Septic arthritis. In Surgery of the Hip Joint, 2nd ed (Tronzo RG, ed), Vol II. New York: Springer-Verlag, 1987, pp 73–84.

38. Griffin PP: Acute septic arthritis of the hip in childhood. In The Hip: Proceedings of the Seventh Open Scientific Meeting of The Hip Society, 1979 (Sledge CB, ed). St. Louis: CV Mosby, 1979, pp 89–104.

39. Johanning K: Coxa vara infantum. I. Clinical appearance and arteriological problems. Acta Orthop Scand 21:273, 1951.

40. Salter RB, Thompson GH: Legg-Calvé-Perthes disease. J Bone Joint Surg [Am] 66:479–489, 1984.

41. Harrison HM, Burwell RG: Perthes' disease: a concept of pathogenesis. Clin Orthop 156:115–127, 1981.

42. Turek SL: Orthopedics: Principles and Their Application, Vols 1 and 2. Philadelphia: JB Lippincott, 1984.

43. Trueta J: The normal vascular anatomy of the femoral head during growth. J Bone Joint Surg [Br] 39:358–394, 1957.

44. Caffey J: The early roentgenographic change in coxa plana: significance of pathogenesis. Am J Roentgenol 103:620–634, 1968.

45. Scoles PV: Developmental disorders of the hip. In Pediatric Orthopedics in Clinical Practice (Scoles PV, ed). Chicago: Year Book Medical, 1988, pp 159–178.

46. Nakamura T, Kawai Y, Nakamura S, et al: Evaluation of the containment and noncontainment treatment of Legg-Calvé-Perthes disease. In The Hip—Clinical Studies and Basic Research (Ueno R, Akamatsu N, Itami Y, et al, eds). Amsterdam: Elsevier Science Publishers, 1984, pp 153–156.

47. King-Echternach D: Hip problems in children and adolescents. In Physical Therapy of the Hip (Echternach JL, ed). New York: Churchill-Livingstone, 1990, pp 191–204.

48. Evans IK, Deluca PA, Gage JR: A comparative study of ambulation-abduction bracing and varus derotation osteotomy in the treatment of severe Legg-Calvé-Perthes' disease in children over 6 years of age. J Pediatr Orthop 8:676–682, 1988.

49. Harrison MHM, Turner MH, Smith DN: Perthes' disease. J Bone Joint Dis 648:3–11, 1982.

50. MacEwen GD: Treatment of Legg-Calvé-Perthes' disease. AAOS Instructional Course Lectures, Vol 30 (Murray GD, ed). St. Louis: CV Mosby, 1981, pp 75–84.

51. Saudek CE: The hip. In Orthopedic and Sports Physical Therapy (Gould JA III, ed). St. Louis: CV Mosby, 1990, pp 347–394.

52. Fackler CD: Nonsurgical treatment of Legg-Calvé-Perthes disease. In AAOS Instructional Course Lectures (Barr Jr JS, ed). St. Louis: CV Mosby, 1989, 38:305–307.

53. Bowen JR, Foster BK, Hartzell CR: Legg-Calvé-Perthes' disease. Clin Orthop 185:97–108, 1984.

54. Spock A: Transient synovitis of the hip joint in children. Pediatrics 24:1042–1049, 1959.

55. Lee DMG: Slipped capital femoral epiphysis (SCFE). In Disorders of the Hip (Lee DMG, ed). Philadelphia: JB Lippincott, 1983, pp 173–192.

56. Katz JF: Legg-Calvé-Perthes disease. In Management of Hip Disorders in Children (Katz JF, Siffert RS, eds). Philadelphia: JB Lippincott, 1983, pp 159–181.

57. Raman D, Haslock I: Trochanteric bursitis—a frequent cause of "hip" pain in rheumatoid arthritis. Ann Rheum Dis 41:602–603, 1982.

58. Kaplan PE, Tanner ED: Hip joint dysfunction. In Musculoskeletal Pain and Disability (Kaplan PE, Tanner ED, eds). Norwalk, CT: Appleton & Lange, 1989, pp 165–181, 1989.

59. Steinberg ME: Avascular necrosis of the femoral head. In Surgery of the Hip Joint, 2nd ed (Tronzo RG, ed), Vol II. New York: Springer-Verlag, 1987, pp 1–30.

60. Graham J, Wood SK: Aseptic necrosis of bone following trauma. In Aseptic Necrosis of Bone (Davidson JK, ed). New York: American Elsevier, 1976, pp 111–146.

61. Calandruccio RA: Classification of femoral neck fractures in the elderly as pathologic fractures. In The Hip: Proceedings of the Eleventh Open Scientific Meeting of The Hip Society, 1983 (Hungerford DS, ed). St. Louis: CV Mosby, 1983, pp 9–33.

62. Ficat RP: Treatment of avascular necrosis of the femoral head. In The Hip: Proceedings of the Eleventh Open Scientific Meeting of The Hip Society, 1983 (Hungerford DS, ed). St. Louis: CV Mosby, 1983, pp 279–295.

63. Nunley JA, Oser ER: Surgical treatment of arthritis of the hip. In Common Disorders of the Hip (Singleton MC, Branch EF, eds). New York: Haworth, 1986, pp 59–83.

64. Echternach JD: Physical Therapy of the Hip. New York: Churchill Livingstone, 1990, p 189.

65. Hielema F: Hip fracture: an epidemic challenging the physical therapist. In Common Disorders of the Hip (Singleton MC, Branch EF, eds). New York: Haworth, 1986, pp 49–58.

66. Sandler, RB: Etiology of primary osteoporosis: an hypothesis. J Am Geriatr Soc 26:209–213, 1978.

67. Laros GS: The role of osteoporosis in intertrochanteric fractures. Orthop Clin North Am 11:525–537, 1980.

## Bibliography

Alavi A: Bone scans in hip disorders. In Hip Disorders in Infants and Children (Chung SMK, ed). Philadelphia: Lea & Febiger, 1981, pp 87–92.

Allwright SJ, Cooper RA, Nash P: Trochanteric bursitis: bone scan appearance. Clin Nucl Med 13:561–564, 1988.

Amstutz HC, Christie J, Mensch JS: Treatment of osteonecrosis of the hip. In The Hip: Proceedings of the Third

Open Scientific Meeting of the Hip Society (Amstute HC, ed). St. Louis: CV Mosby, 1975, pp 19–34.

Ando M, Gotok E: Significance of inguinal folds for diagnosis of congenital dislocation of the hip in infants aged three to four months. J Pediat Orthop 10:331–334, 1990.

Aufranc OE, Harris JM, McKay SJ, et al: Rehabilitation in hip arthroplasty. In Revision Total Hip Arthroplasty (Turner RH, Scheller AD Jr, eds). New York: Grune & Stratton, 1982, pp 379–395.

Berkeley ME, Dickson JH, Cain TE, et al: Surgical therapy for congenital dislocation of the hip in patients who are twelve to thirty-six months old. J Bone Jt Surg [Am] 66:412–420, 1984.

Berquist TH, Coventry MB: The pelvis and hips. In Imaging of Orthopedic Trauma and Surgery (Berquist TH, ed). Philadelphia: WB Saunders, 1986, pp 181–279.

Bobechko WP: Infections of bones and joints. In Pediatric Orthopedics, 2nd ed (Lovell WW, Winter RB, eds), Vol 1. Philadelphia: JB Lippincott, 1986, pp 437–456.

Bomalaski JS, Schumacher HR: Arthritis and allied conditions. In The Hip and Its Disorders (Steinberg ME, ed). Philadelphia: WB Saunders, 1991, pp 501–526.

Boyle KL, DeMarco D: Orthopedia disorders in children and their physical therapy management. In Pediatric Physical Therapy (Tecklin JS, ed). Philadelphia: JB Lippincott, 1989.

Broughton NS, Brougham DI, Cole WG, et al: Reliability of radiological measurements in the assessment of the child's hip. J Bone Jt Surg [Br] 71:6–8, 1989.

Brown ML: Skeletal scintigraphy. In Imaging of Orthopedic Trauma and Surgery (Berquist TH, ed). Philadelphia: WB Saunders, 1986, pp 16–20.

Butt WP: Standard radiographic examination. In Orthopaedic Radiology (Park WM, Hughes SPF, eds). Boston: Blackwell Scientific Publications, 1987, pp 3–44.

Canale ST: Intracapsular fractures. In The Hip and Its Disorders (Steinberg ME, ed). Philadelphia: WB Saunders, 1991, pp 144–159.

Catterall A: The natural history of Perthes' disease. J Bone Joint Surg [Br] 53:37–53, 1971.

Catterall A: Pathology and classification. In The Hip: Proceedings of the Thirteenth Open Scientific Meeting of the Hip Society, 1985 (Fitzgerald RH Jr, ed). St. Louis: CV Mosby, 1985, pp 12–16.

Catterall A: The place of femoral osteotomy in the management of Legg-Calvé-Perthes disease: results of long-term follow-up. In The Hip: Proceedings of the Thirteenth Open Scientific Meeting of the Hip Society, 1985 (Fitzgerald RH Jr, ed). St. Louis: CV Mosby, 1985, pp 24–27.

Catterall A, Chir M: Perthes' disease. In The Hip and Its Disorders (Steinberg ME, ed). Philadelphia: WB Saunders, 1991, pp 419–439.

Chung SMK: Embrology growth and development. In The Hip and Its Disorders (Steinberg ME, ed). Philadelphia: WB Saunders, 1991, pp 3–26.

Collins DN, Nelson CL: Infections of the hip. In The Hip and Its Disorders (Steinberg ME, ed). Philadelphia: WB Saunders, 1991, pp 648–668.

Cooperman DR, Stulberg SD: Ambulatory containment treatment in Legg-Calvé-Perthes disease. In The Hip: Proceedings of the Thirteenth Open Scientific Meeting of the Hip Society, 1985 (Fitzgerald RH, ed). St. Louis: CV Mosby, 1985, pp 38–62.

Crawford A: Neurologic disorders. In The Hip and Its Disorders (Steinberg ME, ed). Philadelphia: WB Saunders, 1991, pp 440–469.

Crawford AH: Osteotomies in the treatment of slipped capital femoral epiphysis. In Instructional Course Lecturers, Vol XXXIII (Murray JA, ed). St. Louis: CV Mosby, 1984, pp 327–349.

Cyriax J: Textbook of Orthopedic Medicine, 8th ed, Vol 1. London: Bailliére Tindall, 1982, pp 376–391.

D'Ambrosia RD: The hip. In Musculoskeletal Disorders (D'Ambrosia RD, ed). Philadelphia: JB Lippincott, 1986, pp 447–489.

Dalinka MK, Neustadter LM: Radiology of the hip. In The Hip and Its Disorders (Steinberg ME, ed). Philadelphia: WB Saunders, 1991, pp 56–71.

de los Reyes AH, Pujalte PM, Yabut SM, et al: A treatment protocol for avascular necrosis of the femoral head. In The Hip—Clinical Studies and Basic Research (Ueno R, Akamatsu N, Itami Y, et al, eds). New York: Elsevier Science Publishers, 1984, pp 171–175.

Doherty M: Common regional pain syndromes II. The Practitioner 233:1467, 1989.

Drummond DS: Congenital and developmental deformities of the hip. In The Hip and Its Disorders (Steinberg ME, ed). Philadelphia: WB Saunders, 1991, pp 372–389.

Dvonch VM, Bunch WH, Scoles PV: The hip. In Pediatric Orthopedics in Clinical Practice (Scoles PV, ed). Chicago: Year Book Medical, 1988, pp 140–158.

Erken EHW, Katz K: Irritable hip and Perthes' disease. J Pediatr Orthop 10:322–326, 1990.

Fackler CD: Nonsurgical treatment of Legg-Calvé-Perthes' disease. In AAOS Instructional Course Lectures, Vol 38 (Barr JS Jr, ed). St. Louis: CV Mosby, 1989, pp 305–307.

Ferguson AB Jr: Orthopedic Surgery in Infancy and Childhood. Baltimore: Williams & Wilkins, 1975.

Ferguson AB Jr: Pathophysiology of Legg-Calvé-Perthes disease. In The Hip: Proceedings of the Thirteenth Open Scientific Meeting of the Hip Society, 1985 (Fitzgerald RH Jr, ed). St. Louis: CV Mosby, 1985, pp 3–11.

Goodman SB, Schurman DJ: Miscellaneous disorders. In The Hip and Its Disorders (Steinberg ME, ed). Philadelphia: WB Saunders, 1991, pp 683–704.

Grogan DP, Sackett JR, Ogden JA: Infection of the hip. In The Hip and Its Disorders (Steinberg ME, ed). Philadelphia: WB Saunders, 1991, pp 354–371.

Henderson RC, Renner JB, Sturdivant MC, et al: Evaluation of magnetic resonance imaging in Legg-Calvé-Perthes disease: a prospective, blinded study. J Pediatr Orthop 10:289–297, 1990.

Hettinga DL: Inflammatory response of synovial joint structures. In Orthopedic and Sports Physical Therapy (Gould JA III, ed). St. Louis: CV Mosby, 1990, pp 87–118.

Jenkins DB: Hollinshead's Functional Anatomy of the Limbs and Back, 6th ed. Philadelphia: WB Saunders, 1991.

Johnson ND, Wood BP, Noh KS, et al: MR imaging anatomy of the infant hip. AJR 153:127–133, 1989.

Kemp HS, Boldero JL: Radiological changes in Perthes' disease. Br J Radiol 39:744–760, 1966.

Kenna C, Murtagh J: Patrick or Fabere test. Aust Fam Physician 18:375, 1989.

Koski JM: Ultrasonographic evidence of hip synovitis in patients with rheumatoid arthritis. Scand J Rheumatol 18:127–131, 1989.

Magee DJ: Orthopedic Physical Assessment. Philadelphia: WB Saunders, 1987, pp 239–265.

Marcus ND, Enneking WF, Massam RA: The silent hip in idiopathic aseptic necrosis. J Bone Joint Surg [Am] 55:1351–1366, 1973.

MacEwen GD: Conservative treatment of Legg-Calvé-Perthes condition. In The Hip: Proceedings of the Thirteenth Open Scientific Meeting of the Hip Society, 1985 (Fitzgerald RH, ed). St. Louis: CV Mosby, 1985, pp 17–23.

Moore FH: Examining infant's hips—can it do harm? J Bone Joint Surg [Br] 71:4–5, 1989.

Morrissy RT: In situ fixation of chronic slipped capital femoral epiphysis. *In* Instructional Course Lectures, Vol XXXIII (Murray JA, ed). St. Louis: CV Mosby, 1984, pp 319–327.

Morrissy RT: Congenital dislocation of the hip. *In* The Hip and Its Disorders (Steinberg ME, ed). Philadelphia: WB Saunders, 1991, pp 313–334.

Mosca VS: Pitfalls in diagnosis. Pediatr Ann 18:12–23, 1989.

Muckle DS: Femoral Neck Fractures and Hip Joint Injuries. New York: John Wiley & Sons, 1977.

Muckle DS: Fractures of the femoral neck, part I. *In* Femoral Neck Fractures and Hip Joint Injuries (Muckle DS, ed). New York: John Wiley & Sons, 1977, pp 55–99.

Mukherjee A, Fabry G: Evaluation of the prognostic indices in Legg-Calvé Perthes disease: statistical analysis of 116 hips. J Pediatr Orthop 10:153–158, 1990.

Nichols JA, Hershman EB: The Lower Extremity and Spine in Sports Medicine, Vol 2. St. Louis: CV Mosby, 1986.

Ogden JA: Development and growth of the hip. *In* Management of Hip Disorders in Children (Katz JF, Siffert RS, eds). Philadelphia: JB Lippincott, 1983, pp 1–32.

Pavlik A: Stirrups as an aid in the treatment of congenital dysplasia of the hip in children. J Pediatr Orthop 9:157–159, 1989.

Peckham R, Dvonch VM: Coxa vara. Orthopedics 12:891–892, 1989.

Phillips EK: Evaluation of the hip. Phys Ther 55:975–981, 1975.

Raman D, Haslock I: Trochanteric bursitis—a frequent cause of "hip" pain in rheumatoid arthritis. Ann Rheum Dis 41:602–603, 1982.

Raney RB, Brashear HR Jr: Shand's Handbook of Orthopedic Surgery, 8th ed. St. Louis: CV Mosby, 1971.

Reckling FW, Mohn MP: Hip and thigh. *In* Orthopedic Anatomy and Surgical Approaches (Reckling FW, Reckling JN, Mohn MP, eds). St. Louis: Mosby Year Book, 1990, pp 307–355.

Rosse C, Clawson DK: The Musculoskeletal System in Health and Disease. Hagerstown, MD: Harper & Row, 1980.

Saito S, Shimizu N, Sakai M, et al: Natural history of idiopathic avascular necrosis of the femoral heads (IANF)—its collapse and prognosis. *In* The Hip—Clinical Studies and Basic Research (Ueno R, Akamatsu N, Itami Y, et al, eds). New York: Elsevier Science Publishers, 1984, pp 167–170.

Salvati EA: Neonatal and infantile septic arthritis. *In* Surgery of the Hip Joint, 2nd ed (Tronzo RG, ed), Vol I. New York: Springer-Verlag, 1984, pp 387–404.

Santore RF: Intertrochanteric osteotomy. *In* The Hip and Its Disorders (Steinberg ME, ed). Philadelphia: WB Saunders, 1991, pp 726–754.

Schoenecker PL, Strecker WB: Congenital dislocation of the hip in children. J Bone Jt Surg [Am] 66:21–27, 1981.

Schuler P, Feltes E, Kienapfel H, et al: Ultrasound examination for the early determination of dysplasia and congenital dislocation of neonatal hips. Clin Orthop 258:18–26, 1990.

Singleton MC: The hip joint: Clinical oriented anatomy—a review. *In* Common Disorders of the Hip (Singleton MC, Branch EF, eds). New York: Haworth, 1986, pp 1–14.

Sorbie C, Zalter R: Bioengineering studies of the forces transmitted by joints. *In* Biomechanics and Related Bioengineering Topics (Kenedi RM, ed). Oxford: Pergamon, 1965, pp 359–367.

Speer DPL: Slipped capital femoral epiphysis. *In* The Hip and Its Disorders (Steinberg ME, ed). Philadelphia: WB Saunders, 1991, pp 390–418.

Springfield DS, Enneking WF: Role of bone grafting in idiopathic aseptic necrosis of the femoral head. *In* The Hip: Proceedings of the Third Open Scientific Meeting of the Hip Society (Amstutz HC, ed). St. Louis: CV Mosby, 1975, pp 3–18.

Staheli LT: Acetabular dysplasia: treatment by pelvic osteotomy. *In* The Hip and Its Disorders (Steinberg ME, ed). Philadelphia: WB Saunders, 1991, 335–353.

Staheli LT, Coleman SS, Hensinger RN, et al: Congenital hip dysplasia. *In* Instructional Course Lectures, Vol XXXIII (Murray JA, ed). St. Louis: CV Mosby, 1984, pp 350–363.

Steinberg ME, Steinberg DR: Avascular necrosis of the femoral head. *In* The Hip and Its Disorders (Steinberg ME, ed). Philadelphia: WB Saunders, 1991, pp 623–647.

Stuberg WA, Koehler A, Wichita M, et al: Comparison of femoral torsion assessment using goniometry and computerized tomography. Pediatr Phys Ther 1:115–118, 1989.

Svenningsen S, Terjesen T, Auflem M, et al: Hip motion related to age and sex. Acta Orthop Scand 60:97–100, 1989.

Tonnis D: Normal values of the hip joint for the evaluation of x-rays in children and adults. Clin Orthop 119:39–47, 1976.

Tronzo RG: Fractures of the hip in adults. *In* Surgery of the Hip Joint (Tronzo RG, ed), Vol II. New York: Springer-Verlag, 1987, pp 163–338.

Tronzo RG: Surgery of the Hip Joint, Vol I. New York: Springer-Verlag, 1984.

Tronzo RG: Surgery of the Hip Joint, Vol II. New York: Springer-Verlag, 1987.

Weinstein SL: Legg-Calvé-Perthes' disease: results of long-term follow-up. *In* The Hip: Proceedings of the Thirteenth Open Scientific Meeting of the Hip Society, 1985 (Fitzgerald RH Jr, ed). St. Louis: CV Mosby, 1985, pp 28–37.

Weinstein SL: Slipped capital femoral epiphysis. In AAOS Instructional Course Lectures, Vol 33 (Murray JA, ed). St. Louis: CV Mosby, 1984, pp 310–318.

Weinstein SL: Background on slipped capital femoral epiphysis. *In* Instructional Course Lectures. Vol XXXIII (Murray JA, ed). St. Louis: CV Mosby, 1984, pp 310–318.

# CHAPTER

# *Eight*

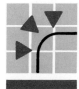

## Knee

### KENT E. TIMM

## INTRODUCTION

This chapter presents orthopaedic physical therapy for the knee in four general sections: anatomy, pathomechanics and differential diagnoses, evaluation, and treatment.The first part of the chapter details the basic clinical sciences of embryology, arthrology, and myology as related to the development and biological construction of the knee and its components. This information is complemented by a presentation of the connective tissues of the knee complex and of the biomechanics that govern its basic functions. The second section expands on the presentation of normal anatomy to describe the principles and manifestations of the pathomechanics of the knee. The specific pathomechanics of knee fractures, ligament sprains, meniscal injuries, tibiofibular instability, degenerative conditions, muscle problems, bursitis, patellar syndromes, reflex sympathetic dystrophy, and amputations are detailed with an emphasis on differential diagnosis.

The third and fourth sections of the chapter are designed to expand the knowledge from the basic sciences into the realm of clinical practice. These sections discuss the process of clinical evaluation of knee disorders with the goal of generating an accurate differential diagnosis. The subjective evaluation components of the patient's history, clinical observation, and medical visualization and the objective evaluation components of clinical neurology, functional mobility testing, structural stability testing, palpation, and performance assessment via isokinetic dynamometry are presented in detail. The fourth section of the chapter reviews the general intervention strategies available to the orthopaedic physical therapist in a clinical setting, with special emphasis on the acute, subacute, and chronic stages of tissue healing, and then presents examples of selected intervention strategies for the management of common knee disorders, specifically cruciate ligament reconstruction, meniscal injury, patellar pain syndromes, and total knee arthroplasty. The chapter concludes with a collection of case studies designed to consolidate the learning experience.

## ANATOMY

### Embryology

The human knee, which has been subjected to the greatest degree of clinical and scientific investigation of any joint in the body,[1] begins to develop during the fourth week of embryonic life as the hind limb buds appear lateral to the primitive L-1 to S-2 vertebral segments. The early limb bud is a mass of mesenchymal cells that arise from the lateral somatopleure and are covered by a layer of ectoderm. The mesenchymal cells are pluripotential and further differentiate into osteoblasts, fibroblasts, myoblasts, or chondroblasts as fetal development continues. The muscles of the limb bud develop in situ rather than by an invasion of myotomal cells from the embryonic somite.

Muscle development results from the differentiation of primitive mesenchymal cells into myoblasts, which then become multinucleate muscle cells. Each muscle typically receives innervation from more than one embryonic vertebral segment and each primitive segmental nerve tends to innervate more than one muscle of a limb bud.

The original orientation of the hind limb bud is such that the hips are externally rotated, the patellae face posteriorly, and the soles of the feet face forward. The limb buds gradually rotate down into the fetal position to become the configuration of normal human lower extremity. The rotational movement of the limb bud toward the anatomic position explains the spiraling nature of the segmental dermatomal, myotomal, and sclerotomal distributions in the human leg and is also responsible for the angles of anteversion and varus of the femoral neck relative to the shaft of the femur and for the magnitude of external torsion of the tibial shaft as compensation for the internal torsion of the femur.

The bones of the lower extremity also develop in situ as the condensation of mesenchymal cells. The mesenchyme first differentiates into chondrocytes that form a cartilage template for the developing bone. The cartilage model is gradually replaced by bone tissue through the process of endochondral ossification. Primary ossification centers are first found in the diathesial regions of the femur and tibia extending toward the proximal and distal ends of each bone. The patella develops as a separate center of ossification. Secondary centers appear at the peripheral edges of the femur and tibia to form the bony epiphyses, which are separated from the diathesial ossification centers by the embryonic epiphyseal plates. The epiphyseal plates are cartilaginous regions that continue to develop chondrocytes for the purpose of endochondral ossification. This process adds new bone to the diathesial ossification centers and the bone continues to grow until the epiphyseal plate closes in response to hormonal changes during the second decade of postpartum life.

The knee joint itself develops as a cleft between the mesenchymal rudiments of the embryonic femur and tibia in the eighth week of life. Vascular mesenchyme becomes isolated within the joint area and serves as the precursor tissue for the components of the articular complex. Layers of interzonal mesenchyme adjacent to the developing epiphyses differentiate into chondrocytes, which secrete cartilage matrix and become the articular cartilage surfaces of the tibia, patella, and femur; fibrochondrocytes, which form the meniscal fibrocartilages; and fibrocytes, which produce the collagen fibers that ultimately become the synovial joint capsule and the knee ligaments. The joint capsule, menisci, and cruciate and collateral ligaments appear as separate and distinct structures within the knee by the 18th week of developmental life. The reader may refer to Williams and Warwick[2] for a more detailed description of the embryology of the knee complex.

## Arthrology

The tibiofemoral joint is a bicondyloid synovial articulation that functions mechanically as a sliding hinge that involves multiple centers of rotation as pivot points for the primary actions of extension and flexion and for the conjunct motions of internal and external rotation.[1,3] The femoral condyles represent segments of a pulley that are convex in both the sagittal and frontal anatomic planes, and the corresponding tibial condyles are relatively flat and require deepening by the meniscal cartilages to form an efficient articular surface.[1,3] The medial tibial condyle is biconcave, and the lateral tibial condyle is concave in the frontal plane and convex in the sagittal plane.[3] The situation of relative incongruence of the tibial and femoral surfaces, with need for the menisci to form a congruent articulation, predisposes to functional instability of the tibiofemoral joint unless the knee musculature can provide dynamic stabilization against external force loads.[1]

The femoral condyles converge anteriorly to form the intercondylar notch, which is the surface for the patellofemoral articulation.[1,3] The articular surface of the patella is divided into seven facets, which exist as proximal, middle, and distal horizontal pairs on the medial and lateral sides of the posterior surface of the patella, along with one medial perpendicular facet known as the "odd" facet (Fig. 8–1).[2,3] The facets serve as efficient joint load distribution mechanisms as the patella tracks superiorly and inferiorly along the intercondylar notch during the motions of knee extension and flexion, respectively.[1,3]

## Muscles

The muscle groups of the knee complex are depicted in Figure 8–2A–I.

### Quadriceps

The quadriceps muscle complex is formed by the rectus femoris, vastus lateralis, vastus intermedius, and vastus medialis muscle groups. The rectus femoris is a large bipennate muscle with two heads. The muscle originates from the anteroinferior iliac spine and from a groove above the edge of the acetabulum and inserts into the superior border of the patella as part of the common quadriceps tendon.[2,4] The rectus femoris is innervated by the femoral nerve, which receives fibers from the second, third, and fourth lumbar nerves.[2,4] By its anatomic nature, the rectus femoris is a biarticular muscle that influences human movement at both the hip and the knee joints.

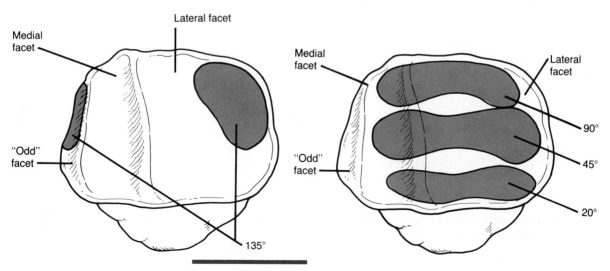

**FIGURE 8–1** ■ Articular surfaces of the patella.

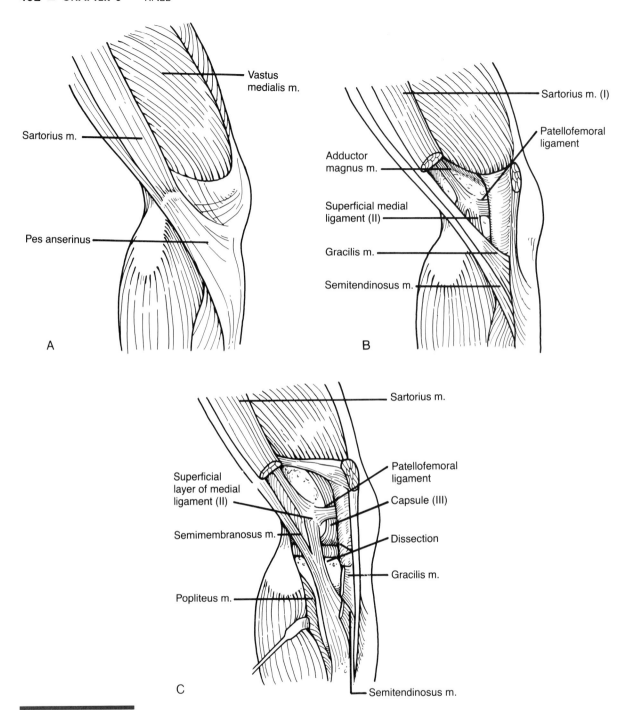

**FIGURE 8-2** ■ (A) Anatomy of the knee complex (medial view). (B) Anatomic dissection—superficial (medial view). (C) Anatomic dissection—deep (medial view).

The muscle is a prime mover for hip flexion and knee extension and a secondary mover for hip abduction.[4]

The vastus lateralis originates from the lateral surface of the femur just below the greater tro-

chanter and from the upper half of the linea aspera.[2,4] The muscle inserts into the lateral and superior borders of the patella as part of the quadriceps tendon.[2,4] The vastus lateralis is innervated by the femoral nerve, which contains

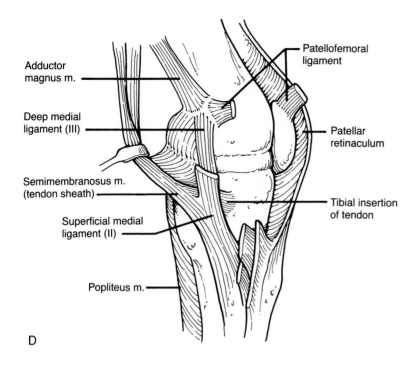

Adductor magnus m.

Deep medial ligament (III)

Semimembranosus m. (tendon sheath)

Superficial medial ligament (II)

Popliteus m.

Patellofemoral ligament

Patellar retinaculum

Tibial insertion of tendon

D

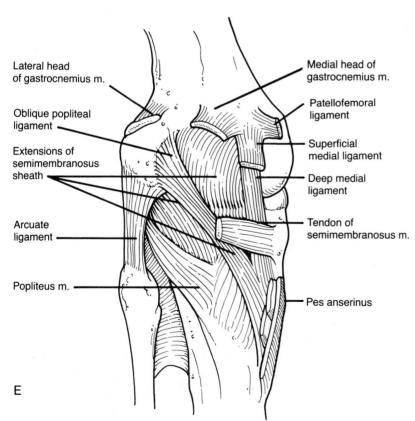

Lateral head of gastrocnemius m.

Oblique popliteal ligament

Extensions of semimembranosus sheath

Arcuate ligament

Popliteus m.

Medial head of gastrocnemius m.

Patellofemoral ligament

Superficial medial ligament

Deep medial ligament

Tendon of semimembranosus m.

Pes anserinus

E

**FIGURE 8-2** ■ *Continued* (D) Anatomic dissection—deep (anteromedial view). (E) Semimembranosus insertions.
*Illustration continued on following page*

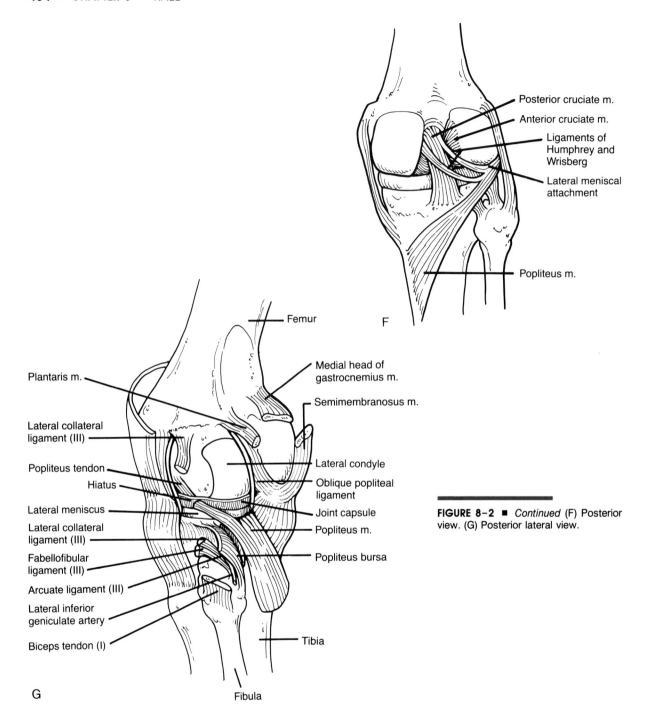

Posterior cruciate m.

Anterior cruciate m.

Ligaments of Humphrey and Wrisberg

Lateral meniscal attachment

Popliteus m.

F

Femur

Medial head of gastrocnemius m.

Semimembranosus m.

Plantaris m.

Lateral collateral ligament (III)

Popliteus tendon

Hiatus

Lateral meniscus

Lateral collateral ligament (III)

Fabellofibular ligament (III)

Arcuate ligament (III)

Lateral inferior geniculate artery

Biceps tendon (I)

Lateral condyle

Oblique popliteal ligament

Joint capsule

Popliteus m.

Popliteus bursa

Tibia

G

Fibula

**FIGURE 8-2** ■ *Continued* (F) Posterior view. (G) Posterior lateral view.

branches of the second, third, and fourth lumbar nerves, and is a prime mover for knee extension.[2,4]

The vastus intermedius lies deep to the rectus femoris and between the medial and lateral vastus muscles. The vastus intermedius stems from the anterior and lateral aspect of the femur and passes to insertion on the superior border of the patella as a part of the quadriceps tendon.[2,4] The muscle is innervated by the femoral nerve, which contains branches of the second, third, and fourth lumbar nerves, and is a prime mover for knee extension.[2,4]

The final component of the quadriceps complex is the vastus medialis (see Fig. 8-2A). It originates from the linea aspera and the supra-

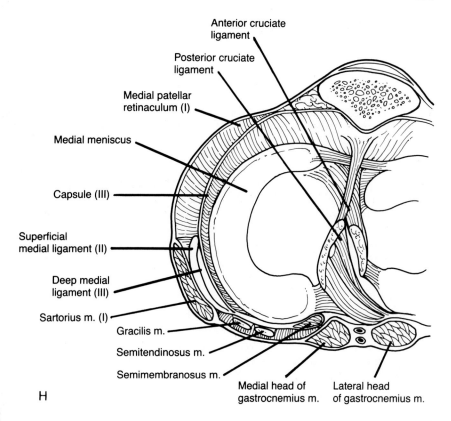

Anterior cruciate ligament

Posterior cruciate ligament

Medial patellar retinaculum (I)

Medial meniscus

Capsule (III)

Superficial medial ligament (II)

Deep medial ligament (III)

Sartorius m. (I)

Gracilis m.

Semitendinosus m.

Semimembranosus m.

Medial head of gastrocnemius m.

Lateral head of gastrocnemius m.

H

**FIGURE  8–2  ■** *Continued*  (H) Cross section of the medial side of the knee. (I) Cross section of the lateral side of the knee.

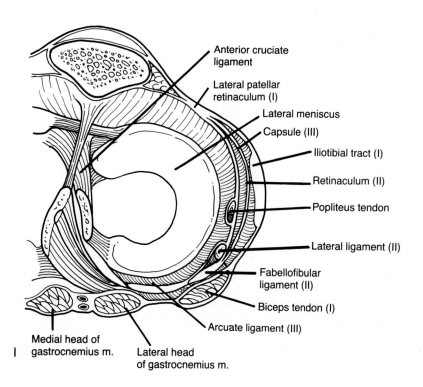

Anterior cruciate ligament

Lateral patellar retinaculum (I)

Lateral meniscus

Capsule (III)

Iliotibial tract (I)

Retinaculum (II)

Popliteus tendon

Lateral ligament (II)

Fabellofibular ligament (II)

Biceps tendon (I)

Arcuate ligament (III)

Medial head of gastrocnemius m.

Lateral head of gastrocnemius m.

I

condylar line of the femur and inserts into the medial border of the patella through the quadriceps tendon.[2,4] As with the other quadriceps muscle, the vastus medialis is innervated by the femoral nerve, which contains branches of the second, third, and fourth lumbar nerves.[2,4] The muscle is a prime mover for knee extension. A subcomponent of the muscle, the vastus medialis obliquus (VMO), has the direct function of pulling the patella medially during the action of knee extension.[2] The ability of the VMO to exert a medially directed force on the patella is vital to the normal arthrokinematics of the patellofemoral joint. This medially directed force counteracts a component lateral force from the vastus lateralis to ensure normal patellar tracking during knee extension.

## Hamstrings

The hamstring complex is formed by the biceps femoris, semitendinosus, and semimembranosus muscle groups, all of which are biarticular muscles that influence movements at both the hip and the knee joints. In an anatomic analogy to the biceps brachii of the upper extremity, the biceps femoris has two heads that originate from the medial facet of the tuberosity of the ischium and from the lateral lip of the linea aspera of the femur.[2,4] The muscle inserts on the lateral condyle of the tibia (see Fig. 8–2I) and the head of the fibula.[2,4] The long head of the biceps femoris is innervated by two branches from the tibial portion of the sciatic nerve complex, which contains fibers from the first, second, and third sacral nerves.[2,4] The short head of the biceps femoris is innervated by branches from the peroneal portion of the sciatic nerve complex, which contains fibers from the fifth lumbar nerve and the first and second sacral nerves.[2,4] Only the long head of the biceps femoris acts at the hip joint, where it is a prime mover for hip extension and external rotation.[4] Both heads of the biceps femoris act as prime movers for knee flexion and external tibial rotation.[4]

The semitendinosus originates from the medial facet of the tuberosity of the ischium, by a common tendon with the long head of the biceps femoris, and inserts on the upper part of the medial surface of the tibia (see Fig. 8–2B, C, E, and H).[2,4] The semitendinosus is also categorized as a unit of the pes anserine functional complex, along with the sartorius and the gracilis muscle groups. The semitendinosus is innervated by two branches of the tibial portion of the sciatic nerve complex, which contains fibers from the fifth

lumbar nerve and the first and second sacral nerves.[2,4] The semitendinosus is a prime mover for hip extension, knee flexion, and internal tibial rotation and is a secondary mover for hip internal rotation.[4]

The semimembranosus stems from the lateral facet of the tuberosity of the ischium and inserts on the posterior medial aspect of the medial condyle of the tibia (see Fig. 8–2C–E, G, and H).[2,4] The muscle is innervated by the tibial portion of the sciatic nerve complex, which includes fibers from the fifth lumbar nerve and the first and second sacral nerves.[2,4] Like the semitendinosus, the semimembranosus is a prime mover for hip extension, knee flexion, and internal tibial rotation and assists the action of internal rotation at the hip.[4]

## Pes Anserine Complex

The pes anserine group (see Fig. 8–2A–D and H) is a functional complex formed by the semitendinosus, sartorius, and gracilis muscles. The group derives its name from a common region of insertion on the tibia whose tendinous arrangement resembles that of the webbed foot of a goose or swan. The sartorius is a biarticular muscle that originates from the anterior superior iliac spine and the upper half of the notch just below it and passes to insertion on the lower anterior part of the medial surface of the tuberosity of the tibia with the tendons of the semitendinosus and gracilis muscles.[2,4] The sartorius is innervated by two branches of the femoral nerve, which contain fibers from the second and third lumbar nerves.[2,4] At the hip the muscle group assists the activities of flexion, abduction, and external rotation.[4] At the knee the sartorius is a secondary mover for internal tibial rotation and may also assist with knee flexion or extension, depending on the exact site of the pes anserine insertion, which may vary between individuals, relative to the instant center of tibiofemoral joint motion.[4] The sartorius is known from ancient anatomic text as the "tailor's" muscle and is also the longest muscle in the human body.[4]

The third member of the pes anserine complex, the gracilis muscle group, originates from the anterior margins of the lower half of the symphysis pubis and from the upper half of the pubic arch.[2,4] The gracilis inserts into the upper portion of the medial surface of the body of the tibia, just below the condyle, with the tendons of the semitendinosus and the sartorius.[2,4] The muscle receives innervation from the anterior division of the obturator nerve, which contains fibers from the third and fourth lumbar nerves.[2,4] The gracilis is a biarticular muscle that is a prime mover for hip adduction and internal rotation and a secondary mover for knee flexion and internal tibial rotation.[4]

### Popliteus

The popliteus (see Fig. 8–2C–G and I) originates as a tripartite tendon from the lateral aspect of the lateral condyle of the femur, from the posteromedial aspect of the head of the fibula, and from the posterior horn of the lateral meniscus.[2,4] The popliteus inserts at the posteromedial side of the tibia, just superior to the origin of the soleus muscle group.[2,4] The muscle group receives innervation from a branch of the tibial nerve, which contains fibers from the fourth and fifth lumbar nerves and from the first sacral nerve.[2,4]

The functions of the popliteus vary in relation to the status of the lower extremity kinetic chain. When the kinetic chain is open, meaning that the lower extremity is non–weight bearing, the popliteus is the prime mover for internal tibial rotation.[4] When the kinetic chain is closed, meaning that the lower extremity is in a weight-bearing state, the popliteus is the prime mover for external rotation of the femur on the tibia.[4] Therefore, the popliteus functions as both a dynamic stabilizer of the tibiofemoral joint and a modulator of the screw-home rotational mechanism during knee extension activities (Fig. 8–3).[4]

### Gastrocnemius

The gastrocnemius (see Fig. 8–2H and I) originates as two heads whose tendons stem from the posterior aspect of the medial and lateral femoral condyles.[2,4] The muscle inserts into the posterior surface of the calcaneus as part of the Achilles tendon.[2,4] The gastrocnemius is innervated by branches of the tibial nerve, which contain fibers from the first and second sacral nerves.[2,4]

As with the popliteus, the actions of the gastrocnemius vary with the status of the lower extremity kinetic chain. In a non–weight-bearing, open chain state, the muscle functions as a prime, mover for plantar flexion at the ankle complex and as a secondary mover for knee flexion.[4] In a weight-bearing, closed chain state, the gastrocnemius becomes a secondary mover for knee joint extension and a prime mover for ankle plantar flexion.[4] The magnitude of the

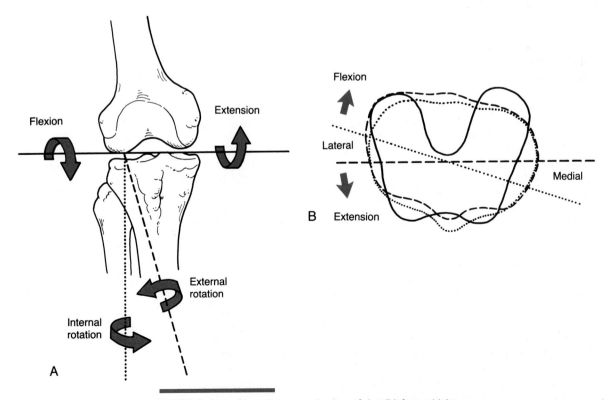

**FIGURE 8–3 ■** Screw-home mechanism of the tibiofemoral joint.

function of the muscle as a knee extensor while weight bearing is in direct proportion to the degree of ankle dorsiflexion; a greater mechanical advantage for knee extension via the gastrocnemius is created with increased ankle dorsiflexion.[4] Technically, the gastrocnemius is quadriarticular because it crosses the axes of the tibiofemoral, patellofemoral, talocrural, and subtalar joints.

## Connective Tissue

### Menisci

The human menisci (Fig. 8–4A–F) are fibrocartilaginous structures situated between the femoral condyles and the tibial plateaus of the tibiofemoral articulation. The menisci, which may be referred to as the genicular semilunar cartilages,[3] serve to increase the area of contact between the femoral condyles and the tibial plateaus but are disproportionate in size. The medial meniscus is smaller and semicircular, and the lateral meniscus is larger and forms a nearly complete circle over the lateral tibial plateau (see Fig. 8–4A and B).[5]

Structurally, the menisci are wedge shaped (see Fig. 8–4C) and composed of a relatively vascular peripheral portion and a nearly avascular inner region. The menisci develop as very cellular and highly vascularized tissue masses in the prenatal stages of life but experience a progressive decrease in vascularity from the central substance to the peripheral margin postnatally.[5,6]

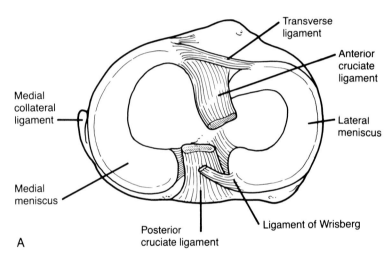

A

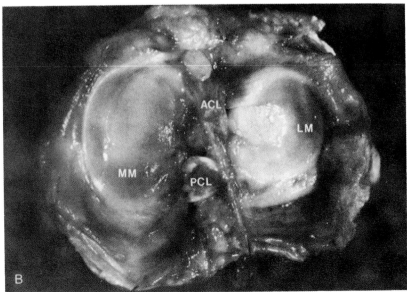

B

FIGURE 8–4 ■ (A) Menisci of the knee—tibial plateau. (B) Tibial plateau—position and shape of medial and lateral menisci. (From Nicholas JA, Hershman EB: The Lower Extremity and Spine in Sports Medicine. St. Louis, CV Mosby, 1986, pp. 686–687.)

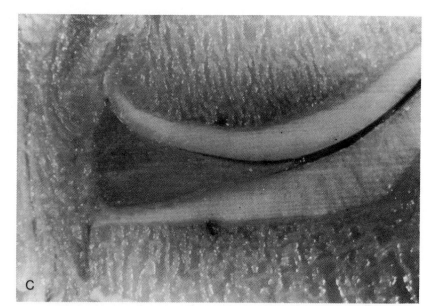

FIGURE 8-4 ■ *Continued* (C) Frontal section of medial compartments of the knee. From Nicholas JA, Hershman EB: The Lower Extremity and Spine in Sports Medicine. St. Louis, CV Mosby, 1986, pp 686–687.) (D) Vascularity of the meniscus. (From Arnoczky SP, Warren RF: Microvasculature of the human meniscus. Am J Sports Med 10(2):90–95, 1982.)
*Illustration continued on following page*

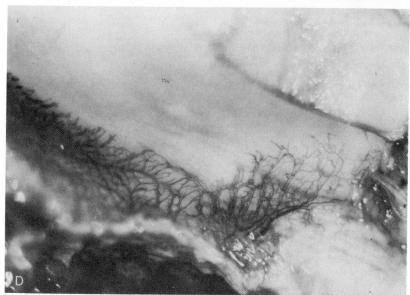

At skeletal maturity the peripheral portion constitutes 10 to 30% of the total structure and is composed of dense connective tissue (type I and II collagen with some elastin), active fibrochondrocytes, and a nonhyaline cartilaginous matrix of proteoglycans (glycosaminoglycan, chondroitin 4-sulfate, chondroitin 6-sulfate, keratin sulfate, and hyaluronic acid).[5] Some studies have discovered the existence in the meniscal matrix of another glycoprotein, thrombospondin, which mediates cell-matrix interactions in the processes of human homeostasis and helps regulate the repair or regeneration of damaged vascular structures.[5]

The peripheral regions of the menisci are serviced by a circumferential capillary plexus that arises from branches of the medial, middle, and lateral geniculate arteries (see Fig. 8–4D–F).[6,7] This plexus affects only the most peripheral 10 to 25% of the meniscus.[6,7] The midsubstance and internal regions of the menisci are avascular and depend exclusively on diffusion of oxygen and nutrients along osmotic gradients from the peripheral regions for tissue maintenance. It is theorized that weight-bearing activities during childhood development are responsible for the progressive degeneration of the vascular supply

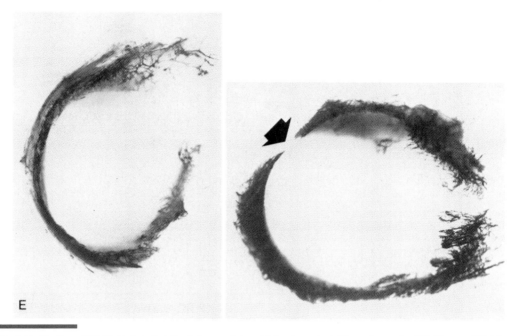

**FIGURE 8-4** ■ *Continued* (E) Superior aspects of the medial and lateral menisci. (From Arnoczky SP, Warren RF: Microvasculature of the human meniscus. Am J Sports Med 10(2): 90–95, 1982.)

to these regions.[7] The meniscal periphery also receives innervation from type I and II nerve endings, whereas the internal regions are completely aneural.[5]

Mechanically, the menisci function as viscoelastic structures, secondary to the composition of the matrix. The matrix exists as two phases: a solid phase (26% wet weight) of the collagen connective tissue and proteoglycan substances and a fluid state (74% wet weight) of water and interstitial electrolytes.[5] The solid phase is essentially a fiber-reinforced composite material that is porous and permeable to allow fluid movement within its internal structure when the menisci are subjected to external forces.[5,6] This biphasic status permits different degrees of controlled tissue deformation in the forms of time-dependent creep, stress relaxation, flow viscosity, and elastic

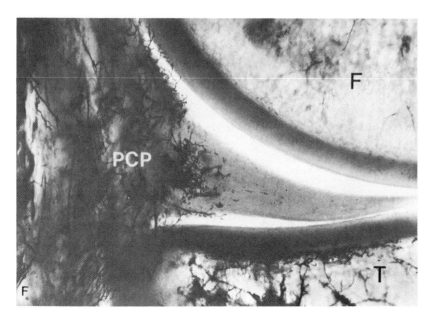

**FIGURE 8-4** ■ *Continued* (F) Frontal section 5 mm thick of the medial compartment of the knee. (From Arnoczky SP, Warren RF: Microvasculature of the human meniscus. Am J Sports Med 10(2):90–95, 1982.)

response, the basis of viscoelastic tissue behavior.[5-7] Such behavior enables the menisci to resist or equilibrate external compression, shear, and tensile forces, so that they function as effective shock-absorbing and load-distributing structures during weight-bearing activities at the tibiofemoral joint.[1,8] The role of physiologic shock absorber is the primary function of the meniscal cartilages.

Anatomically, the menisci are attached to the joint capsule and to several other structures in the knee by various ligament systems. The anterior and posterior horns of both menisci are attached to corresponding regions of the tibial condyle and the intercondylar fossae. The two anterior horns are interconnected by a transverse ligament and by a common ligament that also connects the horns to the patella via the infrapatellar fat pad.[3] The corollary ligaments attach the peripheral margins of both menisci to the corresponding medial and lateral margins of the tibial plateaus.[8] Meniscopatellar fibers stem from the lateral edges of the corollary ligaments to create another route of attachment between the menisci and the patella.[3] The medial meniscus blends with the substance of the medial collateral ligament, receives a fibrous slip from the semimembranosus tendon, and is also attached to the anterior cruciate ligament at the site of the anterior horn.[3,8] The lateral meniscus is attached to the popliteus tendon and to the posterior cruciate ligament by way of a meniscofemoral ligament.[3,8] Whereas the meniscal periphery is fairly stable because of the corollary ligament system, the internal edges of the menisci are unattached and mobile.[1,8]

Although attached to the tibial plateaus, the menisci do move during knee joint activities. The menisci move in coordination with the motions of the femoral condyles as an elastic coupling to transmit joint loading forces.[3] During tibiofemoral flexion, the medial meniscus is pulled posteriorly by the semimembranosus expansion as the lateral meniscus is being moved posteriorly through its connection to the popliteal tendon.[3,8] During knee extension, both menisci are pulled anteriorly by the meniscopatellar ligaments, while the lateral meniscus receives assistance as the structure tightens from the meniscofemoral ligament attachment to the posterior cruciate ligament.[3,8] Rotatory motions of the menisci are directed by the motion of the femoral condyles during actions of tibiofemoral rotation.[3] The femoral condyles also push the menisci anteriorly during knee extension and posteriorly during flexion.[8]

### Collateral Ligaments

The medial collateral ligament (MCL), also known as the tibial collateral ligament, is a broad, flat band which arises from the medial epicondyle of the femur, immediately below the adductor tubercle, and continues distally to insert on the medial condyle and surface of the tibia (Fig. 8–5; see Figs. 8–2D, E, H and 8–4A).[2,3]

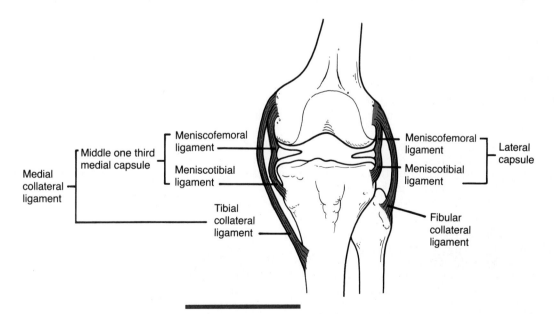

FIGURE 8–5 ■ The collateral ligaments.

The MCL blends with the connective tissue of the knee joint capsule and the medial meniscus along the path from the femur to the tibia.[2,3] It passes below the tendons of the pes anserine muscle complex but covers the medial inferior genicular artery and nerve.[2] Near the tibial insertion just below the medial condyle, the MCL blends with the anterior part of the semimembranosus tendon.[2]

The lateral or fibular collateral ligament (LCL) originates from the lateral epicondyle of the femur, just above a groove for the tendon of the popliteus muscle, and inserts on the head of the fibula at the styloid process (see Figs. 8–2F, G, I and 8–5).[2,3] The LCL is posterior to the axis of tibiofemoral joint motion. It is covered by the tendon of the biceps femoris muscle group, to which it sends a fibrous slip, and covers the popliteus tendon and the inferior lateral genicular vessels and nerve.[2] The LCL does not attach to the lateral meniscal cartilage or to the lateral side of the knee joint capsule and, therefore, is a completely extra-articular structure.[2,3]

### Anterior Cruciate Ligament

The vast majority of contemporary knee literature has been devoted to the structure, function, pathology, and rehabilitation of the anterior cruciate ligament (ACL). The ACL begins to develop along the femoral and tibial condyles between the seventh and eighth weeks of fetal life and is well developed by the ninth week.[9] The normal ACL remains isometric, meaning that it maintains a constant length, as the tibiofemoral joint moves through the normal range of knee joint motion.[10] In tibiofemoral orientation, the ACL attaches proximally to the posterior part of the medial surface of the lateral femoral condyle in the intercondylar fossa, 12 mm inferior to the level of the adductor tubercle (Fig. 8–6A; see Fig. 8–2F).[11–14] The area of origin is crescentic, with the anterior side linear and the posterior side convex, and is directed anteroinferiorly from the posterior aspect of the intercondylar shelf of the femur, along the margin of the articular cartilage of the lateral condyle. It is at an angle of 25 degrees oblique from vertical, for a distance of 23 mm.[11–14] Along the course from proximal to distal attachments, the ACL is partially surrounded by the synovial cavity, the membrane being reflected around it anteriorly, medially, and laterally, so that the ligament lacks capsular attachment along the midsubstance yet is completely intra-articular.[11–14]

The ACL courses obliquely anterior, inferior, and medial from origin to insert on the wide, depressed area in front of and lateral to the inferior aspect of the anterior spine of the medial intercondylar tubercle of the tibia (see Figs. 8–2F, H, I and 8–6B).[11–14] The distal attachment is angled and extends 30 mm posteriorly from an area 15 mm posterior to the edge of the anterior intercondylar area of the tibia, adjacent to the medial condyle, in a triangular fashion.[11–14] The insertion extends fibrous slips to the anterior and posterior horns of the lateral meniscus, to the anterior horn of the medial meniscus, and to the knee joint capsule.[11–14]

The ACL is dense connective tissue that is derived from embryonic mesenchyme and consists of type I collagen fibers similar in nature to the knee joint capsule.[2] An interlacing network of collagen fibrils 150 to 250 nm in diameter is grouped into fibers 1 to 20 $\mu$m in diameter, which are, in turn, grouped into subfascicular bundles 100 to 250 $\mu$m in diameter and enveloped by endotenon loose connective tissue.[11,13,14] Fascicles 250 $\mu$m to 1 mm in diameter are formed from the aggregation of 3 to 20 subfascicular units and are covered with peritenon loose connective tissue.[11,13,14] Although the collagen fibers and connective tissue are continuous, the fascicles are arranged into three distinct bands: anteromedial, posterolateral, and intermediate (Fig. 8–7).[13,14]

The anteromedial band originates posteriorly and superiorly in the crescentic attachment of the ACL on the medial aspect of the lateral femoral condyle and passes to the medial aspect of the intercondylar eminence to form the medial corner of the triangular insertion.[11,13,14] The posterolateral band inserts at the apex of the tibial triangle, just lateral to the midline of the intercondylar eminence, and originates from the anterior and inferior aspects of the femoral attachment.[11,13,14] The intermediate band is juxtaposed between the anteromedial and posterolateral bands to complete the crescentic proximal attachment and inserts in the midline and lateral aspects of the intercondylar eminence, just medial to the posterolateral band attachment, to become the lateral corner of the triangle and complete the tibial attachment.[11,13,14]

The ACL is supplied by segments of the middle and lateral inferior genicular arteries, which are branches of the popliteal artery, that enter at the femoral attachment and descend along the dorsum of the ligament, bifurcating proximal to the tibial spine into intercondylar arteries that supply the tibial condyles.[9,15–17] The artery segments are aligned in parallel to the collagen fas-

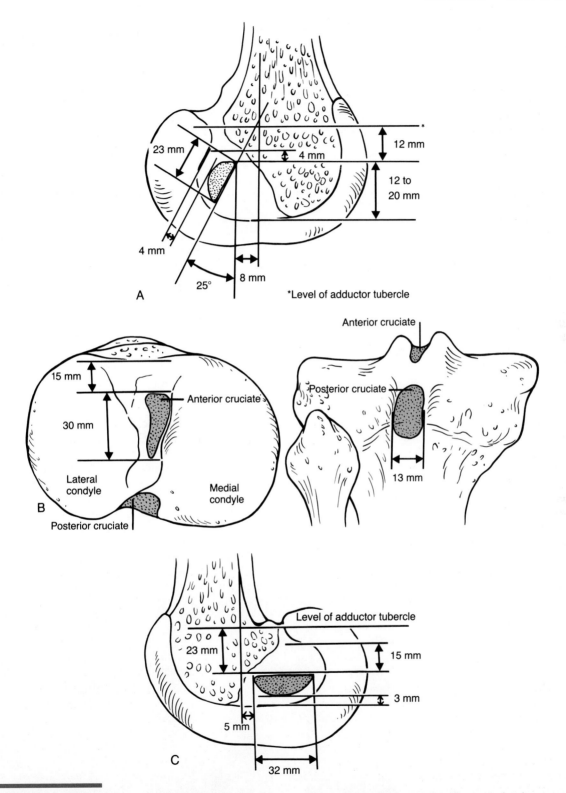

**FIGURE 8–6** ■ Anatomy of the cruciate ligaments. (A) Medial surface of the anterior cruciate ligament showing average measurements and body relations of the femoral attachment of the ACL. (B) Location of cruciate ligaments on the tibial plateau. (C) Lateral surface of the posterior cruciate ligament showing average measurements and body relations of the femoral attachment of the PCL.

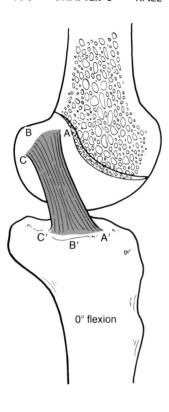

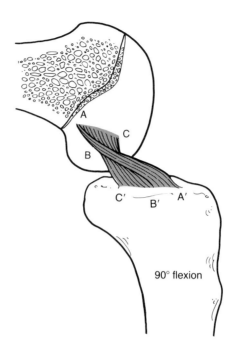

0° flexion

90° flexion

**FIGURE 8-7** ■ Changes in shape and tension of ACL components with flexion and extension. Flexion produces lengthening of the anteromedial band (A–A′) and shortening of the posterolateral aspect of the ligament (C–C′). The intermediate component (B–B′) represents transition between the anteromedial band and the posterolateral bulk.

cicles and give rise to connecting vessels that penetrate the peritenon to perfuse the subfascicular units (Fig. 8–8).[9,15-17] A vascular plexus in the synovial membrane serves as a secondary source of tissue nutrition.[15-17] The ACL is innervated by branches of the tibial nerve that lie parallel to the courses of the arterial segments

and the collagen fascicles.[11,13,14,16] Mechanoreceptors that resemble Golgi tendon organs are present throughout the ligamentous substance and create a reflex network with the knee musculature.[18] This network influences the dynamic stabilization of the knee as muscle firing is initiated whenever the ACL is subjected to excessive

**FIGURE 8-8** ■ Vascularity of the cruciate ligaments (sagittal section). (From Nicholas JA, Hershman EB: The Lower Extremity and Spine in Sports Medicine. St. Louis, CV Mosby, 1986, p 683.)

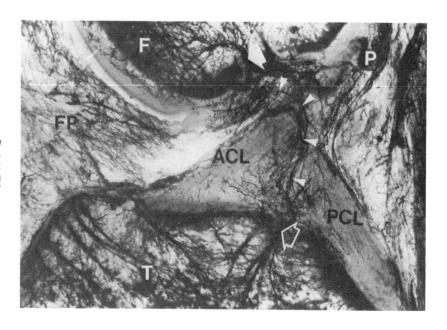

load forces.[18] Other neuronal functions include vasomotor control, nociception, and proprioception.[11,13,14,18]

## Posterior Cruciate Ligament

In contrast to its anterior counterpart, the posterior cruciate ligament (PCL) has received relatively less attention in the professional literature. The PCL is attached to the posterior intercondylar fossa of the tibia and to the posterior horn of the lateral meniscus (see Figs. 8–2F, H, I and 8–6B).[2,3] The ligament passes in an oblique medial, anterior, and superior fashion for attachment to the inner surface of the medial condyle of the femur (see Fig. 8–6C).[2,3] Overall, the PCL is 38 mm long and 13 mm wide and is composed of distinct posterolateral and anteromedial collagen fiber bands.[11,19] Like the ACL, the PCL is supplied by branches of the middle and lateral inferior genicular arteries, by a vascular plexus in the synovial membrane of the joint capsule (see Fig. 8–8), and by branches of the tibial nerve.[2]

## Joint Capsule

The joint capsule (see Fig. 8–2H and I) of the tibiofemoral articulation has been described as a cylinder with a posterior invagination.[3] On the head of the tibia, the capsule is attached to the anterior, medial, and lateral margins of the tibial condyles.[3] On the femur, the anterior margin of the capsule is attached along the edges of a shallow fossa overlying the patella, which provides the recess for the suprapatellar bursa.[3] Medially and laterally from the femur, the capsule is attached to the patella and laterally covers the intracapsular portion of the popliteus tendon.[3] On the posterior aspect of the femur, the capsule is attached at the border of the femoral articular surfaces just distal to the origin of the heads of the gastrocnemius muscle group.[3] Posteriorly, the capsular attachments course in between the intercondylar tubercles of the tibia and into the intercondylar region between the femoral condyles.[3] The capsule is attached to the inner aspect of the medial femoral condyle just below the femoral attachment of the PCL and is attached to the inner aspect of the lateral femoral condyle between the margin of the articular cartilage and the femoral attachment of the ACL.[3] The ACL is also attached to the joint capsule at its tibial insertion.[3] This arrangement of the joint capsule winding around the anterior and posterior ligaments establishes these tissues as being intra-articular but extracapsular structures.

As with all synovial joints, the knee joint capsule is composed of collagenous connective tissue that supports a synovial membrane. The synovial membrane of the knee is the largest in the human body and contains up to three plical folds.[19,20] The most pronounced plica typically runs medially below the quadriceps tendon and continues distally along the medial border of the patella and across the medial femoral condyle to insert into the patellar fat pad.[19,20]

The joint capsule is also reinforced by several extra- and intracapsular structures. The medial aspect of the capsule receives fibers from the semimembranosus, in the form of the oblique popliteal ligament, and blends with the substances of the MCL and the medial meniscus.[19,20] The lateral side of the capsule is reinforced by the popliteus muscle and its tendon and by the arcuate ligament.[19,20] The lateral capsule is also attached to the lateral meniscus. The posterior region of the joint capsule is reinforced by the medial and lateral tendons of the gastrocnemius.[2]

## Patellar Tendon (Patellar Ligament)

The patellar tendon, also referred to as the patellar ligament, is the continuation of the common tendon of the quadriceps femoris muscle group distally from the inferior pole of the patella to the tuberosity of the tibia.[2] The patellar tendon and the quadriceps tendon are actually the same tendinous structure, because the patella is by definition and anatomic derivation a sesamoid bone and does not represent separate components of the knee complex.[2] The difference in terminology reflects an artificial separation of the tendinous region superior to the patella (quadriceps tendon) from the tendinous region inferior to the patella (patellar tendon). Because the patella is a sesamoid bone existing completely within the quadriceps tendon and the connective tissue fibers of the quadriceps tendon and patellar tendon regions are continuous and the same structure, the term "patellar ligament" is inappropriate because the connective tissue region below the patella is not distinct from the quadriceps tendon and, therefore, does not represent a separate tissue connection between the tibia and the patella.

The patellar tendon is 8 cm long and also forms medial and lateral patellar retinacula where it merges with the knee joint capsule.[2] The infrapatellar fat pad separates the patellar tendon from the synovial membrane of the joint capsule.[2] The infrapatellar bursa separates the patellar tendon from the anterior aspects of the tibia proximal to the tendon insertion at the tibial tuberosity.[2]

### Iliotibial Tract

The iliotibial tract, also referred to as the iliotibial band, is the portion of the fascia lata of the thigh that arises from the tensor fascia lata muscle and the tendon of the gluteus maximus and passes distally across the knee joint complex to insert into the lateral condyle of the tibia.[2] Along its course, the iliotibial tract blends with the epimysium of the vastus lateralis muscle and with the lateral patellar retinaculum.[2] The iliotibial tract represents a triarticular (hip complex, patellofemoral joint, and tibiofemoral joint) fascial linkage system between the lower extremity and the pelvic girdle.

### Patellar Fat Pad and Knee Bursae

Several bursae and a large fat pad exist about the patellofemoral and tibiofemoral articulations and serve as shock absorption and joint lubrication structures (Fig. 8–9). The infrapatellar fat pad lies deep to the patellar tendon on the anterior aspect of the intercondylar fossa of the tibia.[3] The fat pad also makes contact with the inferior aspect of the patellar surface of the femur.[3] The fat pad is an encapsulated collection of adipose tissue that remains as a vestige of a median septum that existed in the embryonic knee complex.

The list of bursae about the knee joint includes the subpopliteus, gastrocnemius, prepatellar, suprapatellar, subcutaneous infrapatellar, and infrapatellar bursae. The subpopliteal bursa exists between the popliteus tendon and the lateral tibial condyle at the posterolateral aspect of the tibia.[8] The gastrocnemius bursa is found deep to the medial head of the gastrocnemius muscle and separates it from the medial femoral condyle.[8] The prepatellar bursa is located between the skin and the anterior surface of the patella and allows free movement of the skin over the patella during knee joint motion.[8] The suprapatellar bursa exists between the patella and the knee joint capsule just below the course of the quadriceps tendon.[8] The subcutaneous infrapatellar bursa is found between the skin and the patellar tendon.[8] Finally, the infrapatellar bursa is located between the patellar tendon and the tibial tuberosity.[8] The infrapatellar bursa is separated from the knee joint capsule and cavity by the infrapatellar fat pad.

## BIOMECHANICS

### Kinetics

Although several aspects of the knee have been fully elucidated, kinetic knowledge is complex and still incomplete. Much information is available on the quadriceps muscle group, the hamstrings muscle group, the ACL, and joint reaction forces, but information is scarce on the rotational musculature and on the PCL and collateral ligaments. It is hoped that continuing physical therapy research will correct this information insufficiency problem.

The quadriceps, which has a cross-sectional area of 148 cm[2], shortens up to 8 cm in length during a maximal volitional contraction to generate a force up to 42 kg times body weight, which is three times stronger than that of the corresponding hamstrings musculature.[1,3] Isometrically, the quadriceps produces a mean force of 151 N-m (range 120 to 291 N-m) and is most efficient at a position of 120 degrees flexion as the knee moves toward extension.[1,3] The quadriceps generates an average combined tibiofemoral and patellofemoral compression of 132 kg in knee extension and 274 kg in knee flexion.[1] The quadriceps also produces a maximal shear force

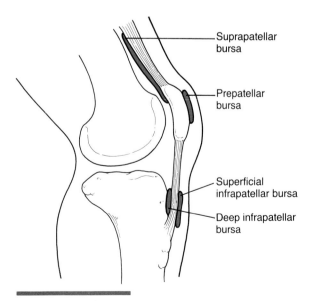

**FIGURE 8–9** ■ Location of the bursa (anterior aspect of the knee).

Suprapatellar bursa

Prepatellar bursa

Superficial infrapatellar bursa

Deep infrapatellar bursa

of 34.7 kg at a position of 15 degrees knee flexion.[1]

In contrast, the hamstrings, as a group, are 49 cm² in cross section and generate an internal contractile force of up to 15 kg times body weight.[1,3] They are most efficient at the position of 30 degrees flexion, as the knee moves toward greater flexion, where it produces an average isometric output of 93 N-m (range 39 to 157 N-m).[1,3] The hamstrings generate an average knee joint compression force of 268 kg in extension but only 10 kg at a position of 90 degrees flexion.[1] The hamstrings also produce an average shear force of 151 kg at 90 degrees knee flexion.[1] The existing information on the tibial rotatory musculature indicates that the lateral tibial rotators produce an internal contractile force of 1.8 kg times body weight and the medial tibial rotators generate an internal contractile force of 2 kg times body weight.[1,3]

Regarding actual joint forces, information is available on tibiofemoral and patellofemoral loading. During closed kinetic chain activities, the tibiofemoral joint is loaded at three times body weight in the stance phase of gait and at four times body weight during the ascension of stairs.[1,3] The patellofemoral joint is loaded at 0.5 times body weight during walking, 3.3 times body weight during stair climbing, and 7.6 times body weight during squatting.[1,3] The actual contact stress at the patellofemoral joint varies from 1.3 to 12.6 N/mm² during normal ambulatory activities.[1]

Some kinetic information is also available on the anterior cruciate ligament and on the patellar tendon. The ACL can withstand tensile forces of up to 1730 N before rupturing; the average tensile load on the ACL is 454 N during normal activities of daily living.[21,22] The ACL can also elongate by 25% before failure and is at minimal strain at 30 to 35 degrees knee flexion and maximal strain at both 0 and 90 degrees flexion.[21,22] Under maximal, volitional, concentric isokinetic loading conditions, the patellar tendon is subjected to a compression force of nine times body weight at a speed of 30 deg/sec, which drops to five times body weight at the speed of 180 deg/sec.[23] Maximal concentric isokinetic activity also imparts a shear force equal to body weight at the speeds of 30 and 60 deg/sec.[23]

## Kinematics

The knee joint is a functional complex whose primary degree of freedom is in the sagittal plane, to allow the motions of flexion and extension, with an accessory degree of freedom in the transverse plane for tibial rotation movements.[1,3,4] Available active mobility at the knee complex includes a range of motion from 10 degrees extension (10 degrees recurvatum) to 145 degrees flexion when the hip is flexed; 0 degrees (terminal knee extension) to 120 degrees flexion when the hip is extended, secondary to the mechanical influence of the hamstrings; and 45 degrees of both medial and lateral rotation when the knee is positioned at 90 degrees flexion.[1,3,4,8] Passive knee motion is possible from 15 degrees extension (15 degrees recurvatum) to 160 degrees flexion.[1,3,4,8] In order to engage in normal, unrestricted functional activities, a knee complex flexion arc of 65 degrees is necessary for walking, 83 degrees for stair climbing, 93 degrees for sitting, and 106 degrees for donning and doffing shoes.[1]

During the motion of knee extension, the femoral condyles first roll and then slide across the surfaces of the tibial plateaus in order to produce the overt limb action of terminal knee extension.[3,4,8] In an open lower extremity kinetic chain state, the motion of knee flexion involves both rolling and sliding of the tibial articular surfaces posteriorly on the femoral condyles in the direction of the limb segment movement.[3,4,8] This is an example of the orthopaedic convex-concave rule: a concave joint surface rolls and slides in parallel directions upon a convex joint surface in order to produce the desired motion pattern. An opposite action occurs in the closed lower extremity kinetic chain state when the foot is planted and the tibia is fixed; the femoral condyles roll posteriorly and slide anteriorly on the tibial condyles in order to flex the knee.[3,4,8] For the motion of lateral rotation, the lateral femoral condyle slides forward as the medial femoral condyle slides backward on the tibial surface, in an open kinetic chain state, or the medial tibial condyle slides anteriorly while the lateral tibial condyle slides posteriorly, in a closed kinetic chain state.[3,4,8] The opposite relationships produce medial rotation of the knee: posterior movement of the lateral femoral condyle coupled with anterior movement of the medial femoral condyle in an open chain state or forward sliding of the lateral tibial plateau with backward sliding of the medial tibial plateau in a closed chain state.[3,4,8]

Because the diameters of the medial meniscus and the medial tibial condyle are larger than the corresponding surfaces of the lateral meniscus and tibial condyle, a conjunct lateral rotation of the tibia occurs as the knee moves toward terminal extension.[1,3,4,8] This is known as the screw-home mechanism of the knee (see Fig. 8–3), which is thought to occur only during weight bearing in closed kinetic chain activities.[1,3,8] The conjunct lateral rotation, which is up to 20 degrees in magnitude, occurs during the last 30 degrees of terminal knee extension.[1,3,8]

From a position of terminal knee extension, the screw-home mechanism is reversed, or the knee is "unlocked," and the motion of flexion initiated through the action of the popliteus muscle. In a closed kinetic chain state, the popliteus unlocks the knee and initiates flexion by causing a lateral rotation of the femoral condyles on the tibia, which directly reverses the screw-home mechanism.[1,3,4,8] In an open kinetic chain state, the popliteus reverses the screw-home mechanism and initiates knee flexion by creating a medial rotation of the tibial surface on the femoral condyles.[1,3,4,8] The popliteal action in the open chain state is assisted by the VMO, which contributes up to 5 to 7 degrees of the medial rotation excursion.[1,3]

The kinematics of the knee are modulated by the restraining effects of the cruciate and collateral ligaments. The ACL becomes taut during knee flexion and guides the anterior sliding movements of the femoral condyles on the menisci and the tibial plateaus (Fig. 8–10A and B).[1,3,4,8] The PCL becomes tight during knee extension and has the opposite effect of guiding the posterior sliding movements of the femoral condyles on the tibial articulations (Fig. 8–10C and D).[1,3,4,8] Together, the cruciate ligaments provide the primary static restraint for anteroposterior stability of the tibiofemoral joint and allow the biomechanical relationship of near constancy of contact by the tibial articular surface with the femoral condyles during the motions of knee flexion and extension.[1,3,4,8]

Static rotatory stability is provided by both the cruciate and collateral ligaments. During medial rotation, the cruciates tighten by winding around themselves and provide medial rotatory stability to the knee, while the collaterals lose tension and become relatively slack (Fig. 8–11).[1,3,4,8] During lateral rotation, the collaterals become taut and provide lateral rotatory stability to the tibiofemoral complex while the cruciate ligaments unwind and become relatively lax (see Fig. 8–11).[1,3,4,8] The collateral ligaments, however, become slack at a position of 90 degrees knee flexion; this state of relative laxity allows medial and lateral rotation of the tibia on the femur in an open kinetic chain state and of the femur on the tibia in a closed lower extremity kinetic chain state.[1,8]

## Functional Stability

The structural integrity of the human knee complex is a function of four factors: joint geometry, compression forces, active restraints, and passive restraints.[24] The anatomic configurations of and mechanical relationships between the tibial plateaus, the medial and lateral menisci, and

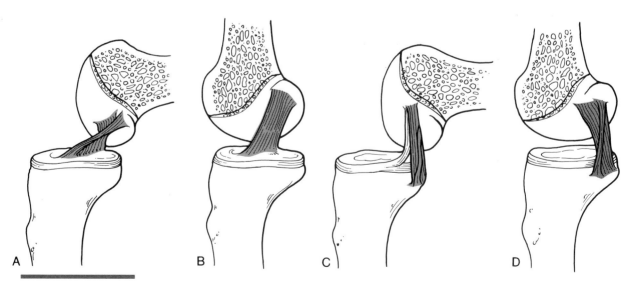

**FIGURE 8–10** ■ Kinematics of the cruciate ligaments. (A) ACL in flexion. (B) ACL in extension. (C) PCL in extension. (D) PCL in flexion.

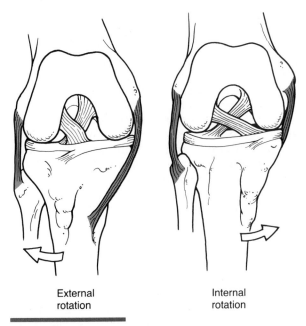

External rotation          Internal rotation

**FIGURE 8-11 ■** Effect of tibial rotation of the cruciate ligaments. The external rotation: collateral ligament is taut and the cruciate ligament is lax. The internal rotation: collateral ligament is lax and the cruciate ligament is taut.

the femoral condyles afford some degree of resistance to external forces and help to prevent disruption of the normal biomechanics of the knee.[1,8] Likewise, the configurations of and the physical interactions between the patella and the anterior surfaces of the distal femur help to prevent malarticulation of the patellofemoral joint.[1,8] An increase in joint compression forces, through active weight-bearing situations, helps to enhance the anatomic relationships of the knee joint components and promote a greater degree of biomechanical stability.[24] However, these degrees of stability are minimal and require reinforcement through the active and passive restraint systems of the knee to maintain the functional integrity of the knee complex.

In order to classify the other restraint systems that are operational at the knee, the supporting structures may be categorized as either active or passive and the knee may be divided into medial and lateral compartments. The medial and lateral compartments may be, in turn, subdivided into anterior, middle, and posterior regions. The active supporting structures are the muscles and related aponeuroses of the knee, which provide dynamic stability, and the passive supporting structures are the capsular and noncapsular ligaments, which provide static stability.[24,25] A plane that transects the patellar tendon and the PCL

divides the knee into the medial and lateral compartments.[24,25]

The anterior portion of both medial and lateral compartments of the knee receives active support from the quadriceps femoris muscle group by way of the extensor retinaculum.[24] The VMO reinforces the stabilization of the anterior portion of the medial compartment through the action on the patella. The middle portion of the lateral compartment receives active support from the iliotibial band; the middle portion of the medial compartment is without a dynamic stabilizing structure.[8,24] The posterior portion of the medial compartment is actively stabilized by the semimembranosus muscle, the pes anserine complex (sartorius, gracilis, and semitendinosus muscle groups), and the medial head of the gastrocnemius muscle.[8,24] On the opposite side of the knee, the posterior portion of the lateral compartment receives active support from the biceps femoris and popliteus muscle groups and from the lateral head of the gastrocnemius.[8,24] The balanced action of the active restraint muscle groups, which is coordinated by the nervous system during performance of the human motor patterns associated with activities of daily living, helps facilitate the functional stability of the knee complex by maintaining the normal anatomic relationships between the tibia, femur, and patella and by modulating the magnitude of joint compression forces, which, in turn, allow the normal kinematics of the knee.

Passively, the anterior regions of both the medial and lateral compartments of the knee receive support from the capsular ligaments of the knee, along with the meniscofemoral and meniscotibial fibers.[8,24] In the medial compartment, the middle region is restrained passively by the MCL and the posterior region by the capsular and posterior oblique ligaments.[8,24] In the lateral compartment of the knee, the middle region is supported by the capsular ligaments and the posterior region receives restraint from the capsular, lateral collateral, and arcuate ligaments.[8,24] Regarding the cruciate ligaments, the ACL, whose anteromedial band resists posterior glide of the femur in knee flexion and whose posterolateral band limits posterior glide of the femur on the tibia in extension, is included with the lateral compartment, and the PCL, which limits anterior glide of the femur on the tibia, is included in the medial compartment.[24] In combination with the active restraints, the ligamentous passive restraints interact to provide the knee with functional stability in both single and multiple planes. Table 8–1 summarizes these relationships.

**Table 8-1.** KNEE STABILITY

| Direction | Active Restraint | Passive Restraint |
|---|---|---|
| Medial | Pes anserine complex<br>Semimembranosus | Medial collateral<br>Capsular complex<br>Posterior cruciate |
| Lateral | Popliteus<br>Biceps femoris<br>Iliotibial band | Lateral collateral<br>Capsular complex<br>Anterior cruciate<br>Posterior cruciate<br>Arcuate complex |
| Anterior | Extensor complex | Anterior cruciate<br>Medial collateral<br>Lateral collateral |
| Posterior | Biceps femoris<br>Gastrocnemius<br>Semimembranosus<br>Popliteus | Posterior cruciate<br>Oblique complex<br>Arcuate complex |
| Rotatory | | Medial collateral<br>Oblique complex<br>Capsular complex<br>Anterior cruciate |

# PATHOMECHANICS AND DIFFERENTIAL DIAGNOSIS

## Fractures

### Femoral Condyle

Femoral condyle fractures are caused by impaction, avulsion, or shearing forces to which the knee is subjected through sports participation, trauma, or activities of daily living.[26] The medial femoral condyle is the most commonly affected site because it is by anatomic design more vulnerable to direct exogenous trauma, especially when the knee is subjected to shear forces in a fall.[26] Femoral condyle fractures are treated surgically by open reduction with internal fixation procedures, which include attempts to repair any osteochondral defects in the articular surface.[26] For surface lesions up to 20 mm in length, regardless of depth, tissue replacement is satisfactory and an acceptable functional result is obtained with surgical correction followed by appropriate rehabilitation techniques.[26]

Postoperative management involves early mobilization activity via the use of a continuous passive motion (CPM) device. This procedure promotes nourishment, revascularization, and healing of the fracture site and of any condylar surface defects. Therapeutic motion also involves the use of a hinged cast brace or controlled motion brace during crutch ambulation activities. The patient walks in a controlled manner with weight bearing to tolerance, depending on the severity of the injury and the extent of the surgical correction, as the magnitude of available knee joint motion is increased through CPM exercise. Isometric knee exercises and straight leg raising (SLR) procedures accompany the motion activities in order to prevent knee muscle atrophy and promote the functional stability of the knee joint. More aggressive rehabilitation procedures may be undertaken when a sufficient degree of healing has been achieved, typically 6 to 12 weeks after surgery.[26]

## Patella

Fractures of the patella most frequently result from a direct blow to the patella, typically in a fall or when the patella is struck against an external object, as seen in motor vehicle accidents.[26] Patellar fractures are managed by (1) closed reduction followed by immobilization or (2) open reduction with internal fixation followed by mobilization procedures. Immobilization is complemented by isometric and SLR exercises for the knee musculature and by crutch ambulation with weight bearing to tolerance. Progressive therapeutic procedures are initiated when the fracture site has healed, usually after 6 to 12 weeks. Mobilization procedures parallel the techniques used in the management of a femoral condyle fracture; CPM and controlled motion brace protection during ambulation lead to advanced muscle strengthening and joint motion techniques.

## Tibial Plateau

Fractures of the tibial plateau may be isolated injuries or may be associated with ligamentous disorders, meniscal tears, and other knee fractures.[26,27] The most common mechanism of injury that produces a fracture of the tibial plateau is a combination of valgus and compression stresses to the knee while the joint is positioned in flexion.[27] In this mechanism the lateral femoral condyle is driven forcibly downward into the posterolateral aspect of the tibial plateau, resulting in fracture and disruption of the normal osseous integrity of the tibial plateau.[27]

Tibial plateau fractures require immobilization and, most often, surgical repair.[26,27] Surgery involves an open reduction with internal fixation procedure using a wedge-shaped bicortical bone graft from the iliac crest.[27] After surgery, the involved lower extremity is immobilized in a cast brace fixed in complete extension for 6 to 12 weeks, depending on the severity of the fracture.[27] Initial therapeutic management involves quadriceps strengthening via isometric and SLR exercises complemented by functional electronic muscle stimulation (EMS) and non–weight-bearing ambulation on crutches.[27] Treatment is advanced to involve progressive range-of-motion (ROM) activities at 14 days after surgery if the fracture existed in the absence of a ligamentous injury; ROM activities are performed in a controlled clinical situation while the patient remains in brace immobilization and on crutch ambulation for other activities of daily living.[27]

Tibial plateau fractures are typically associated with a concomitant ligamentous injury. The most commonly involved structure is the MCL.[26,28] Surgical correction of the ligamentous injury in the process of tibial plateau fracture management is necessary to ensure acceptable functional results for the afflicted patient.[27,28] After surgery for a combined tibial plateau fracture–ligament injury, the patient's knee is immobilized in a controlled motion brace fixed at 45 degrees of knee flexion.[27,28] The patient walks on crutches with a non–weight-bearing status of the affected lower extremity for 6 to 12 weeks.[27] Although CPM activities may be started initially after surgery, more advanced mobilization and rehabilitation procedures are deferred until 4 to 6 weeks after surgery.[27] At this time the patient is gradually progressed toward a normal functional status of joint mobility, musculoskeletal stability, and muscle performance ability.

### Epiphyseal Plate

Epiphyseal plate fractures at the knee are relatively common in adolescents and may strongly resemble an adult's ACL injury.[26] The patient usually presents with a history of a direct blow to the knee resulting in hyperextension or, more commonly, with a noncontact, weight-bearing injury accompanied by a torsional stress, similar to a cutting movement that is a component of many athletic activities.[26] This is the same injury mechanism that produces an ACL rupture. The patient may also experience an audible "pop" in the knee joint followed by a painful hemarthrosis that prevents terminal knee extension.[26] A radiographic examination is necessary to differentiate the osteochondral epiphyseal plate fracture

from the ligamentous ACL rupture.[26] The management of epiphyseal plate fractures directly parallels that used in the rehabilitation of tibial plateau fractures.

### Osteochondritis Dissecans

Osteochondritis dissecans (OD) is an osteochondral fracture that most commonly affects the lateral aspect of the medial femoral condyle (Fig. 8–12A and B).[26,29] The lesion may result from ischemia with loss of circulation to the osseous tissue of the epiphyseal plate, from avulsion of the proximal attachment of the PCL, or from direct trauma transmitted through the patella directly against the medial femoral condyle.[26,29] The fracture results in the development of an intra-articular fragment of articular cartilage and its underlying subchondral bone that may be present in situ, incompletely detached from the medial femoral condyle or completely detached and free within the tibiofemoral joint.[26,29]

Osteochondritis dissecans presents on x-ray films as a rounded or ovoid fragment with an irregular outline that may be misinterpreted as an articular surface cavitation rather than fragmentation.[29] Histologic studies reveal local revascularization, although a displaced fragment is nonvascular.[26,29] Clinically, the patient presents with symptoms of general knee pain, knee joint effusion, and episodes of joint locking, especially in the case of a displaced fragment.[26,29] Treatment involves surgical open reduction and internal fixation or excision of the osseous fragment, strict knee immobilization for 1 week, and then progressive ambulation and muscle-conditioning activities at the patient's level of tolerance.[26,29]

## Ligament Sprains

A sprain is defined as an injury to a ligament that results from hyperpositional mechanical stresses that, in turn, damage the ligamentous collagen fibers.[26] When a force is applied to the knee joint, its ligaments become tense in an effort to maintain the normal degree of joint integrity in resistance to the applied stress. If the mechanical stress exceeds the tensile capacity of the ligament, microtrauma may occur with damage to a limited number of collagen fibers. If the external force is excessive, macrotrauma in the form of complete separation of all collagen fibers (ligament rupture) may occur and the hyperpositional force may drastically alter the normal bio-

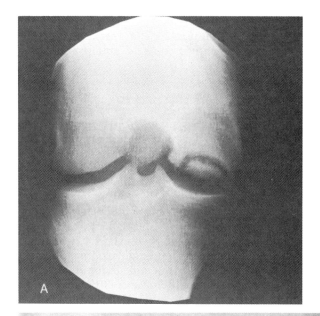

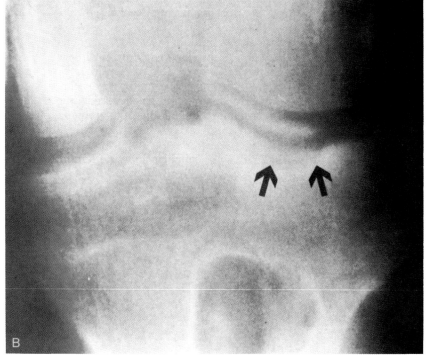

**FIGURE 8-12** ■ (A) Osteochondritis dissecans. (From Nicholas JA, Hershman EB. The Lower Extremity and Spine in Sports Medicine, St. Louis, CV Mosby, 1986, p 686.) (B) Osseous defect in the lateral tibial plateau. (From Lotke PA, Ecker ML: Osteonecrosis-like syndrome of the medial tibial plateau. Clin Orthop 176:148–153, 1983.)

mechanical relationships of the affected joint. When a knee ligament is sprained or ruptured, the knee complex has a limited capacity to maintain a normal degree of operational integrity. A knee that has sustained a ligament injury shows both structural compromise and significant functional disability.

The nature and severity of a knee ligament injury may be classified in several different for-

mats. One system ranks knee ligament disorders as first-, second-, or third-degree sprains. A first-degree, or mild, sprain involves minimal damage to collagen fibers.[26] Although an injury has occurred, there is no loss of ligament function, no discernible loss of strength of the ligament's substance, and only a slight diminution of the ligament's ability to resist external hyperpositional stresses.[26] A second-degree, or moderate, sprain is an injury in which some portion of the ligamentous substance is torn, resulting in a discernible degree of functional compromise of the knee joint.[26] A moderate sprain may heal completely with a proper supportive environment of protective bracing complemented by physical therapy activities that encourage collagen repair and remodeling.[26] A third-degree sprain, which is a complete rupture of the affected ligament, involves complete loss of function of the ligament as a modulator of external forces, resulting in functional disability of the knee complex.[26] Third-degree sprains require surgical correction or reconstruction to restore stability to the knee joint.

## Posterior Cruciate Ligament

Common mechanisms of PCL injury involve an anteromedial blow to the flexed knee or a fall onto the knee accompanied by a hyperextension stress.[30] Typical examples of these specific mechanisms include striking the knee against the dashboard in a motor vehicle accident and having an opponent kick the proximal tibia while attempting to make a tackle in soccer.[31] The common component of all mechanisms of PCL injury is a force directed in a posterior direction on the proximal tibia, which results in a hyperpositional posterior glide of the tibial plateau on the femoral condyles (hyperextension) that, in turn, sprains or ruptures the ligamentous substance of the PCL.[30,31]

A differential diagnosis of PCL injury is made through functional ligamentous testing. The posterior drawer, anterior drawer with internal tibial rotation, varus and valgus in full knee extension, and external rotation recurvatum tests all assess the structural integrity of the PCL.[30] A single positive finding usually indicates a PCL sprain, and multiple positive findings suggest a complete PCL rupture.[30]

PCL ruptures are frequently accompanied by tears of the MCL and of the arcuate ligament complex, resulting in posterolateral rotatory instability (PLRI).[30,31] PLRI of the knee is a posterior rotational subluxation of the lateral tibial plateau in relation to the lateral femoral condyle; it may be masked by a finding of straight posterior instability, indicating PCL rupture, and therefore may be missed during a knee examination.[30,31] The differential diagnosis of PLRI is based on positive posterolateral drawer and external rotation recurvatum ligamentous stress tests.[30,31]

Reconstructive surgery is often necessary for the restoration of functional stability in a knee that has sustained a PCL injury or rupture. Indications for operative repair include a 2+ or greater level of varus instability of the knee at 30 degrees of flexion in conjunction with a positive external rotation recurvatum or posterolateral drawer ligament stress test.[31] Reconstruction of the PCL may be accomplished by transposition of the gracilis and semitendinosus tendons to simulate the anatomical tensile behaviors of the PCL's anterolateral and posteromedial portions.[32] Surgery involves sectioning the tendon at the tibial insertion, freeing it to the level of muscular junctions, pulling it through parallel drill holes made in the anterior aspect of the medial femoral condyle, and then advancing it through additional drill holes for fixation into the posterior aspect of the tibial plateau.[32] This dynamic method of repair is favored over a static, direct repair of the ruptured PCL.[32] Primary surgical repairs of the PCL are possible, however, when an avulsion fracture has occurred in the absence of actual ligament disruption.[30,31] PCL reconstruction is also possible via the Clancy procedure, in which a graft is taken from the central third of the patellar tendon, along with tibial and patellar bone segments, passed through drill holes in the tibia and the femur along a course that parallels the normal anatomic configuration of the intact PCL, and then firmly fixed in the osseous substance of both the tibia and the femur.[32]

Reconstructive surgery may be deferred or precluded in patients with PCL injuries who have a negative posterolateral drawer test, no more than a level 1+ response on varus stress testing of the knee at 30 degrees of flexion, an active knee range of motion of at least 10 to 120 degrees, and minimal osseous changes on joint x-ray films.[31] In addition, it is advisable that such patients also have complete absence of knee swelling, ability to engage in desired functional activities without pain and disability, ability to ascend and descend stairs without difficulty, and ability to squat without limitation or discomfort.[31] Patients who meet these criteria are candidates for a program of active knee rehabilitation.

## Anterior Cruciate Ligament

The most common mechanism of ACL injury involves a combination of valgus and external rotation forces applied to the knee while the foot is firmly planted on the ground.[10,33] Excessive internal rotatory forces or a combination of internal rotation and hyperextension may also injure the ACL.[10,33] As opposed to PCL injuries, which involve some form of external contact with the knee complex, ACL disorders are most frequently noncontact injuries in which sudden limb deceleration accompanied by contraction of the quadriceps muscle group produces the damaging force moments.[10,33] A classic example of the mechanism of ACL rupture occurs in football when a running back plants his foot and attempts to make a cut to avoid being tackled and to gain additional yardage.[10,33] Another example occurs in basketball when a player receives a pass, plants the foot, and then either drives on a dribble toward the basket or quickly pivots to take a jump shot.[10,33] Either activity places valgus and rotational stresses on the knee that may injure the ACL.

Situations involving external contact forces to the tibiofemoral joint may also result in an ACL injury or, more accurately, in combined knee injuries of which an ACL rupture is a component. The classic knee contact injury that results in a combination of knee pathologies is the O'Donoghue "unhappy triad."[10,26,33] The unhappy triad results from a combination of valgus, flexion, and external rotation forces applied to the knee while the foot is planted on the ground and involves damage to the ACL, MCL, and medial meniscus, the three components of the triad (Fig. 8–13).[10,26,33] The classic example of this injury involves a football player who receives a blow to the knee from an opponent as he attempts a cutting motion to avoid being tackled.[10,26,33] This devastating injury frequently results in complete rupture of both the ACL and MCL plus a longitudinal tear of the medial meniscus, all of which require surgical correction.

The differential diagnosis of an ACL injury involves observation of the patient's response to injury and the performance of ligamentous stress tests. A patient with an ACL disorder usually feels or hears a pop at the time of injury, which is followed within 1 hour by knee joint swelling.[10,26,33] Acute hemarthrosis develops within 12 hours.[10,26,33] The Lachman and pivot shift tests (refer to the ACL tests section) are the most reliable noninvasive indicators of ACL damage.[10] The dynamic extension Lachman test may be substituted for the traditional Lachman stress test to reveal ACL laxity. Although not as accurate as the Lachman procedures, the traditional anterior drawer test may also be used to diagnose the presence of ACL sprain.[26] In addition to the pivot shift test, the flexion-rotation drawer test is used to confirm the presence of a lateral pivot shift phenomenon, which is representative of anterolateral rotatory instability (ALRI).[10,33] ALRI is a combined injury of the ACL and the anterolateral joint capsule that results in significant multiplanar instability of the tibiofemoral joint.[10,26,33] The results of manual stress tests may be confirmed objectively by use of an instrumented joint analysis system, magnetic resonance imaging (MRI), or diagnostic arthroscopy.

Reconstructive surgery is often necessary after ACL injury to restore knee stability and normal function. Reconstructions are preferable to direct, primary repairs of the injured ligamentous tissue because the latter has a poor record of long-term success.[10,34] Reconstructive procedures are indicated when an injured patient has a repairable meniscus, has an anterior tibial displacement of more than 5 mm, and has normal life requirements that involve jumping or pivoting movements.[10,33,34] Patients who have not sustained a concomitant meniscal injury, who have an anterior tibial displacement of less than 5 mm, and who are willing to modify their lifestyle to avoid excessive rotational and valgus forces or are willing to wear a protective derotation knee brace

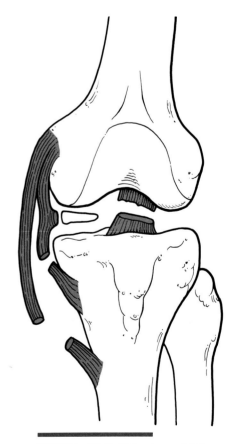

**FIGURE 8–13** ■ The unhappy triad.

during functional activities may avoid surgery.[33,34]

Contemporary reconstructive surgery frequently involves a combination of intra- and extra-articular procedures. The intra-articular procedure of choice, at this time, is a vascular-ized patellar tendon graft (Fig. 8–14A and B) in which a bone-tendon-bone graft is harvested from the central third of the patellar tendon, including osseous tissue from the patellar and tibial insertions for the vascular component, and directed through a drill tunnel in the tibial plateau

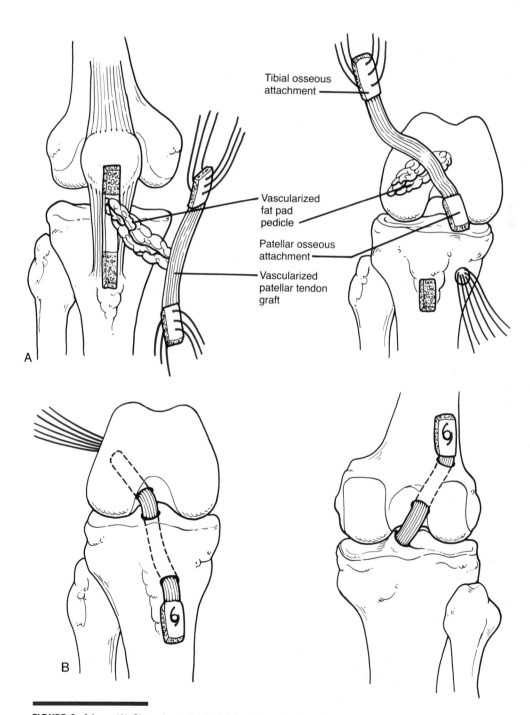

Tibial osseous attachment

Vascularized fat pad pedicle

Patellar osseous attachment

Vascularized patellar tendon graft

**FIGURE 8-14 ■** (A) Clancy's method of ACL reconstruction. (B) Noyes' method of reconstruction.

and femoral condyles along the approximate course of the normal ACL.[10,34–36] A patellar tendon graft is selected as the tissue for ACL reconstruction because it is 1.7 times as strong as the normal ACL.[10] If performed correctly, the reconstructive graft fulfills the normal role of ACL isometry and guards against anterior translation of the tibia on the femur.[33–36] Nonisometric placement results in abnormal knee biomechanics that lead to failure of the repair and knee joint instability.[33–36]

The intra-articular patellar tendon graft procedure is usually complemented by an extra-articular surgical procedure to ensure that the reconstruction techniques effectively compensate for the absence of a functional ACL. A typical extra-articular augmentation involves an Ellison or MacIntosh technique in which the iliotibial band is surgically detached from the normal anatomic insertion into Gerdy's tubercle on the lateral aspect of the proximal tibia, rerouted through a drill tunnel in the lateral femoral condyle (Ellison) or looped under the course of the LCL (MacIntosh), and then reattached to the insertion on Gerdy's tubercle.[10,35,36] If anteromedial rotatory instability, AMRI as opposed to ALRI, is present, the intra-articular reconstruction is reinforced by a distal repositioning of the pes anserine tendinous insertion, which provides both a dynamic and a static restraint against external loading forces.[10]

The reconstructive graft tissues become enclosed by new vascular tissue within 4 to 6 weeks after surgery. During this time the tissues are structurally weakest and, therefore, most vulnerable to failure.[10] At the sixth postsurgical week the process of collagen proliferation begins to occur and the healing tissues begin to become physically stronger.[10] The ligament formation process is complete by the 30th postsurgical week with maximum collagen strength in the newly formed ligamentous structure reached at the 36th week (9 months) after ACL reconstruction.[10] The ultimate success of the ACL reconstruction process is influenced by three factors: isometric placement of the graft during surgery, restoration of normal knee motion early in rehabilitation, and control of tissue loading forces to protect the remodeling structures throughout the treatment process.[10,37] Assuming that these three factors are present and that isometric graft placement is accomplished by the orthopaedic surgeon, the ultimate success of the patient's ACL reconstruction is determined by the physical therapist.

## Collateral Ligaments

The MCL is injured by application of an external valgus force to the knee, typically in a position of extension or of flexion to less than 90 degrees, with the foot planted on the ground.[26] The opposite mechanism, in which a varus stress is applied to an extended or partially flexed knee, damages the LCL.[26] Although isolated injuries are possible, MCL problems are frequently accompanied by damage to the medial meniscus, medial knee joint capsule, and ACL, as in O'Donoghue's unhappy triad (See Fig. 8–13).[26] Isolated LCL injuries are rare because of the ligament's location posterior to the axis of tibiofemoral joint flexion, and the LCL is most commonly injured as a result of a torsional overload that would also affect the cruciate ligaments.[26] The varus and valgus knee ligament stress tests, performed at both terminal extension and 30 degrees of knee flexion, are used to confirm a differential diagnosis of MCL (positive valgus test) or LCL (positive varus test) involvement.

The key to success in the clinical management of collateral ligament injuries is to establish the existence of an isolated lesion with no associated damage to other knee structures, particularly the ACL.[38,39] Isolated MCL and LCL injuries can heal spontaneously, without the need for surgical correction, even in complete ligament ruptures when the fragmented ends of the damaged tissue are not in close approximation.[39,40] However, this situation occurs only when the knee is protected, with controlled motion bracing, against excessive varus and valgus stresses.[39] Surgery is still the primary method for managing collateral ligament ruptures, followed by a rehabilitation program that parallels that used with postsurgical ACL patients, whereas collateral injuries of lesser degree respond positively to conservative physical therapy pain control, ROM promotion, and muscle-conditioning methods.[38,40] Functional rehabilitation and nonsurgical management of nonrupture collateral ligament injuries are effective for returning a patient to pain-free, normal function in an average of 3 weeks.[38]

## Meniscal Injury

Common elements in meniscal injury include force moments of tibiofemoral joint flexion, compression, and rotation that place abnormal shear stresses on the fibrocartilaginous tissue, resulting in peripheral or transverse tears.[26,34,41] Some form of knee joint twisting is thought to be inherent in meniscal injuries.[41] Specifically, injury results when the meniscus fails to follow the excursion path of the femoral condyle during knee motion, which is possible during activities that involve quick knee joint motions.[26,34,41] Transverse or peripheral tears (Fig. 8-15A-F) may result when the meniscus is trapped between the femoral condyle and the tibial plateau and subjected to supranormal compression forces during violent episodes of knee extension.[26,34,41] This action may also result in detachment of the anterior meniscal horn.[34] A longitudinal meniscal tear, also known as a bucket handle tear (see Fig. 8-15A and C), may result from a combination of displacement and rotational forces at the tibiofemoral joint, as when an athlete places a foot and then cuts to change direction quickly.[26,34,41] A bucket handle tear is frequently accompanied by knee joint locking when the patient attempts terminal knee extension.[26,34,41]

Meniscal injuries are differentially diagnosed by evaluating the patient's symptoms and results of knee stress tests, such as the McMurray and Apley procedures (refer to the meniscal tests section). Symptoms of meniscal injury include lateral or medial joint line pain, specific to the involved structure, effusion, sensations of joint crepitus or popping, limitation in the normal knee ROM, joint locking, and demonstrable instability during ambulation.[26,41,42] Anderson and Lipscomb[42] report that some form of joint noise occurs in 43% of patients with a meniscal injury,

effusion or swelling in 51%, and specific joint line pain in 63%. Positive results of the McMurray (58% positive correlation for meniscal tear, 5% false-positive result), Apley compression, and medial-lateral grind (68% positive, 1% false-positive) meniscal stress tests also confirm the diagnosis of meniscal injury.[26,42] However, margins of error exist for these noninvasive clinical procedures, and arthroscopic examination or MRI is often needed to confirm the clinical impression of a meniscal injury.[26] Means of differentiating between meniscal and patellar disorders are summarized in Table 8-2.

Surgery may be necessary for functional correction of meniscal injuries. Total meniscectomy is contraindicated unless a meniscus is totally involved; partial meniscectomy and direct repair of the torn tissue are the surgical procedures of choice.[34,43] Indications for partial meniscectomy or meniscal repair are vertical tears at or near the periphery of the meniscal substance, a generally intact meniscal body, and a total tissue defect length of less than 2 cm.[34,43] Direct repairs of meniscal tears lead to successful healing or nonexcessive scarring of the injured tissue, especially if the defect occurs at the meniscal periphery, where the structure has the greatest vascularity.[43] The object of both repair and partial meniscectomy procedures is to retain as much meniscal tissue as possible in order to preserve the meniscal functions of stability, shock absorption, load transmission, nutrition, lubrication, and motion control in the overall scheme of tibiofemoral joint biomechanics.[34,43]

## Table 8-2. DIFFERENTIATION OF MENISCAL AND PATELLAR DISORDERS

| Factor | Meniscus | Patella |
|---|---|---|
| Frequency | Second most common knee disorder | Most common knee disorder |
| Onset | Twisting injury | Overuse, direct trauma |
| Site of pain | Specific to joint line | Diffuse, anterior |
| Joint locking | Distinct | Not common |
| Weight bearing | Painful | Delayed onset of pain |
| Squatting | Pain at full squat | Pain upon arising |
| Kneeling | No pain | Painful |
| Stairs | Pain on ascending | Pain on descending |
| Sitting | Painless | Delayed onset of pain |
| Effusion | Intermittent | Not common |
| Quadriceps atrophy | Significant | Insignificant |
| Grind test | Painful | Painless |
| X-ray | Joint space narrowing | Articular erosion |
| Surgery | Definitive | Palliative |

From Bloom MH: Differentiating between meniscal and patellar pain. Phys Sports Med 17(8):95–108, 1989. Reproduced with permission of McGraw-Hill, Inc.

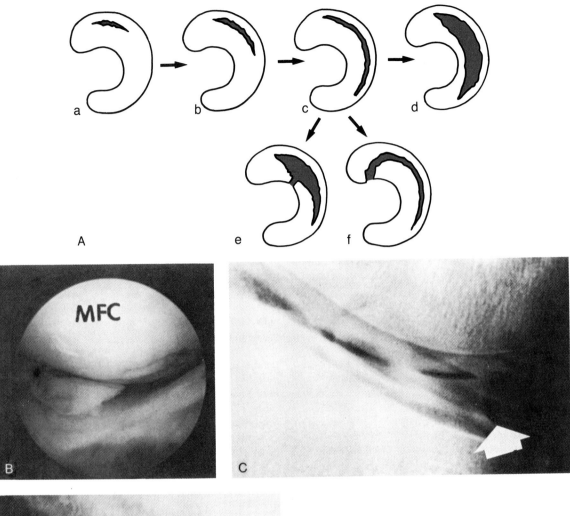

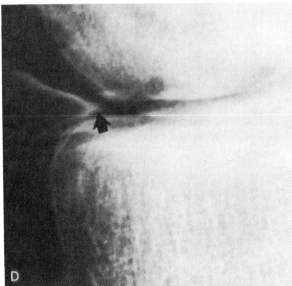

**FIGURE 8–15** ■ (A) Meniscal injuries. The tear can become longer with repeated injuries (a through d) or a split can cause flap tears (e and f). (B) Arthroscopic view of a chondral fracture. (C) Bucket handle tear of the medial meniscus. (D) Anterior horn tear of the medial meniscus. (Parts B–D from Nicholas JA, Hershman EB. The Lower Extremity and Spine in Sports Medicine. St. Louis, CV Mosby, 1986, pp 832–833.)

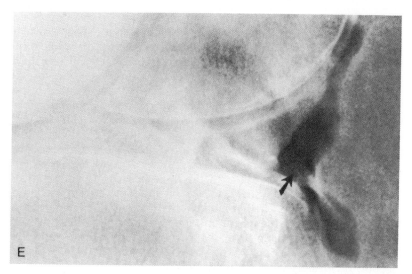

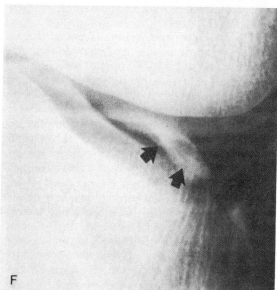

**FIGURE 8-15** ■ *Continued* (E) Posterior horn tear of the lateral meniscus. (F) Crushed posterior horn of the lateral meniscus. (Parts E and F from Nicholas JA, Hershman EB. The Lower Extremity and Spine in Sports Medicine. St. Louis, CV Mosby, 1986, pp 832–833 and 957.)

## Tibiofibular Instability

The superior tibiofibular articulation serves as a functional dissipator for forces that are transferred along the lower extremity kinetic chain from the subtalar and talocrural complexes to the tibiofemoral joint.[1,26] With activities that involve excessive torsional stresses at the ankle, the superior tibiofibular joint becomes subject to sprain, hypermobility, subluxation, or dislocation. Injury, although relatively uncommon, may occur in baseball by sliding feet-first into a base, in basketball by falling on another player's foot when rebounding, and in parachute jumping by using an incorrect landing technique.[44]

The specific mechanism that results in superior tibiofibular joint instability involves a fall on the affected lower extremity with the leg adducted at the hip, flexed at the knee, and inverted at the ankle.[44] In case of a subluxation or a complete dislocation, physical examination reveals an obvious bony prominence because the head of the fibula has been traumatically repositioned from its normal anatomic alignment.[44] As opposed to knee instabilities, which involve some form of ligamentous internal derangement, joint effusion is minimal or completely absent and the tibiofemoral articulation demonstrates complete functional stability.[44] Bilateral comparison of roetgenograms is necessary to confirm a differential diagnosis of superior tibiofibular subluxation or dislocation. An anteroposterior x-ray view demonstrates lateral displacement of the fibular head along with widening of the proximal interosseous space.[44] A lateral view shows greater overlap of the fibula on the tibia when the injured is compared to the noninjured knee.[44]

A superior tibiofibular sprain, which presents as joint hypermobility, is not demonstrated on radiographs and requires functional and mobility tests for a correct differential diagnosis. As a functional test, the patient is asked to stand and balance on the affected leg with the knee flexed 15 to 30 degrees.[44] In the presence of superior tibiofibular sprain or hypermobility, the patient reports pain and a feeling of instability in this position and is not able to maintain the posture for a prolonged period.[44] The knee pain and feeling of instability are removed by having the patient place the instep of the foot of the noninjured lower extremity over the affected superior tibiofibular joint and apply a medial force as counterpressure to the hypermobile joint.[44] A differential diagnosis of superior tibiofibular involvement may also be confirmed through the finding of increased joint movement ability during anterolateral and posteromedial passive motion testing of the afflicted knee complex compared to the noninvolved side. A neurologic evaluation is also necessary to screen for peroneal nerve entrapment, which occurs frequently with superior tibiofibular joint injuries.[44]

Superior tibiofibular joint subluxation or dislocation may be reduced via direct anterolateral or posteromedial manipulation of the displaced head of the fibula back into its normal anatomic position.[44] A superior tibiofibular joint sprain may be treated by local adhesive tape strapping or by use of a circumferential brace, to support the fibular head in its normal position and prevent further damage to the injured support ligaments.[44] Care must be taken to avoid excessive pressure in the joint region, which might compromise the peroneal nerve. When a chronic hypermobility problem does not respond to conservative support measures, surgical resection of the fibular head is the treatment of choice.[44]

## Degeneration

### Osteoarthritis

Osteoarthritis (OA) is a degenerative articular condition characterized by deterioration of the cartilaginous weight-bearing surfaces of joints, presence of sclerotic changes in subchondral bone, and proliferation of new bone at the joint margins.[45] The proliferation of new bone is manifest as osteophytes and spurs, which are evident on radiographs. OA is a localized phenomenon afflicting joints that are frequently subjected to excessive external forces and to musculoskeletal overuse, especially the knee, as opposed to rheumatoid arthritis, which is a systemic disease.[45]

OA is present in 15% of adult females and 11% of adult males in the United States; at least some evidence of the disorder is present in the majority of people age 55 years and older.[45] Repetitive stress to the knee complex from athletic and industrial activities, or from the forces associated with normal activities of daily living magnified over multiple decades, results in the fraying and fibrillation of the tibial, femoral, and patellar articular cartilages with concomitant loss of chondrocytes through pressure necrosis.[45] Cartilage matrix is disrupted and collagen fibers are destroyed, which results in a tissue defect in the articular surfaces. This process produces fragments of dead articular cartilage that dislodge from the patellofemoral and tibiofemoral joint surfaces, enter the synovial fluid in the knee joint capsule, and irritate the synovial membrane.[45] The synovial irritation produces an acute inflammation that is manifest as a general knee pain that worsens with weight-bearing activities.

With continued activity, the rate of articular cartilage degeneration is greater than the rate of tissue healing and the inflammation becomes a chronic condition, which is the basic nature of OA.[45] In the chronic inflammatory situation, OA progresses to a state of decreased articular cartilage thickness, decreased tibiofemoral joint space, increased subchondral bone density, and periarticular bone spurring, all of which are evident on a standard x-ray film.[45] At this point the knee complex loses normal function.

Clinically, a patient with OA presents with a condition of general joint pain, which may be exacerbated by knee motion; a reduction in the normal knee joint ROM; quadriceps muscle weakness; and generally diminished functional capacity.[45] Patients experience knee pain when climbing stairs or standing up from a sitting position and have slight knee joint effusion after prolonged activity.[45] Knee pain caused by OA typically eases or resolves with rest, only to appear again with renewed joint activity. A lower extremity varus (bowleg) or valgus (knock-knee) deformity may also be present in advanced cases of OA.[45] OA is also a long-term sequela of meniscal and ligamentous lesions and failed knee surgery.

The differential diagnosis of OA is based on knee stability and laboratory studies. Clinical observation of knee pain production during extension activities and during flexion actions greater than 90 degrees is indicative of OA.[45] OA presents as knee joint line pain, similar to that of a meniscal lesion, but does not produce a positive McMurray test.[45] Effective laboratory studies for OA include an erythrocyte sedimentation rate (ESR) and a synovial fluid culture. The erythrocyte sedimentation rate is normal in OA but increased in the presence of joint infection and rheumatoid arthritis, and the synovial fluid culture reveals a firm mucin clot, a white blood cell count under 2000 per microliter, and a glucose concentration equal to the patient's circulatory blood level.[45] These findings, plus the degenerative joint changes visualized radiographically, confirm the existence of knee joint OA.

Effective treatment of OA involves pain control and external force control. Pain control is achieved through the standard physical therapy modalities of thermal agents, electronic stimulation, and continuous passive motion (CPM) along with a regimen of nonsteroidal anti-inflammatory drugs (NSAIDs).[45] External force control is accomplished by reduction of the patient's weight, quadriceps muscle strengthening through isometric exercise, and correction of aberrant lower extremity biomechanics through use of orthoses or braces. A program of isokinetic exercise using an inverted velocity spectrum sequence, which is gradually progressed from submaximal toward maximal, also benefits the OA patient by increasing the functional capacities of the knee musculature while facilitating articular cartilage nutrition and knee joint complex decompression.[46]

### Rheumatoid Arthritis

Whereas OA results from musculoskeletal overuse and typically affects only one or a few joints unilaterally, rheumatoid arthritis (RA) is a systemic disease that affects multiple joint systems throughout the body in a symmetric or bilateral presentation.[47] A synovial fluid culture reveals a fragile mucin clot, a white blood cell count of 2000 to 75,000 per microliter, and a glucose titer as much as 25 mg/dL below the patient's serum level.[45] The disease is characterized by inflammation in the synovial lining of joint complexes, which may be either acute or chronic, that results in articular cartilage and bone destruction.[47] Such degenerative changes occur simultaneously in multiple joint systems, resulting in severe pain and limited mobility for activities of daily living.[47] The ultimate result is a general deconditioning via muscle atrophy and loss of aerobic function, which are secondary to the loss of normal joint mobility.[47]

The adverse effects of RA can be controlled through an appropriate exercise program. Aerobic-type exercise for at least 15 minutes performed at least three times per week is sufficient to improve the functional status of patients afflicted with RA.[47] Whereas traditional treatment regimens for RA focused on ROM and isometric muscle-strengthening activities coupled with large amounts of rest, current thought suggests that a program of vigorous aerobic conditioning activities may be more effective for the long-term management of the condition.[47] A prudent approach for effective management of RA would be to utilize aspects of both of these therapeutic philosophies relative to the inflammatory status of the patient's RA.

In the acute stage or during an acute flare-up after a period of chronic RA inflammation, motion activities through the patient's comfortable range help to maintain available joint functions and prevent further degeneration of the joint complex.[47] CPM is also productive for painless healing and regeneration of damaged articular cartilage.[47] Isometric exercises, performed at a pain-free level of intensity, help to maintain muscle strength in order to prevent further deterioration of the patient's functional status.[47]

In the nonacute and chronic stages of RA joint inflammation, total body aerobic activity, such as swimming, walking, cycling, and cross-country skiing, benefits the patient by promoting an increase in systemic condition, functional capacity, and psychologic well-being.[47] However, close control and monitoring are needed to ensure that the exercise is nontraumatic to involved joints. Although weight-bearing activities are necessary for articular cartilage and subchondral bone healing, other aerobic activities, such as running and court games, may place excessive (and intolerable) pressures on the healing joints and thus are contraindicated for the patient with RA.[47] Controlled exercise is an efficient adjunct to traditional physical therapy thermal modalities for the successful management of RA.[47]

## Muscle Injuries

### Contusion

Contusion of the quadriceps is a relatively frequent injury in contact sports, such as football and ice hockey, and results from a direct impact to the anterior aspect of the thigh.[26] Quadriceps contusion injuries may also occur in occupational settings, usually as a result of a fall. Hamstring contusion injuries are rare.[26]

Examination of the injured area reveals diffuse tenderness, with or without a muscle guarding reaction to evaluative palpation, over the region of traumatic impact.[26] Ambulation may be relatively pain free, but the patient's range of comfortable tibiofemoral joint motion is diminished. Passive motion testing reveals a functional loss of knee flexion with muscle guarding or an empty end feel (the limit of motion cannot be reached because of pain). Quadriceps resistive testing shows a strong or weak and painful response, depending on the severity of the contusion, in comparison to the opposite lower extremity; manual muscle testing (MMT) typically demonstrates a 3 to 4 (fair to good) level of response. A hematoma may be present in the area of injury.[26]

The general procedures used for treatment and rehabilitation of muscle contusion injuries include initial use of ice, compression, and elevation followed by progressive ROM activities.[26] Electronic muscle stimulation (EMS) is used to enhance resolution of the hematoma and delay muscle atrophy. Isometric muscle exercises are used to promote restrengthening of the injured muscle and progress from a submaximal to a maximal level of intensity, based on the patient's level of comfort and exercise tolerance. When the knee ROM has normalized, the patient may begin progressive ambulation, muscle performance conditioning, and work conditioning activities.

## Myositis Ossificans

A deep quadriceps contusion, whose traumatic effects include damage to the femoral periosteum, may result in myositis ossificans.[48,49] This is a reaction to chronic or traumatic irritation of a muscle in which the body's reparative response is ossification instead of connective tissue remodeling.[48,49] New bone replaces the normal myofibrillar substance within the affected area, which becomes evident on radiographic studies.

The situation most frequently arises when an existing muscle contusion is treated too vigorously or when a patient is returned to activity before complete muscle healing has occurred.[48,49] The presence in the intramuscular compartments of blood from a nonresolved hematoma that comes in contact with the femoral periosteal surface appears to be the stimulus for the ossification response.[48,49] Management of the problem parallels that used for the treatment of a muscle contusion, but progresses in a conservative, gradual, and gentle fashion to avoid continued irritation of the injured, ossifying tissues. Surgical intervention to remove the extraneous bone mass may ultimately be required if conservative rehabilitation is not successful.

## Muscle Strains

As a pathologic entity, strain is defined as damage to some part of the muscle unit—the muscle belly, the tendon, or the tenoperiosteal junction—caused by chronic overuse or acute overload.[26] Patients may be predisposed to chronic strains because of muscle inflexibility, which may stem from postural faults, deconditioning, or improper body mechanics, and result in general fatigue and decreased performance efficiency of the affected muscle group.[26] Acute strains result from a single episode of hyperpositional stress in which the contractile elements experience physical failure as a result of mechanical overload. Acute strains may also occur when a loaded muscle is acts concentrically, becomes fatigued, and then succumbs to the eccentric, lengthening stimulus of gravity.[26] Although muscle strains may affect any of the muscle groups that influence the knee complex, they most frequently afflict the hamstrings.

Muscle strains are gauged in relative degrees based on the level of functional disability. A first-degree, or mild, muscle strain involves general discomfort in the affected muscle but without a discernible loss of strength on resistive MMT and without a diminution in the normal, functional joint ROM.[26] A second-degree, or moderate, strain is accompanied by severe pain in the affected region, by a distinct diminution in the available, pain-free joint ROM, by a strong and painful resistive test response, and by a decrease in the MMT level from 5 (normal) to as low as 2 (poor). A third-degree muscle strain, which is an actual separation or rupture of the contractile elements, presents as complete functional disability of the affected muscle and of the joints that the muscle may influence.[26] The patient has a weak and painful resistive test response and an MMT level of 0 to 1 (absence to trace). Interestingly, although the patient's active ROM is minimal to nonexistent, the passive ROM may be normal, painless, and hypermobile, secondary to the loss of tissue integrity.

Management of muscle strain injuries involves the common physical therapy treatment modalities of initial ice, compression, and elevation; protective support of the area of injury; ROM normalization activities; systematic muscle reconditioning exercise; progressive ambulation; and activity reintegration procedures. Muscle strains are best managed, however, through prevention; a program of flexibility exercise and body mechanics training limits the extent of muscle strain injury and helps to prevent recurrence. Actual muscle ruptures, third-degree strains, frequently require correction through surgery.

## Bursal Involvement

### Prepatellar Bursitis

The prepatellar bursa may become injured through direct trauma, such as a fall on the flexed knee, or chronic irritation, such as prolonged kneeling, which results in "housemaid's knee" (Fig. 8–16).[26] Any excessive or prolonged irritation of the bursal membrane results in an acute effusion, which in turn causes the characteristic swelling that is commonly associated with bursitis. Besides swelling (tumor), a patient afflicted with prepatellar bursitis demonstrates the other classic signs of soft tissue injury: dolor (pain), calor (heat), and rubor (redness). The patient may also show a small diminution of pain-free knee flexion,[26] a strong and painful quadriceps resistive test, and a grade of 4 to 5 (good to normal) in quadriceps strength MMT. Palpation of the enlarged bursa definitely increases the patient's pain unless the bursitis has become chronic. Long-standing, chronic prepatellar bursitis is essentially a painless, nondebilitating entity that is more of a cosmetic abnormality than a functional disorder.[26]

Prepatellar bursitis is managed through the use of pain and edema control modalities, such as cryotherapy, electronic muscle stimulation, and nonthermal ultrasound, phonophoresis or iontophoresis, and a physician-prescribed course of anti-inflammatory agents. Unresponsive patients may require corticosteroid injections or drainage of the bursa contents in order to resolve the problem.[26] A padded knee support may be utilized for protection of the prepatellar bursa after resolution of the lesion as a guard against recurrence.

### Baker's Cyst

In contemporary terms, Baker's cyst refers to any form of synovial hernia or bursitis involving the posterior aspect of the knee (Fig. 8–17).[26] A cyst may result from irritation of the semimembranosus or medial gastrocnemius bursa or from herniation of the synovial membrane of the

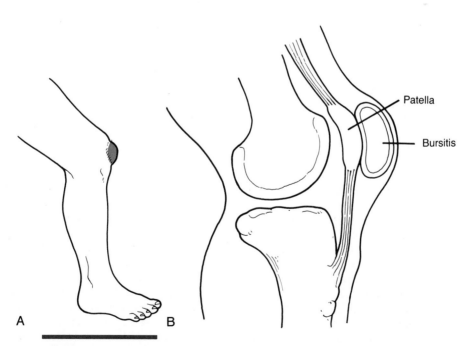

Patella

Bursitis

**FIGURE 8–16** ■ Prepatellar bursitis. (A) Clinical presentation. (B) Underlying problem.

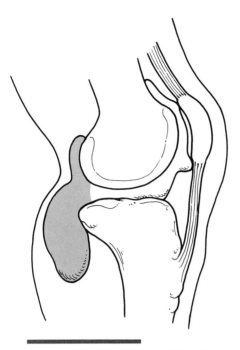

**FIGURE 8-17** ■ Popliteal cyst (Baker's cyst).

semitendinosus tendon sheath or the posterior knee joint capsule.[26] The condition, although benign and usually asymptomatic, must be distinguished from tumor growth and from aneurysm of the popliteal artery.[26] Such a differential diagnosis is made through the use of radiographic procedures and vascular studies. Clinically, the patient has normal knee stability, mobility, and performance ability. The only evidence of a possible disorder is an area of swelling on the posterior aspect of the knee. In the relatively rare instance in which a Baker's cyst becomes symptomatic, surgical removal of the affected tissue is the treatment of choice.[26]

## Patellar Disorders

### Patellar Instability

Instability of the patellofemoral articulation, in the form of patellar subluxation or dislocation, may be associated with a number of factors: direct trauma to the medial or lateral aspect of the patella; a broad configuration of the pelvis, which creates an external force vector at the patellofemoral joint; insufficiency of the VMO; a shallow patellar groove; an abnormally positioned patella; a flattened internal aspect of the lateral femoral condyle; an abnormally posi-

tioned patella; and/or an excessive Q angle.[26] The Q angle is the angle of intersection of the line of pull of the quadriceps muscle group on the patella with the line connecting the center of the patella with the center of the tibial tuberosity (Fig. 8-18A-D).[26] The normal Q angle of the knee is 10 degrees (see Fig. 8-18B),[26] and any larger value may indicate a predisposition to patellar instability (see Fig. 8-18C and D). Thus, measurement of the Q angle is a useful clinical tool in the differential diagnosis of patellar instability disorders.

Subluxation or dislocation of the patella is most often caused by a combination of planting the foot and externally rotating the femur as the affected knee is flexed.[26] A contraction of the quadriceps while the lower extremity is configured in this manner may overcome the resistance of the medial extensor retinaculum, permitting the patella to translate laterally over the lateral femoral condyle, especially if the VMO is weak.[26] The patella may or may not relocate (subluxation versus dislocation) (Figs. 8-19 and 8-20) if the knee is extended from the position of injury. The initial management involves radiographic studies to screen for the presence of concomitant patellar, femoral, or cartilaginous fractures, followed by knee stability testing to detect ligament sprains that may have accompanied the patellar injury.[26] Reduction of a patellar dislocation may require manipulation under anesthesia.

The treatment of a patellar instability may range from simple relocation of the patella to its normal anatomic configuration to complex surgical alteration of the patellofemoral biomechanical relationships. The goal is to prevent future episodes of patellar subluxation or dislocation that, over time, would result in general hypermobility of the patellofemoral articulation and loss of the normal functional stability of the knee. Physical therapy procedures for the management of patellar instability disorders include conditioning of the VMO through exercise or EMS, use of foot orthotics as a lower extremity kinetic chain compensation for biomechanical abnormalities at the knee, and patellar braces to maintain the normal positional alignment of the patella on the femoral groove.

### Synovial Plica

Synovial plicae of the knee are the remnants of three embryonic pouches of synovial membrane that regress to form the singular synovial compartment of the tibiofemoral joint during the processes of development.[50-52] If remission of the

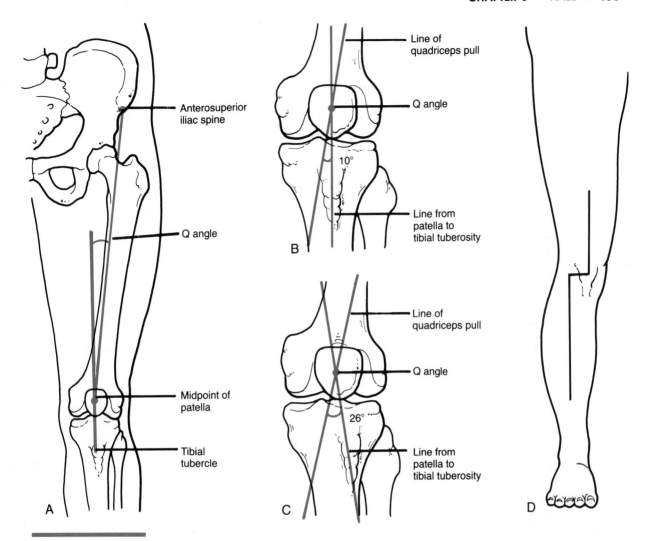

**FIGURE 8-18** ■ Q angle. (A) Quadriceps or Q angle defined. (B) Normal Q angle. (C) Increased Q angle. (D) Increased Q angle.

three developmental synovial chambers is incomplete, plicae may remain within the knee complex as distinct bands of excessive synovial material (Fig. 8–21).[50-52] The most common synovial vestige is the infrapatellar plica, which extends from the intercondylar notch of the tibia to the infrapatellar fat pad.[50] The structure is rarely problematic as a functional disorder of the knee complex.[50] The suprapatellar plica, which is also nonproblematic, is a medial or lateral suprapatellar band in approximately 20% of all human knees.[51] The third form of plica, the medial plica, is usually symptomatic and problematic, in contrast to the other two varieties.

The medial synovial plica originates on the medial surface of the synovial capsule of the knee joint, attaches to either the suprapatellar plica or the medial wall of the knee, and extends distally to the infrapatellar fat pad.[50-52] The plica tightens during knee flexion and causes an alteration in the normal mechanics of the patellofemoral joint, which results in the symptoms of a patellar pain syndrome.[50-52] Patients are predisposed to the plical symptomatology by direct knee trauma, chronic overuse, and quadriceps, especially VMO, muscle insufficiency.[51,52] Plical irritation, again resulting in patellofemoral joint pain, may also be caused by a rotation injury to the knee.[30,53]

Active irritation of the medial plica presents as a pain in the medial aspect of the knee joint, specific to the anatomic path of the synovial remnant; generalized knee swelling, especially after prolonged weight-bearing activities; a click-

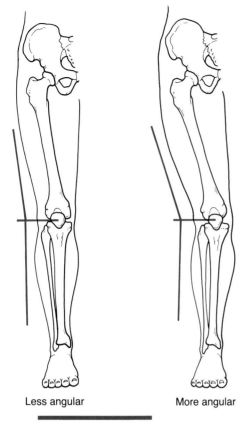

Less angular                    More angular

**FIGURE 8-19** ■ Patellar subluxation.

ing and intermittent locking sensation on the medial side of the knee; and general feelings of quadriceps weakness and knee joint instability.[50-52] A definitive differential diagnosis is often obtained by eliminating other possible knee disorders, as plical syndromes frequently mimic the signs and symptoms of meniscal injuries, ligament sprains, and osteochondral damage.[50,53] However, a classic symptom that is specific to a plical syndrome is inability to sit for prolonged periods because of knee pain.[20] The patellar stutter test, indicating absence or interruption of normal, smooth patellar tracking, may also be used for diagnostic purposes.[20] A high correlation exists between the incidence of symptomatic medial patellar plica and fibrillation of the patellar articular cartilage.[52,53]

Plical syndromes are most commonly managed through a conservative therapeutic approach. Treatment involves a regimen of NSAIDs com-plementing a clinical program of cryotherapy, quadriceps EMS, and gradual progressive resistance exercise for the knee musculature. Transverse friction massage may also be effective for remediation of the patient's symptoms. Conservative measures should completely rectify all functional problems within 6 to 12 weeks; arthroscopic surgery, which provides excellent results in up to 84% of plical cases,[50] is an alternative.

### Osgood-Schlatter Disease

Osgood-Schlatter disease (Fig. 8–22) is a traction apophysitis of the tibial tubercle at the site of the patellar tendon insertion; the term "disease" is a misnomer because the problem is not systemic or infectious but mechanical.[26] The disorder, which mimics patellar tendinitis or a general patellofemoral pain syndrome, may manifest as infrapatellar bursitis, as aseptic necrosis of the tip of the epiphysis of the patellar tubercle of the tibia, or as a true epiphysitis involving the complete extent of the epiphysis of the tibial tubercle.[26] Any of the three possible manifestations may be due to a traumatic incident involving the tibial tubercle, most frequently a fall; the tubercle fails to heal and is constantly reirritated by the traction forces transduced through the patellar tendon from quadriceps muscle group activity.[26] The irritated area tends to enlarge and form a benign osseous tumor over the tibial tubercle.[26]

For differential diagnosis, the irritated, enlarged bony mass on the tibial tubercle is painful upon palpation and resisted knee extension.[26] Manual muscle testing may reveal some diminution of quadriceps strength from a normal grade to a good or a fair grade if the situation is chronic. Radiographs confirm the epiphyseal irritation. Otherwise, the knee complex is normal from an orthopaedic and functional perspective. The problem is best managed by controlling knee loading activities, to allow for epiphyseal healing in the absence of excessive patellar tendon traction forces, and by protective padding and bracing, to guard against impact trauma to the area of injury.[26] A regimen of physician-prescribed NSAIDs and clinical iontophoresis may be helpful for pain and inflammation control. Surgical excision of the excess osseous tissue may be necessary if conservative measures fail.[26]

### Patellar Pain Syndrome

The term patellar pain syndrome (PPS) encompasses the pathologic entities of patellar ten-

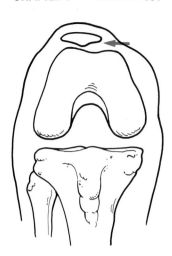
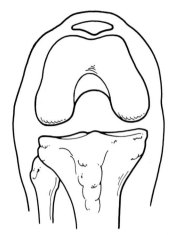

FIGURE 8–20 ■ Patellar dislocation.

dinitis, chondromalacia patellae, and patellar malalignment. Because these problems may be inter-related, may predispose to one another, and have common symptoms, they are frequently designated as PPS. Patellar tendinitis is an over-use injury caused by excessive eccentric loading of the muscle-tendon unit.[54] This occurs during the body deceleration activities that are usually associated with running and jumping.[54] The common sports-related condition known as jumper's knee is, in fact, patellar tendinitis. The patellar tendinitis component of PPS specifically involves pain anteriorly near the inferior pole of the patella, whereas in the other PPS disorders pain is manifested more generally over the entire patella.[54]

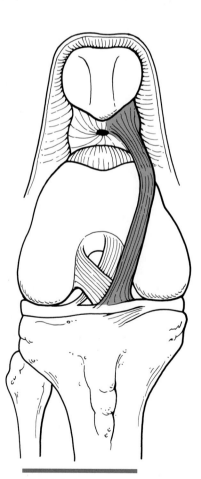

FIGURE 8–21 ■ Synovial plica.

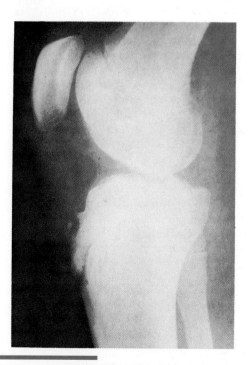

FIGURE 8–22 ■ Osgood-Schlatter disease. (From O'Don-oghue DH: The Treatment of Injuries to Athletes, 4th ed. Philadelphia: WB Saunders, 1984, p 574.)

Chondromalacia patellae, a term formerly applied to any disorder involving general patellar pain, refers to progressive softening, fibrillation, and, finally, degeneration of the articular cartilage on the undersurface of the patella (Fig. 8–23).[55] It is an overuse syndrome that stems from altered patellar biomechanics, which might result from patellar tendinitis or patellar malalignment, repetitive microtrauma, improper athletic or occupational body mechanics, especially running or lifting, or direct trauma to the patella.[55] As opposed to patellar tendinitis and patellar malalignment disorders, the pain of chondromalacia patella is entirely retropatellar.[55]

Patellar malalignment disorders include conditions in which the patella is positioned or tracks abnormally lower or higher in its femoral intercondylar articulation relative to the normal patellofemoral joint. These conditions are known as patella infera or patella baja (tracks lower) and as patella alta (tracks higher), respectively. Patella infera (baja) results in restricted knee extension, which causes abnormal articular cartilaginous

wearing and, ultimately, chondromalacia patellae and osteoarthritis.[56] When it is chronic, patients also present with a knee flexion contracture.[56] Patella alta results in chronic instances of patellofemoral joint subluxation and/or dislocation.[56] Instability is due to the fact that the patella is positioned higher than normal along the articular track and loses mechanical stability from the lateral lip of the femoral intercondylar fossa, the normal osseous deterrent to patellar subluxation or dislocation.[56] Patients with patella alta demonstrate the characteristic "camel back" sign of two "humps" as the knee moves from flexion to extension (Fig. 8–24). The infrapatellar fat pad, which is inferiorly displaced from the patella in cases of patella alta, and the patella form the two visible humps. A normal knee, where the fat pad and the patella are in close approximation, is a "one-hump camel." Surgical correction, via a lateral retinacular release, may be necessary if rehabilitation activities do not remediate the problems of patellar malalignment disorders.

PPS is differentially diagnosed through an ac-

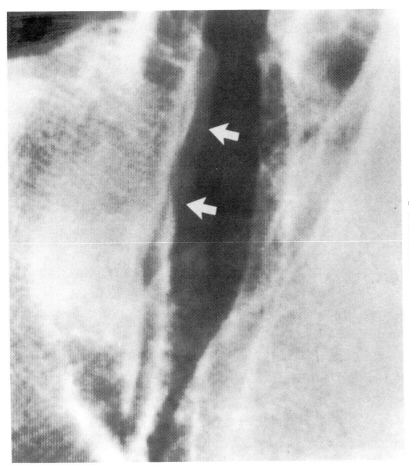

FIGURE 8–23 ■ Chondromalacia patella. (From Pavlov H, Torg JS: The Running Athlete: Roentgenograms and Remedies. Chicago: Mosby-Year Book Inc., 1987, p 190.)

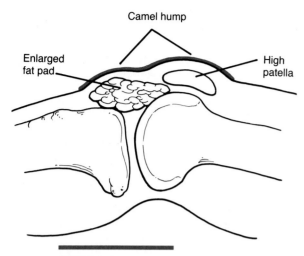

Camel hump

Enlarged fat pad

High patella

**FIGURE 8-24** ■ Camel back sign.

curate history accompanied by clinical tests. The extent of PPS pathology may be classified in four phases, based on the magnitude of the patient's knee pain. Phase I, patellar pain only after extended activity, and phase II, pain during activity that does not interfere with the successful completion of the activity, represent a relatively minor irritation of the joint that usually responds to cryokinetics, therapeutic ultrasound, quadriceps muscle strengthening, specialized strapping (athletic taping) of the patella or use of a patellar stabilizing brace, and a regimen of physician-prescribed NSAIDs.[56,57] Phase III is characterized by patellar pain during activity that interferes with participation in the selected activity and is reflective of advanced patellofemoral joint microtrauma. Treatment involves eliminating stressful activities until tissue healing takes place. Phase IV, patellar pain before, during, and after activity along with patellofemoral joint functional disability, represents tissue macrotrauma that requires remediation through surgery.

The PPS clinical test is used to complement the patient's history and pain response in the differential diagnosis of active PPS. The test involves manual compression of the patella into the intracondylar notch while the knee is extended and the patient contracts the quadriceps muscle group.[56] A painful response is a positive indication of PPS.[56]

## Reflex Sympathetic Dystrophy

Reflex sympathetic dystrophy (RSD) is the manifestation of a microvascular disturbance in which a pain stimulus overloads the internuncial neuronal pool, triggering an efferent response in the sympathetic portion of the autonomic nervous system.[58,59] The sympathetic response affects local circulation through an initial vasoconstriction followed by a secondary vasodilation, which produces a tissue response that is similar to the inflammatory process.[58,59] Capillary stasis results and leads to edema, increased interosseous pressure, decreased local circulation, bone marrow necrosis, and, ultimately, tissue fibrosis.[58,59]

RSD is frequently overlooked in the differential diagnosis of knee disorders because the patient's symptoms are usually perceived as being exaggerated relative to the degree of pathology. Because of this misinterpretation, patients with RSD are often classified as exhibiting inappropriate illness behavior or a psychologic disorder rather than a true neurophysiologic problem. Pain is the most dominant symptom of RSD and is frequently present nocturnally.[58,59] Ambulation and motion activities and superficial pressure, such as from clothing, may be intolerable for the patient.[58,59] Initially, the affected knee is warmer than the noninvolved knee and may present with a rubor color.[58,59] As the condition advances, the affected knee becomes colder to superficial palpation, hyperesthetic to cold, and cyanotic.[58,59] The normal range of knee joint motion diminishes as the connective tissues become fibrotic.[58,59] On x-ray films the knee complex with RSD appears decalcified and osteoporotic.[58,59]

Management of RSD by means of physical therapy is challenging and is often limited in effectiveness. Pain control modalities and counterirritation methods may be used, but only very conservatively and in a relatively nonprogressive manner.[58,59] Treatment may also include ganglionic blocking medications or epidural sympathetic blockade injections.[58,59] Surgical sympathectomy is the final treatment solution if other procedures fail.[58,59]

## Amputation

Removal of some portion of the lower extremity via amputation may be necessary when systemic pathology, such as carcinoma, advanced infection, such as gangrene, or traumatic involvement, such as a crush injury, threatens the life of a patient. Traditional amputation surgeries have included above knee, knee disarticulation, and below knee methods. These procedures are designed to preserve as much lower extremity tissue as possible for the individual patient, including the patellofemoral and tibiofemoral joints, and to provide a reasonable limb stump for fitting of a prosthetic device that will allow the individual maximal functional activity.[60,61] Another surgical procedure is van Ness rotation, in which the knee complex and the calf region are excised from the leg, leaving the neurovascular tree intact, and the ankle complex is rotated 180 degrees and then reattached to the distal remnant of the femur.[62] Through this unusual procedure, the calcaneus becomes a functional patella and the subtalar and talocrural joints become a functional tibiofemoral joint to allow quasi-normal motion.[62] The van Ness procedure is used in the specific cases of proximal tibial, patellar, and distal femoral osteosarcomas because it requires a healthy ankle complex, and it is preferable to a knee disarticulation or above knee amputation because it creates a motorized substitute knee joint that more readily accommodates a functional lower extremity prosthesis.[62]

The postoperative management procedures used after all four amputations are essentially the same.[60–62] A postsurgical dressing is applied to the limb stump to reduce phantom pain and tissue swelling. The dressing is replaced by a postoperative prosthesis, which shapes the stump into a largely conical form that will more easily accommodate a permanent prosthetic limb. The permanent prosthesis must be comfortable, lightweight, and capable of producing an energy-efficient gait pattern for the patient.[61] Ambulation and muscle-conditioning activities are initiated after the first postsurgical week in order to decrease the patient's pain and swelling and are directed toward the goals of prevention of joint contractures and maximization of walking tolerance.

The rehabilitation program is advanced when the patient has been successfully fitted with a permanent prosthetic limb. Because walking with a lower extremity prosthesis may place a 50% greater demand on the aerobic capacities of patients who have undergone an amputation,[61] rehabilitation procedures parallel those used with advanced cardiac rehabilitation patients or cardiovascular conditioning clients. Progressive walking, treadmill exercise, bicycle ergometry, and stationary cross-country skiing simulation are all effective means of combining cardiovascular enhancement and muscle-conditioning exercise. The physical therapist can also employ kinesiologic measurements and objective means of assessing the patient's gait pattern in order to maximize the energy efficiency of ambulation.[61] When rehabilitation is effective, the patient who has experienced a knee amputation can return to activities of daily life with a negligible or even nonexistent degree of functional disability.

## EVALUATION

### History

The patient's history, or subjective interview, is the first step of the clinical process that results in an accurate physical therapy differential diagnosis of a knee disorder. In taking a history, the clinician collects important information about the patient's injury experience that helps with the formation of a clinical impression or clinical hypothesis. This initial hypothesis is then tested through the other components of the clinical evaluation process as the patient's subjective complaints are translated into objective findings of knee pathology.

The history is designed to clarify the occurrence aspects of the knee disorder and outline the patient's present complaints. Information is collected about the onset of the problem (sudden versus gradual) and the duration of the disorder (acute versus chronic).[63–65] The patient's description of the precise location of the problem in the knee complex and of the exact mechanism of injury is beneficial in this phase of clinical evaluation.[63–65] Information is also elicited on the existence and onset of any joint swelling, nearly immediate as with a hemarthrosis versus delayed as with a synovial irritation; any unusual sensations that accompanied the injury, such as an audible pop or a feeling of knee instability; and the patient's performance status, including ambulation ability and any functional disability related to normal daily requirements.[63–65]

The clinical history must also include a thorough description of the patient's knee pain: the nature of the pain (the dull ache of a degenerative situation versus the sharp intensity of a mechanical problem), the effect of changes of position and posture on the pain, and the reaction of the pain to rest (diminution is indicative of a mechanical disorder, whereas presence of pain indicates a nonmechanical, systemic problem).[63–65] A comparison of the history with the information presented in the preceding discussions of knee pathologies helps form the initial clinical impression, which becomes a differential diagnosis when the entire evaluation has been completed. Also, any information regarding previous knee problems (a recurring disorder versus a new injury) helps to guide the course of rehabilitation.

## Observation

This portion of the clinical evaluation focuses on the patient's gait, posture, knee swelling, and lower extremity anthropometric measurements. The patient's ambulation ability and gait pattern are analyzed to detect any deviation from a normal functional condition.[63] Gait assessment helps in gauging the willingness of the patient to move the affected knee and determining the performance of the joint during functional closed lower extremity kinetic chain activities.

The patient's standing posture is observed to compare the injured knee to the noninvolved lower extremity.[63,64] The position of the knee is viewed to screen for the presence of genu varus or genu valgus postural discrepancies, which would affect the normal biomechanics of the knee.[64] The patella is observed to note the existence of any patellar positional problems, such as patella alta or patella infera, and to screen for malalignment problems that would disrupt normal patellar tracking.[63] In addition, the patellar Q angle may be measured to assess the presence of any arthrokinematic abnormality.[63,64]

The extent of knee swelling and the knee's response to swelling provide important information about the patient's problem. Joint swelling and effusion may be highly localized, suggestive of bursal involvement; gradual and generalized, suggestive of a synovial or meniscal irritation; immediate and generalized, suggestive of a hemarthrosis and intra-articular derangement; or apparently absent with extravasation of fluid into the quadriceps, hamstrings, and gastrocnemius muscle groups, suggestive of knee capsule disruption.[63] The knee complex must also be studied for any signs of trauma, such as abrasions, contusions, and ecchymoses, which may indicate the site of tissue stress and provide clues to the mechanism of knee injury.[63]

As an adjunct to the subjective observation of knee swelling, anthropometric measurements are taken to quantify the degree and extent of knee effusion.[63,64] Anthropometric readings are also useful in determining the extent of muscle atrophy accompanying a chronic knee disorder.[63,64] Although specific schemes may vary between clinicians, most take circumferential measurements with a tape measure at the knee joint line, at the suprapatellar region over the VMO, at midthigh, and over the muscle belly of the gastrocnemius.[63] The circumferential measurements

are recorded on a relative scale that may be used to gauge the patient's progress through the rehabilitation process; the joint line circumferential measurement should decrease as the problems of effusion and swelling are resolved, and the other measures should increase as atrophied muscles are conditioned.

## Medical Visualization

### Radiographs

Medical visualization techniques for the assessment of knee disorders include radiography, arthrography, scintolography (bone scans), and MRI. X-ray films are useful for the differential diagnosis of a variety of knee problems. Degenerative joint changes are marked by narrowing of the joint compartment, usually the medial side more than the lateral side, with osteophyte formations along the joint margins and the tibial spines.[66] Ewing's sarcoma is demonstrated by increased density of cortical bone with loss of normal bony trabeculae and periosteal reaction in the proximal metaphysis.[66] Osteoid osteomas are indicated by ovoid, lucent areas in the lateral cortex of the proximal tibia or distal femur (Fig. 8–25).[66] True chondromalacia patellae is visualized as increased radiodensity of the midportion of the patellar cartilage, which identifies the presence of fibrillation and articular degeneration (see Fig. 8–23).[66]

Hoffa's disease, patellar fat pad necrosis, is identified by calcific deposits within the substance of the fat pad, which indicate tissue necrosis (Fig. 8–26).[66] Osgood-Schlatter disease is evidenced by thickening and irregularity of the patellar tendon, soft tissue swelling anterior to the tibial tubercle, and fragmentation or irregularity of the tibial tubercle (see Fig. 8–22).[66] Finally, stress x-ray films of the knee may be used to identify disruption of ligamentous support structures when an increased distance is discovered between the tibial and femoral contact regions, indicating joint laxity.[66] In general, a 5-mm joint opening determined during a stress x-ray study is indicative of a grade 1 ligament injury, an opening between 5 and 8 mm is classified as a grade 2 injury, and a joint displacement greater than 8 mm represents a grade 3 structural disorder or total rupture of the injured ligament.[64]

### Arthrograms

Arthrograms are obtained by injecting a contrast medium into the knee joint cavity and then

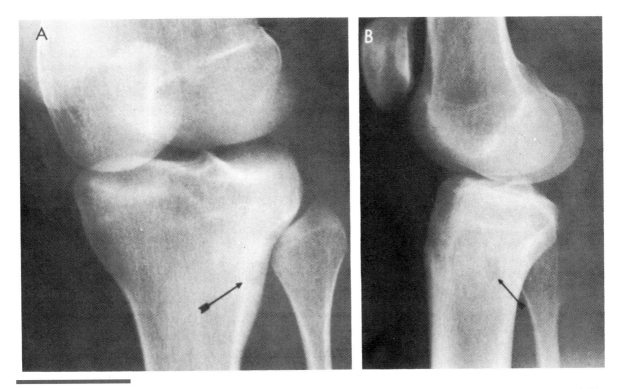

**FIGURE 8-25** ■ Osteoid osteoma (A) Posterior view. (B) Medial view. (Modified from Pavlov H, Torg JS, Hersh A, et al: The roentgen examination of runners' injuries. Radiographics 1:17–34, 1981.)

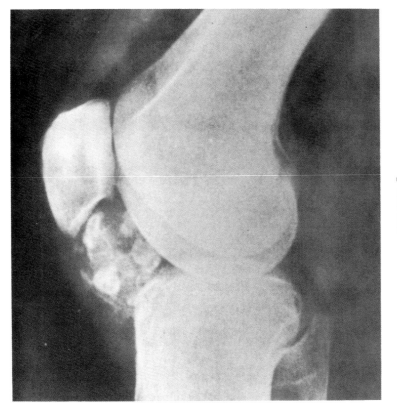

**FIGURE 8-26** ■ Fat pad necrosis. (From Pavlov H, Torg JS: The Running Athlete: Roentgenograms and Remedies. Chicago: Mosby-Year Book Inc., 1987, p 218.)

visualizing the internal environment with x-rays. A torn ACL is indicated by absence of the ligament, by pooling of the contrast medium in the anatomic region of the ligament, or by acute angulation of the anterior portion of the ligament substance.[66] Rupture of the knee joint capsule is evidenced by escape of the contrast medium from the joint cavity.[66] For a popliteal cyst, also known as Baker's cyst, the normal posterior joint compartment is demonstrated by arthrography when the knee is flexed but is absent when the knee is extended (see Fig. 8–17).[66]

### Scintigraphy

Bone scans involve injection of a saline solution containing a radioisotope into the blood stream, followed by visualization of the radioisotope's distribution throughout the skeletal system. This procedure in nuclear medicine typically utilizes a technetium isotope, which is detected by a radiosensitive camera and transformed into a visual image. A lag of 1 to 2 hours usually separates the time of isotope injection from the period of detection; a delay is necessary for appropriate uptake of the visualization medium by the affected area of bone. Relative to the knee, bone scans are frequently used in detecting proximal tibial and distal femoral stress fractures.[66]

### Magnetic Resonance Imaging

MRI is a contemporary imaging tool that has become useful for the detection of knee disorders, especially ligamentous injuries. Although relatively expensive as a diagnostic procedure, MRI has the advantages of being precisely accurate, avoiding invasive procedures, and not subjecting patients to ionizing radiation.[67,68]

MRI is also effective in the detection of osseous lesions. Small occult fractures, which are associated with 62% of all ACL injuries and do not usually appear on x-ray films, such as traumatic medullary lesions, intraosseous fractures, and microtrabecular fractures, are evident upon utilization of standard MRI scanning techniques.[69,70] Epiphyseal plate and osteochondral fractures may also be elucidated through MRI technology.[70]

## Functional Neurology

A neurologic examination of the knee complex includes the assessment of sensory, motor, and reflex functions. The patient's responses to touch, texture, and temperature sensation stimuli are evaluated through the dermatomal regions that cover the knee and its related structures, specifically the L-2, L-3, L-4, L-5, S-1, and S-2 distributions.[64,71] These dermatomes correspond to the skin surfaces covering the midthigh (L-2), lower thigh (L-3), medial side of the lower leg and foot (L-4), lateral side of the lower leg and dorsum of the foot (L-5), lateral side of the foot (S-1), and posterior thigh (S-2) regions.[71] Sensory changes, as compared to the noninvolved knee, point toward a possible neurologic conduction disorder or a neurocirculatory disorder such as RSD.

Motor functions are assessed through resisted testing, or manual muscle testing (MMT), of the myotomal distributions that affect the knee, which are also the L-2 to S-2 regions.[63,64,71] These myotomes correspond to the iliopsoas, quadriceps, tibialis anterior, extensor digitorum longus, peroneus longus, peroneus brevis, and hamstrings muscle groups.[63,71] In turn, the motor function capabilities of these muscles and the corresponding myotomal distributions are assessed by manually resisting the patient's efforts to perform the actions of hip flexion (L-2), knee extension (L-3), ankle and foot inversion (L-4), ankle dorsiflexion with digital extension (L-5), ankle and foot eversion (S-1), and knee flexion (S-2).[64,71] As an alternative to manually resisting the patient's active joint motions, motor integrity may be tested by attempting to "break" the patient's isometric hold against the evaluation patterns of joint motion.

The data collected during the MMT portion of the neurologic examination may be interpreted in two ways: MMT grade and/or strength-pain response. The MMT grades are presented in Table 8–3. As the name implies, the strength-pain response is the relationship between the level of the patient's perceived strength and the level of pain experienced during active resistive testing. Table 8–4 summarizes the interpretations of strength-pain responses.

Reflex testing is used to assess the neurologic integrity of the muscle stretch reflex arc between the muscle spindle, the afferent peripheral neuron, the spinal cord synapse, and the efferent alpha motoneuron.[71] The classic patellar tendon reflex, when the patellar tendon is tapped with a rubber reflex hammer to elicit a knee jerk extensor response by the quadriceps muscle group, is appropriate for neurologic evaluation of the knee complex.[71] The patellar reflex is interpreted by comparing the injured and noninvolved knees

**Table 8-3.** MANUAL MUSCLE TEST GRADES

| Muscle Response | Description of Response |
|---|---|
| 5—normal | Complete joint ROM against gravity against full manual resistance |
| 4—good | Complete joint ROM against gravity against some manual resistance |
| 3—fair | Complete joint ROM against gravity in the absence of manual resistance |
| 2—poor | Complete joint ROM when gravity effects are eliminated |
| 1—trace | Incomplete joint ROM with nominal degree of muscle action |
| 0—zero | Absence of both joint motion and muscle action |

From Hoppenfield S: Orthopaedic Neurology: A Diagnostic Guide to Neurologic Levels. Philadelphia: JB Lippincott, 1977.

and is reported in terms of relatively normal, increased, or decreased magnitude of the response.[71] Whereas a normal reflex response indicates a state of neurologic normalcy, a decreased response, hyporeflexia, indicates the potential existence of a lower motoneuron disorder and an increased response, hyperreflexia, points toward an upper motoneuron lesion.[71]

## Functional Mobility

A patient's functional mobility is assessed by analyzing the active and passive movements available at the knee complex. Active movements of knee flexion and extension are performed to test the integrity of the contractile elements, the muscle, the tendons, and the tenoperiosteal junctions, of the quadriceps, hamstrings, and gastrocnemius muscle groups.[72] Squatting may be used as a quick, overall screen for active mobility because almost all structural components are stressed during some phase of the squatting

**Table 8-4.** STRENGTH–PAIN RESPONSES

| Resisted Test Response | Interpretation |
|---|---|
| Strong and painless | Normal functions |
| Strong and painful | Contractile lesion |
| Weak and painless | Contractile rupture or neurologic disorder |
| Weak and painful | Serious systemic pathology |

Data from Cyriax JH, Cyriax PJ: Illustrated Manual of Orthopedic Medicine. London: Butterworth, 1983.

cycle. The nature of any pain experienced during squatting would require further elucidation through the other phases of the clinical evaluation. Active mobility testing also includes goniometric procedures and the Helfet test. Goniometric readings for knee flexion and extension may be taken to compare the available ROM of an injured knee joint to that of the noninvolved extremity or to the biomechanical range of arthrokinematic normalcy.[63,64] These motion measurements may be used as reference or as intracase normative data to gauge functional improvement of an injured knee during the rehabilitation process.

The Helfet test is used to assess the normalcy of the screw-home mechanism of the knee. The tibial tubercle is normally aligned in the center of the patella but should rotate laterally as the tibia rotates externally during terminal knee extension.[63,64] The Helfet test is performed by marking the center of the patella and the tibial tubercle with the knee held in flexion and then observing the markings as the patient extends the knee (Fig. 8-27).[63,64] Lack of external rotation, visualized as failure of the tibial tubercle mark to move lateral to the mark on the center of the patella as the knee moves into terminal extension, indicates disruption of the normal screw-home mechanism of the knee.[64]

Passive movements are used to assess the structural integrity of the inert tissues, including the knee joint capsule, ligaments, bursae, fascia, and nerve roots, and of antagonist contractile elements.[72] Technically, the special tests used for clinical evaluation of knee stability are also passive movement tests. Passive joint movements impart a variety of specific sensations to the hands of the physical therapist at the end of the available ROM, known as end feels, which have diagnostic significance.[72] The different end feels and their interpretation are presented in Table 8-5.

Related to the capsular end feel is the capsular pattern of the injured knee, which is a partial limitation of extension with a greater limitation of flexion.[72] Cyriax and Cyriax[72] define the capsular pattern of the knee, which is indicative of pathologic involvement for the entire knee joint capsule, as a proportion of 5 degrees of extension limitation equating to 70 degrees of flexion restriction. A noncapsular pattern of knee motion restriction is indicative of a ligamentous sprain or unspecified internal derangement within the knee.[72]

Passive mobility testing also involves evaluation of the accessory motion capabilities of the

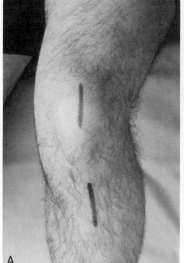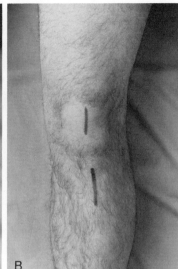

**FIGURE 8-27** ■ Helfet's test. (A) Knee flexed to 90 degrees. (B) Knee fully extended.

patellofemoral, tibiofemoral, and superior tibiofibular joints. The accessory gliding ability of the patellofemoral joint is assessed by manually moving the patella on the femoral articulating surface in medial, lateral, inferior, and superior directions in order to evaluate the relative quantity and quality of and the patient's response to the passive movements (Fig. 8–28). Passive lateral gliding may elicit a positive apprehension test response of a quadriceps muscle guarding reaction or a verbal request to avoid the lateral distraction motion by patients who are susceptible to patellar subluxation and/or dislocation (Fig. 8–29).[64] Tibiofemoral joint accessory motions are assessed indirectly through the special tests for knee joint stability. The accessory motion potentials of the superior tibiofibular joint are examined by manually grasping the superior aspect of the fibula and attempting to glide it in anterolateral and posteromedial directions. This may be accomplished with the patient seated on an examination table with knees flexed to 90 degrees or with the patient positioned in a hands-and-knees configuration. Conclusions about relative hypomobility, normal mobility, or hypermobility are drawn by comparing the injured side to the noninvolved lower extremity for passive mobility testing at all joints of the knee complex.

## Functional Stability

The clinical evaluation of the functional stability of the knee complex involves performing special tests that selectively stress the cruciate and collateral ligaments and the meniscal cartilages. The responses of the knee to each of the stability tests provide significant information for an accurate differential diagnosis of the nature of a patient's knee pathology. Many different knee stress tests exist, but the present discussion focuses on the techniques that can generate the most consistent and reliable responses. Additional information on knee stability tests can be found in the works of Daniel et al.,[73] Davies and

**Table 8-5.** END FEELS[72]

| End Feel | Sensation | Interpretation |
|---|---|---|
| Bone to bone | Abrupt halt of knee motion; contact of bony surfaces | Normal knee extension |
| Muscle guarding | Reflex muscle spasm during motion; protective response | Acute injury |
| Capsular | Stretching thick leather; flexion restricted more than extension | Joint capsule involvement |
| Springy block | Rebound effect at the motion barrier | Meniscal injury |
| Tissue contact | Approximation of muscle groups and soft tissues | Normal knee flexion |
| Empty feel | Motion barrier cannot be assessed because of pain response | Acute injury; indefinable pathology |

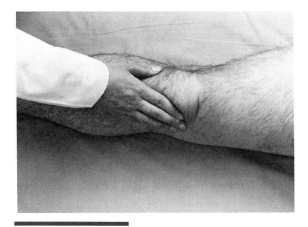

FIGURE 8–28 ■ Assessment of lateral and medial glide motions of the patella.

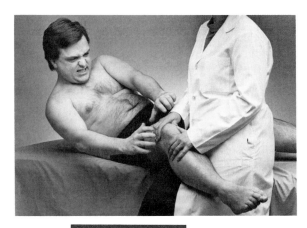

FIGURE 8–29 ■ Apprehension test.

Larson,[63] Feagin,[74] Jensen,[75] and Magee.[64] All tests require a comparison of the responses of the injured and noninvolved knees to ensure accurate interpretation of stability test results.

### Meniscal Tests

Knee stress procedures that assess the stability of the meniscal cartilages include the Apley compression test, the McMurray test, and the medial-lateral grind test. The Apley compression test involves a combination of tibiofemoral compression and rotation forces that are used to check for the presence of a meniscal tear. To perform the test, the patient is placed in a prone-lying position with the knee flexed to 90

degrees. The physical therapist then compresses the tibiofemoral joint by applying manual pressure through the shaft of the tibia by way of the sole of the foot. The foot and tibia are then rotated internally and externally as the compressive force is applied to assess the status of the menisci (Fig. 8–30).

The McMurray test (Fig. 8–31) is performed with the patient supine with hip flexed to 90 degrees and knee flexed to a maximal comfortable position. To assess the integrity of the medial meniscus, the physical therapist stands on the lateral side of the knee that is being tested and places one hand over the anterior aspect of the knee while the other hand grasps the foot around the heel. The proximal hand palpates the

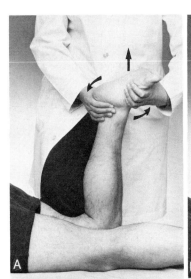

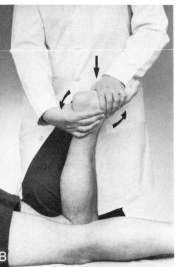

FIGURE 8–30 ■ Apley's test using (A) distraction and (B) compression.

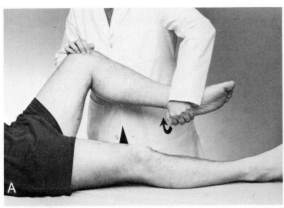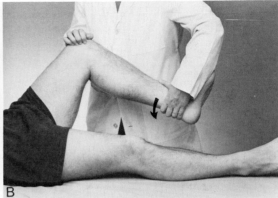

FIGURE 8-31 ■ (A) External rotation of the tibia while extending the knee (medial meniscus). (B) Internal rotation of the tibia to test for lateral meniscus.

medial joint line and the region of the medial meniscus as a valgus force is applied to the knee. The distal hand externally rotates the tibia, by way of the foot and ankle, and then slowly extends the knee from the starting position. The combined motion of valgus, extension, and external rotation produces a palpable or audible clicking response over the medial joint line if the medial meniscus has sustained structural damage. To test the lateral meniscus, the patient assumes the same starting position of hip and knee flexion but the physical therapist stands on the contralateral side of the patient and reaches across the patient's body to hold the affected lower extremity at the knee and foot. The proximal hand palpates the lateral joint line and the region of the lateral meniscus and also applies a varus stress to the knee as the distal hand grasps the heel and ankle and provides an internal rotation force to the knee through the tibia. The knee is then slowly extended; the combination of varus, extension, and internal rotation forces elicits an audible or palpable clicking sensation over the lateral knee joint line if the lateral meniscus has been injured.

The medial-lateral grind test for meniscal integrity is performed with the patient supine on an examining table as the physical therapist supports the knee with one hand, holds the lower leg between the support arm and the side of the body, and places the other hand over the anterior aspect of the knee.[42] The index finger and the thumb of the lead hand are positioned to palpate the medial and lateral joint lines of the knee and the corresponding regions of the medial and lateral menisci.[42] From a starting position of full extension, alternating varus and

valgus stresses are applied as the knee is alternately flexed and extended to and from a position of 45 degrees flexion.[42] A longitudinal meniscal tear produces a grinding sensation along the lateral joint line for a lateral cartilaginous injury and along the medial joint line for medial meniscal involvement.[42] Prolonged grinding is indicative of a complex meniscal tear or of injury to both menisci.[42] The medial-lateral grind test may also produce a pivot shift response if the patient has sustained an ACL injury.[42]

## Collateral Ligament Tests

The functional stability and structural integrity of the MCL and LCL are assessed through the valgus and varus stress tests, respectively (Figs. 8-32 and 8-33). These tests are performed for both terminal knee extension and a position of 30 degrees knee flexion. The injured knee is supported by placing the foot and ankle between the physical therapist's arm and the side of the therapist's body as the hands are placed on the knee to provide either a valgus or varus force to the joint line of the knee. A valgus force is used to gap the medial aspect of the tibiofemoral joint in order to stress the MCL, and a varus force is used to gap the lateral side of the knee complex, thereby stressing the LCL. The performance of the valgus and varus procedures in both full extension and 30 degrees flexion controls for the factor of tibiofemoral stability via the screw-home mechanism of terminal knee extension, which might result in false interpretation of test results. A true MCL or LCL injury yields a positive stress response for knee instability in both test positions.

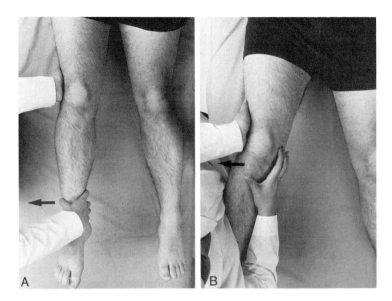

FIGURE 8-32 ■ (A) Valgus stress test. (B) Abduction stress test (medial laxity).

A collateral ligament stress test is positive when the tibia moves away from the femur by an excessive degree when a valgus or a varus stress is applied. In a position of terminal knee extension, a positive valgus test indicates potential damage to several structures besides the MCL: the posterior oblique ligament, ACL, PCL, posteromedial joint capsule, or semimembranosus muscle.[64] A positive varus test in full extension indicates possible injury to the posterolateral joint capsule, arcuate ligament, popliteus muscle, biceps femoris muscle, ACL, or PCL besides the LCL.[64] In a position of 30 degrees flexion, a pos-itive valgus stress test demonstrates MCL and, possibly, posterior oblique ligament or PCL injury, whereas a positive varus stress test shows LCL and, possibly, posterolateral capsule, arcuate ligament, popliteus muscle, iliotibial band, or biceps femoris tendon damage.[64]

## Anterior Cruciate Ligament Tests

ACL injury that results in straight plane instability of the tibiofemoral articulation, where abnormal anterior translation of the tibia on the femur occurs, may be detected through the ante-

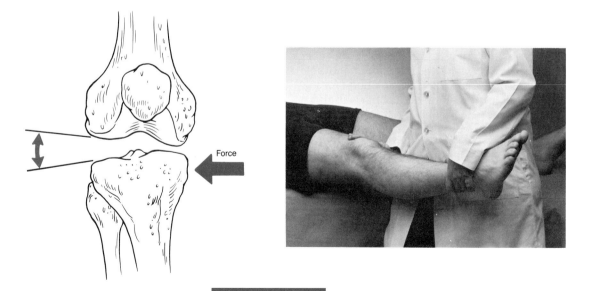

Force

FIGURE 8-33 ■ Varus stress test.

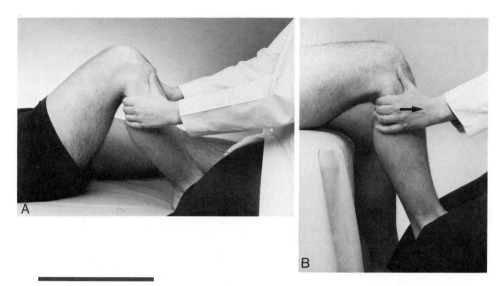

**FIGURE 8-34** ■ Anterior drawer test. (A) Classic test postion. (B) Alternative test position.

rior drawer and Lachman stress tests. The anterior drawer test (Fig. 8–34A and B) is performed with the patient positioned supine on an examining table with the foot placed flat on the table surface and the problem knee flexed to 90 degrees. The physical therapist stabilizes the lower leg by sitting on the patient's foot and then cups his or her hands around the posterior region of the proximal tibia. After the patient is instructed to relax the knee musculature, the physical therapist applies an anteriorly directed translatory force to the proximal tibia to screen for excessive ACL laxity. Abnormal forward translation of the proximal tibia, compared to the noninjured knee, or a palpable reflex muscle guarding reaction by the hamstring muscles indicates a positive finding of ACL injury. Besides ACL involvement, a positive anterior drawer test may point to possible injury to the posterolateral and posteromedial aspects of the knee joint capsule, the MCL, the iliotibial band, the posterior oblique ligament, the arcuate ligament, and the popliteus muscle.[64]

The Lachman test (Fig. 8–35), which is considered the most sensitive test for ACL injury, is performed with the patient positioned supine and the physical therapist supporting the affected knee between terminal extension and 20 degrees of flexion. The distal femur is stabilized by one of the examiner's hands while the proximal tibia is translated forward by the other hand.

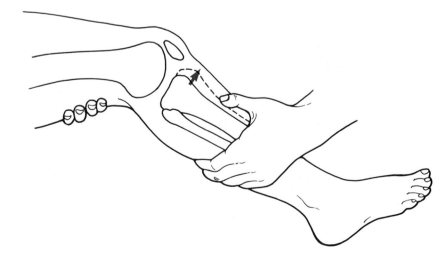

**FIGURE 8-35** ■ Lachman's test.

A normal knee exhibits either minimal anterior movement of the tibia relative to the femur or anterior translation with a firm, distinct end point. An indefinite or soft end point is a positive Lachman test sign representing an ACL injury. When the size of the patient's leg or the size of the examiner's hands precludes an accurate test in the standard examination position, the Lachman test may be modified by using two examiners, by using straps to stabilize the distal femur while both hands are used to stress the proximal tibia, and by positioning the patient prone to stabilize the upper leg while the lower leg and tibia are manually translated forward on the femur. A positive Lachman test is most definitely indicative of ACL injury but may also detect PCL, arcuate ligament, and popliteus muscle involvement.[64]

### Posterior Cruciate Ligament Tests

The functional stability of the PCL may be assessed through use of the posterior drawer test and the posterior sag sign. For the posterior drawer test the patient is positioned in the same configuration used for the anterior drawer test for the ACL: lying supine with the injured knee flexed to 90 degrees and the foot placed flat on the examining surface (Fig. 8–36; see Fig. 8–34A). The physical therapist then sits on the patient's foot in order to stabilize the lower extremity and grasps the proximal tibia with both

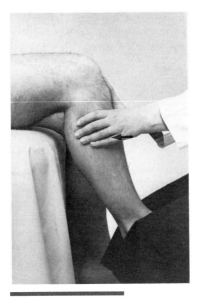

FIGURE 8–36 ■ Posterior drawer test.

hands. Instead of the anterior translation force applied to the proximal tibia in the anterior drawer test, the physical therapist imparts a posteriorly directed force on the proximal tibia in an attempt to displace it posteriorly on the distal femur. Abnormal posterior translation of the proximal tibia on the distal femur, compared to the noninvolved knee, is a positive indication of PCL damage. A positive posterior drawer test may also reflect injury to the posterior aspects of the knee joint capsule, the MCL, the iliotibial band, and the posterior oblique and arcuate ligaments.[64]

If the PCL has been ruptured, the tibia naturally slides back on the femur into a posterior resting configuration when a patient is placed in position for the posterior drawer test. This allows a seemingly excessive amount of anterior translation of the tibia on the femur when an anterior drawer test is performed, resulting in a false-positive sign of ACL injury as opposed to PCL damage. Observation of the posterior sag sign helps to eliminate the possibility of a misdiagnosis. The posterior sag sign (Fig. 8–37), also called the PCL gravity test, is assessed by placing the contralateral leg in the same position as the leg being tested for PCL injury, 90 degrees of knee flexion with the foot flat on the examining surface. The patient is now in a hook-lying position. The patient's knees are approximated so that the relative positions of the bilateral tibial tuberosities can be assessed. In a knee with an intact PCL, the tibial tuberosity appears as a distinct convexity on the anterior surface of the proximal tibia just inferior to the patella. In a knee with a ruptured PCL, the tibial tuberosity may be visually absent as a distinct structure and a relative concavity exists at the anterior margin of the lower leg between the inferior aspect of the patella and the midshaft of the tibia. The relative concavity is caused by gravity, which is normally restrained by an intact PCL, pulling the proximal tibia in a posterior direction. This concavity (compared to the normal position of the tibial tuberosity in the noninvolved knee) reflects posterior sagging of the tibia on the femur because of a damaged PCL and is therefore known as the posterior sag sign.

### Rotatory Instability Tests

Rotatory instability may exist in a knee that has sustained damage to several ligament groups, resulting in multiplanar abnormalities in tibiofemoral joint functioning. Specific instabilities in-

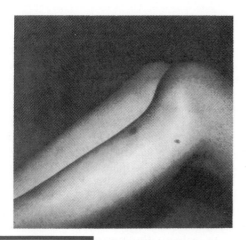

**FIGURE 8-37** ■ Posterior sag sign. (From Nicholas JA, Hershman EB. The Lower Extremity and Spine in Sports Medicine, St. Louis, CV Mosby, 1986, p 972.)

clude anteromedial rotatory instability (AMRI), posteromedial rotatory instability (PMRI), posterolateral rotatory instability (PLRI), and, the most common, anterolateral rotatory instability (ALRI). The presence of these functional instabilities of the knee may be assessed through a number of different tests that are described in the following paragraphs.

AMRI is assessed through the anterior drawer with external rotation test, also called the Slocum test (Fig. 8-38A and B).[64] The test is performed with the patient in the same position used for the anterior and posterior drawer tests: supine with the knee flexed to 90 degrees and the foot flat on the examining surface. The patient's foot is then turned outward for external rotation of the tibia relative to the femur by a factor of at least 15 degrees. The physical therapist then sits on the patient's foot to stabilize the lower leg,

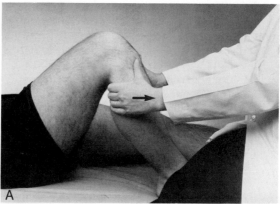

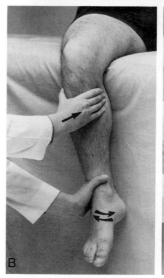

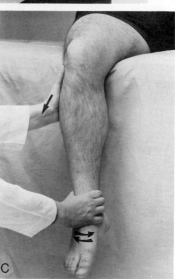

**FIGURE 8-38** ■ Slocum test. (A) Supine. (B) Sitting—posterior shear force. (C) Sitting—anterior shear force.

grasps the proximal tibia with both hands, and exerts an anterior translatory force to the knee by pulling on the tibia. Except for the position of the foot and of the tibia, these are the same actions taken during an anterior drawer test for ACL integrity. By comparison to the uninjured leg, excessive forward translation of the anterior and medial aspects of the tibia on the femur represents a positive test for AMRI and a positive indication for MCL, posterior oblique ligament, posteromedial knee joint capsule, and ACL damage.[64]

Similarly, PMRI and PLRI are assessed using the same basic drawer test position of the patient supine with the knee flexed to 90 degrees and the foot flat on the examining surface and stabilized by the examiner's body weight. Testing proceeds as in a posterior drawer test for PCL instability, the only differences being that the patient's foot and tibia are internally rotated for the assessment of PMRI and externally rotated for the evaluation of PLRI. Excessive posterior and medial and posterior and lateral translations of the tibia on the femur in reference to the uninjured knee are positive signs for PMRI and PLRI and denote damage to the PCL, posterior oblique ligament, MCL, semimembranosus muscle, and posteromedial knee joint capsule and the PCL, arcuate ligament, popliteus muscle, LCL, biceps femoris muscle, and posterolateral knee joint capsule, respectively.[64] These procedures are also known as the Hughston posteromedial and posterolateral drawer tests.[64]

PLRI may also be assessed by performing another knee ligament stress test, the posterolateral drawer test (Fig. 8–39A and B). For this test, the patient is placed in a supine position and the physical therapist manually supports the knee and stabilizes the lower extremity between an arm and the side of the therapist's body.[31] The patient's hip is then passively flexed to 80 degrees and the knee flexed to 45 degrees while the proximal tibia is held in external rotation.[31] The examiner then applies a posterior drawer force to the proximal tibia in an effort to produce a posterolateral translation effect of the tibia on the distal femur.[31] The posterolateral drawer test is positive for PLRI when the physical therapist is able to palpate the posterolateral rotation of the lateral tibial plateau on the femoral condyles as the drawer force is applied to the knee.[31]

ALRI may be diagnosed by use of the Slocum, MacIntosh lateral pivot shift, Hughston jerk, Losee, and flexion-rotation drawer tests. A positive result in any of these knee ligament stress tests is indicative of injury to the ACL, posterolateral knee joint capsule, arcuate ligament, popliteus muscle, LCL, and iliotibial band.[64] The Slocum test for ALRI directly parallels the Slocum test for AMRI (see Fig. 8–38A and B), the only exception being that the foot and tibia are internally rather than externally rotated. All other test positions and mechanics are the same as in the AMRI test.

The MacIntosh lateral pivot shift test (Fig. 8–40) is designed to screen for the presence of the

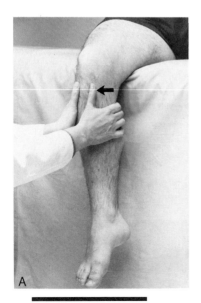
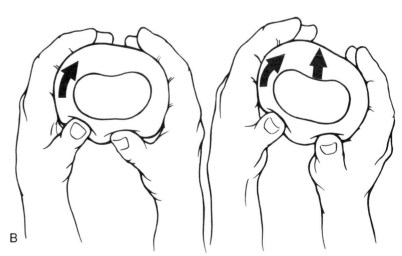

**FIGURE 8–39** ■ Posterolateral drawer test. (A) Test performance. (B) Illustration of posterolateral rotatory instability.

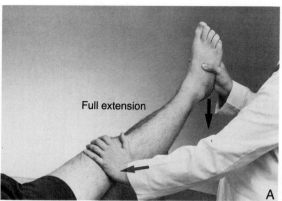
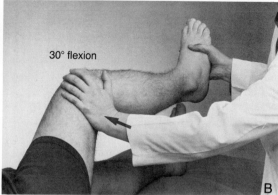

**FIGURE 8-40** ■ MacIntosh's lateral pivot.

pivot shift sign, a component of ALRI. The pivot shift occurs in a knee that is compromised by ALRI as an anterior subluxation of the lateral tibial plateau when the knee approaches terminal extension, followed by a sudden reduction of the tibial subluxation as the knee reaches approximately 40 degrees flexion.[75] The tibia subluxes in an anterolateral direction (anterior translation plus internal rotation) during extension if the ACL has been torn and the posterior capsular structures have been compromised and then reduces with knee flexion secondary to an external rotation force moment from the biomechanical action of the iliotibial band.[75] This pivot shift phenomenon is the clinical manifestation of the sensation of knee instability that frequently accompanies attempts to perform normal functional activities by many knee patients.

The MacIntosh test is performed with the patient lying supine and the physical therapist supporting the ankle of the involved side in one hand and the injured knee in the other hand. In a position of full knee extension, a valgus stress is applied by the hand holding the patient's knee to the lateral aspect of the proximal portion of the tibia as the tibia is internally rotated by the hand holding the patient's foot and ankle. The combined external stress to the knee of valgus and internal rotation may be accomplished by pressure on the head of the fibula if the superior tibiofibular joint is intact. The valgus force is maintained as the knee is slowly flexed toward a position of 40 degrees. The test is positive for ALRI if tension in the iliotibial band causes a sudden reduction of the anterolateral aspect of the tibia, via external rotation of the tibial shaft, at or slightly before a position of 40 degrees knee flexion.

The Hughston jerk test for ALRI elicits a pivot

shift by reversing the order of stresses applied to the knee during the MacIntosh test.[75] With the patient lying supine, the involved lower extremity is passively positioned in 45 degrees of hip flexion and 90 degrees of knee flexion. The tibia is internally rotated via the foot and ankle and through pressure at the head of the fibula as a valgus stress is applied to the lateral aspect of the tibial plateau. The knee is then gradually extended toward the terminal position. In a positive test, the knee begins in a reduced position of 90 degrees of flexion, experiences an anterolateral subluxation of the tibial plateau as it is extended through the position of 40 degrees flexion, and then is reduced again as the screw-home mechanism locks the knee into terminal extension. The sudden subluxation and then reduction that occur as the knee moves from flexion toward extension represent the "jerk" in the name of the test.[75]

The Losee test for ALRI (Fig. 8-41) is similar to the Hughston jerk test in that both tests start in a position of knee flexion when they are performed to detect a pivot shift phenomenon. The tests differ in their starting position for tibial rotation: internal rotation for the jerk test and external rotation for the Losee test.[75] The Losee test starts with the patient supine and the physical therapist supporting the ankle of the involved lower extremity with one hand as the other hand supports the knee in a position of 45 degrees flexion. As the hand on the foot and ankle imparts an external rotatory force through the tibia, the thumb of the other hand hooks the head of the fibula as the fingers are draped over the patella. The hand at the knee then applies a valgus force to the proximal tibia as the thumb lifts upward on the head of the fibula to reverse the tibial rotation moment from an external to an

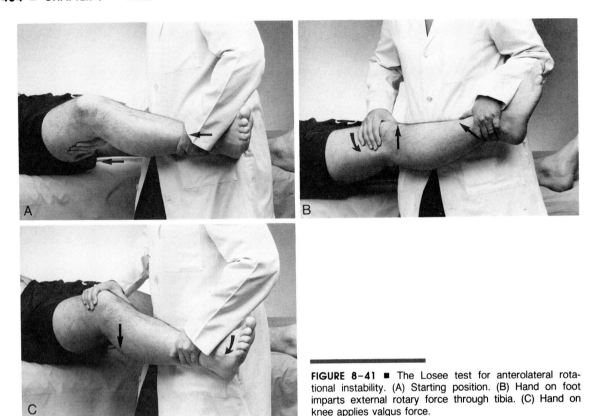

FIGURE 8–41 ■ The Losee test for anterolateral rotational instability. (A) Starting position. (B) Hand on foot imparts external rotary force through tibia. (C) Hand on knee applies valgus force.

internal direction. The knee is then slowly extended; the established situation of forces creates an anterolateral subluxation of the tibial plateau as the knee moves toward full extension in a positive test. The Losee test is used as an alternative to the MacIntosh and Hughston tests because it reproduces the mechanism of functional knee instability that can accompany jumping and deceleration activities.[75]

The flexion-rotation drawer test (Fig. 8–42) is a modification of the MacIntosh test and produces the lateral pivot shift effect of tibial plateau subluxation through the effect of gravity acting on the proximal femur instead of a manually applied valgus force.[75] As the patient lies supine, the examining therapist supports the involved lower extremity with both hands and holds the knee in a position of 20 degrees flexion with neutral tibial rotation. In the presence of ALRI, the pull of gravity causes a posterior displacement of the distal femur relative to the tibial plateau along with an external rotation force moment, which together result in an anterior subluxation of the lateral tibial plateau. The physical therapist then imparts a posterior force to the proximal tibia, as in a posterior drawer test, and the knee is slowly flexed. This combination of forces produces the pivot shift of anterolateral tibial plateau subluxation, which suddenly reduces via the influence of the iliotibial band as the knee reaches a position of 40 degrees flexion.

## Interpretation of Knee Ligament Stability Tests

Knee stability tests may be interpreted in terms of either the degree or grade of ligamentous laxity. Laxity, however, must be differentiated from stability. Laxity refers to the degree of slackness, or state of tension, in a ligament, as determined through the clinical examination process, and may be described as normal, based on arthrokinematics and normal accessory joint motions, or abnormal, indicating physical damage to the restraint structure.[76] The grade or degree of ligamentous laxity is based upon the amount of joint movement present during stability testing.[76] The relative state of ligamentous laxity does not necessarily, however, translate into a situation of

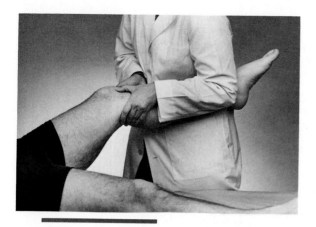

**FIGURE 8–42** ■ The flexion-rotation drawer test.

functional instability. Instability refers to the patient's perception or description of a form of abnormal knee movement that precludes successful participation in or completion of functional activities of daily life.[76] Some patients may have ligamentous laxity at the knee but not demonstrate any appreciable degree of instability; conversely, patients without any degree of laxity may demonstrate functional instability.[76] In the majority of cases, however, abnormal ligamentous laxity develops into functional instability of the knee complex.[76]

Knee injury, secondary to ligamentous laxity and functional instability, may be expressed in terms of three degrees. A first-degree, or mild, injury presents with relatively minor symptoms and represents damage to only a limited portion of a ligament's fibers. The patient demonstrates point tenderness over the injured ligament and a negligible amount of abnormal joint motion. A second-degree, or moderate, injury represents a partial, but incomplete, tear of the affected ligament that results in a moderate loss of functional performance ability and a moderate amount of abnormal knee joint motion. A third-degree, or severe, injury, which is a complete rupture of a ligamentous structure, presents as a total loss of normal knee function accompanied by substantial amounts of abnormal mobility.

A knee injury, or, more precisely, knee ligament laxity, may also be expressed in terms of different grades. A grade one injury presents as knee laxity that allows 0 to 7 mm of joint displacement. This represents disruption of a few fibers of the primary restraint ligaments while the secondary restraints are not affected. For example, if a patient sustains an injury to the medial aspect of the knee from a valgus force

mechanism, a grade one sprain corresponds to some minor involvement of the MCL while the medial knee joint capsule, medial meniscus, and ACL are fully intact. A grade two injury represents partial to a nearly complete tear of the primary restraint ligament accompanied by some degree of damage to the secondary stabilizing structures. This would result in knee laxity and joint displacement of 8 to 10 mm. Compared to the previous example of a valgus stress knee injury, a grade two disorder would involve partial to complete rupture of the MCL along with fiber damage in the knee joint capsule and the ACL plus some form of medical meniscal compromise. A grade three injury presents as ligamentous laxity that allows more than 10 mm of joint displacement, which reflects complete rupture of the primary restraint and partial to complete tearing of the secondary restraining structures. As is true with a third-degree injury, a grade three injury results in significant loss of normal knee joint stability and functional performance ability and typically requires reconstructive surgery. In reference to the example of the valgus stress injury, a grade three knee disorder would involve a complete tear of the MCL, medial capsule, medial meniscus, and ACL and would, in fact, represent the O'Donoghue unhappy triad. The degree or grade of a knee ligament injury may be determined by using a knee arthrometer. An instrumented device can measure precisely the amount of joint displacement in an injured knee, which can quantify the magnitude of the relative degree or grade of the knee problem. Figure 8–43 depicts a relative comparison of the rotatory instabilities of the knee and Table 8–6 presents a classification scheme for ALRI.

### Lysholm's Functional Test

The functional stability of the knee complex may also be assessed through the Lysholm test. The Lysholm testing procedure involves a number of functional activities or specific responses of the patient to attempted functional activities that help to determine the status of the knee relative to the performance of normal activities of daily life.[77] The assessment procedures may be incorporated into a sequence of other functional tests or modified to evaluate the specific functional requirements of a patient as part of a work hardening examination. The Lysholm test scoring scale is presented in Table 8–7; a score of 85/100 or higher indicates a level of functional normalcy for a knee patient.[77]

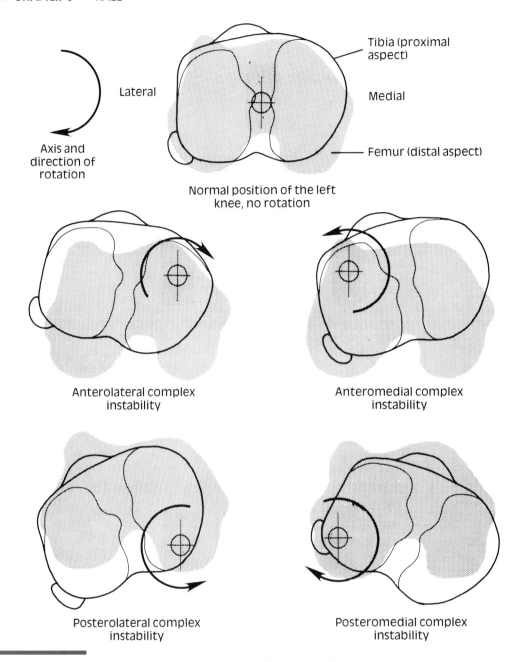

Lateral

Axis and
direction of
rotation

Tibia (proximal
aspect)

Medial

Femur (distal aspect)

Normal position of the left
knee, no rotation

Anterolateral complex
instability

Anteromedial complex
instability

Posterolateral complex
instability

Posteromedial complex
instability

**FIGURE 8-43** ■ Anatomic correlation of various rotatory instabilities. (From Nicholas JA, Hershman EB. The Lower Extremity and Spine in Sports Medicine. St. Louis, CV Mosby, 1986, p 788.)

## Palpation

A palpatory examination may provide additional information about the nature of the patient's knee problem while confirming the results of previous assessment methods. Palpation is typically done near the end of a complete orthopaedic physical therapy clinical examination be-

cause of the relatively limited precision of the information that may be obtained; a McMurray test definitely identifies a meniscal disorder, but palpation reveals only joint line tenderness that may be of osseous or ligamentous as well as meniscal origin. Using palpation at the end of a clinical examination also helps to prevent aggravation of the patient's symptoms.[63]

Palpation methods are designed to examine

**▰▰▰ Table 8-6.** CLASSIFICATION OF ANTEROLATERAL ROTATORY LAXITY

| Severity (Grade) | Amount of Abnormal Tibial Motion | Positive Test* | Comment |
|---|---|---|---|
| Mild (grade I) | 1 + (<5 mm) | Lachman, FRD | May be present with generalized joint laxity (physiologic) |
| Moderate (grade II) | 2 + (5–10 mm) | Lachman, FRD, Losee, ALRI, pivot "slide" but not "jerk" | No obvious jump with jerk and PS |
| Severe (grade III) | 3 + (11–15 mm) | Lachman, FRD, Losee, ALRI, jerk, PS | Obvious jump with jerk and PS and gross subluxation-reduction with test |
| Gross (grade IV) | 4 + (>15 mm) | Lachman, FRD, Losee, ALRI, jerk, PS | Impingement of lateral tibial plateau in subluxated position which requires examiner to back off during pivot shift test to effect reduction |

* FRD, flexion-rotation drawer; ALRI, anterolateral rotatory instability; PS, pivot shift.
Adapted from Noyes FR, Grood ES, Suntay WJ, et al: Classification of anterolateral rotary laxity. Iowa Orthop J 3:32, 1982.

the aspects of tissue temperature, peripheral pulses, joint swelling, and structural pain. The palpable temperature of the affected knee region is compared to that of the noninvolved extremity in order to screen for the presence of increased skin temperature, indicative of an active inflammatory process, or decreased skin temperature, indicative of circulatory problems or advanced RSD. The popliteal, posterior tibial, and dorsalis pedis pulses are palpated to assess the integrity of the peripheral circulation through the knee complex.[63]

In addition to observations and anthropometric measurements, knee joint effusion may be assessed through three palpatory tests. An extensive synovial effusion within the knee joint capsule creates a ballotable patella.[63,64] In this situation, a patella that is manually pressed posteriorly into its normal femoral articulation quickly rebounds anteriorly when released.[63,64] A minor effusion may be assessed by "milking" the contents of the suprapatellar region toward the medial side of the knee, while manual pressure is held against the lateral side, and then percussing the accumulated fluid (Fig. 8–44).[63,64] Effusion is present when a fluid wave is felt on the lateral side of the knee when the medial side is tapped.[63,64] A third palpatory method, the bounce-home test, involves passive extension of a flexed knee. A palpable springy block or muscle-guarding end feel may indicate the existence of a synovial effusion.[63]

Several specific regions of the knee complex may be palpated to determine tissue sensitivity to manual pressure; examples are shown in Figures 8–45 and 8–46. The pain response of a particular structure may serve as a useful confirmation of the results of the other diagnostic methods

employed in the clinical evaluation. Specific tissue structures and possible pathologies that may be identified by a painful palpatory response are listed in Table 8–8.

## Isokinetic Testing

Isokinetic testing is a practical, noninvasive adjunct to the other segments of the clinical evaluation process. By use of computerized isokinetic technology, knee performance may be assessed under the conditions of fixed velocity, which may be adjusted through the course of testing to simulate functional knee joint speeds, and of an accommodating concentric and/or eccentric resistance, which varies throughout an available arc of motion to match precisely the level of applied muscle force.[46] This allows maximal, yet completely safe, dynamic loading of the joint complex at each point through the knee's ROM in order to assess the performance capabilities of all fiber types of all motor units in the knee musculature.[46] These performance capabilities may be quantified in terms of a number of measurement variables that reflect knee muscle strength, power, and endurance functions, such as peak torque or force, average power, total work, performance as a percentage of the patient's body weight, agonist/antagonist and ipsilateral/contralateral performance ratios, acceleration energy, and endurance ratios.[46] Through the objective and accurate measurement of knee muscle performance abilities, isokinetic testing enables the physical therapist to draw reliable and valid conclusions regarding the functional status of a patient's knee.[46]

Although clinically practical, isokinetic testing

■■■■ **Table 8–7.** LYSHOLM'S KNEE SCORING SCALE

| | |
|---|---:|
| Limp (5 points) | |
| None | 5 |
| Only with excessive activity | 4 |
| Slight or periodic | 3 |
| Severe and constant | 0 |
| Support (5 points) | |
| None | 5 |
| Cane or crutches | 2 |
| Weight bearing impossible | 0 |
| Locking (15 points) | |
| No locking or catching sensations | 15 |
| Catching sensation without locking | 10 |
| Occasional locking | 6 |
| Frequent locking | 2 |
| Locked joint on examination | 0 |
| Instability (25 points) | |
| Never giving way | 25 |
| Rarely giving way during exertion | 20 |
| Frequently giving way during exertion | 15 |
| Occasionally in daily activities | 10 |
| Frequently in daily activities | 5 |
| With every step | 0 |
| Pain (25 points) | |
| None | 25 |
| Slight during severe exertion | 20 |
| Marked during severe exertion | 15 |
| Marked on or after walking >2 km | 10 |
| Marked on or after walking <2 km | 5 |
| Constant | 0 |
| Swelling (10 points) | |
| None | 10 |
| On severe exertion | 6 |
| With daily activities | 2 |
| Constant | 0 |
| Stair climbing (10 points) | |
| No problems | 10 |
| Slightly impaired | 6 |
| One step at a time | 2 |
| Impossible | 0 |
| Squatting (5 points) | |
| No problems | 5 |
| Slightly impaired | 4 |
| Not beyond 90 degrees flexion | 2 |
| Impossible | 0 |
| Threshold for normalcy: | 85/100 |

Data from Gillon J: Comparative validity of a functional knee test with isokinetic and arthrometer testing in anterior cruciate ligament deficient patients. Isokinetic Continuing Education Course and MERAC Workshop, Cedar Rapids, IA, August 24-26, 1990.

does have limitations. As a noninvasive procedure, isokinetic testing of knee muscle function and knee joint stability cannot approach the precision of invasive procedures, such as direct needle electromyography, muscle biopsy, arthroscopic visualization, or MRI. Also, isokinetic testing of the knee depends largely on a bilateral comparison of the injured side to the contralat-eral, noninvolved side or to an established data base and, therefore, depends on the presence of a normal range of knee motion to yield completely accurate test results. In addition, isokinetics is still a relatively young branch of medical science, having been founded in the late 1960s through the work of James Perrine.[46] Its rate of evolution parallels the ongoing advances in computer science and technology, but a thorough and comprehensive set of clinical procedures and measurement standards that is accepted throughout the field of physical therapy has not yet been completely developed. Furthermore, many different companies manufacture isokinetic dynamometers, with the individual devices representing variations on a common theme. Even though each device demonstrates appropriate levels of intrarater or intra-device species and measurement reliability, an acceptable level of inter-rater reliability does not yet exist between the devices made by different companies. This is the isokinetic paradox: high-technology equipment exists that is both accurate and practical for the objective clinical measurement of joint performance capabilities, yet its clinical potential is limited by the lack of standardization and diversity of equipment options in the field. This paradox should be solved as more knowledge is gained through clinical and laboratory research.

Although differences exist between specific devices, the majority of isokinetic protocols for testing the knee complex share the same principles. These principles, which are based on both scientific research and long-term clinical experience, include pretest preparation, stabilization of the patient, testing sequence, prespeed preparation, and data collection format. Pretest preparation involves instruction of the patient in all the aspects of the upcoming isokinetic experience, in order to reduce measurement error resulting from the learning effect, and preparation of the cardiovascular system for a relatively intense exercise effect, which may be accomplished through any aerobic-type activity that raises the patient's core temperature.

Stabilization involves relative isolation of the knee joint, which is interfaced to the computerized isokinetic dynamometer, onto which the patient is firmly strapped. The straps are designed to eliminate or at least minimize extraneous movements that might occur at the ankle, knee, hip, and pelvic complexes and might alter muscle recruitment patterns, thereby clouding the quadriceps and hamstrings performance data to be collected. Straps across the chest and shoulder and hand grips may also be used to minimize

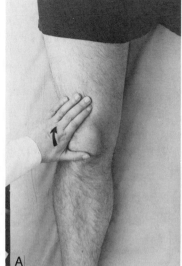
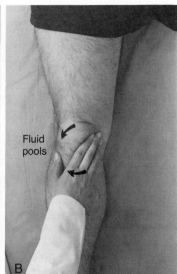

FIGURE 8–44 ■ Assessment of effusion: (A) medial and (B) lateral.

effects of the torso and upper body muscles and joints on the test signal.

Based on clinical research and experience, testing proceeds in a sequence of low to high isokinetic speeds for the noninvolved joint, followed by the injured knee. Progressing from lower to higher isokinetic velocities is thought to ease the accommodation of the patient to the demands of the test and to facilitate an optimal neuromuscular reaction of both the agonist and antagonist muscles so that accurate and stable performance data may be collected.[46] Testing the noninvolved knee before the involved knee allows the accurate collection of data on the con-

tralateral quadriceps and hamstrings muscle groups, which serve as a reference for the corresponding muscle groups of the ipsilateral, involved knee for the data interpretation process, and also facilitates accommodation of the patient to the demands of isokinetic knee testing.[46] Another aspect of the isokinetic testing sequence is that the knee begins from a position of flexion and then moves through reciprocal cycles of extension followed by flexion to assess the quadriceps and hamstrings performance capabilities. The same sequence may be followed with reciprocal concentric or eccentric agonist and then antagonist muscle testing, with concentric quadri-

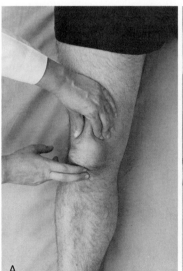
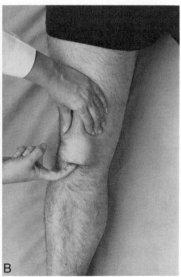

FIGURE 8–45 ■ Palpation of the patellar tendon (A) Midsubstance. (B) Patellar attachment.

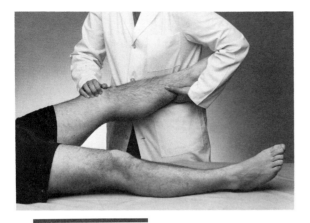

**FIGURE 8-46** ■ Examination for suprapatellar plica.

ceps followed by eccentric quadriceps or with eccentric hamstrings followed by concentric hamstrings testing formats.

In addition to the pretest period of cardiovascular preparation, a prespeed warm-up of isokinetic activity is used to ensure accuracy and reliability of the collected muscle performance data.[46] An effective warm-up involves at least three gradient submaximal repetitions followed by at least one maximal effort for the reciprocal motion of knee extension and then flexion before collecting data at each isokinetic test speed. The patient moves through at least three cycles of knee extension and then flexion, with the cycles becoming progressively more intense. This is followed by at least one cycle at maximal muscle intensity before testing at each isokinetic velocity. This warm-up activity is thought to control for the possible extraneous effects of the motor learning phenomenon and to allow maximal po-

tentiation of muscle performance abilities during formal testing at each isokinetic speed.[46]

Isokinetic performance data are collected across a variety of speeds, also known as a velocity spectrum, that simulate the movement speeds at the knee complex during normal human activities.[46] It is possible to perform an isokinetic test at many speeds, but relatively few need to be utilized to generate accurate performance data. Also, the speeds used should be relatively comfortable for the patient, have reference to the dynamic physiology of the knee complex, and correspond to a data base that has been established through professional research. The customary starting speed for isokinetic assessment of the knee is 60 degrees per second. This velocity approximates the joint speed and forces associated with isotonic muscle activity, so it provides a functional estimate of knee strength capacities. This is the lowest speed that can be generated under isokinetic loading conditions that does not create excessive compression forces in the patellofemoral joint.[46] The next speed typically used in an isokinetic knee testing sequence is 180 degrees per second. This velocity is selected because a physiologic overflow phenomenon exists under isokinetic conditions and its magnitude may be at most 120 degrees per second both faster and slower than the muscle testing or training velocity.[78] Because of the existence of the overflow phenomenon between 60 and 180 degrees per second, it is not necessary to include an isokinetic test speed between these two velocities.[78]

The selection of isokinetic test speeds higher than 180 degrees per second is largely dependent on the performance capabilities of the different versions of isokinetic dynamometers. Additional test speeds of 210, 240, 300, 400, 420, 450, and 500 degrees per second are possible choices. Specific information on the higher-speed measurement capabilities of the different isokinetic systems is given by Malone.[79] Table 8–9 shows an example isokinetic knee testing protocol using 300 and 420 degrees per second as higher test velocities beyond 180 degrees per second. This selection is based on the 120 degrees per second physiologic overflow effect.[78]

**Table 8-8.** PALPATION RESPONSES

| Structure | Pathology |
|---|---|
| Quadriceps tendon | Strain or rupture |
| Suprapatellar pouch | Synovial effusion |
| Prepatellar bursa | Prepatellar bursitis |
| Patellar tendon | Patellar tendinitis |
| Tibial tubercle | Osgood-Schlatter disease |
| Patellar facets | Patellar pain syndrome |
| Medial-lateral joint line | Meniscal injury |
|  | Capsular sprain |
|  | Collateral sprain |
| Superior tibiofibular joint | Joint instability |
| Popliteal fossa | Popliteal cyst |
| Hamstring tendons | Tendinitis |

**Table 8-9.** ISOKINETIC TESTING FORMAT

| Speed (deg/sec) | 60 | 180 | 300 | 420 |
|---|---|---|---|---|
| **Repetitions** | 4 | 4 | 20 | 20 |
| **Rest (seconds)** | 20 | 20 | 20 | 20 |

Table 8-9 also shows the suggested number of repetitions at each test speed and the suggested minimum rest interval used to separate the isokinetic test speeds. Clinical research has demonstrated that a minimum of four test repetitions is necessary to generate accurate and stable isokinetic performance data.[46] Also, a minimum of 20 repetitions has been used at higher test speeds to generate reliable data on knee muscle endurance capabilities under isokinetic loading conditions.[46] A minimum rest interval of at least 20 seconds is necessary between test speeds to allow physiologic regeneration of the bioenergetic sources adenosine triphosphate and creatinine phosphate in the muscles being tested; these are the primary contractile fuels used during the high-intensity, short-duration activity of isokinetic testing. Table 8-9 is not intended to replace any other isokinetic knee testing protocols that may be used to meet the clinical needs of the practicing physical therapist or the specific functional needs of the individual patient. Regardless of the isokinetic testing protocols employed in a clinical setting, it is strongly suggested that such protocols be standardized across testing clinicians and across the patients being tested.

Specific data on various muscle performance parameters are collected for both the noninvolved and involved knees for the quadriceps and hamstrings muscle groups at each test speed used during an isokinetic knee testing protocol. These data are then compiled for interpretation of any performance differences between the tested knee complexes. The specific parameters that are part of an isokinetic assessment include peak torque, expressed in foot-pounds or newton-meters; average power, expressed in joules; total work, expressed in watts; and endurance ratio, which is the ratio of the work performance between the first and last 20% of the test at the higher test speeds.[46] Table 8-10 summarizes a data collection format that may be used during an isokinetic knee test.

When specific information has been collected for all indicated parameters for the quadriceps and hamstrings muscle groups of both legs, the data may be reduced for interpretation and bilateral comparison via mathematical processes utilizing statistical means and percentages. For each muscle group, the numbers that correspond to the appropriate isokinetic performance parameters are totaled and then divided by the number of parameters to determine a mean score for each muscle group. The muscle groups, quadriceps or hamstrings, are then compared bilaterally

**Table 8-10.** ISOKINETIC DATA COLLECTION

| | | | | |
|---|---|---|---|---|
| **Noninvolved Quadriceps** | | | | |
| **Speed (deg/sec)** | 60 | 180 | 300 | 420 |
| **Parameters\*** | PT | PT | PT | PT |
| | AP | AP | AP | AP |
| | TW | TW | TW | TW |
| | | | ER | ER |
| **Noninvolved Hamstrings** | | | | |
| **Speed (deg/sec)** | 60 | 180 | 300 | 420 |
| **Parameters** | PT | PT | PT | PT |
| | AP | AP | AP | AP |
| | TW | TW | TW | TW |
| | | | ER | ER |
| **Involved Quadriceps** | | | | |
| **Speed (deg/sec)** | 60 | 180 | 300 | 420 |
| **Parameters** | PT | PT | PT | PT |
| | AP | AP | AP | AP |
| | TW | TW | TW | TW |
| | | | ER | ER |
| **Involved Hamstrings** | | | | |
| **Speed (deg/sec)** | 60 | 180 | 300 | 420 |
| **Parameters** | PT | PT | PT | PT |
| | AP | AP | AP | AP |
| | TW | TW | TW | TW |
| | | | ER | ER |

\* PT, peak torque; AP, average power; TW, total work; ER, endurance ratio.

to determine the level of performance of the involved versus the noninvolved knee. This is done by dividing the mean score for the involved side by that for the noninvolved side. The result is a percentage statistic for the involved versus the noninvolved side, which is termed the performance level. The performance deficit of the muscle group of the involved side versus the noninvolved side is determined by subtracting the performance level percentage from 100%. Table 8-11 shows an example of the data reduction and interpretation process; actual test scores have been substituted for the performance parameter variables that appeared in Table 8-10.

Based on the data reduction and interpretation that were applied in Table 8-10, the physical therapist would report that the patient demonstrated a 64% level of quadriceps muscle performance capability and a 51% level of hamstrings muscle performance ability or, conversely, a 36% quadriceps muscle performance deficit and a 49% hamstrings performance deficit for the involved joint compared to the noninjured knee complex. Muscle performance levels below 90%, or muscle deficits greater than 10%, are generally accepted as problematic for functional

■■■■■ **Table 8-11.** ISOKINETIC DATA REDUCTION AND INTERPRETATION

| Noninvolved Quadriceps | | | | |
|---|---|---|---|---|
| **Speed (deg/sec)** | 60 | 180 | 300 | 420 |
| **Parameters** | 150 | 100 | 80 | 65 |
| | 100 | 120 | 210 | 300 |
| | 75 | 80 | 70 | 65 |
| | | | 80 | 75 |

Factor total = 1570
Performance score (1570/14) = 112

| Noninvolved Hamstrings | | | | |
|---|---|---|---|---|
| **Speed (deg/sec)** | 60 | 180 | 300 | 420 |
| **Parameters** | 90 | 75 | 55 | 40 |
| | 70 | 95 | 110 | 200 |
| | 55 | 65 | 60 | 50 |
| | | | 90 | 80 |

Factor total = 1135
Performance score (1135/14) = 81

| Involved Quadriceps | | | | |
|---|---|---|---|---|
| **Speed (deg/sec)** | 60 | 180 | 300 | 420 |
| **Parameters** | 110 | 80 | 65 | 40 |
| | 70 | 95 | 110 | 150 |
| | 40 | 55 | 50 | 35 |
| | | | 65 | 40 |

Factor total = 1005
Performance score (1005/14) = 72

| Involved Hamstrings | | | | |
|---|---|---|---|---|
| **Speed (deg/sec)** | 60 | 180 | 300 | 420 |
| **Parameters** | 65 | 55 | 40 | 25 |
| | 30 | 45 | 55 | 60 |
| | 25 | 40 | 40 | 15 |
| | | | 50 | 30 |

Factor total = 575
Performance score (575/14) = 41

| Bilateral comparison: Performance scores | | |
|---|---|---|
| | Noninvolved | Involved |
| Quadriceps | 112 | 72 |
| Hamstrings | 81 | 41 |

Performance levels: involved/noninvolved
Quadriceps = 72/112 = 0.64 = 64%
Hamstrings = 41/81 = 0.51 = 51%
Performance deficits: 100% − performance level
Quadriceps = 100% − 64% = 36%
Hamstrings = 100% − 51% = 49%

stability of the knee complex. Such performance deficits or insufficiencies in performance levels are a positive indication that the patient is a candidate for therapeutic intervention.

## TREATMENT: GENERAL PRINCIPLES

In order to be effective, any strategy used in physical therapy to treat a knee disorder must adhere to the physiologic constraints of the body's inflammatory response to tissue injury.

Therapeutic approaches that deviate from the body's healing response or from the suggested course of rehabilitation after a specific surgical procedure for the knee could have an adverse effect on the treatment outcome and delay the patient's return to normal function. The physiologic processes of which the physical therapist must be cognizant are the acute, subacute, and chronic tissue responses of the inflammatory process.

## Acute Phase

The acute phase of inflammation begins at the onset of a knee injury and lasts up to the first 72 hours after injury.[2,72] The body's response to tissue damage is a nonspecific reaction with humoral and cellular components. The humoral response includes the intrinsic blood coagulation system, a protective mechanism to minimize circulatory blood and fluid loss at the site of injury that is triggered by immune system contact with exposed and torn collagen fibers; the fibrinolytic system modification of the intrinsic coagulation system, which prevents systemic clotting of blood; the kinin system, which vasodilates the local capillary bed, increasing tissue permeability and, as an offshoot, producing edema; and the complement system, which stimulates the processes of phagocytosis and chemotaxis to remove cellular debris and attract inflammatory cells, respectively.[2,72] The cellular response of acute inflammation involves degranulation of mast cells, which in turn release histamine and serotonin, and release of prostaglandin by granulocytes, which magnifies the humoral responses of vasodilatation and chemotaxis.[2,72] The combined humoral and cellular effects are responsible for production of the characteristic signs of acute tissue injury and inflammation: tumor (swelling), rubor (redness), calor (warmth), and dolor (pain).[2,72]

During the acute phase of tissue inflammation, the goals of physical therapy are to protect the area of injury, delimit the extent of swelling and tissue damage, and control the patient's knee pain. These goals are accomplished through the use of supportive splints or knee braces (Fig. 8-47A-C) complemented by ambulation on crutches. Such measures provide control against abnormal motion and weight-bearing forces that might prolong the inflammatory process. Cryotherapy accompanied by joint compression and elevation, which limits swelling and reduces joint pain through cold-induced anesthesia, and EMS (Fig. 8-48), which elicits a muscle-pumping ef-

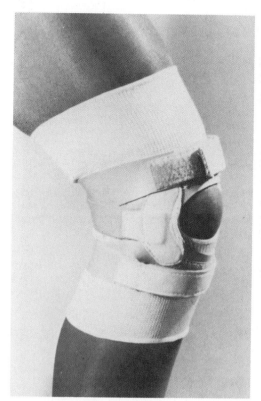

A

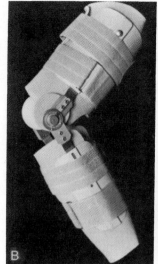

B

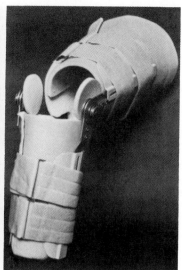

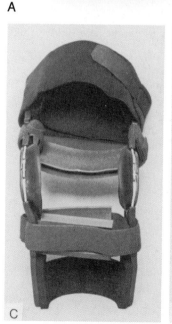

C

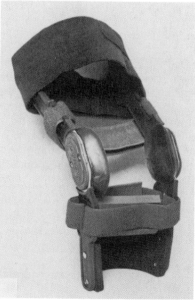

FIGURE 8–47 ■ Dynamic braces. (A) Palumbo patellar stabilization brace. (From Nicholas JA, Hershman EB. The Lower Extremity and Spine in Sports Medicine, St. Louis, CV Mosby, 1986, p 1031.) (B) Controlled motion brace. (C) Sports brace. (From Millet CW, Drez DJ: Principles of bracing for the anterior cruciate ligament–deficient knee. Clin Sports Med 7:827–833, 1988.)

fect to evacuate edema fluid from the injury area, are also efficacious therapeutic methods. Other types of transcutaneous electronic stimulation, such as classic transcutaneous electrical nerve stimulation, high-voltage galvanic stimulation, or microamperage electronic nerve stimulation, may also be effective for pain control. CPM may also be used, but more aggressive joint mobility procedures, such as active exercise and manual mobilization, are typically delayed until

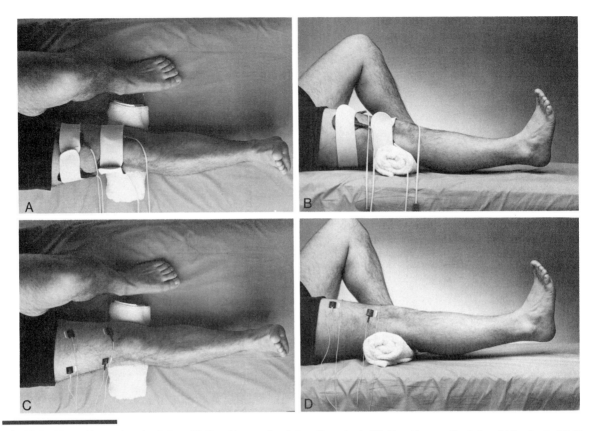

**FIGURE 8-48** ■ Electronic stimulation. (A) Quadriceps stimulation (top view). (B) Quadriceps stimulation (side view). (C) Biofeedback (top view). (D) Biofeedback (side view).

at least the subacute inflammatory phase. Isometric muscle setting and cocontraction exercise may be performed by the quadriceps and hamstrings muscle groups, if tolerated by the patient. This complements the EMS muscle-pumping effect for edema fluid evacuation. In addition to physical therapy, a course of physician-prescribed NSAIDs or other pain and anti-inflammatory medications may be useful.

## Subacute Phase

The subacute phase, or repair stage, of tissue inflammation may begin as early as 48 hours after injury, depending on the severity of the knee disorder, and may last through the sixth week after injury.[2,72] This phase is characterized by synthesis and deposition of new collagen fibers to replace the structures that have been damaged through injury. First, macrophages are mobilized to remove the by-products of the acute phase of inflammation, and then fibrocytes are activated to lay down an immature matrix of

new collagen fibers at the site of injury.[2,72] The new collagen fibers are termed immature because of their random orientation; proper alignment of the fibers is necessary to avoid the development of an inflexible scar that might detract from the normal mechanics of the knee complex.[2,72]

The treatment goals during the subacute phase of injury response are as follows:

1. Protect the healing site from excessive external forces, which might damage the maturing collagen and thereby reactivate the acute phase of inflammation.
2. Facilitate early remodeling of the deposited collagen.
3. Restore normal arthrokinematics of the knee joint complex.
4. Begin the process of muscle reconditioning.
5. Progress to normal ambulatory status.

The injury site may be protected by use of a motion control knee brace, which permits some functional joint movement while controlling against excessive external forces that might lead to reinjury. The processes of collagen fiber production and orientation may be facilitated by use of gentle transverse friction massage (TFM) and joint mobilization activities; the latter are also used to restore normal joint arthrokinematics.[72,80] Submaximal TFM across the normal anatomic course of healing tissues increases the efficiency of collagen production by fibrocytes and helps prevent the development of abnormal scar tissue.[72] Maximal, strenuous TFM, which is effective for collagen remodeling and the normalization of collagen fiber alignment, is reserved for the chronic phase of inflammation because it may damage the maturing tissues.[72] Orthopaedic manual mobilization procedures are a useful complement to TFM for facilitation of collagen production and maturation.[80]

Orthopaedic joint mobilization (OJM) procedures also promote restoration of the normal arthrokinematics of the patellofemoral and tibiofemoral joints. If CPM has not been successful for normalization of joint mobility, OJM is necessary to prevent abnormal tissue scarring, which would result in a knee joint contracture.[80] Restricted motion of knee flexion may require mobilization of the patella on the femoral articulation. This is accomplished by manually applying a caudal glide to the patella along the normal course of movement on the distal femur in an effort to enhance tissue mobility and, therefore, knee movement ability.[80] The OJM caudal patellar glide action may also be beneficial in the situation of patella alta. Concomitant treatments of medial and lateral gliding of the patella may be necessary to restore all normal accessory patellofemoral joint motions.[80] A cranial glide of the patella may be necessary if the patient has a deficit of knee extension of patellofemoral joint origin or has a patella infera (patella baja) prob-

lem. OJM is also often necessary at the tibiofemoral joint to restore normalcy of knee joint arthrokinematics and movement. Hypomobility of the knee may be managed through manual longitudinal traction techniques, which provide a general elongation stimulus to the collagenous tissues of the knee, the anterior translatory gliding of the proximal tibia on the distal femur, or the posterior translatory gliding of the distal femur on the proximal tibia, which enhances knee extension but should be avoided after ACL injuries. The posterior gliding of the proximal tibia on the distal femur, or the anterior gliding of the distal femur on the proximal tibia, can assist the development of knee flexion capabilities.[80] Medial and lateral manual translations of the tibia on the femur may also be necessary OJM procedures in restoring the normal accessory motions of the tibiofemoral joint.[80] All OJM techniques that may be used during the subacute phase require a controlled, submaximal level of application to avoid placing excessive load pressures on the healing collagen fibers.[80]

Muscle conditioning is promoted during the subacute phase of tissue inflammation by muscle setting, leg raising, and isometric exercise procedures. Muscle setting of the quadriceps or hamstring muscle groups, either singly or together via a cocontraction activity, by way of a maximal volitional isometric action defends against the effects of muscle atrophy that may follow knee injury or surgery. Muscle isometrics may also be used to complement straight leg raising (Fig. 8–49) or bent leg raising, the latter being used if, for some reason, the knee is not permitted to reach terminal extension. Straight leg raising and bent leg raising are typically performed in the four quadrants of the hip joint and consist of

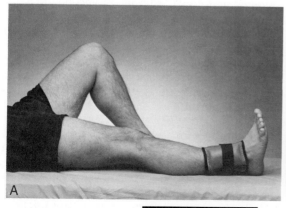
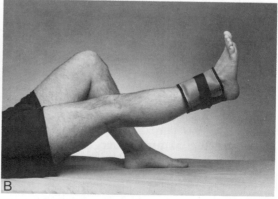

**FIGURE 8–49** ■ Straight leg raises. (A) Neutral. (B) Elevated.

isolated hip flexion, extension, abduction, and adduction movements while the quadriceps and/or hamstrings sustain an isometric hold. This procedure may be advanced to an isotonic progressive resistance exercise by adding external loads via weights at the distal femur, proximal tibia, or ankle region of the lower extremity.

Another useful exercise procedure that combines proprioceptive and joint motion development influences with the muscle-strengthening effect of knee exercise is known as multiple-angle isometrics (MAI). MAI involves the performance of isometric contractions by the quadriceps and the hamstrings, reciprocally, at various positions within the patient's available range of knee joint motion.[46] MAI exercise conforms to the isometric rule of tens with each joint position: 10 seconds of muscle contraction, consisting of a 2-second interval when volitional muscle force is recruited from a resting to a maximal level followed by a 6-second maximal isometric hold followed by a 2-second gradual force release back to the resting state of the muscle; 10 seconds of rest between repetitions; 10 repetitions for the quadriceps; and 10 repetitions for the hamstrings. MAI is then applied within the available or safe limits of ROM at intervals that are separated by a maximal position of 20 degrees. The 20-degree interval conforms to the physiologic overflow effect that accompanies isometric muscle activity.[46,78] Table 8–12 presents an example of MAI exercises. MAI complements the other therapeutic methods that are used during the subacute phase because it promotes joint mobility and muscle development and provides a proprioceptive stimulus that may assist progressive ambulation activities.[46] Treatment may also include the pain and edema control procedures used during the acute phase for effective care of the individual patient.

## Chronic Phase

Not to be confused with chronic pain or disability, the chronic phase of tissue inflammation, also known as the remodeling stage, may begin as early as 3 weeks after knee injury and may last through the 12th month after injury.[2,72] Physiologically, this period of tissue healing involves remodeling and anatomic alignment of collagen fibers to increase the functional capabilities of the affected knee structures to withstand the stresses associated with joint loading and to allow return of the patient to normal daily activity.[2,72] Treatment is advanced progressively dur-

**Table 8–12.** MULTIPLE-ANGLE ISOMETRIC EXERCISE (Example: 80 degrees knee ROM)*

| Flexion Position (deg) | Quadriceps Repetitions | Hamstrings Repetitions |
|---|---|---|
| 80 | 10 | 10 |
| 60 | 10 | 10 |
| 40 | 10 | 10 |
| 20 | 10 | 10 |
| 0 | 10 | 10 |

* Sequence: 10 seconds isometric action, 10 seconds rest; 10 seconds isometric action 2 seconds force increase, 6 seconds maximal hold, 2 seconds force release.

ing this phase of rehabilitation in order to prepare the knee for a successful return to function with a minimal chance of structural failure and reinjury. The philosophy of treatment is one of specific adaptation to imposed demand, whereby the individual's precise functional needs are addressed and fulfilled in order to restore normal levels of knee joint mobility and stability and permit maximal functional performance. To accomplish this, advanced mobilization, protection, and exercise procedures are used.

During the chronic phase, OJM and TFM are progressed as necessary from the controlled submaximal techniques applied during the subacute phase toward maximal levels of force application.[80] Such procedures ensure complete maturation of the new collagen fibers that have been deposited at the injury site through the healing process, promote proper collagen fiber alignment, and prevent inflexible scar tissue formation. In addition, the procedures re-establish the normal arthrokinematics of the patellofemoral and tibiofemoral joints.[80] However, such conditions may require additional external protection of a force or motion control knee brace, depending on the severity and conditions of the patient's knee injury or surgery, for the patient to resume normal life activities with a modicum of safety.

Progressing from the MAI procedures of the subacute phase, therapeutic exercise is advanced through short-arc isotonic and isokinetic activities (SAI), full-range activities (FRA), and isokinetic velocity spectrum rehabilitation program (VSRP) exercise. All forms of treatment progress from a submaximal to a maximal level of exercise intensity, directed by the patient's level of comfort and tolerance. SAI may be undertaken throughout any pain-free range of knee motion but is best reserved for conditions of at least 50% of

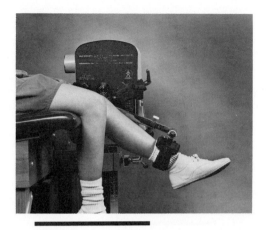

**FIGURE 8-50** ■ Isokinetic knee extension.

the patient's normal motion capability and of the chronic phase when collagen is capable of withstanding external joint loading forces.[46] Isotonic SAI exercise progresses at the patient's rate of comfort and performance tolerance in a general passive resistance exercise approach.[46] Isokinetic SAI (Fig. 8-50) is performed through the available knee ROM, which is blocked by 5 degrees at each end point for safety, through a spectrum of exercise velocities ranging from 60 to 180 degrees per second.[46] Exercise occurs in a velocity spectrum format progressing from the lower speeds to the higher speeds and then back down to the lower speeds. Table 8-13 illustrates the sequence and configuration of the isokinetic SAI approach.

FRA involves isotonic muscle activity throughout a complete, safe range of knee motion complemented by weight training activities for the other major muscle groups of the patient's body. This total-body conditioning philosophy is designed to promote an optimal state of musculoskeletal health, for the knee and for all of the patient's major joint systems. FRA includes advanced proprioceptive (Fig. 8-51A and B) and ambulation activities designed to simulate the patient's specific skills used during normal life activities. Such a functional progression, which parallels the work conditioning philosophy used in industrial physical therapy, is the direct application of the principles of specific adaptation to imposed demand to an individual patient's case and should help ensure the patient's successful return to a normal functional state.

The isokinetic VSRP approach is used during the final stages of knee rehabilitation, when motion has been normalized and joint protection is under a state of control. VSRP is designed to restore functional normalcy of the quadriceps and hamstring muscle performance capabilities.[46] As with the isokinetic SAI approach, exercise progresses along a velocity spectrum from a lower to a higher speed and then regresses back to a lower speed. However, VSRP is different in that speed advancement occurs up to the highest speed that can be achieved on an individual isokinetic dynamometer system. Flexibility is possible in programming a VSRP regimen, as some clinicians prefer to only use exercise speeds above 180 degrees per second[46] whereas others may choose to incorporate both lower and higher isokinetic speeds. Table 8-14 illustrates a fast high-speed VSRP protocol; a combined low- and high-speed VSRP program is presented in Table 8-15.

When patellofemoral pathology or excessive compression forces may aggravate a patellar pain syndrome, it is also appropriate to reverse the order of isokinetic exercise speeds. Known as inverted VSRP, exercise begins at a higher velocity, moves down to a lower speed, and then progresses up to a higher speed. Table 8-16 presents an example of an inverted high-speed VSRP format. The final level of regression for the isokinetic speed spectrum would be determined by the patient's level of comfort. This allows the velocity to be increased to permit exercise that is totally pain free throughout the range of knee motion. The general principles of VSRP and of all therapeutic approaches which may be used throughout the acute, subacute, and chronic phases of tissue healing may require modification for application to the rehabilitation challenge presented by a variety of knee problems. The remainder of this chapter describes

**■ Table 8-13.** SHORT-ARC ISOKINETIC EXERCISE

| Speed* (deg/sec) | Repetitions | Rest† (seconds) |
|---|---|---|
| 60 | 10 | 20 |
| 90 | 10 | 20 |
| 120 | 10 | 20 |
| 150 | 10 | 20 |
| 180 | 20 | 20 |
| 150 | 10 | 20 |
| 120 | 10 | 20 |
| 90 | 10 | 20 |
| 60 | 10 | |

* Speed = isokinetic exercise velocity.
† Rest = interval (seconds) between speeds.

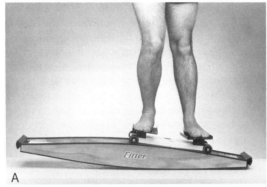

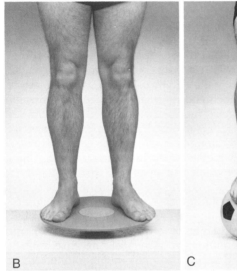

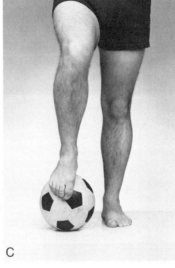

**FIGURE 8–51** ■ Proprioceptive exercises. (A) Dynamic balance. (B) Ankle platform for rehabilitation. (C) Use of soccer ball.

specific therapeutic intervention strategies for various knee injuries and surgeries.

## TREATMENT: SELECTED STRATEGIES

### Posterior Cruciate Ligament Rehabilitation

Rehabilitation of PCL injuries, both nonsurgical and those that require reconstruction, may be descriptively classified as occurring in distinct phases. The phases are meant to categorize various rehabilitation procedures and to serve as a general guide for management of the patient. These are only guidelines for PCL rehabilitation. The individual nature of each patient's injury, surgery, and response to therapeutic intervention dictates the course of actual rehabilitation procedures. PCL rehabilitation progresses through preoperative, maximal protection, controlled mo-

tion, moderate protection, minimum protection, and return to activity phases.

### Preoperative Phase

This phase of rehabilitation precedes the surgical repair of a PCL injury and is applicable only to patients scheduled to undergo knee surgery. However, the procedures and principles are important aspects of many nonsurgical contemporary physical therapy regimens. The primary focus of this phase is education of the patient. The patient is instructed about the nature of the surgery, the postsurgical experience, the importance of postsurgical rehabilitation, and the necessity of compliance with the rehabilitation process to ensure a successful surgical outcome. The patient is also familiarized with the aspects of neuromuscular stimulation as a therapeutic modality, the nature and usage of a controlled-motion cast brace, and the muscle conditioning activities that will encompass the individualized

**▰▰▰▰ Table 8–14.** HIGH-SPEED VELOCITY SPECTRUM REHABILITATION PROGRAM

| Speed* (deg/sec) | Repetitions | Rest† (seconds) |
|---|---|---|
| 180 | 10 | 20 |
| 210 | 10 | 20 |
| 240 | 10 | 20 |
| 270 | 10 | 20 |
| 300 | 20 | 20 |
| 270 | 10 | 20 |
| 240 | 10 | 20 |
| 210 | 10 | 20 |
| 180 | 10 | 20 |

\* Speed = isokinetic exercise velocity.
† Rest = minimum interval (seconds) between speeds.
Data from Davies GJ: A Compendium of Isokinetics in Clinical Usage, 3rd ed. LaCrosse, WI: S&S Publishers, 1987.

**▰▰▰▰ Table 8–15.** COMBINED SPEED VELOCITY SPECTRUM REHABILITATION PROGRAM

| Speed* (deg/sec) | Repetitions | Rest† (seconds) |
|---|---|---|
| 60 | 10 | 20 |
| 120 | 10 | 20 |
| 180 | 10 | 20 |
| 240 | 10 | 20 |
| 300 | 10 | 20 |
| 360 | 10 | 20 |
| 420 | 10 | 20 |
| 500 | 20 | 20 |
| 420 | 10 | 20 |
| 360 | 10 | 20 |
| 300 | 10 | 20 |
| 240 | 10 | 20 |
| 180 | 10 | 20 |
| 120 | 10 | 20 |
| 60 | 10 | |

\* Speed = isokinetic exercise velocity.
† Rest = minimum interval (seconds) between speeds.

postsurgical home exercise program. Finally, the patient is introduced to continuous passive motion (CPM) as a postsurgical treatment device and instructed in the use of ambulatory devices for mobility.

## Maximal Protection Phase

The maximal protection phase begins immediately after a patient's PCL surgery and lasts until 6 weeks after surgery. The goals of this period are to

1. Protect the articular cartilage of the healing knee.
2. Reduce the possibility of scar tissue adhesion formation.
3. Ensure adequate circulation to the surgery site and the remodeling tissues.
4. Re-establish normal tibiofemoral and patellofemoral arthrokinematics.
5. Attain voluntary control over joint forces through muscle reconditioning.

These goals are accomplished first through a program of CPM and protective bracing.

CPM is initiated immediately after surgery and continues on a home basis after discharge from the hospital. It is performed for 8 to 12 hours per day for the first 6 weeks after surgery. The first, second, and third postsurgical weeks involve a CPM protocol of 15 degrees extension to 70 degrees knee flexion which is progressed to a range of 0 degrees extension to 90 degrees flexion for postsurgical weeks 4 to 6. The CPM is programmed at the rate of 5 cycles per minute and is accompanied by continuous electronic neuro-

muscular stimulation to the quadriceps femoris muscle group. CPM may be complemented by ice, elevation, and cryocompression pumping of the knee to help decrease joint swelling. This is complemented by a home program of isometric muscle setting, cocontraction exercises, and leg raising activities to facilitate knee muscle reconditioning.

Also immediately after surgery, the patient is fitted with a long-leg cast brace. The brace is a cross between traditional cast immobilization and a protective knee support that is designed to

**▰▰▰▰ Table 8–16.** INVERTED HIGH-SPEED VELOCITY SPECTRUM REHABILITATION PROGRAM

| Speed* (deg/sec) | Repetitions | Rest† (seconds) |
|---|---|---|
| 300 | 10 | 20 |
| 270 | 10 | 20 |
| 240 | 10 | 20 |
| 210 | 10 | 20 |
| 180 | 20 | 20 |
| 210 | 10 | 20 |
| 240 | 10 | 20 |
| 270 | 10 | 20 |
| 300 | 10 | |

\* Speed = isokinetic exercise velocity.
† Rest = minimum interval (seconds) between speeds.

allow a controlled degree of joint motion while protecting the healing tissues from excessive, deleterious joint forces. The brace worn by the patient when not actively involved with CPM is initially set to allow knee motion through a range of 30 to 70 degrees knee flexion. Use of the brace also allows the patient to begin crutch ambulation as early as 2 days after knee surgery, using a completely non-weight-bearing status on the surgical side.

After discharge from the hospital, the patient continues all previous programs, progressing in the home program at an individual rate of comfort and tolerance through the third postsurgical week. During this time the patient is also involved in active exercise activities for the uninvolved leg and for the trunk and upper extremities in order to preserve an optimal level of systemic health. From the fourth week through the sixth postoperative week, the patient begins crutch ambulation with touch-down weight-bearing status, still using the cast brace set for 30 to 70 degrees flexion mobility. At this time MAI exercises are initiated. MAI is progressed gradually from a submaximal to a maximal level of intensity and may be accomplished through manual or isokinetic means or with assistance from the noninvolved leg. The isometric rule of tens is used for MAI activities.

### Controlled-Motion Phase

The controlled-motion phase of PCL rehabilitation lasts from the 7th through the 12th week after knee surgery. The treatment goals for this phase are to:

1. Control external forces while protecting the healing knee.
2. Nourish the articular cartilage surfaces of the knee joints.
3. Decrease and eliminate knee complex fibrosis.
4. Stimulate collagen fiber maturation and remodeling.
5. Promote complete revascularization of the repair site.
6. Obtain a normal, functional range of knee joint motion.
7. Normalize muscle force production ability (strength).

At the seventh week, the patient begins crutch ambulation with a 25% weight-bearing status and also begins active mobility exercises within the limits of the controlled-motion brace, the arc of which is progressed to limits of 20 and 80 degrees of knee flexion. The patient also begins progressive resistance isotonic exercises, including eccentric activities and SAI exercises.

At the ninth postsurgical week the program is progressed to allow ambulation with a 50% weight-bearing status plus mobility activities within controlled-motion brace limits of 10 and 90 degrees knee flexion. At the 11th week after surgery, ambulation with a 75% weight-bearing status is allowed and exercises are permitted within brace limits of 0 degrees extension and 110 degrees flexion. CPM, electronic quadriceps neuromuscular stimulation procedures, isometric exercises, and the controlled-motion brace are discontinued during the 12th week, assuming that knee joint motion goals have been attained and the patient is prepared to progress toward a full weight-bearing ambulatory status.

### Moderate Protection Phase

This phase of PCL rehabilitation begins with the 13th week after knee surgery and lasts through the 24th postoperative week. The goal of this phase is to prepare the patient for full weight-bearing activities. The criteria for the attainment of this goal are as follows: 1) an active range of knee joint motion from 0 degrees extension to at least 90 degrees flexion, 2) quadriceps functional performance ability (strength, power, and endurance) that is at least 70% that of the noninvolved lower extremity, 3) bilateral equivalence in the performance abilities (strength, power, and endurance) of both hamstring muscle groups, and 4) complete absence of knee joint effusion.

Beginning with the 13th postsurgical week, the patient is removed from the controlled-motion cast brace and fitted with a functional derotation brace, which continues knee protection until the end of the rehabilitation program. Depending on the nature of the repair, success of the treatment process, long-term functional goals of the patient, and opinions of the physician, physical therapist, and patient, use of the derotation knee brace may continue beyond the point of discontinuance of treatment procedures and into the patient's general lifestyle as a preventative measure. When fitting of the derotation brace has been completed, the patient progresses to ambulation with just one crutch, positioned for use by the contralateral upper extremity, until the criteria for full weight-bearing ambulation have been accomplished. The patient then walks without assistive devices while wearing the derotation knee brace.

From the 13th week through the 24th week of the moderate protection phase, the patient's therapeutic exercise program is advanced to include more endurance-type activities, such as swimming, stationary cycling, and power-type activities, through isokinetic training. When the patient becomes fully weight bearing, isokinetic training is progressed from SAI to VSRP, which emphasizes the higher isokinetic speeds. This high-speed exercise complements the program of eccentric isokinetic training, which continues for the development of knee muscle strength.

When the patient is fully weight bearing and can walk without the need for assistive devices, the treatment program is also modified to include advanced weight training and proprioceptive activities. Although weight training was initiated as an early part of the PCL rehabilitation process in the form of leg raising exercises, it is now advanced through the use of weight machines and a passive resistance exercise conditioning program. A leg press device is an important part of the process because it allows the combined therapeutic effect of concentric and eccentric knee muscle conditioning in the presence of a closed lower extremity kinetic chain. This effect complements other possible proprioceptive activities, such as balance training on the affected leg and proprioceptive neuromuscular facilitation patterns, to ensure effective reintegration of the patient's neuromuscular system. Exercise is not limited to the affected knee; total body conditioning is advocated to promote a state of overall systemic health in the PCL-injured patient. All treatment modes are gradually progressed at the patient's level of comfort until the 25th postsurgical week, when the minimum protection phase is initiated.

### Minimum Protection Phase

This rehabilitative period ranges from the 25th through the 36th postoperative week and includes the treatment goal of complete normalization of the patient's neuromusculoskeletal functions in the affected knee. The combined treatment program of cardiovascular endurance, progressive resistance, isokinetic, and proprioceptive training methods is advanced vigorously so that the patient demonstrates normal levels of muscle strength, power, and endurance; cardiovascular conditioning; proprioceptive balance; and functional joint stability by the 36th postoperative week. Treatment advancement involves frequent measurement of the patient's functional capabilities using objective clinical means. Although a complete functional balance between lower extremities is desirable, in bilateral comparison of the affected and unaffected quadriceps and hamstring muscle groups, a performance deficit of less than 10% is generally assumed to be a nominal index of normalcy.

The patient also begins a vigorous walking program to facilitate gradual weaning from the derotation knee brace. Such weaning may not be indicated, however, if the patient is returning to athletic activities or to heavy work situations. If appropriate for the patient's employment situation, vigorous work hardening activities would be an appropriate part of this phase of PCL rehabilitation. The work hardening philosophy of introducing the recovering patient to a functional progression of activities specific to the physical demands in the patient's work environment may be effectively applied to all rehabilitation situations.

### Return to Activity Phase

If an equilibrium between the nature and extent of the knee surgery, the methods of treatment, and the patient's response to rehabilitation has been reached, the patient should be a candidate for a return to normal activities of daily living by the ninth month after surgery. Any factor that detracts from optimal rehabilitation might delay a successful return to activity until the 12th postoperative month; further delays may compromise the patient's functional reintegration. The return to activity phase consists of various activities that are used to "fine-tune" the patient's functional status in preparation for discharge from the physical therapy program.

Because the patient has attained a normal, or nearly normal, functional status before entering this rehabilitative phase, treatment emphasizes bridging clinical activities with the patient's real-life activities. For an athlete this would mean a gradual de-emphasis on the clinic-based treatment program and emphasis on a maintenance exercise program as the patient begins to practice, scrimmage, and then play in a particular sport. For a worker this would also mean a gradual de-emphasis on the clinical program and initiation of a continuing home program as the worker progresses from light duty or part-time work to a normal duty, full-time occupational status. When the patient can demonstrate normal functional capacity in the affected knee along with successful reintegration into normal activities of daily living, the PCL rehabilitation program is ended and the former patient, now a healthy individual, is discharged from physical therapy.

## Anterior Cruciate Ligament Rehabilitation

Directly paralleling the program of PCL rehabilitation, the course of ACL rehabilitation occurs in a sequence of treatment stages: preoperative, maximum protection, moderate protection, minimum protection, and return to activity. These stages allow minimization of surgical and immobility effects in the affected knee complex and permit controlled tissue loading as a stimulus to remodeling of the reconstructed ligament. Assuming that isometric placement of the ligament substitute graft has been achieved through surgery, the rehabilitation scheme allows efficient and effective return of a patient who has sustained an ACL rupture to normal activity within 6 to 9 months. As in the PCL rehabilitation section, the material is presented as general guidelines for ACL management and not as a "cookbook recipe" for physical therapy.

### Preoperative Phase

The presurgical period of therapeutic management includes instruction in the use of crutches for postsurgical ambulation, education and training in the program of muscle-strengthening exercises to be used after surgery, and fitting of a controlled motion or cast brace that will be used to protect the knee complex from overload forces during the initial phases of rehabilitation. The patient is also fitted for a CPM unit, whose operation begins immediately after surgery, and is instructed in its nature and operation. This phase emphasizes education to prepare the patient for successful completion of the other ACL rehabilitation phases.

### Maximum Protection Phase

The goals of this rehabilitative period are to minimize the effects of surgery and of limited knee mobility, control stresses placed on the healing ligament reconstruction, maintain normal patellofemoral joint mechanics, prevent atrophy of the knee musculature, and reduce the patient's postsurgical joint pain and edema. This phase begins immediately after surgery and lasts for the first six postsurgical weeks. Activity begins in the surgical recovery room, where the patient is placed in CPM. Instituting CPM immediately

after surgery helps maintain a normal articular surface and prevent degenerative changes that might occur as a result of ACL reconstruction. CPM proceeds at the rate of five cycles per minute for 8 to 12 hours per day. During the first 3 weeks after ACL reconstruction, the CPM range allows knee motion from complete extension (0 degrees) to 70 degrees flexion. The CPM range is increased to a motion arc of complete extension to 120 degrees knee flexion for the fourth through sixth weeks after surgery. If CPM is not effective in restoring normal knee ROM, patellofemoral joint mobilization procedures may be necessary to re-establish the normal arthrokinematics of the knee complex.

Maximum protection activities also include controlled ambulation and active muscle-strengthening exercise. The patient is allowed to walk with crutches while wearing a controlled motion brace, whose ROM is limited to an arc of 20 to 70 degrees knee flexion. The patient walks with a non–weight-bearing status for the first week after surgery and may then progress to weight-bearing activities as tolerated. Crutches are used throughout this phase as a protective measure, even if the patient achieves full weight-bearing status.

Therapeutic exercises include quadriceps, hamstrings, and gastrocnemius cocontraction muscle-setting activities plus leg-raising exercises while wearing the controlled-motion brace. Quadriceps EMS is used to complement these muscle-strengthening procedures. MAI exercises are used at 20-degree intervals through the range of available knee motion as a specific activity for hamstring strengthening. This activity helps to empower the hamstrings as a dynamic stabilizer against anterior tibial translation forces, which helps to protect the healing ACL reconstruction tissues. In addition to these procedures, controlled proprioceptive neuromuscular facilitation exercises at a submaximal intensity of quadriceps action may be attempted within the limits of the motion brace. Also, the patient is given total body conditioning exercises and activities to maintain a sufficient level of overall physical fitness.

### Moderate Protection Phase

This stage lasts from the 7th through the 12th postsurgical week. By this time the patient is ready for progressive ambulation activities and begins the accommodation process of walking without dependence on crutches and the controlled-motion brace. However, unassisted and unprotected walking depends on the patient's ability to achieve a pain-free, unrestricted knee ROM of at least 0 to 120 degrees from the maximum protection phase procedures. Failure to achieve this milestone requires a delay of the moderate protection phase activities until sufficient knee motion can be restored.

The patient is maintained on the program of therapeutic exercises that were introduced during maximum knee protection but is also given several new activities. SAI exercises that advance toward isokinetic VSRP are introduced for the hamstrings, as are proprioception procedures. Balance training is especially important in light of the ACL's function as a proprioceptive structure. The patient may also begin activities that selectively stress the quadriceps by swimming, walking, or exercising in a pool and by riding a stationary bicycle. Stationary cycling begins with the seat positioned low and the knee in flexion and gradually progresses toward a normal bicycle height, which allows knee extension. The cycling activity allows gradual, controlled stressing of the healing structures, which assists in collagen maturation and remodeling. As will all phases of ACL rehabilitation, treatment includes exercises directed toward the goal of total body conditioning.

### Minimum Protection Phase

This phase encompasses postsurgical weeks 13 to 16 and emphasizes the normalization of quadriceps muscle performance capabilities. In addition to the progressive ambulation, hamstring exercise, and total body conditioning activities from the prior stages of treatment, the quadriceps muscle group is gradually progressed through MAI and isotonic and isokinetic SAI procedures toward isokinetic VSRP work. Isokinetic exercise requires the use of an antishear device or a proximally positioned input pad to protect the reconstructed ACL against excessive anterior tibial translation forces. VSRP work is permitted when the quadriceps reaches a level of performance ability that is 70 to 80% of that for the noninvolved extremity.

As complementary activities, the quadriceps and knee complex may be subjected to unrestricted proprioceptive neuromuscular facilitation exercises and to eccentric isotonic muscle training. Procedures involving a closed lower extremity kinetic chain may be instituted as exercises that simulate normal functional activities, thereby reintroducing the person to the usual demands of life. Work conditioning or work hardening may

also be initiated at this time as an effective bridge to the return to activity phase.

### Return to Activity Phase

The return to activity phase, which may begin as early as the 17th week after ACL surgery, involves a progression of activities so that the patient can safely resume normal activities of daily living with a stable knee complex. The functional progression may encompass skill acquisition, work hardening, and high-intensity exercise procedures or any activity that would be suitable for the patient's individual requirements for normal life function. The emphasis in this phase is on the ability of the affected knee and of the patient's total body to return to the activities that were performed routinely before ACL injury without further risk of joint disability.

Physical therapy procedures that are commonly used to enhance a patient's return to activity include VSRP isokinetics, progressive total body conditioning via weight training, and eccentric isotonic exercises for the quadriceps. Patients are also involved in functional skill drills, such as progressive running and cutting for an athlete and work conditioning for an industrial worker, that are specific to their life demands. The return to activity phase concludes when objective clinical measurements demonstrate that the previously disabled knee has a normal level of joint mobility along with a sufficient level of static and dynamic joint stability to allow resumption of daily activities at a level of ability that is normal for the patient. The patient who does not achieve these levels of normalcy requires additional and prolonged rehabilitation activities in order to achieve joint mobility and muscle performance ability and use of a derotation knee brace or additional knee surgery to achieve joint stability. Otherwise, there is a risk of knee complex degeneration and functional disability. The reader may refer to the works of Engle and Canner,[81] Indelicato,[33] Noyes et al.,[82,83] Sachs et al.,[84] Seto et al.,[85] and Shelbourne and Nitz[86] for additional detailed information about ACL rehabilitation.

## Meniscal Injury Rehabilitation

A rehabilitation program for management of a meniscal injury may be divided into four phases: maximum protection, moderate protection, minimum protection, and return to activity. The rehabilitation phases are based on the time required for healing of the meniscal tissue. The individual patient's treatment program depends on the anatomic site of the injury, whether it occurred peripherally (vascular tissue) or centrally (nonvascular tissue); the use of sutures for meniscal repair, which may fail if rehabilitation is pursued too vigorously; and the presence of other intra-articular pathology, such as ACL or PCL injury, which would compound the rehabilitation protocol.

### Maximum Protection Phase

The maximum protection phase begins immediately after surgery and lasts through the third postoperative week. As with PCL and ACL rehabilitation, the patient is subjected to CPM and is also fitted with a motion-control brace. The motion restraints for both modalities are determined by the site of the lesion: 0 to 90 degrees knee flexion with a peripheral defect in the middle portion of the meniscus, 20 to 90 degrees with a peripheral defect in either the anterior or posterior horn of the meniscus, and 20 to 70 degrees flexion with a meniscal defect in the central, nonvascular region. Isometric MAI and cocontraction exercises plus straight leg raising (SLR) maneuvers are used to limit knee muscle atrophy and may be complemented by EMS. Ambulation is limited to crutch walking with a toe-touch status. As with any contemporary regimen of therapeutic exercise and with all phases of meniscal rehabilitation, the patient is also engaged in total body conditioning activities in order to preserve a sufficient level of systemic physical fitness.

### Moderate Protection Phase

This phase encompasses the fourth through eighth weeks after meniscal surgery. The patient's exercise program is advanced to include isotonic loading of the SLR exercises, short-arc isotonic and submaximal isokinetic exercise, and proprioception techniques. The patient may also begin ergometry on a stationary bicycle; tension is kept minimal and then progressed gradually at the patient's level of comfort when the minimum protection phase has been reached.

The patient's ambulation activities are progressed, dependent on the vascularity of the repair site. After the repair of a peripheral defect (vascular tissue), the patient reaches a weight-bearing status of one half of body weight at the fourth postsurgical week and then advances to three quarters of body weight in the fifth week and full weight bearing in the sixth week. With a central repair (nonvascular tissue), however, ambulation progresses more conservatively: one quarter of body weight in the fifth week, one half of body weight in the sixth week, three quarters of body weight in the seventh week, and then full body weight bearing in the eighth week after meniscal surgery.

### Minimum Protection Phase

This phase is oriented toward muscle strength and endurance gains in preparation for resumption of normal functional activities and encompasses the 9th through the 20th weeks after meniscal surgery. Therapeutic exercise procedures are progressed gradually from submaximal to maximal for isotonic full-range activities and isokinetic VSRP. Flexibility procedures are now emphasized to ensure normalcy of tibiofemoral and patellofemoral joint ROMs. Proprioception activities are continued and closed kinetic chain exercises are introduced to ensure reintegration of the neuromuscular system for the affected lower extremity. Cardiovascular and cardiomuscular endurance is emphasized by progression of the patient's program of bicycle ergometry and by including swimming, extended walking, and/or work conditioning or work hardening activities. Athletic patients are started on plyometrics as a preparation for the joint-loading situations associated with many athletic activities.

### Return to Activity Phase

This phase emphasizes restoration of the functional skills necessary for return of the patient to normal life activities. Preventing a recurrence of the patient's meniscal problem is an obvious component of this emphasis. Functional simulation activities, athletic skill drills, and occupational work hardening or work conditioning procedures are the mainstay of this phase of meniscal injury management. All previous therapeutic activities are also continued and progressed until the patient demonstrates normalcy of knee functions and structural integrity of the healing meniscus on objective clinical measurements. When normal knee mobility, meniscal stability, and overall functional performance ability have been reattained, the patient is appropriate for discharge from the program of physical therapy.

## Patellar Injury Rehabilitation

Patellar rehabilitation may be categorized as nonsurgical or surgical. Rehabilitation after patellar surgery may be subcategorized as lateral retinacular release, distal realignment, and proximal realignment procedures. All categories share common aspects of therapeutic intervention at some point during the rehabilitation process.

### Nonsurgical Rehabilitation

The initial phase of treatment involves controlled-motion activities to restore a normal, pain-free arc of motion to the patellofemoral and tibiofemoral articulations complemented by muscle-conditioning activities directed toward the VMO specifically and the quadriceps complex in general. Procedures may include MAI and SLR exercises within the available range of comfortable motion, short-arc activities to emphasize terminal knee extension, and quadriceps EMS.[87] Submaximal isokinetic exercise performed at relatively high velocities may be used to facilitate normal patellar arthrokinematics and joint nourishment. Total body conditioning activities are also undertaken to ensure maintenance of an appropriate level of physical fitness.

Rehabilitation is progressed when the knee ROM becomes functional and pain free. The therapeutic exercise program is advanced to include isotonic activities and procedures that involve functional simulation in a closed lower extremity kinetic chain.[87] Reciprocal concentric-eccentric quadriceps exercise is accomplished via leg press and quarter-squat weight training.[87] Isokinetic exercises are gradually progressed toward maximal intensities and a complete velocity spectrum; any recurrence of patellofemoral pain is a contraindication to isokinetic activity.

Patients recovering from nonsurgical patellar disorders are advanced through functional simulation and work conditioning activities based on the objective clinical measurement of quadriceps performance ability compared to that of the noninvolved lower extremity. Such progression requires the maintenance of a normal, pain-free knee ROM.[87] Patients may begin extended ambulation and jogging activities at a 50 to 60% level of quadriceps function, cutting and pivot drills at the 75% level, controlled practice of normal life activities at the 85% level, and a full return to normal function at the 95%+ level of quadriceps muscle function.[87] Patients are encouraged to become involved in a maintenance program of knee exercises after formal discharge from physical therapy services in order to prevent a recurrence of patellar problems.[87]

### Lateral Retinacular Release

Surgical release of the lateral patellar retinaculum is indicated for correction of patellar malalignment or the long-standing pain of PPS. The procedure involves excision of the lateral retinaculum and the distal vastus lateralis muscle fibers to allow a normal degree of patellar tracking. The surgery may be accomplished as an open or an arthroscopic procedure.

The postoperative rehabilitation program for patellar disorders that require lateral retinacular release involve motion control and muscle-conditioning activities that are chronologically based. Starting immediately after knee surgery, treatment involves quadriceps EMS, isometric muscle setting and SLR exercises, and crutch ambulation (one quarter of full weight bearing). Ambulation and weight-bearing activities are progressed as tolerated starting on the third day after surgery and active ROM procedures are added to the exercise regimen. Joint mobilization is started in all planes of patellar motion.

Muscle-conditioning exercises, such as short-arc isotonic and isokinetic procedures, are initiated during the second postsurgical week and are progressed as tolerated within the available range of comfortable knee motion. Stationary bicycle ergometry and swimming activities may be used to facilitate a normal knee ROM. When the patient demonstrates a normal range of painless knee motion, the exercise program is advanced toward maximal-intensity isotonic, closed kinetic chain, and isokinetic procedures. Paralleling the nonsurgical patellar rehabilitation program, the patient is then progressed into functional simulation and work conditioning activities toward the eventual resumption of normal life skills based on the level of quadriceps muscle performance. Successful rehabilitation and successful return to normal function may be accomplished in as little as 8 weeks or as much as 24 weeks after knee surgery.

### Distal Realignment

Distal repositioning of the patellar tendon insertion is indicated to correct extensor mechanism malalignment or reduce an excessive patellar Q angle. Surgery involves excision of the patellar tendon via the tibial tubercle, repositioning of these structures in an area on the proximal tibia that will allow enhanced patellofemoral biomechanics, and fixation of the excised tissues via surgical screws. Surgery may also be limited to a swing transfer, where only a portion of the tibial tubercle is repositioned.

After surgery, patients who have undergone distal repositioning of the patellar tendon are placed in a controlled-motion brace, which allows a 0 to 60 degree arc of knee movement, and can walk on crutches with a non–weight-bearing status. Treatment involves isometric knee muscle exercises, quadriceps EMS, and joint mobilization of the patella. During the third postsurgical week, ambulation is progressed to one quarter of body–weight bearing within a 0 to 90 degree controlled knee ROM. SLR and stationary cycling activities are added to the exercise regimen. Treatment is gradually progressed until the sixth postsurgical week, when the use of crutches and the controlled-motion brace is usually discontinued. The patient then begins muscle conditioning, work conditioning, and functional progression activities that lead to the point of patellofemoral normalcy. A successful return to normal function may be expected by the 20th to the 24th week after knee surgery.

### Proximal Realignment

Proximal realignment of the quadriceps extensor mechanism may be necessary when there is inadequate dynamic restraint to lateral tracking, subluxation, or dislocation of the patella. The surgical procedure involves a transfer of the VMO distally into the patella from the normal proximal insertion. The surgery is designed to increase the resting length tension in the VMO, which prevents lateral excursion of the patella on the femur.

Postoperative rehabilitation initially involves immobilization in a controlled-motion brace, which permits a 0 to 30 degree arc of knee movement, and non–weight-bearing ambulation activities. Isometric exercises, quadriceps EMS, and patellar mobilization procedures complement this early stage of treatment. During the third week after knee surgery, brace motion is increased to an arc of 0 to 60 degrees, ambulatory activities are progressed to one quarter of body–weight bearing, and SLR exercises are added to the program. During the fourth through the sixth weeks after surgery the motion brace limits are increased to allow a 0 to 90 degree knee ROM and weight bearing during ambulation is pro-

gressed as tolerated. Use of crutches and of the controlled-motion brace is gradually discontinued during postsurgical weeks 7 and 8 and muscle-conditioning activities are initiated. As in the other programs of postsurgical patellar rehabilitation, muscle training and functional progression techniques are used as a final phase of rehabilitation until normal patellar functions have been restored. Return to normal activities of daily life is usually accomplished by the 24th week after knee surgery.

## Total Knee Arthroplasty

Total knee arthroplasty (TKA), also known as total joint replacement, is a surgical attempt to salvage a knee complex that has become dysfunctional as a result of extensive degenerative changes or trauma. The rehabilitation of patients who have undergone TKA surgery takes place in three phases based on postsurgical chronology: early motion, moderate protection, and return to activity. The goal of these phases is to promote a maximal degree of knee joint mobility while allowing sufficient bone ingrowth within the intra-articular prosthesis to ensure sufficient knee joint stability.

### Early Motion Phase

This phase begins immediately after surgery and emphasizes muscle re-education, initiation of knee joint motion, and reduction of postsurgical joint swelling. Muscle-conditioning activities include quadriceps and hamstrings cocontraction exercises, complemented by active EMS, MAI within the available pain-free knee ROM, and SLR procedures. CPM is started in the postoperative recovery period and is used to reduce the magnitude of joint swelling and to facilitate an increase in comfortable joint motion. Strength is emphasized to enable patients to control the limb in space independently. Patients who cannot perform SLR independently are at high risk of being unable to ambulate and, in some cases, even transfer safely.

The patient's ambulatory status is based on the type of prosthesis used in the TKA procedure. For a cemented knee prosthesis, weight bearing is allowed to the level of the patient's tolerance. For a cementless knee prosthesis, ambulation gradually progresses from non–weight bearing to toe touch and then to one quarter of body–weight bearing across the duration of the rehabilitation phase. For both prostheses, assistive devices, such as crutches, canes, or walkers, are used during ambulation. The early motion phase ends in the sixth week after TKA surgery and treatment is advanced to the moderate protection phase.

### Moderate Protection Phase

This phase, which encompasses postsurgical weeks 7 to 12, continues the processes of muscle conditioning and joint mobilization but also emphasizes progressive ambulation activities based on the stages of tissue healing. Patients with cemented prostheses may be gradually weaned from dependence on assistive devices for ambulatory activities and may be advanced to bicycle ergometry and aquatic therapeutic procedures. Patients with a cementless knee prosthesis, whose rehabilitation must parallel the time frame of fracture healing, are progressed from one-quarter weight bearing in the early motion phase to 50% weight bearing by the end of week 8, 75% by the end of week 10, and then to 100% weight bearing without use of an assistive device by the end of the phase in week 12.

### Return to Activity Phase

This phase, which begins in the 13th week after TKA and lasts until the patient's knee functions have been normalized or optimized, emphasizes maximizing full activity for the rehabilitating patient. Muscle conditioning may advance through short-arc, isotonic, and isokinetic activities to ensure sufficient performance ability and therefore sufficient dynamic stability of the knee complex. Joint motion and progressive ambulation activities, such as bicycling, swimming, aquatic therapy, and fitness walking, help to maximize both the available degree of knee joint motion and cardiovascular fitness. Proprioception activities in a closed lower extremity kinetic chain along with functional simulation and work conditioning procedures are incorporated to prepare the patient for a successful return to activities of daily life.

Although TKA surgery may produce radical changes in the normal biomechanics of the tibiofemoral and patellofemoral joints, a patient's recovery may be complete enough to permit a full return to desired functional activities without a significant degree of disability. The reader is directed to the works of Hungerford et al.,[88] Romness and Rand,[89] and Vince and Insall[90] for further information on rehabilitation after TKA. As in all programs of knee rehabilitation, success is based on appropriate use of clinical measurement procedures and progressive therapeutic techniques by the contemporary physical therapist.

## SUMMARY

This chapter has presented basic anatomic, pathomechanical, clinical diagnostic, and treatment knowledge concerning the knee complex from the viewpoint of orthopaedic physical therapy. Such knowledge should help to prepare the physical therapy student for the demands of the clinical environment as well as assist the practicing clinician in providing high-quality health care services. However, this information is simply a review of the knowledge that has been acquired to date through research and practice in the fields of orthopaedic medicine and physical therapy and is not a complete discussion of the knee. The reader is reminded that this chapter is only a starting point, because clinical and professional competence in orthopaedic physical therapy for the knee, or any other area, requires ongoing education, research, and literature review to ensure an optimal level of care.

### CASE STUDY 1: ANTERIOR CRUCIATE LIGAMENT RECONSTRUCTION

▼ A 17-year-old male high school basketball player sustained a complete rupture of the ACL of his right knee during participation in a game. He became injured while duplicating the classic ACL injury mechanism of planting the foot to make a cut motion in order to change direction. Specifically, the player was dribbling down court toward the top of the free throw circle at the opposing team's basket, quickly planted his right foot firmly on the court, and then attempted to cut to the left to make an unguarded jump shot. The lower extremity actions of planting and then cutting involved a rapid deceleration of the knee complex, accompanied by a large-magnitude contraction of the quadriceps, followed by a combined valgus and external rotation stress to the knee complex, which resulted in the rupture of the ACL. There was a loud, audible pop, followed by functional instability of the right knee, which caused the player to fall to the floor in pain.

The initial examination at courtside revealed positive Lachman's and flexion-rotation drawer tests accompanied by a subjective anterior displacement of the tibial plateau on the femoral condyles of greater than 10 mm. The battery of functional stability tests failed to reveal involvement of the PCL, the collateral ligaments, and the menisci. The player had bilaterally equivalent sensation and deep tendon reflex responses in both lower extremities, grade normal manual muscle text (MMT) responses in the L-2 and L-5 to S-2 myotomal distributions of the injured leg, grade normal MMT responses in the L-2 to S-2 myotomes of the left leg, but a grade fair MMT response for the L3-4 myotomes of the right leg, which was also very painful. The player's knee was immobilized in a knee splint, with ice packs and a compressive bandage, and he was taken to the hospital by ambulance under the instructions of the team physician. The initial diagnosis, made by the physical therapist and the team physician, was a rupture of the ACL accompanied by ALRI of the right knee.

This diagnosis was confirmed at the hospital by the finding of similar functional evaluative responses by an orthopaedic surgeon and by an MRI scan, which revealed complete rupture of the ACL without involvement of the other ligaments or menisci of the right knee. The various options for management of the player's situation were described by the team physician and the orthopaedic surgeon to the player and his parents. All parties eventually agreed that reconstructive surgery was the best choice for the player because he was relatively young, physically fit, and had a goal of eventual participation in athletic activities at the college or university level. ACL reconstructive surgery was scheduled for 3 weeks after the injury to allow time for remediation of the effects of the acute and subacute stages of tissue inflammation after the injury and for optimization of the preoperative phase of ACL rehabilitation.

For the preoperative phase, the patient was fitted with a controlled-motion brace and allowed to walk with the assistance of crutches. Knee ROM was limited to the arc of 30 to 60 degrees, which was the comfortable range for the patient, with an ambulatory status of weight bearing as tolerated. The patient was also treated with an intermittent compression cryogenic pump device designed to relieve the effects of the inflammatory process and to resolve the hemarthrosis at the right knee, which had begun to develop within the first 12 hours after injury. This treatment was complemented by EMS of the knee musculature, to elicit a cocontraction effect by the quadriceps, hamstrings, and gastrocnemius muscle groups, and by volitional isometrics for the ankle, knee, and hip muscle groups. Upper body ergometry was used to maintain the patient's preinjury level of cardiovascular fitness. The patient was also fitted for the CPM device to be used after surgery and instructed in the nature of the postsurgical rehabilitation process. Presurgical functional assessment revealed a Lysholm score of 34.

Surgery consisted of an uncomplicated arthroscopy-assisted reconstruction of the ACL using a vascularized bone-tendon-bone graft from the central third of the patient's right patellar tendon. The maximum protection phase of ACL rehabilitation was initiated in the recovery room with the institution of CPM procedures. The CPM format consisted of five cycles per minute for 8 hours a day and was complemented by use of an intermittent compression cryogenic pump and by EMS for knee muscle cocontraction. A submaximal level of muscle contraction was used to avoid possible

interference with the CPM activity, which occurred through a 0 to 70 degree ROM for the first week after surgery and then a 0 to 120 degree ROM until the beginning of the moderate protection phase. Actively, the patient was allowed to walk with crutches, bearing weight to his tolerance, and exercised via volitional cocontractions of the knee muscle groups, SLR through the four quadrants of hip motion, and MAI for knee flexion. The controlled-motion brace was configured to allow an active arc of 20 to 70 degrees during ambulatory activities. The patient was also involved in upper body ergometry for general physical conditioning and was treated at the patella with grade II and III OJM to ensure a functional level of patellofemoral joint mobility. Treatment consisted of three clinical sessions per week and continuation of the clinical program by the patient at home.

After the fifth postsurgical week, the moderate protection phase of ACL rehabilitation was begun. Progression was allowed because the patient had an active and passive knee ROM of 0 to 120 degrees, had no complaints of excessive knee pain or patellofemoral joint problems, and could demonstrate a good MMT response for the L3-4 myotomal levels accompanied by coordinated contractions of the hamstrings and quadriceps muscle groups. The motion stops were removed from the patient's brace and he was allowed to walk while wearing the brace, but without crutches, to his tolerance. The knee brace was removed completely by the 10th postsurgical week because the patient had a normal, functional gait pattern and did not report any knee pain or feelings of joint instability. Therapeutic exercise was progressed to include isokinetic bicycle ergometry using both legs; SAI for the knee muscle groups, progressed from a submaximal status based on the patient's comfort and the Daily Adjustable Progressive Resistance Exercise (DAPRE) protocol; functional balance and proprioceptive activities; and submaximal isokinetic VSRP exercise. Exercise encompassed open and closed kinetic-kinematic chain activities that simulated the patient's daily living requirements but not athletic demands. The patient was also engaged in PRE activities for his opposite leg, trunk, and upper extremities to maintain his overall level of total body muscular fitness.

The minimum protection phase of ACL rehabilitation was begun at the 11th week after knee surgery. Progression was based on the normalization of the patient's knee ROMs, his ability to ambulate with a normal gait and without complaints of pain and instability, and his responses to therapeutic exercise and functional simulation activities. Exercise was progressed to isotonic FRA and isokinetic VSRP regimens, which were developed from submaximal to maximal levels of training intensity; functional eccentric and isotonic eccentric exercises for the right leg and right quadriceps muscle group; and advanced levels of ADL functional simulation. At the 14th postsurgical week, the patient demonstrated bilateral equivalence in sensation, myotomal, and deep tendon reflex responses; MMT grade levels; and tibiofemoral and patellofemoral movement ability between both lower extremities. Manual functional stability tests failed to reveal abnormalities for the right knee; the Lachman and flexion-rotation drawer tests were negative. An isokinetic test revealed only a 4% performance deficit for the knee extensor muscle group of the right leg compared to the left leg and equal performance levels for the bilateral knee flexor muscle groups. The Lysholm functional battery revealed a performance score of 90, a normal level. Based on these findings, the patient was progressed to the return to activity phase of ACL rehabilitation.

For the return to activity phase, the patient was discharged from the formal clinical program but rehabilitation activities continued under the supervision of the athletic trainer and the consultant supervision of the physical therapist at the patient's high school. Activities during this phase consisted largely of basketball skill drills, such as dribbling, shooting, rebounding, and simulation of offensive and defensive plays, and total body conditioning exercises, such as circuit training passive resistance exercises, running, sprinting, and low-impact plyometrics, designed to return the patient to his preinjury level of competence as a basketball player. These activities continued until the preseason basketball practice activities of the next school year; rehabilitation had successfully changed into normal activities of daily living. The player was able to return to his athletic activities without a further episode of ACL or knee dysfunction.

## CASE STUDY 2: LATERAL MENISCUS REPAIR

▼A 33-year-old female carpenter sustained a bucket handle tear of the lateral meniscus of her left leg while climbing a ladder during construction work at an industrial site. During her climb, a rung of the ladder broke as she attempted to step on it with her left foot. Her attempt to compensate for the sudden absence of support involved an internal rotation action at the tibiofemoral joint accompanied by a violent extension of the knee in order to regain balance. This action produced an audible pop along the lateral aspect of the left knee, which was immediately accompanied by pain.

The patient descended the ladder and sought the support of the corporate physical therapist who served as the entry point for the company's occupational health system. The patient experienced a catching-locking sensation and had to limp to avoid pain as she walked into the on-site clinic. Examination showed generally diminished active and passive tibiofemoral ROMs secondary to pain along the lateral margin of the joint line and proximal tibial plateau. Functional stability tests for compromise of the collateral and cruciate ligaments were negative. However, the McMurray, Apley compression, and medial-lateral grind tests for involvement of the left lateral meniscus were all positive. Sensory, reflex, and myotomal tests revealed equivalent responses of the bilateral lower extremities, although a painful grade fair MMT was found

for the L3-4 myotomes and the knee extensor muscle group of the left leg. The Helfet test revealed a normal functional screw-home mechanism for the left knee compared to the right knee. An initial Lysholm functional battery revealed an overall score of 19. The physical therapist made a differential diagnosis of left lateral meniscus injury.

The diagnosis was confirmed by the corporate orthopaedic surgeon, who performed the same clinical tests and also ordered an MRI scan of the patient's left knee, which revealed a bucket handle tear of the lateral meniscus. After discussions with the surgeon, the patient elected to undergo surgery for the direct repair of the injured meniscus. Surgery was scheduled for 1 week after the patient's injury. Preoperatively, the patient was instructed in the use of crutches for assistance with ambulation, in the use of a controlled motion brace, in the mechanics of postsurgical CPM, and in the general concepts of postsurgical rehabilitation activities. Surgery consisted of an arthroscopic direct repair of the bucket handle lesion. The actual tissue defect was only a 15-mm tear in the midsubstance of the left lateral meniscus. The surgical procedure was successful and uncomplicated.

After surgery, the maximal protection phase of rehabilitation was begun for the lateral meniscus problem. CPM was initiated in the recovery room through a motion arc of 0 to 90 degrees, complemented by use of an intermittent compression cryogenic pump and by EMS for the knee flexor and extensor muscle groups. CPM consisted of five cycles per minute for 8 hours a day. The patient was allowed to walk with crutches while wearing a controlled-motion brace but was not allowed to bear weight on the affected leg. The brace permitted active knee motion through the arc of 0 to 90 degrees. Therapeutic exercise activities consisted of MAI for the quadriceps and hamstring muscles, SLR through the four quadrants of the hip for the leg and hip muscles, and upper body ergometry for maintenance of cardiovascular fitness. All activities were increased from a submaximal toward a maximal level of exercise intensity, based on the patient's comfortable response during rehabilitation. Treatment consisted of three clinical sessions per week complemented by continuation of the clinical program on a self-treatment basis at home.

At the fourth week after surgery, the patient was started on the moderate protection phase of lateral meniscus rehabilitation. SLR exercise continued, but treatment progressed to include SAI exercise through the patient's comfortable ROM. The motion constraints on the patient's brace were modified during each treatment session to accommodate the comfortable increases in the patient's tibiofemoral ROM. The patient also began cycling on an isokinetic bicycle ergometer through her comfortable range of knee motion. For ambulation, the patient was progressed to one half body weight bearing during the fifth postsurgical week, three quarters body weight bearing during the sixth postsurgical week, and then full weight bearing during the seventh week after surgery. The patient was allowed to walk without crutches during the eighth post-surgical week because she had no knee pain or feelings of joint catching-locking during ambulation, was initiated on progressive functional balance and proprioception activities, and advanced to the minimum protection phase of treatment.

At the ninth week after surgery, the program progressed to include isotonic FRA exercise for the lower extremity joints and muscle groups, using the DAPRE protocol; isokinetic VRSP exercise for the tibiofemoral joint, using an inverted velocity spectrum approach; and work conditioning exercises, using activities that simulated her usual job requirements and activities that incorporated eccentric exercise at the knee in a closed kinetic-kinematic chain. Treatment also included PRE activities for the opposite leg, the trunk, and the upper extremities plus aerobic training on bicycle and upper body ergometers to maximize musculoskeletal and cardiovascular fitness. Activity always proceeded at the patient's reported level of comfort and absence of knee pain.

At the beginning of the 12th week after surgery, an isokinetic test showed a 5% deficit of left knee extensor and 2% deficit of left knee flexor performance compared to that of the corresponding muscle groups of the opposite leg and a Lysholm functional test score of 95, which is in the range of normal. Clinical examination did not reveal any swelling or pain at the proximal tibial plateau and along the lateral joint line, and negative results were obtained in the McMurray, Apley, and medial-lateral grind meniscal integrity tests. The tibiofemoral and patellofemoral ROMs and sensory, reflex, and myotomal responses of the lower extremities were equivalent. The patient was discharged from the clinical program and was able to return to work without any knee problems.

## References

1. Soderberg GL: Kinesiology: Application to Pathological Motion. Baltimore: Williams & Wilkins, 1986.
2. Williams PL, Warwick R, eds.: Gray's Anatomy, 36th British ed. Philadelphia: WB Saunders, 1980.
3. Kapandji IA: The Physiology of the Joints, Vol II, Lower Limb, 2nd ed. New York: Churchill-Livingstone, 1970.
4. Rasch PJ, Burke RK: Kinesiology and Applied Anatomy, 6th ed. Philadelphia: Lea & Febiger, 1978.
5. McDevitt CA, Webber RJ: The ultrastructure and biochemistry of meniscal cartilage. Clin Orthop 252:8–18, 1990.
6. Swiontkowski MF, Schlehrf R, Sanders R, et al: Direct real-time measurement of meniscal blood flow. Am J Sports Med 16:429–433, 1988.
7. Arnoczky SP, Warren RF: Microvasculature of the human meniscus. Am J Sports Med 10:90–95, 1982.
8. Norkin C, Levangie P: Joint Structure and Function: A Comprehensive Analysis. Philadelphia: FA Davis, 1983.
9. King S, Butterwick DJ, Cuerrier JP: The anterior cruciate ligament: a review of recent concepts. J Orthop Sports Phys Ther 8:110–122, 1986.
10. Pascale MS, Indelicato PA: Anterior cruciate ligament insufficiency of the knee. Adv Sports Med Fitness 1:183–216, 1988.
11. Girgas FG, Marshall JL, Al Monajem ARS: The cruciate ligaments of the knee joint. Clin Orthop 106:216–231, 1975.
12. Kennedy JC, Weinberg HW, Wilson AS: The anatomy and function of the anterior cruciate ligament. J Bone Joint Surg [Am] 56:223–235, 1974.
13. Norwood LA, Cross MJ: The anterior cruciate ligament: functional anatomy of its bundles in rotatory instabilities. Am J Sports Med 7:23–26, 1979.
14. Norwood LA, Cross MJ: The intercondylar shelf and the anterior cruciate ligament. Am J Sports Med 5:171–176, 1977.
15. Dunlap J, McCarthy JA, Joyce ME, et al: Quantification of the perfusion of the anterior cruciate ligament and the effects of stress and injury to supporting structures. Am J Sports Med 17:808–810, 1989.
16. Ginsburg FG, Whiteside LA, Piper TL: Nutrient pathways in transferred patellar tendon used for anterior cruciate ligament reconstruction. Am J Sports Med 8:15–18, 1980.
17. Skyhar MJ, Danzig LA, Hargens AR, et al: Nutrition of the anterior cruciate ligament: effects of continuous passive motion. Am J Sports Med 13:415–418, 1985.
18. Dvir Z, Koren E, Halparin N: Knee joint position sense following reconstruction of the anterior cruciate ligament. J Orthop Sports Phys Ther 10:117–120, 1988.
19. Blackburn TA, Craig E: Knee anatomy: a brief review. Phys Ther 60:1553–1557, 1980.
20. Blackburn TA, Eiland WG, Bandy WD: An introduction to the plica. J Orthop Sports Phys Ther 3:171–177, 1982.
21. Dye SF, Cannon WD: Anatomy and biomechanics of the anterior cruciate ligament. Clin Sports Med 7:715–725, 1988.
22. Markolf KL, Gorek JF, Kabo JM, et al: Direct measurement of resultant forces in the anterior cruciate ligament. J Bone Joint Surg [Am] 72:557–561, 1990.
23. Nisell R, Ericson MO, Nemeth G, et al: Tibiofemoral joint forces during isokinetic knee extension. Am J Sports Med 17:49–54, 1989.
24. Grood ES, Noyes FR, Butler DL, et al: Ligamentous and capsular restraints preventing straight medial and lateral laxity in intact human cadaver knees. J Bone Joint Surg [Am] 63:1257–1269, 1981.
25. Butler DL, Noyes FR, Grood ES: Ligamentous restraints to anterior-posterior drawer in the human knee. J Bone Joint Surg [Am] 62:259–270, 1980.
26. O'Donoghue DH: Treatment of Injuries to Athletes, 4th ed. Philadelphia: WB Saunders, 1984.
27. Waldrop JI, Macey TI, Trettin JC, et al: Fractures of the posterolateral tibial plateau. Am J Sports Med 16:492–498, 1988.
28. Delamarter RB, Hohl M, Hopp E: Ligament injuries associated with tibial plateau fractures. Clin Orthop 250:226–233, 1989.
29. Schwarz C, Blazina ME, Sisto DJ, et al: The results of operative treatment of osteochondritis dissecans of the patella. Am J Sports Med 16:522–529, 1988.
30. Baker CH, Norwood LA, Hughston JC: Acute combined posterior cruciate and posterolateral instability of the knee. Am J Sports Med 12:204–208, 1984.
31. Delee JC, Riley MB, Rockwood CA: Acute posterolateral rotatory instability of the knee. Am J Sports Med 11:199–206, 1983.
32. Wirth CJ, Jager M: Dynamic double tendon replacement of the posterior cruciate ligament. Am J Sports Med 12:39–42, 1984.
33. Indelicato PA: Treatment of the anterior cruciate ligament–deficient knee. Clin Sports Med 7:700–770, 1988.

34. Clancy WG, Keene JS, Goletz TH: Symptomatic dislocation of the anterior horn of the medial meniscus. Am J Sports Med 12:57–64, 1984.

35. Hartar RA, Osternig LR, Singer KM: Instrumented Lachman test for the evaluation of anterior laxity after reconstruction of the anterior cruciate ligament. J Bone Joint Surg [Am] 71:975–983, 1989.

36. Penner DA, Daniel DM, Wood P, et al: An in vitro study of anterior cruciate ligament graft placement and isometry. Am J Sports Med 16:238–243, 1988.

37. Sapega AA, Moyer RA, Schneck C, et al: Testing for isometry during reconstruction of the ACL. J Bone Joint Surg [Am] 72:259–267, 1990.

38. Holden DL, Eggert AW, Butler JE: The nonoperative treatment of grade I and II medial collateral ligament injuries to the knee. Am J Sports Med 11:340–344, 1983.

39. Woo S, Inoue M, McGurk-Burleson E, et al: Treatment of the medial collateral ligament injury. II. Structure and function of canine knees in response to differing treatment regimens. Am J Sports Med 15:22–29, 1987.

40. Hart DP, Dahners LE: Healing of the medial collateral ligament: the effects of repair, motion, and secondary stabilizing ligaments. J Bone Joint Surg [Am] 69:1194–1220, 1987.

41. Bloom MH: Differentiating between meniscal and patellar pain. Phys Sports Med 17(8):95–108, 1989.

42. Anderson AF, Lipscomb AB: Clinical diagnosis of meniscal tears: description of a new manipulative test. Am J Sports Med 14:291–293, 1986.

43. Carlsen TJ: The rationale behind meniscus repair. Postgrad Adv Sports Med 2(3):3–12, 1987.

44. Turco VJ, Spinella AJ: Anterolateral dislocation of the head of the fibula in sports. Am J Sports Med 13:209–215, 1985.

45. Hoaglund FT: Confirming the diagnosis of osteoarthritis. J Musculoskel Med 7(3):32–45, 1990.

46. Davies GJ: A Compendium of Isokinetics in Clinical Usage, 3rd ed. LaCrosse, WI: S & S Publishers, 1987.

47. Harkcom TM, Lampman RM, Banwell BG, et al: Therapeutic value of graded aerobic exercise training in rheumatoid arthritis. Arthritis Rheum 28:32–39, 1985.

48. Estwanik JJ, McAlister JA: Contusions and the formation of myositis ossificans. Phys Sports Med 18(4):53–64, 1990.

49. Lipscomb AB, Thomas ED, Johnston RK: Treatment of myositis ossificans traumatica in athletes. Am J Sports Med 4:111–120, 1976.

50. Calvo RD, Steadman JR, Sterling JC, et al: Managing plica syndrome of the knee. Phys Sports Med 18(7):64–74, 1990.

51. Hardaker WT, Whipple TL, Bassett FH: Diagnosis and treatment of the plica syndrome of the knee. J Bone Joint Surg [Am] 62:221–225, 1980.

52. Hughston JC, Stone M, Andrews JR: The suprapatellar plica: its role in internal derangement of the knee. J Bone Joint Surg [Am] 55:1318, 1973.

53. Nottage WM, Sprague NF, Auerbach BJ, et al: The medial patellar plica syndrome. Am J Sports Med 11:211–214, 1983.

54. Percy EC, Strother RT: Patellalgia. Phys Sports Med 13:43–59, 1985.

55. Rintala P: Patellofemoral pain syndrome and its treatment in runners. Athl Train 25(2):107–109, 1990.

56. Malek MM, Mangine RE: Patellofemoral pain syndromes: a comprehensive and conservative approach. J Orthop Sports Phys Ther 2:108–116, 1981.

57. Villar RN: Patellofemoral pain and the infrapatellar brace. Am J Sports Med 13:313–315, 1985.

58. Barrack RL, Skinner HB, Buckley SL: Proprioception in the anterior cruciate deficient knee. Am J Sports Med 17:1–6, 1989.

59. Fahrer H, Rentsch HU, Gerber NJ, et al: Knee effusion and reflex inhibition of the quadriceps: a bar to effective retraining. J Bone Joint Surg [Br] 70:635–638, 1988.

60. Duerksen F, Rogalsky RJ, Cochrane IW: Knee disarticulation with intercondylar patellofemoral arthrodesis: an improved technique. Clin Orthop 256:50–57, 1990.

61. Lane JM, Kroll MA, Rossbach PG: New advances and concepts in amputee management after treatment for bone and soft-tissue sarcomas. Clin Orthop 256:22–28, 1990.

62. Krajbich JI, Carroll NC: Van Nes rotationplasty with segmental limb resection. Clin Orthop 256:7–13, 1990.

63. Davies GJ, Larson R: Examining the knee. Phys Sports Med 6(4):49–67, 1978.

64. Magee DJ: Orthopedic Physical Assessment. Philadelphia: WB Saunders, 1987.

65. Ritter MA, Gioe TJ, Gosling C: Examination of the acutely injured knee. Phys Sports Med 8(10):41–49, 1980.

66. Pavlov H, Torg JS: The Running Athlete: Roentgenograms and Remedies. Chicago: Mosby-Year Book Inc., 1987.

67. Glashow JL, Katz R, Schneider M, et al: Double-blind assessment of the value of magnetic resonance imaging in the diagnosis of anterior cruciate and meniscal lesions. J Bone Joint Surg [Am] 71:113–119, 1989.

68. Silva I, Silver DM: Tears of the meniscus as revealed by magnetic resonance imaging. J Bone Joint Surg [Am] 70:199–202, 1988.

69. Wirth CR, Yao L, Lee JK: Magnetic resonance imaging of meniscal tears. Phys Sports Med 18(3):76–79, 1990.

70. Yao L, Lee JK, Wirth CR: Magnetic resonance imaging of osseous lesions of the knee. Phys Sports Med 18(5):81–84, 1990.

71. Hoppenfeld S: Orthopaedic Neurology: A Diagnostic Guide to Neurologic Levels. Philadelphia: JB Lippincott, 1977.

72. Cyriax JH, Cyriax PJ: Illustrated Manual of Orthopedic Medicine. London: Butterworth, 1983.

73. Daniel DM, Stone ML, Barnett P, et al: Use of the quadriceps active test to diagnose posterior cruciate-ligament disruption and measure posterior laxity of the knee. J Bone Joint Surg [Am] 70:386–391, 1988.

74. Feagin JA, ed: The Crucial Ligaments. New York: Churchill-Livingstone, 1988.

75. Jensen K: Manual laxity tests for anterior cruciate ligament injuries. J Orthop Sports Phys Ther 11:474–481, 1990.

76. Noyes FR, Grood ES, Torzilli PA: Current concepts review: the definition of terms for motion and position of the knee and injuries of the ligaments. J Bone Joint Surg [Am] 71:465–472, 1989.

77. Gillon J: Comparative validity of a functional knee test with isokinetic and arthrometer testing in anterior cruciate ligament deficient patients. Isokinetic Continuing Education Course and MERAC Workshop, Cedar Rapids, IA, August 24–26, 1990.

78. Timm KE: Investigation of the physiological overflow effect from speed-specific isokinetic activity. J Orthop Sports Phys Ther 9:106–110, 1987.

79. Malone TR: Evaluation of Isokinetic Equipment. Baltimore: Williams & Wilkins, 1988.

80. Quillen WS, Gieck JH: Manual therapy: mobilization of the motion-restricted knee. Athl Train 23:123–130, 1988.

81. Engle RP, Canner GG: Proprioceptive neuromuscular fa-

cilitation and modified procedures for anterior cruciate ligament instability. J Orthop Sports Phys Ther 11:230–236, 1989.

82. Noyes FR, Bassett RW, Grood ES, et al: Arthroscopy in acute traumatic hemarthrosis of the knee. J Bone Joint Surg [Am] 62:687–695, 1980.

83. Noyes FR, Mangine RE, Barber S: Early knee motion after open and arthroscopic anterior cruciate ligament reconstruction. Am J Sports Med 15:149–160, 1987.

84. Sachs RA, Daniel DM, Stone ML, et al: Patellofemoral problems after anterior cruciate ligament reconstruction. Am J Sports Med 17:760–765, 1989.

85. Seto JL, Brewster CE, Lombardo SJ, et al: Rehabilitation of the knee after anterior cruciate ligament reconstruction. J Orthop Sports Phys Ther 11:8–18, 1989.

86. Shelbourne KD, Nitz P: Accelerated rehabilitation after anterior cruciate ligament reconstruction. Am J Sports Med 18:292–299, 1990.

87. Woodall W, Welsh J: A biomechanical basis for rehabilitation programs involving the patellofemoral joint. J Orthop Sports Phys Ther 11:535–541, 1990.

88. Hungerford DS, Krackow KA, Kenna RV: Total Knee Arthroplasty. Baltimore: Williams & Wilkins, 1988.

89. Romness DW, Rand JA: The role of continuous passive motion following total knee arthroplasty. Clin Orthop 226:34–37, 1988.

90. Vince KG, Insall JN: Long-term results with cemented total knee arthroplasty. Orthop Clin North Am 19:575–580, 1988.

## Bibliography

Galway HR, MacIntosh DL: The lateral pivot shift: a symptom and sign of anterior cruciate ligament insufficiency. Clin Orthop 147:45–50, 1980.

Gould JA, Davies GJ: Orthopaedic and Sports Physical Therapy. St. Louis: CV Mosby, 1985.

Lee JK, Yao L, Wirth CR: Magnetic resonance imaging of major ligamentous knee injuries. Phys Sports Med 18(4):97–100, 1990.

Polly DW, Callaghan JJ, Sikes RA, et al: The accuracy of selective magnetic resonance imaging compared with the findings of arthroscopy of the knee. J Bone Joint Surg [Am] 70:192–198, 1988.

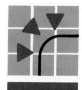

# CHAPTER *Nine*

## Foot and Ankle

### DANIEL L. RIDDLE

## INTRODUCTION

The examination and treatment of patients with disorders of the foot and ankle have recently undergone a metamorphosis, primarily because of the work of Manter,[1] Hicks,[2] and Inman.[3] The work of these researchers was completed many years ago, but the concepts so beautifully illustrated in their studies have only recently affected physical therapy practice on a large scale. Manter,[1] for example, was the first to determine the location of the axis of rotation of the subtalar joint. As a result of the work of Manter,[1] Hicks,[2] and Inman,[3] therapists now have a working knowledge of the kinematics of the foot and ankle. Many therapists are currently treating patients with foot and ankle disorders in ways that are drastically different from those used a few years ago. For example, patients with plantar fasciitis might have received diathermy treatments several years ago but may now be treated with custom-made orthoses. A question we must ask ourselves and eventually answer is, Are our patients any better off with these new treatments?

One of the purposes of this chapter is to provide a comprehensive terminology guide for the reader. A key issue when communicating with colleagues is whether they understand the terms that are used. Effective communication cannot occur if terminology is ill defined or ambiguous. The terminology used to describe motions, positions, and deformities of the foot and lower leg has been a source of confusion for many readers of literature on the foot and ankle.

The classic example of confusing terminology is the use of the terms supination (inversion) and pronation (eversion). The orthopaedic surgery literature uses the terms inversion and eversion to describe the primary motions of the entire foot and ankle, whereas the podiatric and physical therapy literature most commonly use the terms pronation and supination to describe these motions. The result of this overlapping terminology is miscommunication among clinicians. This chapter clarifies the terminology used for the foot and ankle and can serve as a guide for clinicians when discussing the foot and ankle with their colleagues.

A second purpose of this chapter is to describe what is known about the structure and function of the joints and associated soft tissues of the foot and ankle. The classic works of the authors mentioned previously are discussed, as well as some of the more recent work. The primary purpose of reviewing the original and more recent work is to provide a foundation of knowledge about the structure and function of the foot and ankle. This knowledge provides an anatomic and kinesiologic basis for critical examination of the methods used to assess and treat patients with foot and ankle problems.

A third purpose of this chapter is to review the examination procedures for the foot and ankle. Many of the procedures used are described and discussed. We now have a substantial amount of data to guide us in determining which examination procedures provide meaningful information and which provide error-ridden information. This ability to use deductive reasoning in clinical decision making is new and is a result of recent research on the foot and ankle. Before research data were available to support clinical decisions, the decisions were based solely on experience, either our own or that of the "experts." This new research provides a scientifically sound basis for making clinical decisions related to examination and treatment of the foot and ankle.

Throughout this chapter the literature is used to make arguments in support of or in opposition to examination or treatment techniques advocated for the foot and ankle. An effort is made to summarize what we know about scientific clinical practice related to the foot and ankle. The hypothesis-oriented algorithm for clinicians (HOAC),[4] a scientifically based method for solving patients' clinical problems, is reviewed in the examination section of the chapter. The HOAC serves as the link between science and clinical practice.

A fourth purpose of the chapter is to discuss foot and ankle pathologies and their treatments. Volumes have been written on the foot and ankle, and it is not possible in one chapter to elaborate on all the pathologies and treatments that may be encountered. However, the more common pathologies are discussed and the treatments designed to address them are critically examined. For example, part of the standard treatment of patients with lateral ankle sprains has included strengthening of the peroneal muscle group. What is the theoretical basis for this treatment? More important, are there any data to support the effectiveness of this form of treatment?

This chapter provides the physical therapy student with some of the content needed to examine and treat effectively the more common foot and ankle disorders. In addition, it provides the student with some scientifically based clinical problem-solving skills that should be generalizable to other types of problems. After reading this chapter, practicing physical therapists will also gain new insights into the bases for the examination and treatment of the foot and ankle.

## TERMINOLOGY

**Abduction and Adduction.** Abduction and adduction refer to motions of the forefoot in the horizontal plane about a superior-inferior axis.[5]

**Plantar Flexion and Dorsiflexion.** Plantar flexion and dorsiflexion are motions of the foot and ankle in the sagittal plane about a medial-lateral axis.[5] The term *leg extension* is synonymous with the term dorsiflexion and *leg flexion* is synonymous with plantar flexion.

**Triplane Motion.** Triplane motion is motion about an obliquely oriented axis through all three body planes.[6]

**Supination.** When the foot is non–weight bearing, supination is a combination of plantar flexion, adduction, and inversion. Inversion is defined as frontal plane motion of the foot about an anterior-posterior axis in which the lateral aspect of the sole of the foot moves in a plantar direction. Williams and Warwick define supination as a downward rotation of the lateral part of the forefoot when the foot is on the ground.[5]

**Pronation.** When the foot is non–weight bearing, pronation is a combination of dorsiflexion, abduction, and eversion. Eversion is defined as frontal plane motion of the foot about an anterior-posterior axis in which the medial aspect of the sole of the foot moves in a plantar direction.[1] Williams and Warwick define pronation as a downward rotation of the medial part of the forefoot when the foot is on the ground.[5]

**Inversion and Eversion.** These are motions of the foot in the frontal plane about an anterior-posterior axis. According to Williams and Warwick, inversion is a triplane motion consisting of supination, adduction, and plantar flexion. Eversion is then a triplane motion consisting of pronation, abduction, and dorsiflexion.[5] Clinically, the terms pronation and supination are more commonly used to describe the triplane motions that occur in the foot and ankle.

**Subtalar Joint.** The subtalar joint consists of the articulations between the talus and the calcaneus and the talus and navicular.[1] Williams and Warwick define the subtalar joint as the articulation between the talus and the calcaneus.[5]

**Talocalcaneonavicular Joint.** This is the articulation between the talus and the navicular and the talus and calcaneus.[2]

**Transverse Tarsal Joint.** The transverse tarsal joint is the complex articulation between the talus and navicular and the calcaneus and cuboid. Terms that have been used synonymously for transverse tarsal joint are *Chopart's joint* and *midtarsal joint.*[7]

**Open Kinetic Chain.** In an open kinetic (kinematic) chain the distal segment terminates free in space. Steindler defines open kinetic chain as a series of joints in which the terminal joint is free.[9]

**Closed Kinetic Chain.** In a closed kinetic chain the end segments are united to form a ring or a closed circuit.[8] Steindler defines closed kinetic chain as one in which the terminal joint meets with some considerable external resistance that prevents or restrains free motion.[9]

**Proprioception.** Proprioception refers to the systems involved in the transmission of information from all the receptors located in muscles, tendons, joints, and the vestibular apparatus (Sherrington as reported by Sage).[10]

**Kinesthesia.** Kinesthesia refers to the perceptual experiences that arise from the transmission of the proprioceptive receptors.[9] Newton has defined kinesthesia as the ability to discriminate joint position: relative weight of body parts and joint movement including direction, amplitude, and speed.[11]

**Somatosensory System.** This is the system that provides sensations from the body. Somatic sensory receptors are located in the skin, muscles, tendons, joints, and vestibular apparatus. The two categories of receptors included are cutaneous receptors and proprioceptive receptors. Collectively, the receptors of this system are sensitive to stimuli of various kinds that impinge on the exterior surface of the body and to stimuli arising from various structures within the body. Receptors within the somatosensory system include the cutaneous receptors and the receptors in the muscles, tendons, joints, and vestibular apparatus.[10]

**Varus and Valgus.** These terms denote structural deformities and are used to describe the limb or part of the limb that is abnormally angulated inward (varus) or outward (valgus) with respect to the midsagittal plane of the body. They should be used only to describe irreversible pathology in a joint or segment and not motions that allow reversible changes in position.[8]

**Subtalar Joint Neutral.** The neutral position is the position of the subtalar joint that is neither pronated nor supinated. Elveru et al. define the subtalar joint neutral position operationally as the relative zero position of the subtalar joint where the following two conditions are met:[12]

- With the patient positioned prone, the forefoot is passively pronated and the ankle dorsiflexed until a soft end feel is encountered.
- The head of the talus cannot be palpated or is felt to extend equally at the medial and lateral borders of the talonavicular joint.

**Tibial Torsion.** Tibial torsion is the horizontal plane relationship between the position of the proximal tibia and the distal tibia. The normal amount of tibial torsion in the adult is 25 degrees of external rotation.[13]

**Tibial Varum.** Tibial varum is the frontal plane angle of the tibia with respect to the floor while the subject is weight bearing equally with bilateral feet approximately the shoulder width apart. Normally, the tibia should be aligned vertically with respect to the floor during standing.

## ANATOMY

Entire textbooks have been devoted to describing the anatomy of the foot and ankle.[14,15] These books and other sources[5,16] provide detailed descriptions of many aspects of the anatomy of the foot and ankle that are not covered in this chapter. The anatomy section of this chapter examines aspects of the anatomy of the foot and ankle that are essential for effective clinical practice. The bony architecture of the foot and ankle and its impact on foot function are reviewed. In addition, this section examines how joint surface shapes may influence commonly used clinical tests. The attachments of ankle and foot ligaments are thoroughly reviewed. Issues related to palpation and stress testing of these ligaments are addressed.

The structure, function, and maintenance of the arches of the foot are described. Clinical issues related to interventions designed to affect the position of the arch during weight bearing are also discussed.

The attachments and innervations of the muscles of the leg and foot are reviewed. Foot and leg muscle function during weight-bearing and non–weight-bearing activities are discussed. Because most "overuse syndromes" of the foot and ankle are directly related to muscle function, a thorough understanding of foot and leg muscle structure is a prerequisite to effective treatment.

The nervous and vascular supplies of the foot and ankle are described. The anatomic arrangement of the soft tissues and bone in relation to the nervous and vascular supplies of the foot and ankle is reviewed. These tissues frequently contribute the development of the more common pathologies affecting the nerves and vascular structures of the foot and ankle.

This section is not designed to provide a comprehensive review of the anatomy of the foot and ankle. The reference list at the end of the chapter is designed to furnish the resources needed for a thorough anatomic review. This section does provide clinically useful information related to the anatomy of the foot and ankle.

## Bones

The 3 bones that make up the ankle and the 26 bones that make up the foot serve many functions. When considering the bones of the

ankle and foot, major emphasis must be placed on the fact that the foot functions most of the time in a weight-bearing position. During weight bearing, the position of the bones of the foot is affected by gravitational forces, ground reaction forces, and forces produced by soft tissues in the foot and ankle. Understanding the osteology of the ankle and foot is prerequisite to understanding how weight bearing affects foot function.

### Distal Tibia and Fibula

The distal end of the tibia is quadrangular in shape. The medial surface has an apophysis, the medial malleolus, that is attached to its distal aspect. The lateral aspect of the medial malleolus is covered with articular cartilage, and the medial surface serves as an attachment site for the deltoid ligament. Posteriorly, the medial malleolus has a groove that is the site of attachment for the fibrous tunnel of the posterior tibialis tendon.

The lateral malleolus is longer and narrower and descends farther posteriorly and inferiorly than the medial malleolus. The articular surface of the lateral malleolus slants laterally and inferiorly and is smaller than the corresponding facet of the talus. Only the proximal half of the lateral malleolus is covered with articular cartilage.[17]

The inferior aspects of the distal tibia and fibula form the ankle mortise (Fig. 9–1). The mortise is bordered by three malleoli. The lateral

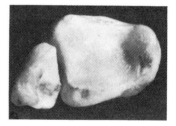

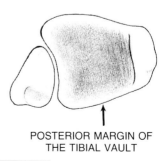

POSTERIOR MARGIN OF
THE TIBIAL VAULT

**FIGURE 9–1 ■** Distal articulating surfaces of the tibia and fibula. (From Kelikian H, Kelikian AS: Disorders of the Ankle. Philadelphia: WB Saunders, 1985, Fig. 1–8A and E.)

malleolus forms the lateral border of the mortise, the medial malleolus forms the medial border of the mortise, and the posterior malleolus of the tibia forms the posterior border of the mortise. The posterior malleolus is sometimes described as the third malleolus and extends approximately 8 mm inferiorly.[17]

## Talus

Because the talus (astragalus) plays a crucial role in the function of the three main joints of the ankle and foot (ankle, subtalar, and midtarsal joints), its anatomy is described in detail. The talus has many sites for ligamentous attachments but has no tendinous attachments. The talus is commonly described as having three parts: the body (trochlea), the neck, and the head (Fig. 9–

2). The body is defined as the part of the bone posterior to an imaginary line in the frontal plane that passes through the anterior border of the trochlea of the talus. The neck is the segment of the talus anterior to this imaginary line and posterior to the head of the talus. The head of the talus is the articular surface of the anterior aspect of the talus. This surface articulates with the navicular anteriorly and the calcaneus inferiorly.[14]

Unlike other tarsal bones, the talus has no muscular attachments. Because muscular attachments are a major source of vascularity for bones, the talus has a limited blood supply. The talus is susceptible to delayed union or nonunion as a result of this poor vascularity. This issue is addressed in greater detail in the section on disorders of the ankle and foot.

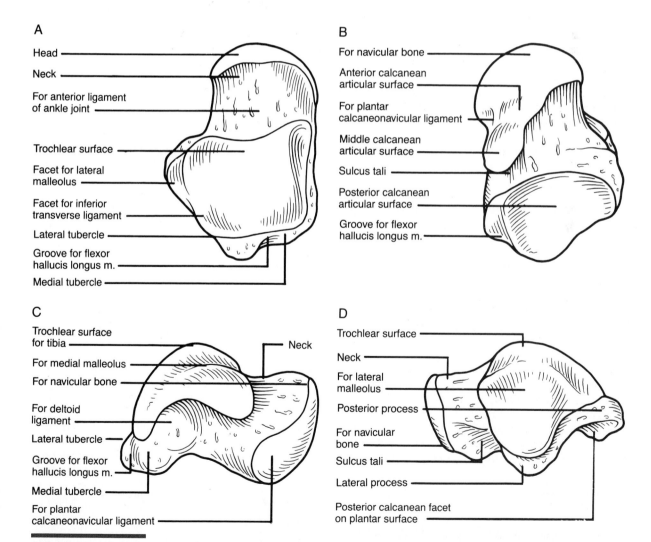

**FIGURE 9–2** ■ Articular surfaces of the talus. (A) Dorsal (superior) aspect. (B) Plantar inferior aspect. (C) Medial aspect. (D) Lateral aspect.

**Body of the Talus.** The superior aspect of the body of the talus is pulley or saddle shaped and is also called the dome of the talus. This saddle-shaped trochlear surface is approximately 2.5 mm wider anteriorly than posteriorly.[6] The medial and lateral surfaces of the talar body are composed primarily of smooth articular surfaces for the medial and lateral malleoli. The posterior aspect of the medial surface also has a flat or slightly raised surface that gives rise to the insertion of the deep portion of the deltoid ligament.

The anteroposterior (AP) dimension of the lateral facet of the dome of the talus is greater than that of its medial facet. Therefore, the radius of curvature of the lateral side of the talus is greater than that of its medial side.[6] According to Inman, the implication of this anatomic arrangement is that the malleoli separate a negligible amount when the ankle moves through a range of plantar flexion to dorsiflexion.[6]

The posterior surface of the talar body is made up primarily of the posterolateral and posteromedial tubercles. These tubercles serve as attachment sites for ligaments and retinacula. The os trigonum, an accessory bone, is present in approximately 6% of the population and articulates with the posterolateral tubercle.[18] The inferior surface of the talar body is made up almost exclusively of articulating surfaces. There may be as few as one or as many as four separate articular facets on the inferior aspect of the talar body. These surfaces articulate with the calcaneus posteriorly and anteriorly and the calcaneonavicular ligament anteriorly.[14]

**Neck of the Talus.** The neck is the part of the talus between the body posteriorly and the head anteriorly. The neck is approximately 17 mm long on average and is directed anteriorly and slightly medially and inferiorly.[14] Inferior to the neck of the talus is the tarsal sinus, which is formed by the sulcus tali and the sulcus calcanei.

**Head of the Talus.** The talar head has three facets: one for the navicular, one for the calcaneus, and one for the plantar calcaneonavicular ligament. The head of the talus is rotated on a longitudinal axis relative to the talar body so that the articular surface is higher laterally than medially. The rotation is approximately 45 degrees and is clockwise on the right and counterclockwise on the left.[14]

### Calcaneus

The calcaneus (os calcis) is the largest bone in the foot and is rectangular in shape (Fig. 9–3). For the purposes of description, the dorsal surface is divided into thirds. The posterior third of the calcaneus provides the site of attachment for the triceps surae muscle. The middle third contains the large posterior facet for the talus. The anterior third of the dorsal surface of the calcaneus begins with the floor of the sinus tarsi. The remainder of the anterior third is covered by one or more articular surfaces. The number of articular facets on the dorsal surface of the calcaneus is variable, much like that of the corresponding facets on the talus. Sarrafian states that, most commonly, two facets are present on the dorsal surface of the calcaneus.[14] Less frequently three facets are present, and least frequently one facet is present.

The inferior surface of the calcaneus has a base posteriorly and an apex anteriorly. The base of the calcaneus has a medial and a lateral tuberosity. The medial tuberosity is larger and is thought to bear more weight than the lateral tuberosity during weight bearing.[14] The plantar aponeurosis and the flexor digitorum brevis muscle attach to both tuberosities. The abductor hallucis muscle attaches to the medial tuberosity and the abductor digiti minimi attaches to the lateral tuberosity.

The most important structure on the medial side of the calcaneus is probably the sustentaculum tali. This bony projection protrudes anteromedially and is tilted downward at an average angle of 46 degrees.[14] This structure gives rise to the deltoid ligament and the plantar calcaneonavicular ligament. The sustentaculum tali serves as the pulley to allow efficient function of the flexor hallucis longus and flexor digitorum longus muscles. This structure also acts as a buttress to impede inferior movement of the talus during weight bearing.

### Navicular

The navicular (scaphoid) is positioned between the head of the talus posteriorly and the three cuneiforms anteriorly (Fig. 9–4). It also articulates with the cuboid laterally. It is wedge shaped with the apex pointing inferomedially and the base pointing superolaterally. The tibialis posterior and the plantar calcaneonavicular ligament attach on the inferior surface. Various intertarsal ligaments attach to the dorsal, plantar, medial, and lateral surfaces of the navicular.

### Cuboid

The cuboid is positioned between the calcaneus posteriorly and the base of the fourth and fifth metatarsals anteriorly (see Fig. 9–4). It ar-

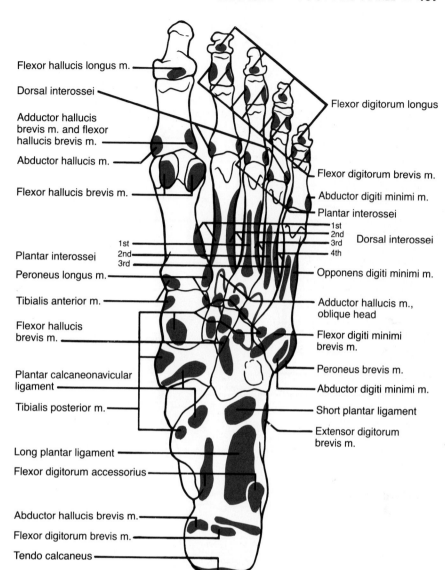

Flexor hallucis longus m.

Dorsal interossei

Adductor hallucis brevis m. and flexor hallucis brevis m.

Abductor hallucis m.

Flexor hallucis brevis m.

Plantar interossei
1st
2nd
3rd

Peroneus longus m.

Tibialis anterior m.

Flexor hallucis brevis m.

Plantar calcaneonavicular ligament

Tibialis posterior m.

Long plantar ligament

Flexor digitorum accessorius

Abductor hallucis brevis m.

Flexor digitorum brevis m.

Tendo calcaneus

Flexor digitorum longus

Flexor digitorum brevis m.

Abductor digiti minimi m.

Plantar interossei
1st
2nd
3rd
4th    Dorsal interossei

Opponens digiti minimi m.

Adductor hallucis m., oblique head

Flexor digiti minimi brevis m.

Peroneus brevis m.

Abductor digiti minimi m.

Short plantar ligament

Extensor digitorum brevis m.

**FIGURE 9–3** ■ Plantar view of the skeleton of the left foot.

ticulates medially with the lateral cuneiform and, at times, can articulate with the navicular. The cuboid is also somewhat wedge shaped with the apex facing inferolaterally and the base facing superomedially. Inferiorly and laterally the cuboid has a groove through which the tendon of the peroneus longus muscle passes. The cuboid serves as a pulley that increases the mechanical efficiency of the peroneus longus much as the sustentaculum tali does for the flexor hallucis longus muscle.

### Cuneiforms

The three cuneiforms are wedge shaped (see Fig. 9–4). The lateral and middle cuneiforms are positioned such that the inferior surface of each

bone serves as the apex and the superior surface serves as the base of a wedge. The medial cuneiform is reversed, with the superior surface forming the apex and the inferior surface the base. The medial cuneiform is also the largest of the three cuneiforms and protrudes farther distally than the other two. The configuration of the cuneiforms contributes to the formation of the transverse arch, which is discussed later in this section. The wedge shape of these bones also provides a cavity for the neurovascular and musculotendinous structures of the foot. The cuneiforms articulate with the first, second, and third metatarsals anteriorly and the navicular posteriorly. The lateral cuneiform also articulates with the cuboid laterally. The medial and lateral cuneiforms protrude farther anteriorly than the

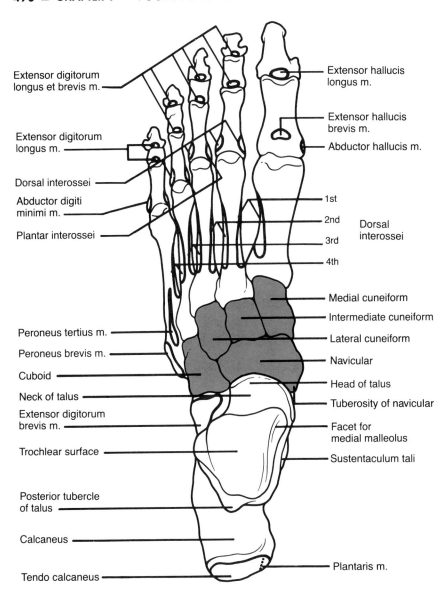

Extensor digitorum
longus et brevis m.

Extensor digitorum
longus m.

Dorsal interossei

Abductor digiti
minimi m.

Plantar interossei

Peroneus tertius m.

Peroneus brevis m.

Cuboid

Neck of talus

Extensor digitorum
brevis m.

Trochlear surface

Posterior tubercle
of talus

Calcaneus

Tendo calcaneus

Extensor hallucis
longus m.

Extensor hallucis
brevis m.

Abductor hallucis m.

1st
2nd    Dorsal
3rd    interossei
4th

Medial cuneiform

Intermediate cuneiform

Lateral cuneiform

Navicular

Head of talus

Tuberosity of navicular

Facet for
medial malleolus

Sustentaculum tali

Plantaris m.

**FIGURE 9-4** ■ Dorsal view of
the skeleton of the left foot.

middle cuneiform. The notch created by this design is thought to contribute to the bone stability
of the midfoot by creating a lock-and-key type of
arrangement.[19]

## Metatarsals

Each metatarsal consists of a base, a shaft, and
a head. The base is proximal and the head is
distal. The medial three metatarsal bases are approximately planar and are wider superiorly than
inferiorly. The bases of metatarsal four and five
are approximately quadrilateral. The base of the
fifth metatarsal is also largely made up of a sty-

loid process that gives rise to the insertion of the
peroneus brevis tendon.

The five metatarsals articulate anteriorly with
the phalanges for each digit. Posteriorly, the
metatarsals articulate with the three cuneiforms
(medial three metatarsals) and the cuboid (lateral
two metatarsals). The articulations between the
metatarsal and the cuneiforms and cuboid form
the tarsometatarsal or Lisfranc's joint. The bases
of the metatarsals form a transverse arch that is
higher medially than laterally. The heads of the
metatarsals do not normally form an arch; instead, the heads lie in the same plane. In a normal foot, this plane is approximately parallel to
the plane formed by the medial and lateral tu-

berosities of the calcaneus. The metatarsals are also plantar flexed relative to the tarsals. This plantar flexed position contributes to the formation of the longitudinal arch of the foot.

The shaft of the first metatarsal is reported to be the shortest and structurally strongest of the five metatarsals. The lengths of the metatarsals are usually considered to be in the proportions $2 > 3 > 1 > 4 > 5$.[14]

The head of the first metatarsal is the largest head and is quadrilateral in shape. Its inferior surface also articulates with two sesamoid bones. The tibial (medial) and fibular (lateral) sesamoids lie within the bifurcated tendon of the flexor hallucis brevis muscle. The tibial sesamoid is usually slightly larger than the fibular sesamoid. The heads of metatarsals two through four are also quadrilateral in shape.

### Phalanges

The large toe has a proximal and a distal phalanx, and each of the remaining toes has a proximal, a middle, and a distal phalanx (see Fig. 9–4). The phalanges of each toe tend to become shorter from posterior to anterior. The middle and distal phalanges of the fifth toe are sometimes fused.[20]

### Accessory Bones

Accessory bones are anomalous bones that are usually formed because of lack of fusion between two ossification sites during development.[21] The three most commonly occurring accessory bones of the foot are the os trigonum, the accessory navicular (os tibiale), and the os intermetatarseum (Fig. 9–5). The os trigonum is located on the posterolateral aspect of the body of the talus. It is reported to be present in 1.7 to 7.7% of the population.[14] The accessory navicular is located on the posteromedial aspect of the navicular tuberosity and its frequency of occurrence is reported to be 3 to 12%.[14] The os intermetatarseum is located between the medial cuneiform and the base of the first and second metatarsal and its frequency of occurrence is reported to be 1.2 to 10%.[14]

## Joints and Ligaments

In this section, particular attention is paid to the shapes of the joint surfaces because they determine, in part, the arthrokinematics at the joint. Knowledge of joint surface shapes is needed to

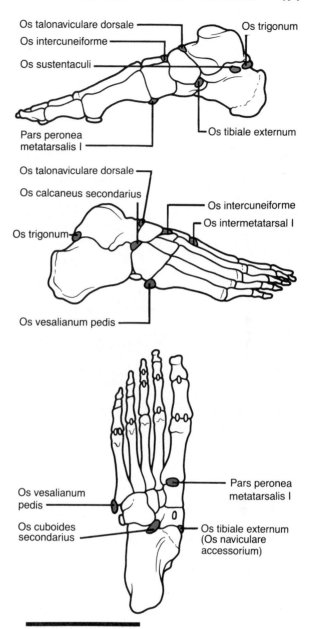

**FIGURE 9–5** ■ Common accessory bones of the foot.

determine the direction of forces used to assess the accessory motion of these joints. Tables are used extensively in this section to summarize information related to joint structure and function that is relevant to clinical practice. The joints of the ankle and foot and their associated ligaments are summarized in Table 9–1.

### Distal Tibiofibular Joint

The distal tibiofibular joint consists of the articulation between a convex fibular surface and a

■■■■ **Table 9–1.** ANKLE AND FOOT JOINTS AND ASSOCIATED LIGAMENTS

| Joint | Associated Ligament | Fiber Direction | Motions Limited |
|---|---|---|---|
| Distal tibiofibular | Anterior tibiofibular | Distolateral | Distal glide of fibula<br>Plantar flexion |
| | Posterior tibiofibular | Distolateral | Distal glide of fibula<br>Plantar flexion |
| | Interosseous | | Separation of tibia and fibula |
| Ankle | Deltoid (medial collateral)<br>Superficial | | |
| |   Tibionavicular | Plantar-anterior | Plantar flexion, abduction |
| |   Tibiocalcaneal | Plantar, plantar-posterior | Eversion, abduction |
| |   Posterior tibiotalar | Plantar-posterior | Dorsiflexion, abduction |
| | Deep | | |
| |   Anterior tibiotalar | Anterior | Eversion, abduction, plantar flexion |
| | Lateral or fibular collateral | | |
| |   Anterior talofibular | Anterior-medial | Plantar flexion<br>Inversion<br>Anterior displacement of foot |
| |   Calcaneofibular | Posterior-medial | Inversion<br>Dorsiflexion |
| |   Posterior talofibular | Horizontal (lateral) | Dorsiflexion<br>Posterior displacement of foot |
| | Lateral talocalcaneal | Posterior-medial | Inversion<br>Dorsiflexion |
| | Anterior capsule | | Plantar flexion |
| | Posterior capsule | | Dorsiflexion |
| Subtalar | Interosseous talocalcaneal | | |
| |   Anterior band | Proximal-anterior-lateral | Inversion<br>Joint separation |
| |   Posterior band | Proximal-posterior-lateral | Inversion<br>Joint separation |
| | Lateral talocalcaneal | (See ankle) | |
| | Deltoid | (See ankle) | |
| | Lateral collateral | (See ankle) | |
| | Posterior talocalcaneal | Vertical | Dorsiflexion |
| | Medial talocalcaneal | Plantar-anterior | Eversion |
| | Anterior talocalcaneal (cervical ligaments) | Plantar-posterior-lateral | Inversion |
| Main ligamentous support of longitudinal arches | Long plantar | Anterior, slightly medial | Eversion |
| | Short plantar | Anterior | Eversion |
| | Plantar calcaneonavicular | Dorsal-anterior-medial | Eversion |
| | Plantar aponeurosis | Anterior | Eversion |
| Midtarsal or transverse | Bifurcated | | Joint separation |
| |   Medial band | Longitudinal | Plantar flexion |
| |   Lateral band | Horizontal | Inversion |
| | Dorsal talonavicular | Longitudinal | Plantar flexion of talus on navicular |
| | Dorsal calcaneocuboid | Longitudinal | Inversion, plantar flexion |
| | Ligaments supporting the arches | | |
| Intertarsal | Numerous ligaments named by two interconnected bones (dorsal and plantar ligaments) | | Joint motion in direction causing ligamentous tightness |
| | Interosseous ligaments connecting cuneiforms, cuboid, and navicular | | Flattening of transverse arch |
| | Ligaments supporting arches | | |
| Tarsometatarsal | Dorsal, plantar, and interosseous | | Joint separation |

**■ Table 9–1.** ANKLE AND FOOT JOINTS AND ASSOCIATED LIGAMENTS *Continued*

| Joint | Associated Ligament | Fiber Direction | Motions Limited |
|---|---|---|---|
| Intermetatarsal | Dorsal, plantar, and interosseous | | Joint separation |
| | Deep transverse metatarsal | | Joint separation<br>Flattening of transverse arch |
| Metatarsophalangeal | Fibrous capsule | | |
| | Dorsally, thin—separated from extensor tendons by bursae | | Flexion |
| | Inseparable from deep surface of plantar and collateral ligaments | | Extension |
| | Collateral | Plantar-anterior | Flexion, abduction, or adduction in flexion |
| | Plantar, grooved for flexor tendons | | Extension |
| Interphalangeal | Collateral | | Flexion, abduction, or adduction in flexion |
| | Plantar | | Extension |
| | Extensor hood replaces dorsal ligaments | | Flexion |

From Riegger CL: Anatomy of the ankle and foot. Phys Ther 68:1802–1814, 1988. Reprinted from PHYSICAL THERAPY with the permission of the American Physical Therapy Association.

concave tibial surface (Table 9–2). This joint is classified as a syndesmotic joint and allows only slight amounts of movement. The ligaments of the distal tibiofibular joint are the anterior tibiofibular, posterior tibiofibular, and interosseous ligaments. The interosseous membrane between the tibia and fibula is also thought to provide stability for this joint.[22] According to Barnett and Napier, the fibula rotates externally slightly during dorsiflexion of the foot.[23]

A controversial aspect of the function of the distal tibiofibular joint is whether the joint space gaps or increases during dorsiflexion. Inman argues that separation of the distal tibiofibular syndesmosis during dorsiflexion amounts to only 1 or 2 mm and is not necessary for full dorsi-

**■ Table 9–2.** SHAPES OF THE JOINT SURFACES OF THE LEG AND FOOT

| Joint | Proximal Bone and Shape of Its Joint Surface | Distal Bone and Shape of Its Joint Surface |
|---|---|---|
| Superior tibiofibular | Tibia—planar | Fibula—planar to convex |
| Inferior tibiofibular | Tibia—concave | Fibula—convex |
| Talocrural | Tibia—concave in anteroposterior direction and concave-convex-concave in mediolateral direction | Fibula—convex in anteroposterior direction and convex-concave-convex in mediolateral direction |
| Talocalcaneal | Talus—posterior facet biconcave, middle facet biconvex, anterior facet convex | Calcaneus—posterior facet biconvex, middle facet biconcave, anterior facet concave |
| Talonavicular | Talus—biconvex | Navicular—biconcave |
| Calcaneocuboid | Calcaneus—convex in mediolateral direction and concave in superoinferior direction (saddle shaped) | Cuboid—concave in mediolateral direction and convex in superoinferior direction (saddle shaped) |
| Cuboideonavicular | Navicular—planar | Cuboid—planar |
| Cuneonavicular | Navicular—slightly convex | Cuneiforms—slightly concave |
| Intercuneiform | Cuneiforms (medial and middle) planar | Cuneiforms (middle and lateral) planar |
| Cuneocuboid | Lateral cuneiform—planar | Cuboid—planar |
| Tarsometatarsal | Cuneiforms and cuboid—planar to slightly convex | Bases of metatarsals—planar to slightly concave |
| Metatarsophalangeal | Metatarsals—biconvex | Proximal phalanges—biconcave |
| Interphalangeal | Proximal phalanges—convex in superoinferior and concave in mediolateral direction | Middle phalanges—concave in superoinferior and convex in mediolateral direction |

flexion range of motion.[6] This issue is addressed in the section on biomechanics. However, if the ligaments joining the distal tibia and fibula are abnormally shortened, it could be hypothesized that they restrict dorsiflexion motion. Abnormally shortened ligaments may limit the ability of the talus to move within the mortise and result in restricted dorsiflexion.

### Talocrural Joint

The talocrural (ankle) joint is classified as a synovial saddle-shaped uniaxial joint. The distal tibia and fibula form the mortise or superior surface of the ankle joint and the trochlea of the talus forms its inferior surface. Both the talus and the mortise are slightly wider anteriorly than

posteriorly, which may explain why there is a snug fit between these joint surfaces throughout the entire range of motion.[6] The ankle mortise is concave in an anteroposterior direction but is concave-convex-concave in a mediolateral direction. The trochlea has a reciprocating joint surface shape. These complex joint surface shapes allow a large surface area of contact during weight bearing.[24] The relatively large surface area of contact probably explains why osteoarthrosis is reported to be uncommon in this joint.[25]

The capsule of the talocrural joint is thin anteriorly and posteriorly but is thickened medially and laterally by ligaments. The medial collateral (deltoid) ligament is most commonly described as having a variable number of deep and superficial bands (Fig. 9–6). The medial collateral ligament attaches proximally to the distal aspect of the

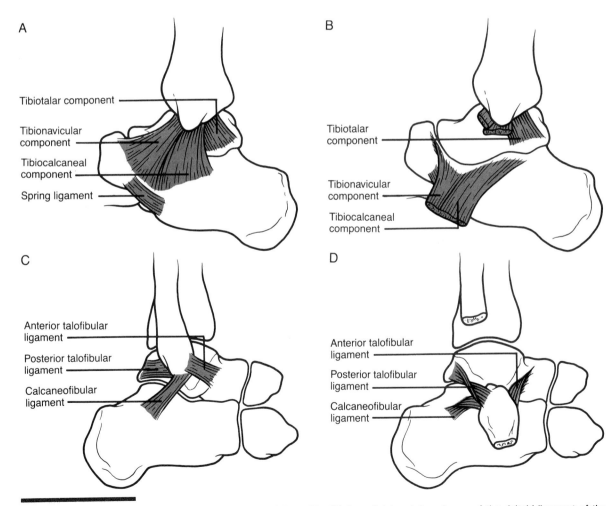

**FIGURE 9–6** ■ Tibial and fibular collateral ligaments of the ankle. (A) Superficial and deep layers of the deltoid ligament of the right ankle. (B) Deep layer of the deltoid ligament. (C) Right fibular collateral ligament. (D) Right fibular collateral ligaments with the fibular malleolus turned down.

medial malleolus and distally to the sustentaculum tali, the medial surface of the talus, and the medial tubercle of the talus. This ligament is broad and fan-like in shape, much like the medial collateral ligament of the knee. The tensile strength of the medial collateral ligament of the ankle greatly exceeds that of the lateral collateral ligament, which may help explain why the medial collateral ligament is injured so infrequently.

The lateral collateral ligament of the ankle is actually a trio of ligaments that cross the lateral side of the talocrural joint (see Fig. 9-6). The broad, flat anterior talofibular ligament attaches to the anterior margin of the fibula, passes anterior and medially, and attaches to the lateral aspect of the neck of the talus. The rope-like calcaneofibular ligament attaches to the apex of the lateral malleolus, passes inferiorly and posteriorly, and attaches to a tubercle on the lateral aspect of the calcaneus. The structurally strong posterior talofibular ligament attaches to the posterior aspect of the lateral malleolus, passes posteriorly and horizontally, and attaches to the posterior surface of the body of the talus. The anterior talofibular and posterior talofibular ligaments are intra-articular, and the calcaneofibular ligament is extra-articular.

## Subtalar Joint

From an anatomic standpoint, the subtalar joint is defined as the articulation between the talus and the calcaneus.[5] Two articulations exist between the talus and the calcaneus: one between the posterior aspect of the talus and the calcaneus and another between the anterior aspect of the talus and the calcaneus. According to Williams and Warwick, the posterior talocalcaneal articulation forms the subtalar joint, and the anterior talocalcaneal joint is part of the talocalcaneonavicular joint.[5] The posterior talocalcaneal joint (subtalar joint) is formed by the biconcave surface on the inferior aspect of the talus and the biconvex posterior calcaneal facet. These two bones are connected by a joint capsule and four ligaments; the medial talocalcaneal, lateral talocalcaneal, interosseous talocalcaneal, and cervical ligaments.

The posterior subtalar joint capsule has no connections to other tarsal joint capsules. The medial talocalcaneal ligament attaches on the medial tubercle of the calcaneus and passes posterior to the sustentaculum tali and the medial surface of the calcaneus. This ligament blends with the medial collateral ligament of the ankle.

The lateral talocalcaneal ligament attaches on the lateral process of the talus, passes inferiorly and posteriorly, and attaches to the lateral surface of the calcaneus just anterior and superior to the calcaneofibular ligament. The broad, flat interosseous talocalcaneal ligament passes transversely in the sinus tarsi. The cervical ligament attaches to the upper surface of the lateral aspect of the calcaneus, passes superiorly and medially, and attaches to a tubercle on the lateral aspect of the neck of the talus.

## Talocalcaneonavicular Joint

Williams and Warwick define the talocalcaneonavicular joint as the articulation between the middle and anterior facets of the talus and the calcaneus and the articulation between the talus and the navicular and upper surface of the plantar calcaneonavicular ligament.[5,26] A single joint capsule surrounds the talocalcaneonavicular joint. Using functional rather than anatomic terms, Sarrafian defines the talocalcaneonavicular joint as all of the joints that allow movement between the talus and navicular and the talus and calcaneus. According to Sarrafian, the calcaneus and the navicular move as a unit around the talus.[14] Sarrafian argues that the subtalar joint and the anterior talocalcaneal joint act as a unit during functional movements of the talocalcaneonavicular joint. In contrast, Williams and Warwick argue that the posterior subtalar joint functions independently of the talocalcaneonavicular joint.[5] Sarrafian[14] also argues that when thinking of the rear foot in functional terms it is more useful to think of the calcaneus and navicular as moving on a relatively fixed talus.

The posterior facet of the talus is biconcave and articulates with the biconvex surface of the calcaneus. The middle and anterior facets of the talus can be either convex or biconvex. The corresponding surfaces of the calcaneus can be either concave or biconcave. The biconvex or convex middle and anterior facets of the talus articulate with biconcave or concave facets on the calcaneus. The biconvex head of the talus articulates with the biconcave posterior surface of the navicular.

Ligamentous support for the talocalcaneonavicular joint is fairly extensive. A ligament that is thought to be of major importance during function is the plantar calcaneonavicular ligament. This ligament attaches to the anterior margin of the sustentaculum tali of the calcaneus, runs anteriorly and inferiorly, and attaches to the plantar surface of the navicular. Because of its plantar position in the foot, this ligament has been termed the spring ligament. No data exist to suggest that this ligament has unique properties that make it spring-like.

### Calcaneocuboid Joint

The articular surfaces of the calcaneocuboid joint are saddle shaped (see Table 9–2). The primary ligaments of this joint are the bifurcate ligament (ligament of Chopart), the short plantar ligament, and the long plantar ligament. The bifurcate ligament is made up of the lateral calcaneonavicular ligament and the medial calcaneocuboid ligament. Both attach to the os calcis of the calcaneus and fan out in the shape of a V.

The short plantar ligament is also known as the plantar calcaneocuboid ligament. It attaches to the anterior tubercle of the calcaneus and the plantar surface of the cuboid. This ligament is deep to the long plantar ligament. The long plantar ligament attaches on the posterior surface of the calcaneus, runs anterolaterally, and attaches to the anterior aspect of the cuboid and the bases of the second through fifth metatarsals.[14] Both the long and short plantar ligaments are thought to be important stabilizers of the lateral longitudinal arch of the foot. The calcaneocuboid joint and the talonavicular joint form the midtarsal or Chopart's joint.

### Remaining Tarsal Joints

The other tarsal joints and their surfaces are summarized in Table 9–2. Because these joints are not frequently affected by pathology and do not contribute significantly to foot motion, they are not described individually.

**Tarsometatarsal Joints.** From a superior view of the foot, the tarsometatarsal (Lisfranc's) joint line runs posteriorly and laterally. Many dorsal, plantar, and interosseous ligaments connect the metatarsals to each other and to the adjacent tarsals. The proximal surfaces of the metatarsals are planar or slightly concave.

The first metatarsal articulates with the medial cuneiform. The second articulates with all three cuneiforms. The second tarsometatarsal joint is positioned slightly more posterior than the first and third tarsometatarsal joints. This configuration is thought to enhance the stability of the second tarsometatarsal joint and facilitate efficient propulsion during the stance phase of gait. The third metatarsal articulates with the lateral

cuneiform. The fourth metatarsal articulates with the lateral cuneiform and cuboid, and the fifth metatarsal articulates with the cuboid.

**Metatarsophalangeal Joints.** The metatarsophalangeal joint line also runs posteriorly and laterally. However, the second metatarsal head typically extends farther anteriorly than the head of the first metatarsal. The metatarsal heads are biconcave and articulate with the biconvex articular surfaces of the proximal phalanges. In addition to the joint capsules, many ligaments bind these joints together (see Table 9–1). The plantar and collateral ligaments are the ligaments thought to contribute the most to joint stability.

**Interphalangeal Joints.** The interphalangeal joints are hinge joints with the proximal surfaces of the phalangeal heads articulating with the distal phalangeal bases. The articular surfaces of the phalangeal heads are concave in a medial-lateral direction and convex in a superior-inferior direction. The articular surfaces of the bases of the phalanges are convex in a medial-lateral direction and concave in a superior-inferior direction. Each interphalangeal joint has a joint capsule and two collateral ligaments. The plantar aspect of the joint capsule is thickened to form a fibrous plate, much like the plantar aspect of the metatarsophalangeal joint capsule.

### Calcaneal Fat Pad

The plantar aspect of the heel consists of a layer of specialized fat and connective tissue 18 mm (range 13 to 21 mm) thick.[27] This pad covers and is anchored by the tuberosity of the calcaneus. Structurally, the heel pad is made of specialized fat divided into chambers (Fig. 9–7). These fascial chambers are highly organized and are classified into superficial microchambers and deep macrochambers.

The heel pad is divided into internal and external layers called cups. The internal cup is attached to the periosteum of the calcaneus via many septa. These septa seal the chambers of fat and serve as a mechanism for shock absorption.[28]

The functions of the calcaneal fat pad are to accept large loads and energies at heel strike and to reduce impact forces.[29] The calcaneal fat pad is the first of many tissues that must function to reduce impact forces associated with weight bearing. Shock absorption and peak force reduction are essential in preventing injuries to the musculoskeletal system.

Some researchers have suggested, on the basis

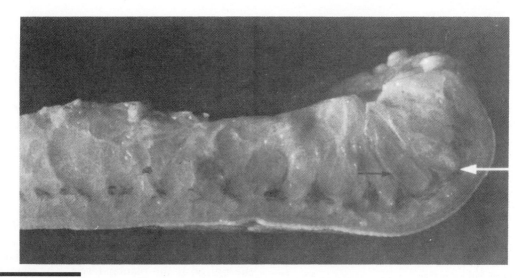

**FIGURE 9-7** ■ Longitudinal section through the heel pad illustrating deep chambers that are especially well developed in the posterior aspect of the heel, the area where large forces are applied during gait. White arrow shows the inner cup ligament. Black arrow shows the ligamentous septum. (From Jahss MH, ed: Disorders of the Foot and Ankle: Medical and Surgical Management, 2nd ed, Vol 1. Philadelphia: WB Saunders, 1991, Fig. 20-8.)

of histologic studies, that the calcaneal fat pads of patients with heel pain are less capable of absorbing forces than the fat pads of subjects without heel pain.[30] Jorgenson suggested that some runners with unilateral overuse injuries of the lower extremity have softened and therefore ineffective calcaneal fat pads.[31] Jorgensen based his determinations on a comparison of the calcaneal fat pads of the involved and uninvolved sides in these runners.

Tietze determined that the thickest part of the calcaneal fat pad is in the area of the calcaneal tuberosity and the lateral aspect of the posterior heel.[32] The septa also provided the greatest reinforcement in these areas. The calcaneal fat pad is optimally designed to absorb forces on the posterior and lateral aspects of the heel, where the greatest pressures are developed during gait (Fig. 9-8).

Bojsen-Moller states that the calcaneal fat pad is softer than normal when the calcaneal tuberosity can be felt easily during palpation.[28,33] Bojsen-Moller does not define what he means by the term "felt easily."[28,33] Jahss et al. suggest, based on biomechanical and clinical examination, that calcaneal fat pads can be classified into

**FIGURE 9-8** ■ When the heel pad is confined by external support, the thickness of the pad is increased, which increases shock absorbence. (Modified from Jahss MH, ed: Disorders of the Foot and Ankle: Medical and Surgical Management, 2nd ed, Vol 1. Philadelphia: WB Saunders, 1991, Fig. 20-10.)

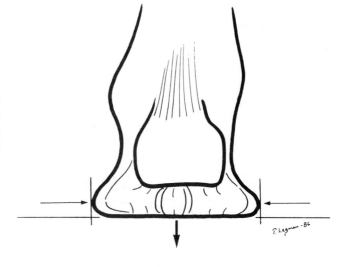

three types.[34] The first type is the normal pad, which is thick and resilient and absorbs most of the forces associated with weight bearing in a fairly small area of the posterior aspect of the heel. The second type is seen in patients with peripheral neuropathy. The pad is soft, pliable, and mildly atrophic. The weight-bearing forces are distributed fairly evenly over a wider area during weight bearing. The third type is a very thin, atrophied pad, with the weight-bearing forces distributed over a very small area in the posterior heel during weight bearing.

## Arches of the Foot and Their Maintenance

The arches allow the foot to vary its function during weight bearing from that of a rigid lever to that of a compliant series of joints. The key to understanding foot function is understanding how the arches of the foot vary in shape depending on the forces applied to the foot or the pathology that is present.

The three main arches of the foot are concave in a plantar direction (Fig. 9–9). Two of these arches are oriented longitudinally and one is oriented transversely. The sole of the foot, therefore, is a biconcave structure.

The three arches of the foot are the medial longitudinal, lateral longitudinal, and transverse arches (see Fig. 9–9). During weight bearing, the only arch that can be seen in most patients is the medial longitudinal. Each arch consists of a keystone (the peak of the arch) and two pillars (opposing ends of the arch that make contact with the supporting surface). Each arch also has a tie rod that prevents the bases of the pillars from separating.[35]

The keystone of the medial longitudinal arch is the talar head. Its pillars are the calcaneus posteriorly and the sesamoids of the great toe and heads of the first, second, and third metatarsals anteriorly. The tie rod is the plantar fascia. The keystone of the lateral longitudinal arch is the cuboid. The pillars are the calcaneus and the heads of the fourth and fifth metatarsals, and the tie rod is the plantar fascia. The plantar fascia serves as the tie rod for both the medial and lateral longitudinal arches, a function more commonly known as the "windlass" phenomenon. The windlass phenomenon is thought to be important clinically; it is partially responsible for moving the foot into a supinated position during the later part of the stance phase of gait.

The transverse arch is present in the tarsals and the metatarsals when the foot is non–weight bearing. In a weight-bearing position the transverse arch is present only in the tarsals and at the bases of the metatarsal. The keystone of the transverse arch is the middle cuneiform and

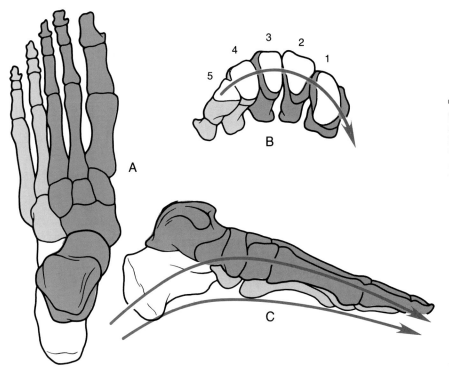

FIGURE 9–9 ■ The three main arches of the foot. (A) Medial longitudinal arch with lines illustrating the active portion of the arch, and lateral longitudinal arch with dots illustrating the passive portion of the arch. The calcaneus is common to both arches. (B) Curve illustrating the shape of the transverse arch. (C) Curves illustrating the shape of the medial and lateral longitudinal arches.

the pillars are the cuboid and the medial cuneiform. The tie rod for the transverse arch is considered to be the peroneus longus muscle.

Many clinicians and researchers have argued that the medial longitudinal is functionally the most important of the arches. It is the most mobile and appears to have the greatest impact on the movement of and the forces applied to the foot and, secondarily, the lower quarter.

The arches of the foot are formed and are maintained primarily by four factors:

■ The architecture of the tarsal bones
■ The orientation of the joints and supporting ligaments
■ The forces produced by contracting muscles
■ The structurally strong plantar ligaments (Fig. 9–10)

The extent to which each of these factors contributes to the maintenance of the medial longitudinal arch is controversial. Most clinicians agree, however, that arch maintenance is an important consideration in the treatment of many types of patients. Therefore, the literature that examines the relative contribution of each of these factors to arch maintenance is reviewed.

Hicks has probably done the most work on the relative contributions of the four factors mentioned previously to maintaining the medial longitudinal arch.[2,35–38] Hicks' data suggested the following. The medial longitudinal arch is maintained because it functions most like a curved beam and a truss. The arch behaves like a curved beam (a solid structure) because bending forces in the arch result in tensile loads being applied to the plantar intersegmental ligaments. The arch also behaves like a truss (a curved multisegmental structure with the plantar fascia connecting the two pillars). Compressive forces are present in the bones of the arch and tensile loads are applied to the plantar fascia.

The clinical implications of these conclusions are that the bony and ligamentous structures of the foot work in combination to absorb and transmit weight-bearing forces. The truss action of the foot becomes more important as the body weight shifts anterior to the foot. That is, when the patient moves from a foot-flat to a toe-off

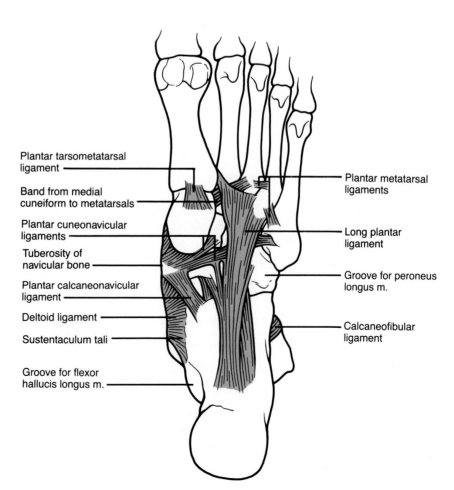

**FIGURE 9–10 ■** Ligaments on the plantar aspect of the left foot.

Plantar tarsometatarsal ligament

Band from medial cuneiform to metatarsals

Plantar cuneonavicular ligaments

Tuberosity of navicular bone

Plantar calcaneonavicular ligament

Deltoid ligament

Sustentaculum tali

Groove for flexor hallucis longus m.

Plantar metatarsal ligaments

Long plantar ligament

Groove for peroneus longus m.

Calcaneofibular ligament

■■■■■ **Table 9–3.** MUSCLES OF THE LOWER LIMB, ANKLE, AND FOOT: THEIR ACTION, INNERVATION, AND NERVE ROOT DERIVATION OF THE PERIPHERAL NERVES

| Action | Muscles Involved | Innervation | Nerve Root Deviation |
|---|---|---|---|
| Plantar flexion (flexion) of ankle | 1. Gastrocnemius[a] | Tibial | S1, S2 |
| | 2. Soleus[a] | Tibial | S1, S2 |
| | 3. Plantaris | Tibial | S1, S2 |
| | 4. Flexor digitorum longus | Tibial | S2, S3 |
| | 5. Peroneus longus | Superficial peroneal | L5, S1, S2 |
| | 6. Peroneus brevis | Superficial peroneal | L5, S1, S2 |
| | 7. Flexor hallucis longus | Tibial | S2, S3 |
| | 8. Tibialis posterior | Tibial | L4, L5 |
| Dorsiflexion (extension) of ankle | 1. Tibialis anterior | Deep peroneal | L4, L5 |
| | 2. Extensor digitorum longus | Deep peroneal | L5, S1 |
| | 3. Extensor hallucis longus | Deep peroneal | L5, S1 |
| | 4. Peroneus tertius | Deep peroneal | L5, S1 |
| Inversion | 1. Tibialis posterior | Tibial | L4, L5 |
| | 2. Flexor digitorum longus | Tibial | S2, S3 |
| | 3. Flexor hallucis longus | Tibial | S2, S3 |
| | 4. Tibialis anterior | Deep peroneal | L4, L5 |
| | 5. Extensor hallucis longus | Deep peroneal | L5, S1 |
| Eversion | 1. Peroneus longus | Superficial peroneal | L5, S1, S2 |
| | 2. Peroneus brevis | Superficial peroneal | L5, S1, S2 |
| | 3. Peroneus tertius | Deep peroneal | L5, S1 |
| | 4. Extensor digitorum longus | Deep peroneal | L5, S1 |
| Flexion of toes | 1. Flexor digitorum longus | Tibial | S2, S3 |
| | 2. Flexor hallucis longus | Tibial | S2, S3 |
| | 3. Flexor digitorum brevis | Tibial (medial plantar branch) | S2, S3 |
| | 4. Flexor hallucis brevis | Tibial (medial plantar branch) | S2, S3 |
| | 5. Flexor accessorius | Tibial (lateral plantar branch) | S2, S3 |
| | 6. Interossei | Tibial (lateral plantar branch) | S2, S3 |
| | 7. Flexor digiti minimi brevis | Tibial (lateral plantar branch) | S2, S3 |
| | 8. Lumbricals (metatarsophalangeal joints) | Tibial (1st by medial plantar branch; 2nd–4th by lateral plantar branch) | S2, S3 |
| Extension of toes | 1. Extensor digitorum longus | Deep peroneal | L5, S1 |
| | 2. Extensor hallucis longus | Deep peroneal | L5, S1 |
| | 3. Extensor digitorum brevis | Deep peroneal (lateral terminal branch) | S1, S2 |
| | 4. Lumbricals (interphalangeal joints) | Tibial (1st by medial plantar branch; 2nd–4th by lateral plantar branch) | S2, S3 |
| Abduction of toes | 1. Abductor hallucis | Tibial (medial plantar branch) | S2, S3 |
| | 2. Abductor digiti minimi | Tibial (lateral plantar branch) | S2, S3 |
| | 3. Dorsal interossei | Tibial (lateral plantar branch) | S2, S3 |
| Adduction of toes | 1. Adductor hallucis | Tibial (lateral plantar branch) | S2, S3 |
| | 2. Plantar interossei | Tibial (lateral plantar branch) | S2, S3 |

[a] The gastrocnemius and soleus muscles are sometimes grouped together as the triceps surae muscles.
From Magee DJ: Orthopedic Physical Assessment, 2nd ed. Philadelphia: WB Saunders, 1992, p 336.

position in the stance phase of gait, the plantar fascia takes on a larger role in dissipating the forces. Theoretically, if the plantar fascia is unable to perform its function the plantar ligaments of the tarsal joints and the supporting muscles have to provide the support for the arch. A test for assessing the length of the plantar fascia was proposed by Hicks and is known as the Hicks test.[39] It has yet to gain much popularity in the clinical setting.

Other factors considered important in maintaining the arches of the foot are the forces produced by contracting muscles. Basmajian and Stecko used needle electrodes to examine the electrical activity of several major extrinsic muscles of the foot and of the flexor digitorum brevis.[40] Recordings were taken while loads were applied to the superior aspects of the knees of seated subjects. Results suggested that muscle activity was not present while the limb was loaded. Mann and Inman showed that essentially no activity was present in the intrinsic foot muscles during quiet standing.[41] It would appear that muscle activity is not required to maintain the shape of the arch during static weight bearing. However, during walking and other activities the forces produced by these muscles appear to assist in the maintenance of the arch. For example, much of the literature suggests that the arches of patients are severely flattened during weight bearing after tibialis posterior tendon ruptures.[42-45] This appears to contradict the findings of Mann and Inman[41] and others suggesting that muscles such as the tibialis posterior are inactive during standing. If these muscles were inactive during standing, they would contribute little to the stability of the arch. However, posterior leg muscles are active during activities such as walking[46] and probably provide dynamic stability to the medial longitudinal arch during these activities.

According to Hicks, the arches of the foot are supported in two ways.[36,47] First, the pillars of the arch can be tied together via the plantar ligaments and fascia. Second, the keystone of the arch is supported on its plantar surface by the wedge shape of the bones, their associated joints, and the supporting ligaments and muscles.

## Muscles of the Leg and Foot

The actions of muscles of the leg and foot are described in Table 9–3 and are pictured diagrammatically in Figure 9–11. The origins and insertions of the leg and foot muscles are summarized in Table 9–4.

## Nerves and Blood Supply

The innervations of the muscles of the leg and foot are described in Table 9–3. Nerve roots that contribute to the innervation of these muscles are also listed in Table 9–3. The dermatomal and peripheral nerve innervation of the skin of the ankle and foot is illustrated in Figure 9–12.

The arterial supply to the ankle and foot is provided by the anterior and posterior tibial arteries, which are divisions of the popliteal artery. The anterior tibial artery supplies the anterior compartment of the leg and terminates in the foot as the dorsalis pedis artery. The dorsalis pedis artery supplies the dorsum of the foot and the digits. The posterior tibial artery has several branches that supply the posterior and lateral compartments of the leg. A main branch of the posterior tibial artery, the peroneal artery, supplies the lateral compartment as well as many hindfoot structures. The posterior tibial and dorsalis pedis arteries provide the branches that form the arterial network for the plantar aspect of the foot.

## BIOMECHANICS

This section reviews what is currently known and what is speculated about the biomechanics of the ankle and foot. Much of the biomechanics of the foot and ankle is based on speculation primarily for two reasons. First, the bony and soft tissue architecture of the foot and ankle is complex. The shapes of the joint surfaces are extremely variable, and many of the approximately 30 joints that make up the foot and ankle function as a group. Second, the movements of the foot and ankle occur rapidly during function. Our methods of studying the movements and forces within the joints of the foot and ankle have yet to be adequately developed. Therefore, much of the treatment for many patients with foot and ankle problems is based primarily on unsubstantiated theory.

The purpose of this section is to summarize and integrate the studies that have examined the biomechanics of the foot and ankle. Papers that have attempted to develop theoretical constructs related to foot function are also summarized.

*Biomechanics* is a general term that is related to both kinematics and kinetics. Kinematics is defined as the study of movements without regard to the forces that caused the movements. The issues related to kinematics addressed in this chapter are the locations of the axes of rotation of the joints of the ankle and foot and the movements that occur about these axes. Most of the fundamental literature on the kinematics of the ankle and foot was published decades ago.

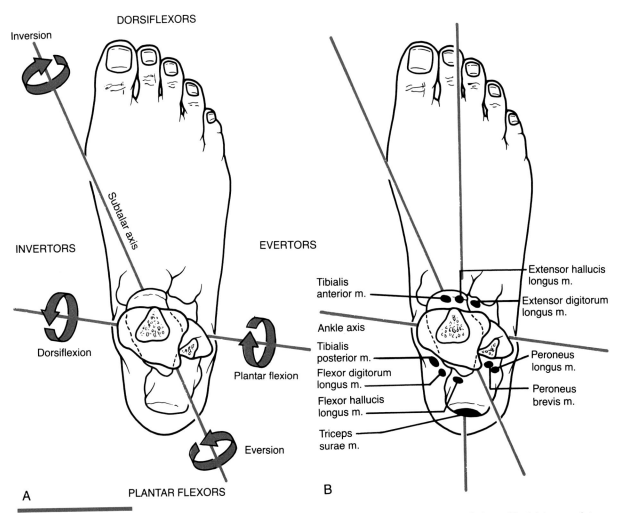

**FIGURE 9–11** ■ (A) Approximate positions of the subtalar and ankle joint axes. (B) Position of the ankle joint musculature relative to the subtalar and ankle joint axes.

The questions asked in some of these earlier studies have been re-examined and in some cases the conclusions of previous studies have been substantiated. However, most of the studies of the biomechanics of the ankle and foot have been in vitro studies. In vivo studies are, for the most part, lacking. This section reviews the earlier as well as the more recent studies.

The axes of rotation of the joints of the ankle and foot provide some of the theoretic basis for many forms of treatment currently advocated for lower extremity problems. Therefore, the literature concerning the positions of these axes is thoroughly examined and the implications of these studies for clinical practice are discussed.

Many studies have attempted to describe the position of the axes of motion for the joints of the foot and ankle and the movements at the various joints. The kinematics of the foot and

ankle in a weight-bearing position have also been studied in living subjects.[48–50] These studies are thoroughly reviewed.

The effectiveness of some treatments of patients with lower extremity complaints is determined, in part, by assessing the kinematics of the patients' lower extremity before and after treatment. A thorough understanding of the kinematics is essential for effective clinical practice.

Kinetics is defined as the study of forces applied to the body.[25] During ankle and foot movements, forces are applied to the ankle and foot by muscles and other external forces. An understanding of the type and magnitude of these forces can aid in determining when abnormal forces may be produced by or applied to patients. Few studies have measured in vivo the forces in and around the ankle and foot. Most studies have used force platforms and mathe-

**Table 9-4.** ORIGINS AND INSERTIONS OF THE MUSCLES OF THE LEG AND FOOT

| Muscle | Origin | Insertion |
|---|---|---|
| Tibialis anterior | Lateral condyle and upper two thirds of lateral aspect of tibia and interosseous membrane | Medial aspect of medial cuneiform and base of first metatarsal |
| Extensor hallucis longus | Middle half of anterior fibula and interosseous membrane | Base of distal phalanx of great toe |
| Extensor digitorum longus | Lateral condyle of tibia and upper half of anterior fibula and interosseous membrane | Dorsal aspect of middle and distal phalanges of lateral four toes |
| Peroneus tertius | Distal one third of anterior fibula | Dorsal surface of the base of fifth metatarsal |
| Gastrocnemius | (Medial head) medial condyle of posterior femur and posterior knee joint capsule; (lateral head) lateral condyle of posterior femur and posterior knee joint capsule | Posterior aspect of calcaneus |
| Soleus | Posterior aspect of head and upper shaft of fibula, middle third of posterior tibia | Posterior aspect of calcaneus |
| Plantaris | Lateral supracondylar line of the femur and oblique popliteal ligament of the knee joint | Medial side of posterior aspect of calcaneus |
| Popliteus | Lateral condyle of femur and oblique popliteal ligament of knee | Posterior surface of tibia proximal to soleal line |
| Flexor hallucis longus | Distal half of posterior aspect of fibula and interosseous membrane | Base of distal phalanx of great toe |
| Flexor digitorum longus | Posterior surface of middle half of tibia | Plantar surface of base of distal phalanx of the lateral four toes |
| Tibialis posterior | Posterior surface of proximal third of tibia, proximal half of posterior fibula and interosseous membrane | Tuberosity of navicular, plantar surface of cuneiforms, plantar aspect of base of second, third, and fourth metatarsals, plantar surface of cuboid and sustentaculum tali |
| Peroneus longus | Lateral condyle of tibia, proximal two thirds of lateral surface of fibula | Lateral aspect of medial cuneiform, base of first metatarsal |
| Peroneus brevis | Lower half of lateral aspect of fibula | Lateral aspect of base of fifth metatarsal |
| Extensor digitorum brevis | Dorsal aspect of lateral surface of calcaneus | Dorsal surface of base of proximal phalanx of great toe and lateral sides of tendons of extensor digitorum longus |
| Abductor hallucis | Medial process of calcaneus and plantar aponeurosis | Medial side of base of proximal phalanx of great toe |
| Flexor digitorum brevis | Medial process of calcaneus and plantar aponeurosis | Middle phalanx of lateral four toes |
| Abductor digiti minimi | Lateral and medial processes of calcaneus and adjacent fascia | Lateral aspect of base of proximal phalanx of the small toe |
| Quadratus plantae | (Medial head) medial surface of calcaneus and long plantar ligament; (lateral head) lateral border of plantar surface of calcaneus and lateral border of long plantar ligament | Tendons of flexor digitorum longus |
| Lumbricals | The four lumbricals arise from the tendons of flexor digitorum longus | Along with the interossei and tendons of extensor digitorum longus into bases of terminal phalanges of the lateral four toes |
| Flexor hallucis brevis | Plantar and medial aspect of cuboid, lateral cuneiform and posterior tibialis tendon | Medial and lateral aspect of proximal phalanx of great toe |
| Adductor hallucis | (Oblique head) bases of second, third, and fourth metatarsals and peroneus longus sheath; (transverse head) capsules of lateral four metatarsophalangeal joints | Lateral aspect of proximal phalanx of great toe |
| Flexor digiti minimi brevis | Base of fifth metatarsal, sheath of peroneus longus | Lateral aspect of base of proximal phalanx of small toe |
| Dorsal interossei | The four dorsal interossei via two heads arise from adjacent metatarsal shafts | The first inserts into the medial aspect of proximal phalanx of the second toe. The second inserts into the lateral aspect of the proximal phalanx of the second toe. The third inserts into the lateral aspect of the proximal phalanx of the third toe. The fourth inserts into the lateral aspect of the proximal phalanx of the fourth toe. |
| Plantar interossei | The three plantar interossei arise from the bases and medial aspects of the third, fourth, and fifth metatarsals | Medial aspects of bases of the proximal phalanges of the third, fourth, and fifth toes |

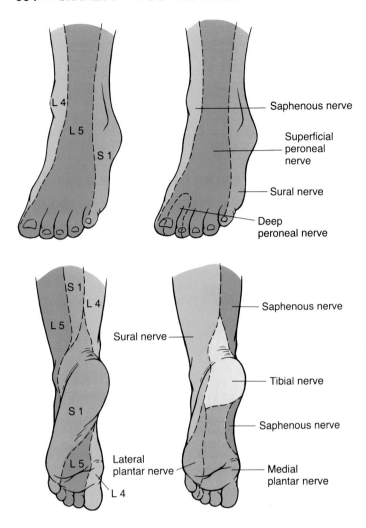

**FIGURE 9-12** ■ Sensory innervation of the surfaces of the foot.

matical equations to aid in predicting forces in the joints and soft tissues of the ankle and foot. Some studies of the kinetics of the ankle are reviewed briefly in this section. The kinetics of the ankle and foot are most commonly studied during gait, and the clinician must have a working knowledge of the forces about the ankle and foot during gait. The reader should study the chapter on gait in conjunction with the material reviewed in this section.

## Kinematics

The kinematics of the ankle and foot are clinically important for several reasons. Our understanding of how the foot functions is based, in part, on the positions of the joint axes and the movements about these axes. The axes and their positions in space indicate the type of motion expected at each joint. These axes are used by therapists to anticipate the type of compensatory lower extremity movement seen in patients. The variability of the positions of these axes has also been used to explain why different foot types are present in the population.[51]

Many methods have been used to quantify the position of the axes of rotation of the ankle and foot. Most of the earlier researchers used cadaver specimens in their studies and relied on ingenuity to develop unique methods of determining axis position. For example, Manter,[1] Elftman,[52] and Isman and Inman[51] developed different types of jigs to stabilize cadaver specimens while mapping out the location of the axis of rotation. Studies of the position of the ankle axis concluded that this axis was fixed in space and did not move when movement occurred at the joint.

The findings of these studies were impressively consistent. However, because cadaver specimens were used, their relevance has always been in question. More recently, a number of studies have examined the kinematics of the ankle and foot in vivo.

The axes of motion for lower extremity joints have been studied in vivo from two-dimensional and three-dimensional perspectives. Two-dimensional methods typically require radiographs to be taken at various positions throughout the range of motion with the x-ray plate positioned parallel to the plane of motion. Studying the movements of joints from a two-dimensional perspective involves the important assumption that the two bones that make up a joint move almost exclusively in one plane.[53] The movements occurring in most foot and ankle joints are typically three-dimensional and violate this assumption.

Studies of the two-dimensional movement of joints attempt to identify what is described as the instant center of motion. The instant center of motion is defined as the pivot point of relative motion between two articulating bones.[54] Implicit in the term "instant center" is that the center of motion moves when movement occurs at the joint. Contrary to the studies of Elftman[52] and Isman and Inman,[51] the researchers who have examined the axis of motion in vivo have found that it does indeed move. A further limitation of studies of the two-dimensional instant center of motion of the ankle[55,56] is that the ankle joint moves in multiple planes simultaneously.

A literature review found only one study that examined in vivo the three-dimensional axis of rotation of the ankle joint.[57] This study showed that the position of the axis for the ankle joint is extremely variable during movement and among subjects. The strength of this study is that the position of the three-dimensional axis of motion can be described using the three cardinal planes. The limitation of two-dimensional methods (i.e., the assumption of planar motion) does not hold true for three-dimensional analysis. Lundberg et al. were the first to attempt to determine the location of the axes of rotation for the ankle joint in three dimensions using living subjects.[57] Unfortunately, no in vivo studies have been published that describe the location of the three-dimensional axis of motion for the subtalar joint or the transverse tarsal joint.

The clinical implications of knowing whether a joint has a fixed or an instantaneous axis of motion may seem subtle. However, muscle and ligament function vary depending on the distance between these tissues and the axis of motion. If one could predict the location of the axis of rotation during movement, the function of muscles and ligaments during different activities could be better elucidated. Clearly, knowing the function of muscles and ligaments during movement would be useful clinically. Knowing the position of the axis of rotation could also be very useful in understanding the effects of disease or injury on joint function. For example, Frankel and colleagues suggested that the position of the instant center of rotation for the knee could be used to predict whether articular cartilage damage was occurring in patients with previous knee injuries.[58] Sammarco et al. examined the locations of the instant centers of rotation of the ankle joints of normal subjects and subjects with diseased ankles.[55] They concluded that the locations of the instant centers in the patients were abnormal and resulted in abnormal compressive forces across the ankle joint.

### Ankle Joint

The primary function of the talocrural joint has been believed to be that of allowing plantar flexion and dorsiflexion motion. Hence, the joint has been referred to as a single-axis hinge joint by many experts.[6,59,60] Much data exist, however, to refute the precept that the ankle joint is uniaxial.

Inman has probably contributed the most to our understanding of the function of the ankle (talocrural) joint.[6] In a series of studies of cadaver specimens, Inman found the ankle axis to lie approximately at the tips of the medial and lateral malleoli. The variability in the position of this axis was quite high among the specimens tested (Fig. 9–13). The direction of this axis is from anteromedial and superior to posterolateral and inferior. Many other researchers have investigated the position of the axis of motion of the ankle joint. Descriptions of the positions of these axes are summarized in Table 9–5. As can be seen from the table, the earlier investigators described a fixed axis of rotation but later investigators described an instantaneous axis of rotation. Barnett and Napier[23] and Hicks[2] were probably the first to infer that the axis of the ankle joint was not fixed. They concluded that the axis for dorsiflexion was different from the axis for plantar flexion. Barnett and Napier demonstrated that the dorsiflexion axis ran from an anteromedial and superior direction to a posterolateral and inferior direction. The plantar flexion axis ran from an anteromedial and inferior direc-

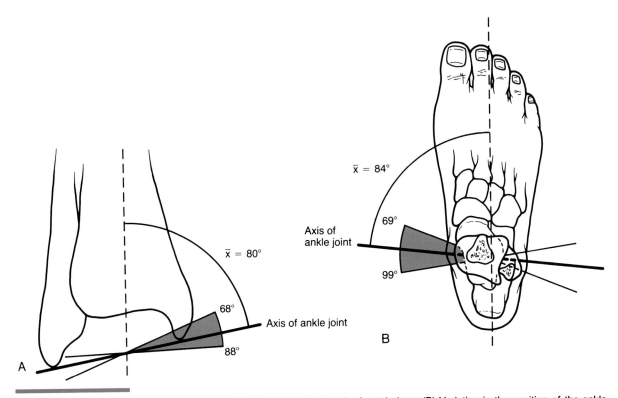

**FIGURE 9-13** ■ (A) Variation in the position of the ankle joint axis in the frontal plane. (B) Variation in the position of the ankle joint axis in the horizontal plane.

tion to a posterolateral and superior direction. The resultant motion produced by these axes is illustrated in Figure 9–14.

Sammarco and colleagues carried out an extensive study of the instant center of rotation of the ankle.[55] They determined the positions of the center of motion in 26 ankles of normal subjects and 14 ankles of patients with ankle disease. As mentioned previously, they used a two-dimensional method to determine the location of the center of motion, so the results should be interpreted cautiously. The results, however, suggest that the center of rotation of the ankle does move during motion. The extent of the movement varies among subjects, but pathology appears to result in even greater movement of the center of rotation. The data of Sammarco et al. provide further evidence that the ankle joint does not function like a simple hinge as some of the earlier investigators suggested.[55]

Lundberg and colleagues were the first to undertake an in vivo study of the instantaneous axis of rotation of the ankle joint.[57] They inserted 0.8-mm metal marker beads into the bones of the ankles and feet of eight subjects positioned in an apparatus. The subjects were asked to move in several directions while orthogonal ra-

diographs were taken. The researchers were able to determine the location of the axes from the radiographs. They found that the axis of the talocrural joint moves during motion and varies among subjects. The change in the position of the axis was similar to that described by Barnett and Napier[23] and Hicks.[2] The results also suggested that the talocrural joint can contribute a significant amount of motion during horizontal plane motion of the tibia. Specifically, approximately 5 degrees of horizontal plane external rotation of the talus occurred relative to the tibia when the tibia moved from a neutral to an internally rotated position. These results suggest that the ankle joint is capable of contributing a fairly large amount of horizontal motion to the foot when the foot moves into a pronated position. That is, the talocrural joint can account for some of the horizontal plane motion that occurs in the lower limb during gait.[61,62] This function has, in the past, been attributed primarily to the subtalar joint.

Knowledge of the locations of the instant axis of rotation of the ankle joint has several clinical implications. Perhaps most important to physical therapists, the positions of these axes allow the therapists to infer the type and amount of talo-

■■■■■■■ **Table 9–5.** TYPE AND POSITION OF THE AXIS OF ROTATION OF THE ANKLE

| Axis[a] | Investigators | Position with Respect to Anatomic Planes | | |
| --- | --- | --- | --- | --- |
| | | Frontal | Sagittal | Transverse |
| Fix. | Elftman (1945) | | 67.6° ± 7.4° | |
| Fix. | Isman and Inman (1969) | | 84° ± 7° | 10° ± 4° |
| | | 8 mm anterior, 3 mm inferior to the distal tip of the lateral malleolus to 1 mm posterior, 5 mm inferior to the distal tip of the medial malleolus | | |
| Fix. | Inman and Mann (1979) | | 79° (68–88°) | |
| Fix. | Allard and associates (1987) | 95.4° ± 6.6° | 77.7° ± 12.3° | 17.9° ± 4.5° |
| Ins. | Sammarco and colleagues (1973) | Inside and outside the body of the talus | | |
| Ins. | D'Ambrosia and coworkers (1976) | No consistent pattern | | |
| Ins. | Parlasca and colleagues (1979) | 96% within 12 mm of a point 20 mm below the articular surface of the tibia along the long axis | | |
| Ins. | van Langelaan (1983) | At an approximate right angle to the longitudinal direction of the foot, passing through the corpus tali, with a direction from anterolaterosuperior to posteromedioinferior | | |
| Q—I. | Barnett and Napier (1952) | Dorsiflexion: down and lateral | | |
| | | Plantar flexion: down and medial | | |
| Q—I. | Hicks (1953) | Dorsiflexion: 5 mm inferior to tip of lateral malleolus to 15 mm anterior to tip of medial malleolus | | |
| | | Plantar flexion: 5 mm superior to tip of lateral malleolus to 15 mm anterior, 10 mm inferior to tip of medial malleolus | | |

[a] Fix. = fixed axis of rotation; Ins. = instantaneous axis of rotation; Q—I. = quasi-instantaneous axis of rotation.

From Jahss MH, ed: Disorders of the Foot and Ankle: Medical and Surgical Management, 2nd ed, Vol 1. Philadelphia: WB Saunders, 1991, p 438.

crural joint motion occurring in the three cardinal planes. For example, although talocrural joint motion occurs primarily in the sagittal plane, a significant amount of motion also appears to occur in the horizontal plane. This horizontal plane motion appears to be greatest during internal rotation of the tibia. In addition, because the axis of motion of the ankle joint moves, some muscle force tests for the ankle joint should be questioned. This issue is addressed in a later section.

## Subtalar Joint

The functions of the subtalar joint have been described by many authors:

■ Force attenuation during the beginning of the stance phase of gait
■ Maintenance of full foot contact with the ground, which may vary in shape and texture
■ Conversion of horizontal plane motion of the lower limb during gait into frontal plane motion of the foot

These various functions require the subtalar joint to be a shock absorber with joint surface shapes that allow motion in three planes simultaneously. In addition, to achieve the third function, most of the motion allowed by the subtalar joint should be in the frontal plane. The subtalar joint is indeed designed to accomplish these three functions.

Perhaps the least understood of the functions is the conversion of horizontal plane limb motion into frontal plane foot motion. Levens and colleagues measured the amount of horizontal plane rotation of the lower limb of 12 normal subjects during ambulation.[62] The tibias of these subjects rotated through a mean arc of approximately 20 degrees during one gait cycle. This horizontal plane rotation, then, must be accounted for by the foot and ankle. Some of this motion is absorbed by joints distal to the subtalar joint[50] and by the talocrural joint.[57] However, a significant portion of the motion is converted, at the subtalar joint, into frontal plane motion of the foot.

The functions of the subtalar joint are complex

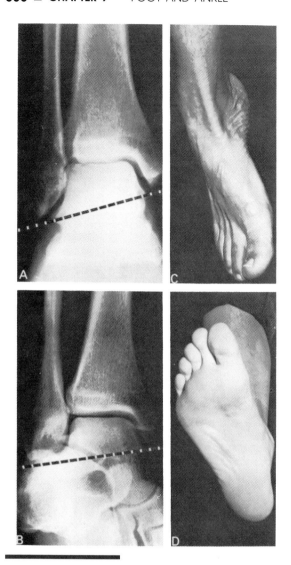

**FIGURE 9–14** ■ (A) Anteroposterior view and (B) ankle mortise view radiographs of the right ankle showing the position of the axis of rotation. (C) Plantar flexed and (D) dorsiflexed right ankle illustrating movement around the oblique ankle axis. (From Kelikian H, Kelikian AS: Disorders of the Ankle. Philadelphia: WB Saunders, 1985, Fig. 2–4A–D.)

and varied, which may help explain why the anatomy of this region is so complex. The subtalar joint is capable of performing these complex functions primarily because of the position of its axis of rotation.

Manter was the first to quantify the position of the axis of rotation of the subtalar joint.[1] He designed a jig that was used to stabilize the feet of 16 cadaveric specimens. A series of rods were placed in the specimens and used to determine the plane in which the joint moved. However, Manter did not describe how movement of the foot in the jig was achieved.

Through a process of trial and error, Manter was able to determine the location of the axis of rotation.[1] The assumption inherent in Manter's method is that the movements of joints are determined solely by the shapes of the articular surfaces. A weakness of this assumption is similar to the weakness of many in vitro studies of the kinematics of joints. Movements of living subjects' joints are produced by muscular, gravitational, and other external forces. These forces are in many ways different from the forces that produce the motion measured in in vitro studies. Because of this difference in the factors that produce the joint motions, the results of in vivo and in vitro studies may be different. Until in vivo studies are done to support or refute in vitro studies, the latter must be interpreted with caution.

Results of Manter's study suggested that the mean average position of the axis was 42 degrees from horizontal and 16 degrees medial to the midsagittal plane.[1] The range was 8 to 24 degrees for the midsagittal plane and 29 to 47 degrees for the horizontal plane. According to Manter, the subtalar joint axis is oriented obliquely relative to the cardinal planes, similar in some ways to the ankle joint axis. The general direction of both the talocrural and subtalar joint axes is from posterolateral and inferior to anteromedial and superior.

Manter also suggested that the subtalar joint axis functions like a screw in that translation of the talus occurs in conjunction with rotation. Inman et al. found that approximately half of the specimens they studied demonstrated a screw-like motion.[63] The amount and type of translation varied in both studies. The position of the subtalar axis and the translation that occurs about the axis vary considerably. Clinicians must keep this variability in mind when examining patients with foot or ankle problems.

Hicks,[2] Isman and Inman,[51] and Root et al.[64] determined the position of the subtalar joint axis and reported findings similar to those of Manter. They all suggested that the axis was fixed and therefore did not move during movement of the subtalar joint (Table 9–6).

Inman and Mann attempted to explain this phenomenon by likening the subtalar joint axis to an oblique mitered hinge.[65] The hinge is able to convert horizontal plane tibial motion into primarily frontal plane foot motion because of the position of the oblique axis in space (Fig. 9–15). Movement about this axis occurs through the three cardinal planes simultaneously. The axis is therefore described as a triplanar axis.

**Table 9-6.** TYPE AND POSITION OF THE AXIS OF ROTATION OF THE SUBTALAR JOINT

| Axis[a] | Investigators | Position with Respect to the Anatomic Planes | | |
| --- | --- | --- | --- | --- |
| | | Frontal | Sagittal | Transverse |
| Fix. | Manter (1941) | | 16° (8°–24°) | 42° (29°–47°) |
| Fix. | Shephard (1951) | Tuberosity of the calcaneus to the neck of the talus | | |
| Fix. | Hicks (1953) | Posterolateral corner of the heel to superomedial aspect of the neck of the talus | | |
| Fix. | Root and coworkers (1966) | | 17° (8°–29°) | 41° (22°–55°) |
| Fix. | Isman and Inman (1969) | | 23° ± 11° | 41° ± 9° |
| Fix. | Kirby (1947) | Extends from the posterolateral heel, posteriorly, to the first intermetatarsal space, anteriorly | | |
| Ins. | Rastegar and coworkers (1980) | Instant centers of rotation pathways in posterolateral quadrant of the distal articulating tibial surface, varying with applied load | | |
| Ins. | van Langelaan (1983) | A bundle of axes that make an acute angle with the longitudinal direction of the foot passing through the tarsal canal having a direction from anteromediosuperior to posterolateroinferior | | |
| Ins. | Engsberg (1987) | A bundle of axes with a direction from anteromediosuperior to posterolateroinferior | | |

[a] Fix. = fixed axis of rotation; Ins. = instantaneous axis of rotation.

From Jahss MH, ed: Disorders of the Foot and Ankle: Medical and Surgical Management, 2nd ed, Vol 1. Philadelphia: WB Saunders, 1991, p 439.

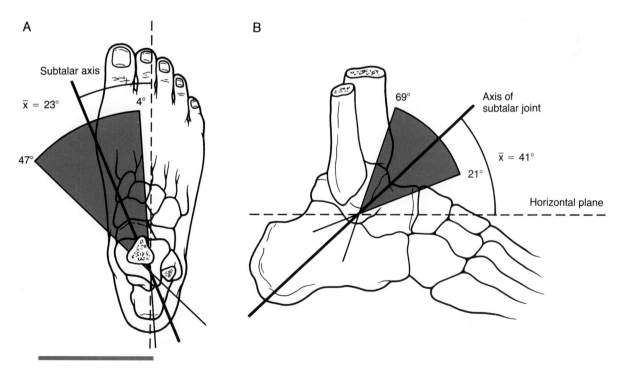

**FIGURE 9-15** ■ Variation in the position of the subtalar joint axis in (A) the horizontal plane and (B) the sagittal plane.

Because motions about the axis do not occur purely in the frontal plane, they are defined as supination and pronation.

Most data suggest that the mean position of the subtalar joint axis is approximately 45 degrees upward from the horizontal plane and approximately 25 degrees medial from the midsagittal line of the foot. Using simple trigonometry, one can approximate the relative amount of motion that would appear to occur in each cardinal plane for every degree of pronation and supination.

Based on Inman and Mann's mitered hinge theory,[65] one could also estimate the amount of cardinal plane subtalar joint motion occurring for every degree of internal and external rotation of the tibia. Because of the fit of the talus within the mortise, the talus probably "follows" the tibia during horizontal plane tibial motion.

Considering a foot with a subtalar axis position of 45 degrees upward, for every degree of horizontal plane tibial motion there is approximately 1 degree of frontal plane subtalar joint motion. A foot with an axis position of 30 degrees upward would demonstrate approximately 2 degrees of frontal plane subtalar joint motion for every degree of tibial motion. A foot with an axis position of 60 degrees upward would demonstrate approximately 1 degree of frontal plane subtalar joint motion for every 2 degrees of horizontal plane tibial motion. These relationships hold true whether the movement is initiated from the foot or from the tibia.

Inman and Mann also suggested that the angle or pitch of the subtalar joint axis can be used to predict the shape of the foot.[65] For example, they stated that an axis with a pitch of approximately 30 degrees upward from the horizontal plane is associated with a flat foot type, whereas an axis pitch of around 60 degrees is associated with a high arch or cavus foot type. This seems valid because patients with flat feet tend to have a large amount of frontal plane subtalar joint motion and those with cavus feet tend to have a small amount of frontal plane subtalar joint motion. No other good experimental data exist to support this concept.

Novick suggested that patients with cavus feet require a greater than normal amount of tibial rotation to achieve contact of the medial side of the forefoot with the ground.[66] Implicit in Novick's hypothesis is the idea that patients with cavus feet who participate in repetitive weight-bearing activities may be predisposed to developing knee pain. The knee pain would be attributable to the excessive horizontal plane tibial

motion. This hypothesis is consistent with the mitered hinge theory of Inman and Mann, but no data currently exist to support this contention.

The subtalar joint, like the talocrural joint, has been considered a uniaxial joint with a fixed axis.[1,2,51] However, data clearly demonstrate that the subtalar axis moves during subtalar joint movement.[67,68] van Langelaan[67] and Benink[68] both showed, using cadaveric specimens, that the position of the axis varies during movement. These data cast some doubt on Inman and Mann's mitered hinge theory.[65] The relationship between subtalar motion and horizontal plane tibial motion is probably more complex than Inman and Mann's mitered hinge theory would imply. However, the general positions of these axes approximate the position of the fixed axis described by Manter,[1] Hicks,[2] and Isman and Inman.[51] That is, the instantaneous axes run from a posterolateral and inferior position to an anteromedial and superior position. The positions of these axes are summarized in Table 9–6.

Whether the subtalar joint axis is fixed or constantly moving during joint movement is worthy of discussion. Another important topic is how the kinematics of the subtalar joint differ in a weight-bearing and in a non-weight-bearing position. In a non-weight-bearing position, the movement of pronation at the subtalar joint consists of the combined foot movements of dorsiflexion, abduction, and eversion. Supination consists of the combined movements of plantar flexion, adduction, and inversion.

During weight bearing, ground reaction forces and balance requirements maintain the foot in contact with the ground. As a result, pronation and supination during weight bearing must be defined differently than during non–weight bearing. Donatelli defines weight-bearing pronation or closed kinetic chain pronation as adduction and plantar flexion of the talus and eversion of the calcaneus.[69] Weight-bearing supination is defined as abduction and dorsiflexion of the talus and inversion of the calcaneus. Apparently, movements are described relative to specific bones because the ground prevents the classic cardinal plane movements of the foot from occurring around the subtalar joint axis. Although these definitions describe what occurs with individual bones, no description of movements at the subtalar joint or talocrural joint is provided. Knowing what motions occur at these joints during supination and pronation would provide the clinician with a more thorough description of the kinematics of the foot during function.

Lundberg et al. determined the amount and

type of three-dimensional movement at each major joint in the feet of eight living subjects.[48-50] Before taking measurements, they inserted 0.8-metal markers surgically into each of the tarsals, the tibia, and the first metatarsal of each subject. Orthogonal radiographs were taken at 10-degree intervals while the subject moved the foot through a range of 20 degrees of eversion to 20 degrees of inversion. These motions were used to simulate those that would occur when the foot is pronated and supinated.

Joint motions that occurred were described as movement of the distal bone relative to the proximal bone. For example, when discussing the talocalcaneal joint, dorsiflexion occurs when the calcaneus attains a more dorsiflexed position relative to the talus. When the feet were moved from a neutral to an everted (pronated) position the talocalcaneal joints dorsiflexed, everted (externally rotated) slightly, and abducted. When the feet were moved from a neutral to an everted (pronated) position the talocrural joints plantar flexed, adducted (internally rotated), and everted slightly. When the feet were moved from a neutral to an inverted (supinated) position the talocalcaneal joints plantar flexed, inverted, and adducted. When the feet were moved from a neutral to an inverted (supinated) position the talocrural joints dorsiflexed, inverted very slightly, and abducted.

An interesting finding of Lundberg and colleagues is that in almost all planes of motion the talonavicular joint moved through a larger range than all other foot or ankle joints. The talonavicular joint appears to move more than other joints of the foot during pronation and supination. It may therefore be a better indicator of foot function and position than the subtalar joint. This is discussed further in the examination section.

Subtalar joint pronation and supination have a direct effect on the movement of proximal structures. Because of the fit of the talus within the mortise, the tibia follows the talus during weight bearing. The talocrural joint rotates internally during pronation and externally during supination (Lundberg and associates).[48-50,57] Therefore, the tibia rotates internally during pronation and externally during supination.[62] The position of the knee in the sagittal plane is also affected by the position of the subtalar joint. Tibial internal rotation results in knee flexion, whereas tibial external rotation results in knee extension.[70] Tiberio has hypothesized that excessive internal femoral rotation is also associated with excessive pronation and secondarily produces symptoms in

some patients with knee pain.[71] The excessive internal femoral rotation is thought to result in malalignment of knee joint structures and excessive patellofemoral compressive forces.

There is little doubt that subtalar joint movements affect proximal structures. However, as Sims and Cavanaugh have stated, the relationship between the kinematics of the subtalar joint and knee or patellofemoral dysfunction has yet to be clearly elucidated.[72] The degree to which subtalar joint motion affects proximal structures is most likely related to foot type. The relationship between lower limb kinematics and foot type is certainly fertile ground for clinical research.

### Transverse Tarsal Joint

The transverse tarsal joint consists of the talonavicular joint and the calcaneocuboid joint. Only a few studies have attempted to determine the location of the axes of rotation of the transverse tarsal joint. These studies have many limitations because they used small numbers of cadaver specimens.

The function of the transverse tarsal joint is to provide the foot with an additional mechanism for raising and lowering the arch.[73] Lundberg and colleagues also imply that the transverse tarsal joint is designed to absorb some of the horizontal plane tibial motion that is transmitted to the foot during stance.[48-50]

To understand these functions, one must understand the anatomy of the transverse tarsal joint. As described in the anatomy section, the calcaneocuboid joint is saddle shaped. The saddle-shaped joint is typically described as having two axes of rotation. The talonavicular joint is condyloid in shape and therefore also has two axes of rotation.[73] According to Elftman, the positions of these two sets of axes are dependent on the position of the talocalcaneal joint.[73] When the talocalcaneal joint is pronated, the two sets of axes are parallel to one another and allow the maximal amount of motion at the transverse tarsal joint. When the talocalcaneal joint is supinated, the two sets of axes become divergent and little motion is allowed (Fig. 9-16). In addition, Mann suggests that the bony stability of the talonavicular joint is enhanced in the supinated position.[74] The talocalcaneal joint therefore apparently determines the extent to which movement is allowed at the transverse tarsal joint.

Manter[1] and Hicks[2] determined the locations of the axes of rotation for the transverse tarsal joint using cadaver specimens (Table 9-7). Metal

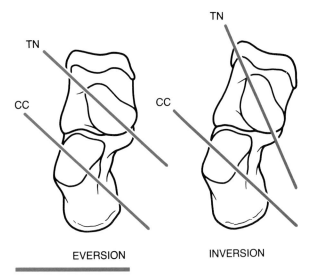

TN
TN
CC
CC
EVERSION
INVERSION

**FIGURE 9-16** ■ Approximate positions of the axes of rotation of the talonavicular (TN) and calcaneocuboid (CC) joints.

and inferior direction to an anteromedial and superior direction, much like the axes of the subtalar and talocrural joints.

Manter[1] and Hicks[2] used cadaveric specimens of the entire foot and moved the specimens in various ways to determine the location of the axes of rotation. Elftman based his descriptions of the axes of rotation for the transverse tarsal joint on an anatomic argument.[73] It appears that the axes described by Elftman are different from the axes described by Manter[1] and Hicks.[2] However, the functional implications of these differences are not clear.

rods were inserted into the specimens, which were placed in a jig and moved by the investigator. Movement of the rods determined the location of the axes of rotation. Both researchers determined that two separate fixed triplanar axes existed for the transverse tarsal joint.

Manter was the first to describe a longitudinal and an oblique triplanar axis for the transverse tarsal joint. Hicks found similar axes. The longitudinal axis allowed primarily frontal plane motion and the oblique axis permitted primarily sagittal plane motion. Both investigators determined that these axes ran from a posterolateral

### The First Ray

The first ray is defined as the articulation between the medial cuneiform and the first metatarsal.[2] The first ray is important functionally because it must achieve and maintain contact with the ground during stance to allow for a normal push-off. Hicks is the only investigator who has attempted to determine the location of the axis of rotation of the first ray.[2]

In a study described previously, Hicks mounted five cadaveric specimens' feet in a jig and determined the location of the axis of rotation of the first ray.[2] This triplanar axis ran approximately horizontally from posteromedial to anterolateral. This axis should allow primarily sagittal and frontal plane motion and little horizontal plane motion. First-ray plantar flexion and inversion are coupled, as are first-ray dorsiflexion and eversion.

**Table 9-7.** LOCATION OF THE CENTERS AND AXES OF ROTATION FOR THE TRANSVERSE TARSAL AND RAYS

| | Transverse Tarsal | | | | | |
| | Longitudinal | | Oblique | | | |
| Investigators | SAGITTAL | TRANSVERSE | SAGITTAL | TRANSVERSE | 1st Ray | 5th Ray |
|---|---|---|---|---|---|---|
| Manter (1941) | 9° | 15° | 57° | 53° | | |
| Shephard (1951) | One axis located, not identified | | | | | |
| Hicks (1953) | Superior aspect of navicular between midline and medial aspect of foot to posterolateral aspect of heel | | Superomedial aspect of head of talus to inferolateral surface of heel | | Mid-dorsum over base of third metatarsal to navicular tuberosity | Superomedial border at tarsometatarsal joint to 15 mm above and behind styloid of fifth metatarsal |

From Jahss MH, ed: Disorders of the Foot and Ankle: Medical and Surgical Management, 2nd ed, Vol 1. Philadelphia: WB Saunders, 1991, p 439.

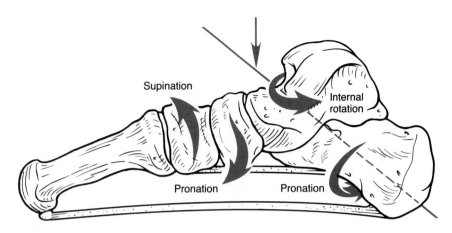

**FIGURE 9–17** ■ Pronation of the foot produced by internal rotation of the tibia. The rear foot and midfoot pronate and the forefoot supinates on the midfoot.

## Foot as a Unit

The work of Lundberg and colleagues[48–50,57] clearly illustrates the importance of considering the foot as a functioning unit during weight-bearing activities. The once commonly held belief that the subtalar joint accounted for most of the motion of the foot greatly oversimplifies foot function. Lundberg and colleagues elegantly demonstrated that the joints of the foot function in synchrony, and not in isolation, during movement.

The foot functions as a force absorber during the early part of the stance phase of gait and as a force transmitter during the push-off phase of gait. The foot can change its architecture to allow absorption of forces by the joints and ligaments during early stance. Conversely, during the push-off phase of gait, the foot behaves as a rigid beam that can efficiently convert muscular forces into a forward propulsion of the body.

Sarrafian provided a thorough description of how the foot achieves these contrasting functions during weight bearing.[39] During the early part of the stance phase of gait, internal rotation of the tibia results in pronation of the hindfoot and of the midfoot (Fig. 9–17). Supination of the forefoot occurs to maintain contact of the metatarsal heads with the ground (see Fig. 9–17). Because the first metatarsal head is moved farther away from the heel in this position, the plantar fascia and ligaments are relatively taut. The joints and soft tissues of the foot are in an optimal position to absorb forces.

Figure 9–18 illustrates how the major joints of the foot permit arch raising when the tibia is externally rotated. Sarrafian uses slightly different terminology to describe the movements, but

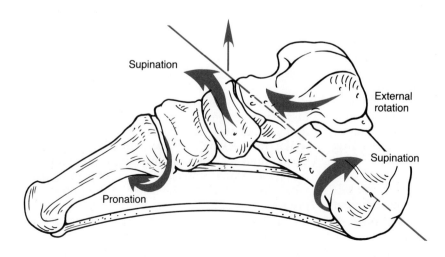

**FIGURE 9–18** ■ Supination of the foot produced by external rotation of the tibia. The rear foot and midfoot supinate and the forefoot pronates on the midfoot.

the description is clear.[39] According to Sarrafian, a sequence of motions occurs in the foot just before the heel-off phase of gait. When the tibia rotates externally, the hindfoot supinates, the transverse tarsal joint supinates, and the forefoot pronates in order to maintain contact of the first metatarsal with the ground (see Fig. 9–18). Because the first metatarsal head is brought closer to the heel in this position, the plantar fascia and ligaments are lax. The foot now behaves as a rigid beam because the bones of the feet are essentially locked on each other. Later, during the stance phase after heel-off, dorsiflexion of the great toe results in the plantar fascia becoming taut. The tautness of the plantar fascia also contributes to raising of the arch. The foot is therefore beautifully designed to function either as a force absorber or a force transmitter.

## Kinetics

Kinetics is the study of forces applied to the body. An understanding of the magnitude and direction of these forces would be useful in understanding normal function as well as the impact of abnormal forces on disease. Unfortunately, few data have been collected on the kinetics of the ankle and foot. Most of the work that has been done has examined the forces present in the foot and ankle during gait, which is discussed in Chapter 11.

An area that has been examined concerns the joint contact area and compressive force for the ankle joint. The compressive force on the ankle during standing is approximately one half of body weight. During the stance phase of gait this force increases to approximately five times body weight.[75] During running the compressive forces have been estimated to be approximately 13 times body weight.[76]

The talocrural joint appears to have a fairly large surface area of contact, which results in a relatively low force per unit area.[77] The shape of the talar dome is such that as the load on the ankle increases, the load-bearing area increases. At low loads the talus makes contact with the ankle mortise on the medial and lateral eminences of the talar dome. As the load increases, the area of contact increases to include the area between the lateral and medial eminences.[78] This mechanism of increasing the surface area of contact with increasing load, combined with the relatively low force per unit area and the inherent bony stability, may explain why the incidence of ankle joint osteoarthrosis is so low.

## EVALUATION

This section describes an approach to the history taking and examination of a patient with a disorder of the ankle or foot. The evaluation approach described is not meant to be an all-inclusive list of history taking and examination procedures. The more commonly used examination techniques are included.

The examination of a patient is made up of a series of tests that can be broken down into several categories. For example, the anterior drawer test and Homans' sign are examples of special tests. Each of the main categories of tests is discussed. The test categories comprise observational data, active and passive range-of-motion (ROM) tests, resistive tests, special tests, and palpation tests. Data on the use of instrumented muscle testing of patients with disorders of the foot and ankle are discussed. Invasive diagnostic tests are discussed briefly also. Evaluation of a patient's gait is covered in the chapter on gait. In describing each test category, the literature concerning the reliability or validity of measurements obtained with each test is reviewed. The literature review is designed to acquaint the reader with data that support or refute the more common clinical tests used for patients with foot and ankle problems. Because reliable and valid measurements should provide the basis for sound clinical problem solving, a major thrust of this section is to review studies of the usefulness of examination procedures for the foot and ankle.

At the end of this section, the hypothesis-oriented algorithm for clinicians (HOAC), a systematic method for clinical problem solving, is summarized.[4] The HOAC can be used by new and experienced clinicians as a model to guide scientifically based clinical practice.

## History

The primary purposes of taking the history are to identify patients who may have serious pathology, identify the patient's problem or reason(s) for seeking care, and obtain a thorough background of information about the patient's problem. Many clinicians have recommended what they consider the most appropriate approach to taking a history. Maitland, for example, describes an elaborate series of questions designed to determine the area, nature, and behavior of a patient's pain symptoms.[79] Cyriax advocates taking a history for the purpose of determining which tissues cause the patient's symptoms.[80] The basic elements of the various history-taking approaches, however, are similar.

A typical patient's history includes a description of the current problem, a description of the past medical history, the family and social history, and a systems review. Perhaps most important for physical therapists is the patient's description of the current problem. The current problem or chief complaint is essentially the answer to the question, What symptoms or problems brought you here? The answer to this question directs the examination and determines its extent and vigor. The answer also lays the groundwork for the hypotheses the therapist may generate about the causes of the patient's complaint. For example, if the patient complains of pain in the area of the plantar surface of the calcaneus after activity, the therapist may consider inflammatory processes as contributing to the problem.

Important aspects of the patient's description of the problem are the site and severity of the pain symptoms. The visual analog scale has been used to attempt to quantify the intensity of pain reported by patients.[81] Body diagrams are also used to map the perimeter of the pain or changes in sensation reported by the patient.[82] Perhaps most crucial is the determination of how the patient's symptoms vary with activity or changes in position. Classically, clinicians have been taught that when movement or activity does not change the intensity of symptoms, serious pathology may be present. This may not always be true and should be determined after all the data have been collected.

Patients with overuse or repetitive-use syndromes of the foot or ankle are often seen clinically. In taking the history of these patients it is important to obtain a thorough description of the activities that aggravate the symptoms and those that relieve the symptoms. Patients with repetitive-use syndromes are among the most challenging to examine because the etiology of the complaint is frequently multifactorial. A thorough history can help greatly in determining the most efficient and sound approach to examining and subsequently treating these patients.

Leading questions about the nature and behavior of symptoms must be avoided. Biased questions regarding pain behavior tend to elicit biased responses. For example, the question Does the pain increase when you walk? tends to bias the patient toward saying "yes." Answers to questions such as these often do not accurately reflect the true nature of the patient's symptoms.

Physical therapists frequently do not go into detail when questioning the patient about past medical or family history. However, the therapist should keep in mind that some pathologies of the foot and ankle may be genetically linked. Many patients with collagen diseases, for example, appear to have a genetic predisposition to the disease.

Information related to the patient's history comes from a variety of sources. These include the patient, the patient's medical chart, the patient's family, and physicians. The therapist should use these sources when planning an examination for a patient with a problem in the foot or ankle.

At the conclusion of the history, the therapist should always ask, Is there anything else that you think I should know? An open-ended question such as this provides an opportunity to obtain the patient's impression of the cause of the disorder. In addition, asking which problem concerns the patient most assists the therapist in ranking the patient's problems when setting goals.

After taking the history, the therapist should have a fairly clear direction for the examination and subsequent treatment. The therapist should have begun the process of generating hypotheses about why the patient has this problem(s). In addition, the therapist should have a general sense of how vigorous to be during the examination.

The following examination form may be used as a guide when reading the material that follows. The procedures that are typically part of a lower quarter scanning examination such as a neurologic examination are not included on this form. Therapists should first determine that the patient's complaints are not due to pathology of proximal structures before examining specific structures of the foot and ankle.

## Examination

### Observational Data

The primary purpose of the observational data section of the examination is to obtain a global assessment of the patient's alignment in frequently maintained postures. For most patients, this posture is a standing position. For some patients the postures they assume at work may be of clinical significance. For example, a patient

# EXAMINATION FORM

## History

History of present illness:
For example, is the patient able to:

> Put on shoes and socks without difficulty?
> Stand comfortably with weight evenly distributed on both feet?
> Walk on level surfaces?
> Walk on uneven surfaces?
> Walk downhill without difficulty?
> Walk uphill without difficulty?
> Wear all types of shoes without change in symptoms?

Assessment of the magnitude of the patient's pain or other symptoms:

Relevant past medical history:

Chart review, if applicable:

Results of invasive diagnostic tests:

Questions to family members, if applicable:

Medications:

Previous treatment for present problem:

What is the patient's chief complaint?

Establish goals:


## Examination

Observational data
  Standing alignment (anterior, posterior and lateral views)
  Shoe wear
  Swelling and/or effusion
  Skin color, texture, moisture, temperature, scars, calluses
  Assessment of gait

Range-of-motion tests

| TESTS | ACTIVE ROM | | PASSIVE ROM | | END FEEL |
|---|---|---|---|---|---|
| Dorsiflexion | P | M | P | M | |
| Plantar flexion | P | M | P | M | |
| Supination | P | M | P | M | |
| Pronation | P | M | P | M | |

| | | | |
|---|---|---|---|
| STJN | XXXXX | | XXXXX |
| Eversion positive | XXXXX | | |
| Inversion positive | XXXXX | | |
| FF to RF | XXXXX | | XXXXX |
| Tibial varum | XXXXX | | XXXXX |
| Tibial torsion | XXXXX | | XXXXX |
| First toe extension | XXXXX | | |
| Hip internal rotation | XXXXX | | |
| Hip external rotation | XXXXX | | |

P, pain; M, motion; STJN, subtalar joint neutral position; FF, forefoot; RF, rearfoot.

Other range-of-motion tests:

Accessory motion tests

Talocrural joint
    Anterior glide
    Posterior glide
First metatarsophalangeal joint
    Superior glide
    Inferior glide
Other accessory motion tests

Resistive tests

| | ISO | | CON | | REP CON | | ECC | | REP ECC | |
|---|---|---|---|---|---|---|---|---|---|---|
| **MUSCLE** | F | P | F | P | F | P | F | P | F | P |
| Gastrocnemius/soleus | | | | | | | | | | |
| Peroneals | | | | | | | | | | |
| Anterior tibialis | | | | | | | | | | |
| Posterior tibialis | | | | | | | | | | |
| Extensor hallucis longus | | | | | | | | | | |
| Extensor digitorum longus | | | | | | | | | | |
| Flexor hallucis longus | | | | | | | | | | |
| Flexor digitorum longus | | | | | | | | | | |

ISO, isometric; CON, concentric; REP CON, repetitive concentric; REP ECC, repetitive eccentric; F, force; P, pain.

Other muscles:

Special tests

Anterior drawer test
Thompson test
Homans' sign
Tinel's sign
Pulses
    Dorsalis Pedis
    Posterior Tibialis
Leg Lengths
Other:

Palpation tests:
Reassessment of goals:

### Working Hypotheses

### Treatment Strategy

### Treatment Tactics

who works on an assembly line and must push a lever with the foot repetitively should be observed while simulating this posture. Alignment of the joints of the lower limb should be observed from anterior, posterior, lateral, and inferior views. A patient's shoes should be examined for wear patterns that are abnormal or asymmetric. Involved areas of the patient's limb(s) are observed for evidence of effusion or swelling, skin color changes, scars, or calluses.

An important part of the examination of a patient with a foot or ankle problem is the gait assessment. See the chapter on gait for a description of the assessment of gait.

### Range-of-Motion Tests

ROM tests encompass a variety of tests that are frequently used by physical therapists. For the purposes of this chapter, tests that are designed to assess some aspect of joint movement are classified as ROM tests. Types of ROM tests that are used by therapists are active ROM (AROM) tests, passive ROM (PROM) tests, and accessory motion tests. When doing PROM tests and accessory motion tests, therapists frequently assess the end feel that is present. End feel is the type of resistance the examiner perceives to be present at the end of the ROM.

In this chapter, accessory motion is defined as movement between joint surfaces that is produced by forces applied by an examiner. Accessory motion tests are procedures used by the examiner to assess the movements between joint surfaces. Examples of accessory motion tests are glide, gap, traction, rotation, and compression tests. These are done in order to assess the arthrokinematics at the joint.

The three types of ROM tests, active, passive and accessory, are used for different reasons. AROM tests are used to make inferences about the patient's ability to move the limbs through an ROM. In other words, AROM tests are used to determine whether the patient is able to produce the muscle forces necessary to move the limb. However, patients may not be able to move their limbs through an ROM for reasons other than lack of muscle force production. The soft tissues crossing the joint may be abnormally shortened, or there may be a bone block.

Passive ROM tests are used to make inferences about whether the bone and soft tissues crossing the joint are of suitable length or configuration to allow motion to occur at the joint. If a limitation of PROM is identified, the ROM is noted and usually the type of end feel is also noted. End feels are classified as soft, firm, or hard. A soft end feel is a gradual increase in resistance perceived by the examiner at the end range. A firm end feel is an abrupt increase in resistance at the end range, and a hard end feel is an immediate stoppage to movement at the end range. PROM measurements can be useful, but they can also be misleading because they do not necessarily indicate why the patient's joint cannot move through the needed ROM. In other words, PROM or AROM measurements in isolation provide an incomplete picture of why the patient may have a functional problem. For example, a patient may report a chief complaint of inability to walk without a limp. During the examination the patient is found to have a decreased dorsiflexion PROM in addition to an even greater limitation in active dorsiflexion. These findings suggest that the patient has a problem with muscle force production in addition to shortened soft tissue structures. Measurements of the ability of the tissues to allow ROM (PROM measurements) and of the ability of muscles crossing the joint to produce the forces (AROM measurements) required to achieve a functional AROM are necessary. Both active and passive ROM measurements are necessary for therapists to make sound hypotheses about why patients have functional deficits.

Accessory motion tests are used to assess whether the amount of joint surface movement is adequate to allow a normal amount of physiologic ROM. They also indicate whether inflammatory processes may be present in tissues crossing the joint in question. A patient's report of an increase in pain during an accessory motion test may suggest that inflammation is one cause of the patient's complaints.

Studies have examined the usefulness of many of the different types of ROM tests. The reliability of PROM measurements of patients with disorders of the foot and ankle has been discussed.[83,84]

Elveru et al. examined the reliability of PROM measurements taken by a large group of therapists for patients with a variety of diagnoses.[83] All patients were considered by their therapists to require PROM measurements as part of the examination. A unique aspect of this study is that the therapists were trained in a newly proposed method for taking subtalar joint measurements. The therapists were selected because they reported seldom taking subtalar joint measurements during examinations. Data were collected after following a brief training period and are summarized in Table 9–8. The intratester reliability for most subtalar and ankle joint measurements was fairly good and suggests inexperi-

**Table 9–8.** SUMMARY OF THE RELIABILITY OF GONIOMETRIC MEASUREMENTS OF THE FOOT AND ANKLE OBTAINED IN CLINICAL SETTINGS

**Elveru et al[83] [a]**

| Joint | Motion | ICC[b] | n |
|---|---|---|---|
| | Intratester Reliability | | |
| Ankle | Dorsiflexion | .90 | 98 |
| | Plantar flexion | .86 | 98 |
| Subtalar | Subtalar neutral | .77 | 100 |
| | Inversion (unref.)[c] | .74 | 100 |
| | Eversion (unref.) | .75 | 100 |
| | Inversion (ref.)[d] | .62 | 100 |
| | Eversion (ref.) | .59 | 100 |
| | Intertester Reliability | | |
| Ankle | Dorsiflexion | .50 | 49 |
| | Plantar flexion | .72 | 49 |
| Subtalar | Subtalar neutral | .25 | 50 |
| | Inversion (unref.)[c] | .32 | 50 |
| | Eversion (unref.) | .17 | 50 |
| | Inversion (ref.)[d] | .15 | 50 |
| | Eversion (ref.) | .12 | 50 |

**Diamond et al.[84] [e]**

| Joint | Motion | ICC | SEM | n |
|---|---|---|---|---|
| | Intratester Reliability | | | |
| Ankle | Dorsiflexion (left) | .96 | 1 | 25 |
| | Dorsiflexion (right) | .89 | 3 | 25 |
| Subtalar | Inversion (left) | .96 | 2 | 25 |
| | Inversion (right) | .92 | 2 | 25 |
| | Eversion (left) | .96 | 1 | 25 |
| | Eversion (right) | .96 | 1 | 25 |
| | Neutral (left) | .96 | 1 | 25 |
| | Neutral (right) | .74 | 0 | 25 |
| Other | Forefoot to rear foot (left) | .93 | 1 | 25 |
| | Forefoot to rear foot (right) | .91 | 1 | 25 |
| | Tibial varum (left) | .84 | 1 | 25 |
| | Tibial varum (right) | .86 | 1 | 25 |
| | Intertester Reliability | | | |
| Ankle | Dorsiflexion (left) | .87 | 2 | 31 |
| | Dorsiflexion (right) | .74 | 3 | 31 |
| Subtalar | Inversion (left) | .89 | 3 | 31 |
| | Inversion (right) | .86 | 3 | 31 |
| | Eversion (left) | .78 | 4 | 31 |
| | Eversion (right) | .79 | 2 | 31 |
| | Neutral (left) | .79 | 2 | 31 |
| | Neutral (right) | .62 | 3 | 31 |
| Other | Forefoot to rear foot (left) | .58 | 3 | 31 |
| | Forefoot to rear foot (right) | .77 | 2 | 31 |
| | Tibial varum (left) | .66 | 1 | 31 |
| | Tibial varum (right) | .62 | 1 | 31 |

[a] In the study of Elveru et al., 14 therapists were randomly paired and took measurements of patients with a variety of diagnoses.
[b] ICC = Intraclass correlation coefficient.
[c] These measurements were not referenced to the subtalar joint neutral position.
[d] These measurements were referenced to the subtalar joint neutral position.
[e] In the study of Diamond et al., two therapists took measurements of patients with a diagnosis of diabetes.

enced therapists can replicate their measurements at an acceptable level. The intertester reliability for most measurements was poor, suggesting that inexperienced therapists should probably not base clinical decisions on these measurements.

Diamond et al. also examined the intratester and intertester reliability of some subtalar and ankle joint measurements.[84] Their study was different from the study of Elveru et al. in that they used two highly experienced therapists to take measurements on a group of patients with a diagnosis of diabetes. The patients in the study required foot and ankle PROM measurements as part of their diabetic foot evaluation. Diamond et al. found that the intratester and intertester reliability for the measurements was high. Experienced therapists appeared to do a much better job of replicating their measurements than therapists who had little experience in taking subtalar measurements. Based on the study of Diamond et al.,[84] clinics should standardize their methods of taking subtalar joint measurements. Therapists should also practice these measurements on many patients before using them to make clinical decisions.

Most of the conflict in the results of Elveru et al.[83] and Diamond et al.[84] could be explained by the fact that the therapists in the two studies had different amounts and types of training before participating in the study. Therapists in the Elveru et al. study had little training in using a standardized procedure to take subtalar measurements. They had much past experience in taking ankle measurements, but the procedures used to take these measurements were not standardized. The therapists in the Diamond et al. study had much experience in using standardized procedures to take all measurements. The differences in the amount of training of the therapists in the two studies, therefore, are probably related only to the subtalar measurements. The therapists in the two studies probably had approximately equal amounts of experience in taking ankle measurements.

The study by Elveru et al.[83] suggests that measurements of dorsiflexion by different testers are not reliable. The study by Diamond et al.[84] suggests that these measurements are reliable. Although the therapists in both studies were experienced in taking ankle measurements, those in the Diamond et al. study used a standardized measurement procedure. Based on these studies, ankle measurement procedures should also be standardized in clinics to ensure the highest possible level of reliability.

Many different accessory motion tests have been described for most major joints of the foot and ankle.[79,85] This chapter does not attempt to review all of these tests. However, the more commonly used tests are described briefly.

All accessory motion tests should be done by examining the uninvolved side first. The amount of motion present on the uninvolved side should be assessed first, and then the involved side should be classified as hypomobile, normal, or hypermobile compared to the uninvolved side. Similarly, the interpretation of the type of end feel present on the involved side should be based on a comparison with the uninvolved side. The end feel is classified in the same way as end feel measurements are classified during PROM tests, as either soft, firm, or hard.

The accessory motion of the talocrural joint is probably assessed more frequently than that of other foot or ankle joints. The two most common tests for the talocrural joint are anterior glide and posterior glide. Anterior glide of the talocrural joint is defined as anterior translation of the talus within the mortise. Posterior glide is defined as posterior translation of the talus within the mortise. Talocrural joint anterior glide should be assessed with the knee in approximately 30 degrees of flexion to place the gastrocnemius in a slackened position. If the test is done while the gastrocnemius is in a taut position, the amount of anterior translation of the talus may be affected. The talocrural joint on the uninvolved side is assessed first.

To assess anterior glide, the examiner places one hand on the distal tibia to stabilize the tibia during the test. The examiner's other hand is placed around the area of the patient's talus and calcaneus. The examiner applies an anterior force to the patient's talus and calcaneus and assesses the amount of anterior talar translation within the ankle mortise and the end feel.

Posterior glide is assessed in a similar fashion except that the hand that grasps the talus and calcaneus applies the force posteriorly during the test. The amount of motion and the end feel are then determined.

Accessory motion of the first metatarsophalangeal joint is also frequently assessed. The two tests most commonly used are superior (dorsal) and inferior (ventral) glide. Superior glide of the metatarsophalangeal joint is assessed by grasping the distal aspect of the first metatarsal with one hand and the proximal phalanx with the other hand. The proximal phalanx is moved superiorly relative to the first metatarsal and the amount of motion and end feel are classified. The same hand positions are used to assess inferior glide.

The proximal phalanx is moved inferiorly relative to the first metatarsal and the amount of motion and end feel are classified.

### Resistive Tests

Resistive tests of the foot and ankle are done primarily for two reasons. The most common reason for resistive testing is to assess the muscle force production capability of a muscle or a group of muscles. The second reason for resistive testing at the foot or ankle is to determine whether inflammatory processes are present in the belly or tendon of the tested muscle. For example, therapists commonly infer that Achilles tendinitis is present when resisted plantar flexion reproduces a patient's posterior heel pain.

Many methods have been advocated in the literature for assessing the force production capability of muscles crossing the ankle and subtalar joints. The force produced is most commonly assessed using the manual muscle test. Muscles can be tested manually in an isometric, concentric, or eccentric mode. Studies have been done to examine the reliability of manual muscle test assessments. Some have suggested that manual muscle tests above the grade of fair are unreliable.[86] Few studies have examined the reliability of manual muscle test assessments of the foot and ankle of patients.

Perry and colleagues examined the validity of manual muscle tests of the leg for inferring the amount of muscle activity required for ambulation in normal subjects.[87] An issue of concern for therapists is whether manual muscle test results can be used to predict functional ability, and Perry and colleagues hoped to address this issue. However, they used normal subjects and had the subjects simulate poor, fair, and normal muscle contraction while needle electromyographic (EMG) recordings were taken from each of the major leg muscles. They then had the subjects walk at a slow, normal, and fast walking pace while EMG recordings of most of the calf muscles were taken. The authors concluded that walking at a slow pace required poor leg muscle strength, walking at a normal pace required fair muscle strength, and walking at a fast pace required fair to normal strength.

Many limitations can be found in the study of Perry et al.[87] One important issue is whether simulated poor, fair, and normal contractions of normal subjects can be used to mimic muscle tests of patients. Many factors that can affect the results of muscle tests of patients (e.g., pain) do not affect those of normal subjects. Although the authors considered both the amplitude and frequency of EMG recordings in their calculations, EMG data provide no information regarding muscle length–associated changes in tension. In addition, muscle force production is not the only factor that determines a patient's ability to walk. Balance responses, muscle contraction timing, and psychologic factors also play a role. Therefore, it is questionable whether EMG data alone can be used as a valid dependent measure of how closely manual muscle test results are related to contractions during gait in normal subjects. In addition, the authors provided no data to support the reliability of many of their measures. Their study, therefore, appears to have questionable clinical usefulness.

Another issue of importance in muscle testing of patients with foot or ankle problems is whether motorized dynamometers should be used to measure forces produced during dynamic contractions. Rothstein and colleagues argue that the instantaneous center of motion of the ankle moves a relatively large amount during movement.[88] The ankle axis is no longer congruous with the axis of the machine. The measurement error that results from this misalignment of the machine and joint axes negates the usefulness of these measurements. The data of Sammarco et al.[55] and Lundberg et al.[57] support the contention that significant movement of the ankle joint axis occurs in patients during movement. Data of Lundberg et al.[49] suggest that the subtalar and other tarsal joint axes also move during joint movements. Based on the literature, it appears that therapists should take isometric measurements when they are interested in quantifying foot or ankle muscle performance. Dynamic measurements are probably invalid because the force measurements obtained do not represent muscularly generated forces.

### Special Tests

Special tests are those designed to allow the therapist to make a specific inference about a structure or disease. The special tests most commonly done on the foot and ankle are the anterior drawer test, the Thompson test, Homans' sign, Tinel's sign, the assessment of pulses, and measurements of leg length inequality.

**Anterior Drawer Test.** The anterior drawer test is a test of the integrity of the lateral ankle ligaments (Fig. 9–19). More specifically, it is designed to assess the integrity of the anterior talofibular ligament. The examiner stabilizes the pa-

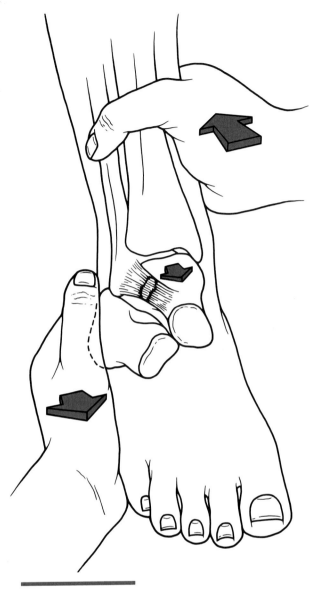

**FIGURE 9–19** ■ Anterior drawer test for injury to the lateral collateral ligaments of the ankle.

ankles and those subjected to sequential resection of the anterior talofibular ligament, the calcaneofibular ligament, and the posterior calcaneofibular ligament.[89] Measurements were taken with the ankles in neutral, plantar flexed, and dorsiflexed positions. The authors applied an anterior force simulating that in an anterior drawer test, an inversion force simulating a talar tilt, and an internal rotation force simulating that in an anterolateral drawer test. In the anterolateral drawer test an attempt is made to move the lateral aspect of the talus anteriorly. The resultant movement is internal rotation of the talus within the mortise. The authors found that the increased motion present when the ligaments were resected was most pronounced during the anterolateral drawer test in the plantar flexed position. The increased motion was less consistent during the anterior drawer test. This study suggests that if the examiner is attempting to assess the integrity of the lateral ankle ligaments, an anterolateral drawer test should be done in the plantar flexed position.

**Anterolateral Drawer Test.** The anterolateral drawer test should be done in the following way. The subject is sitting. The examiner stabilizes the distal tibia with the hand on the medial side of the limb to be tested. The examiner's other hand grasps the lateral and posterior aspect of the patient's calcaneus. The ankle joint is then positioned in slight plantar flexion. The force is applied to the posterior calcaneus so as to produce anterior translation and medial rotation of the talus. The examiner should perform the test first on the patient's uninvolved side to assess the amount of motion and the end feel. The involved side is judged to have a positive anterolateral drawer test when the motion on that side is greater or the end feel is softer than that of the uninvolved side. A positive test may also be obtained when the patient's pain is reported to be reproduced during the test.

**Thompson's Test.** The Thompson test was designed to determine whether the patient's Achilles tendon is ruptured. Thompson and Doherty originally described this test after observing that squeezing the calf of a patient with a ruptured Achilles tendon did not produce a plantar flexion motion.[91] They also reported that the test was positive in 100% of patients who had a surgically confirmed Achilles tendon rupture. They did not report the incidence of false-positive or false-negative test results.

The patient is positioned lying prone while the examiner squeezes the middle third of the pa-

tient's tibia with one hand and applies forces to move the talus anteriorly within the mortise. If the lateral ankle ligaments are torn, the lateral aspect of the dome of the talus translates farther anteriorly than the medial talar dome. The medial talar dome does not translate an excessive amount because it is stabilized by the deltoid ligament. Therefore, when assessing the integrity of the anterior talofibular ligament the examiner is actually assessing for the presence of an anterolateral rotational instability of the ankle.[89,90]

Rasmussen and Tovborg-Jensen measured the amount of motion present in intact cadaveric

tient's posterior leg. The test is positive if the foot does not plantar flex passively when the calf is squeezed (Fig. 9–20).

**Homans' Sign.** Homans' sign was designed to determine whether a deep vein thrombophlebitis is present. The examiner passively dorsiflexes the patient's foot while the knee is extended. The test is positive if the patient reports pain in the posterior leg during the test.

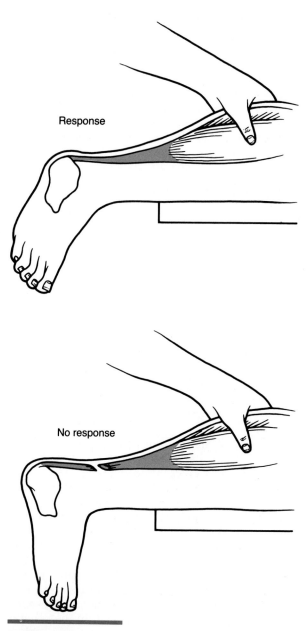

Response

No response

**FIGURE 9–20 ■** The Thompson test for the integrity of the Achilles tendon.

**Tinel's Sign.** Tinel's sign for the foot was designed to determine whether tarsal tunnel syndrome, a nerve compression syndrome, is present. The examiner uses his or her fingers to tap the area of the flexor retinaculum posterior and inferior to the medial malleolus. The test is positive when the patient reports pain or paresthesias either locally or in the distribution of the medial or lateral plantar nerves during the test. These symptoms must be similar in quality and distribution to the pain reported by the patient.

**Assessment of Pulses.** A patient's pulses are typically assessed when the examiner thinks the patient's circulatory system may be affected by disease or iatrogenic causes. Two arteries in the foot are most commonly palpated. The dorsalis pedis artery, a distal branch of the anterior tibial artery is palpated just lateral to the extensor hallucis longus tendon at the level of the tarsals. The posterior tibial artery is palpated posterior to the medial malleolus.

**Measurements of Leg Lengths.** A patient's leg lengths are frequently measured and compared for a variety of reasons. Authors differ in what they consider a clinically significant leg length difference (LLD). For example, Subotnik[92] argues that an LLD as small as 3 mm can cause injury to runners, whereas Anderson believes that an LLD of as much as 19 mm does not require treatment.[92a] Most experts seem to agree that differences in leg length may contribute to a patient's symptoms.

Many methods have been reported in the literature for assessing whether a patient has an LLD. However, many of these methods have not been examined for reliability or validity or have inherent methodologic flaws. Beattie et al. proposed a method for determining the difference in a patient's leg lengths and assessed its reliability and validity.[93]

The following procedure was used to obtain measurements. The patient is positioned supine in the anatomic position and the examiner identifies the inferior portion of the anterior superior iliac spine and the medial malleolus where it slopes inferiorly and laterally. The tape measure is then placed on these two landmarks and the distance is measured. The same procedure is followed for the opposite limb and a difference is calculated. Using this method, Beattie et al. found that the mean of two repeated measurements of the LLD was most reliable and most closely approximated the LLD obtained from radiographs.[93] The intraclass correlation coefficient of Shrout and Fleiss[94] for reliability of the mean of two LLD measurements was .91 and for the comparison of LLD measurements to those obtained from radiographs was .85. Beattie et al. used only one examiner to obtain measurements of LLD.[93] However, these data suggest that the method described by Beattie et al. can be used to obtain highly reliable measurements of LLD that also closely agree with a patient's actual difference in leg length.

### Palpation Tests

Palpation tests are usually done to make inferences about the presence of inflammatory processes. The theoretic basis for these inferences is that when forces are applied to inflamed tissues (via palpation) the patient responds by reporting pain during palpation. When attempting to reproduce a patient's pain during palpation, the examiner should ask the patient, in an unbiased way, about the quality and location of the pain reported. The pain reported by the patient during palpation should be similar in location and quality to the pain associated with the patient's chief complaint.

The therapist should describe in the patient's chart the anatomic location of the area reported by the patient to be painful during palpation. Clear documentation of the anatomic areas of tenderness to palpation can assist therapists who subsequently treat the patient in identifying these areas of tenderness. Palpation tests are typically done at the end of the examination because they tend to exacerbate some patient's symptoms. If the patient's symptoms are exacerbated early in the examination, completion of the examination may be difficult.

### Hypothesis-Oriented Algorithm for Clinicians

The HOAC is a useful and powerful tool for physical therapists. In this author's opinion, no other model for clinical problem solving is as good in describing the steps required to (1) hypothesize why the patient has the functional problems and (2) determine a scientifically based plan of treatment.

Some evaluation approaches are intrinsically linked to a specific type of treatment. For example, Cyriax would claim that if a patient had pain with resisted isometric ankle plantar flexion, pain with passive dorsiflexion, and no pain with passive plantar flexion, a contractile lesion of the gastrocnemius-soleus tendon is present.[80] The

treatment would then be deep friction massage to the tendon. The documentation problems that may result from this form of decision making are significant. For example, therapists not trained in use of the Cyriax approach may not understand the basis for the treatment that was described for this patient.[80] In addition, therapists trained in methods that emphasize joint mobility and manual therapy may find much information lacking in the example just described. The information provided by someone who is Cyriax[80] trained may not be interpretable by someone who is Maitland[79] trained, for example.

The second documentation problem is that some of these evaluation and treatment approaches may have inherent assumptions about causality, the appropriateness of which cannot be tested. For example, a therapist may assume that a patient who complains of posterior heel pain and has a forefoot varus developed the symptoms because of the forefoot deformity. The HOAC places the responsibility on the therapist to define goals, generate hypotheses about the patient's functional problems, and subsequently test the appropriateness of these hypotheses. The HOAC also places the responsibility on the therapist to define operationally terms used during documentation so that all therapists in the clinic understand their meaning.

The HOAC consists of two parts. The first part is a step-by-step guide to examination and treatment planning (Fig. 9–21). The second part is a step-by-step guide to help determine why goals are not being met if that is the case (Fig. 9–22).

Part One of the HOAC guides the therapist during the examination. Immediately before the examination, the therapist collects the initial data from the patient, the patient's family, and chart reviews. All of these data are collected in the context of the patient's reason(s) for seeing the therapist.

The second step requires the therapist to generate problem statements that are used in the development of goals. Problems are listed in the problem-oriented format and stated in terms of the patient's reason(s) for seeking help. Patients usually seek a physical therapist's help because of some type of functional loss. Problems that are anticipated by the therapist are also identified.

After the problem statements, the next step is to identify goals for the patient. This step should be easy if the problem statements are appropriate. The goals should be stated in behavioral terms that are measurable and functional with a temporal component. The reasons for making

## HYPOTHESIS-ORIENTED ALGORITHM FOR CLINICIANS

### PART ONE

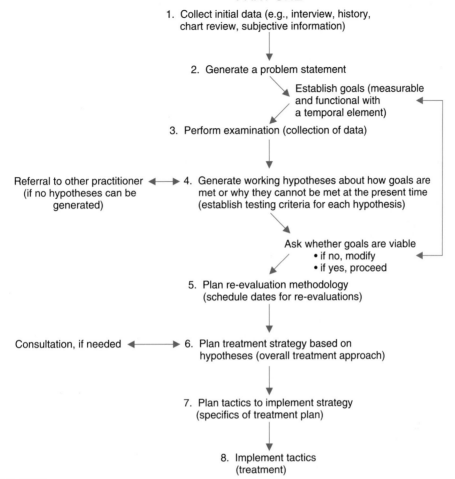

**FIGURE 9-21** ■ Part One of the hypothesis-oriented algorithm for clinicians. (From Rothstein JM, Echternach JL: Hypothesis oriented algorithm for clinicians: a method of evaluation and treatment planning. Phys Ther 66:1388–1394, 1986. Reprinted from PHYSICAL THERAPY with the permission of the American Physical Therapy Association.)

problem statements and setting goals before examining the patient are the following:

1. The therapist is more likely to state problems and goals that are consistent with the patient's reports.

2. The patient and therapist are more likely to communicate more effectively.

3. The therapist can evaluate and treat the patient more effectively if he or she fully understands the patient's expectations.

The temporal element of the goals can be used by the therapist to collect data related to the effectiveness of a type of treatment. To make the temporal element of the goal more realistic, it is set after the patient is examined.

After the goals have been established, the examination is done. The extent and vigor of the examination are determined by the data collected up to this point.

Based on all the data collected during the history and examination, the therapist makes hypotheses about the causes of the patient's problems. A hypothesis is really a clinical impression of the underlying cause of the problem and is based on an assumption of causality. That is, the hypothesis is a testable idea about why the patient has the particular functional problems.

More than one hypothesis can be generated for a patient. The hypotheses provide the rationale for all treatment that follows. Therefore, the therapist must justify all treatment that follows.

## HYPOTHESIS-ORIENTED ALGORITHM FOR CLINICIANS
### PART TWO

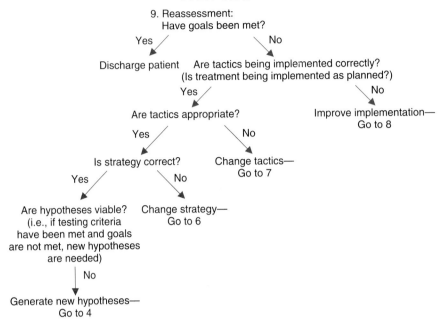

9. Reassessment:
Have goals been met?

Yes / — Discharge patient

No \ — Are tactics being implemented correctly?
(Is treatment being implemented as planned?)

Yes / — Are tactics appropriate?

No \ — Improve implementation—
Go to 8

Yes / — Is strategy correct?

No \ — Change tactics—
Go to 7

Yes / — Are hypotheses viable?
(i.e., if testing criteria
have been met and goals
are not met, new hypotheses
are needed)

No \ — Change strategy—
Go to 6

No ↓

Generate new hypotheses—
Go to 4

**FIGURE 9–22** ■ Part Two of the hypothesis-oriented algorithm for clinicians. (From Rothstein JM, Echternach JL: Hypothesis oriented algorithm for clinicians: a method of evaluation and treatment planning. Phys Ther 66:1388–1394, 1986. Reprinted from PHYSICAL THERAPY with the permission of the American Physical Therapy Association.)

What happens when a therapist cannot generate a hypothesis for a patient? Referral is the appropriate action.

For each hypothesis, the therapist must establish at least one testing criterion to determine whether the hypothesis was correct. Therefore, the testing criteria must be measurable and operationally defined.

Next, the therapist must plan re-evaluation methodology to determine whether the patient has met the goals. Ideally, a schedule should be determined for when the patient will be re-evaluated. The overall treatment strategy and specific treatment tactics are then determined.

### Part II Branching Program

The branching program simply provides a re-checking system for the therapist if the patient has not achieved the goals (see Fig. 9–22).

## Invasive Diagnostic Tests

Some of the more common radiographic views of the foot and ankle are illustrated in Figures 9–23 to 9–25. Therapists may find these helpful when viewing the foot and ankle radiographs of their patients.

## DIFFERENTIAL DIAGNOSIS

This section describes the more common disorders that affect the foot and ankle. It is organized according to the type of tissue that is primarily affected by the disorder.

### Disorders That Affect the Bones

#### The Salter System for Classifying Fractures

Salter has described a system for classifying fractures that is systematic, thorough, and relatively simple.[95] According to Salter, to describe a fracture completely you must determine the site, extent, and configuration of the fracture. In addition, you must determine the relationship of the fracture fragments to each other, the rela-

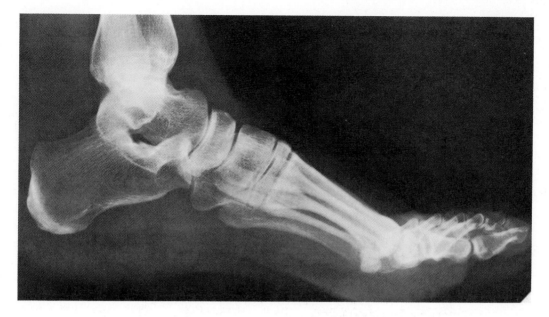

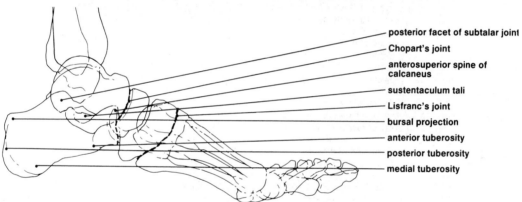

posterior facet of subtalar joint
Chopart's joint
anterosuperior spine of calcaneus
sustentaculum tali
Lisfranc's joint
bursal projection
anterior tuberosity
posterior tuberosity
medial tuberosity

FIGURE 9-23 ■ Lateral radiograph of a normal foot and ankle. (From Greenspan A: Orthopedic Radiology: A Practical Approach. Philadelphia: JB Lippincott, 1988, Fig. 7–14B.)

tionship of the fracture fragments to the external environment, and the presence or absence of complications.

The following six criteria are used to classify a fracture:

**Site.** A fracture may be diaphyseal, metaphyseal, epiphyseal, or intra-articular. If a dislocation occurs in conjunction with the fracture, it is a fracture-dislocation.

**Extent.** Fractures can be either complete or incomplete. Types of incomplete fractures are crack, hairline, buckle, and greenstick fractures.

**Configuration.** Complete fractures can have a transverse, oblique, or spiral arrangement. When more than two fragments result from the fracture it is described as a comminuted fracture.

**Relationship of fracture fragments to each other.** The fragments resulting from a fracture can either be displaced or nondisplaced. Displaced fragments may be shifted sideways, angulated, rotated, distracted, overriding, and/or impacted.

**Relationship of fracture fragments to the external environment.** Fractures can be closed or open. A closed fracture is one in which the overlying skin is intact. An open fracture is one in which the skin in the area

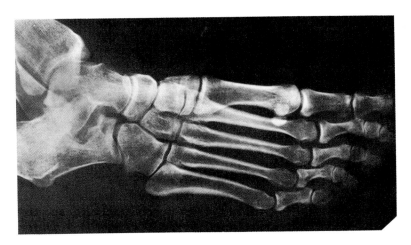

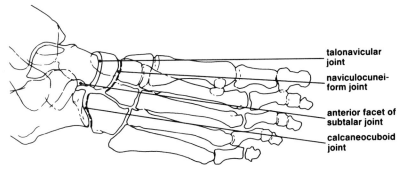

talonavicular
joint

naviculocunei-
form joint

anterior facet of
subtalar joint

calcaneocuboid
joint

**FIGURE 9-24** ■ Oblique radiograph of a normal foot and ankle. (From Greenspan A: Orthopedic Radiology: A Practical Approach. Philadelphia: JB Lippincott, 1988, Fig. 7-15.)

of the fracture is not intact. The fracture fragment may have penetrated the skin, or an object may have penetrated the skin to cause the fracture. Closed fractures have been referred to as simple fractures and open fractures as compound fractures.

**Complications.** A fracture can be complicated or uncomplicated. A complicated fracture is one in which a local or systemic complication results from either the fracture itself or its treatment. An uncomplicated fracture is one that does not immediately result in a local or systemic complication and heals uneventfully.

### Fractures of the Ankle

Ankle fractures are common and result from forces applied directly to the ankle or, more commonly, forces applied indirectly through the foot. Many classification systems exist for frac-

tures resulting from indirect forces. According to Pankovich,[96] the Lauge-Hansen[97] system is one of the more common classification systems used.

**Lauge-Hansen Classification System.** The Lauge-Hansen classification system is based on studies done using cadavers.[97] In these studies, the feet of cadavers were moved into various positions until a fracture occurred. Fractures were classified on the basis of the position of the foot at the time of the fracture. The system utilizes terms to describe these positions. Supination was defined as the combined movement of internal rotation of the foot, adduction of the rear foot, and inversion (internal rotation about an AP axis) of the forefoot. Pronation was defined as the combined movement of external rotation of the foot, abduction of the rear foot, and eversion (external rotation) of the forefoot. The seven types of fractures in this classification system are as follows.

**Supination-adduction fracture.** A transverse

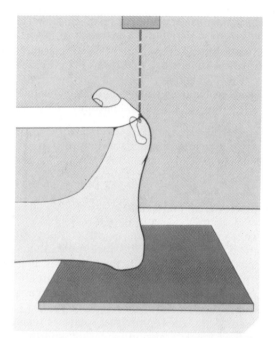

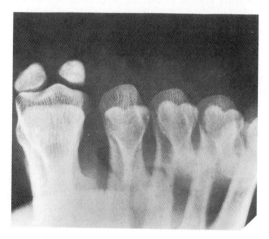

**FIGURE 9–25** ■ Tangential view of the sesamoid bones of the first metatarsal. (From Greenspan A: Orthopedic Radiology: A Practical Approach. Philadelphia: JB Lippincott, 1988, Fig. 7–18A.)

fracture of the fibula below the syndesmosis, followed by a fracture of the medial malleolus. Avulsion of the deltoid ligament or rupture of the lateral collateral ligaments may be seen.

**Pronation-abduction fracture.** Avulsion of the medial malleolus or rupture of the deltoid ligament followed by avulsions of the anterior and/or posterior tibiofibular ligaments. A supramalleolar fracture of the fibula may also occur.

**Supination-eversion fracture.** A spiral or oblique fracture of the fibula at the level of the syndesmosis, always followed by a rupture or avulsion of the anterior talofibular ligament. The posterior tibiofibular ligament may rupture or avulse. The deltoid ligament may also rupture. Finally, the medial malleolus may fracture.

**Pronation-eversion fracture.** A fibular fracture above the syndesmosis, always followed by rupture of the deltoid ligament or fracture of the medial malleolus and damage to the tibiofibular ligaments.

**Supination-inversion fracture.** Rupture of the anterior talofibular ligament followed by avulsion of the calcaneocuboid ligaments.

**Pronation-inversion fracture.** Fractures of the tibia and fibula.

**Pronation-dorsiflexion fracture.** Compression fractures of the tibial plafond.

Fractures of the ankle can also be classified according to the anatomic structure that is fractured (Fig. 9–26).

## Epiphyseal Fractures

The epiphyseal plate is structurally weaker than bone. However, because only shear and tensile forces can separate the epiphysis, epiphyseal plate separations are less common in children than fractures of bone. Compressive forces probably produce fractures more commonly.

Trauma to the epiphyseal plate is classified into four types: avulsion, shearing, splitting, and crushing. The classification system most commonly used to describe epiphyseal plate fractures is the Salter-Harris[98] classification (Fig. 9–27).

### Salter-Harris Classification

The Salter-Harris classification is as follows.

**Type I.** The epiphysis completely separates from the metaphysis. The bone does not fracture. These epiphyseal fractures are most commonly seen in newborns and very young children. Closed reduction is usually routine and prognosis is typically excellent provided the blood supply is intact.

**Type II.** The fracture line extends along the epiphyseal plate and then through the metaphysis to produce a triangular fragment of bone. This is the most common type of epiphyseal plate fracture and results from a combination of shearing and bending forces. Type II injuries are more commonly seen in the older child. Closed reduction is usually the treatment of choice and the prognosis is excellent assuming the vascularity of the plate is intact.

**Type III.** The fracture line extends from the joint surface to the epiphyseal plate and then continues to the outer edge of the bone. These are intra-articular fractures. They are uncommon but are sometimes seen in the distal tibia. Open reduction of the fracture fragment is usually required. The prognosis is usually good if the blood supply to the

displaced fragment has not been compromised.

**Type IV.** The fracture line extends from the joint surface through the entire epiphyseal plate and through a portion of the metaphysis. These fractures require open reduction unless they are nondisplaced. Perfect reduction is necessary to ensure symmetric bone growth.

**Type V.** These fractures are uncommon and result from a large compressive force applied to the joint. They are seen most commonly in the ankle and knee. Prognosis for bone growth is usually poor.

Many complications can occur as a result of an epiphyseal plate fracture. The most common complications are limb length discrepancy, partial growth arrest, varus angulation, and valgus angulation.[99]

Because the distal tibial epiphysis contributes to 43% of tibial length, the age of the child at the time of injury determines the extent of the leg length discrepancy that may result. Type III and type IV fractures most commonly result in limb length discrepancies. The discrepancies can be avoided in some cases by accurate open reduction.[100]

After an epiphyseal fracture, a bony bridge may extend across the epiphysis and inhibit normal growth. The location of the bridge determines the type of growth disturbance that is seen. Most bony bridges result in an angulation deformity.

The varus deformity that occurs as a result of an epiphyseal plate fracture affects the medial side of the distal tibia. Type III and type IV fractures that are not adequately reduced can produce a varus angulation.

The valgus deformity occurs as a result of an epiphyseal fracture of the lateral aspect of the ankle. If the fracture is not adequately reduced, fibular shortening occurs, resulting in a valgus angulation.

### Common Fractures of the Foot

Fractures of the foot are typically described as being in one of three areas; the hindfoot, the midfoot, and the forefoot. Fractures of the calcaneus and/or talus are considered to be hindfoot fractures. Midfoot fractures are confined to the navicular and cuboid. Forefoot fractures occur in the metatarsals, phalanges, or sesamoids.

**Hindfoot Fractures.** Fractures of the calcaneus are classified as extra-articular or intra-articu-

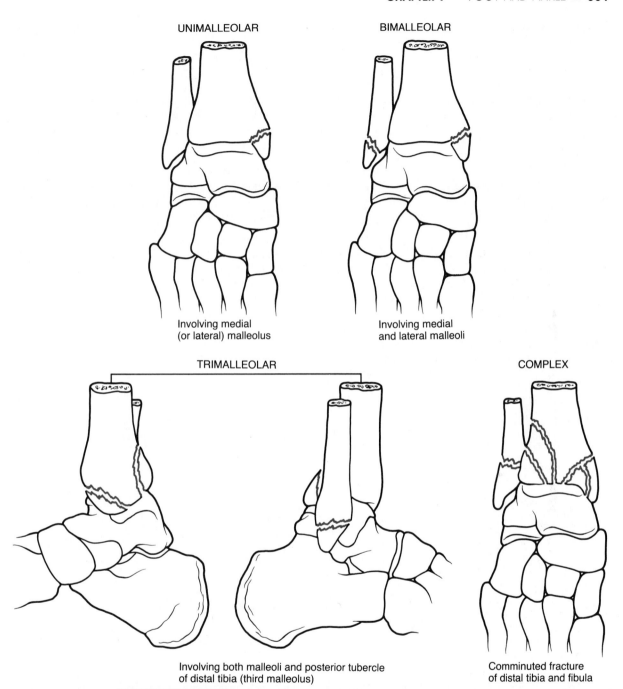

UNIMALLEOLAR

Involving medial
(or lateral) malleolus

BIMALLEOLAR

Involving medial
and lateral malleoli

TRIMALLEOLAR

Involving both malleoli and posterior tubercle
of distal tibia (third malleolus)

COMPLEX

Comminuted fracture
of distal tibia and fibula

**FIGURE 9-26** ■ Ankle fractures classified according to the location of the fracture.

lar.[101] Common extra-articular fractures are the anterior process fracture, the posterosuperior tuberosity fracture, and the fracture of the body of the calcaneus. An anterior process fracture can occur when the foot is forcefully plantar flexed and inverted. The attachments of the bifurcate and interosseous ligaments avulse from the calcaneus, producing the fracture. Anterior process fractures are often diagnosed initially as lateral ankle sprains. Posterosuperior tuberosity fractures most commonly result from an avulsion of the triceps surae tendon from the calcaneus.

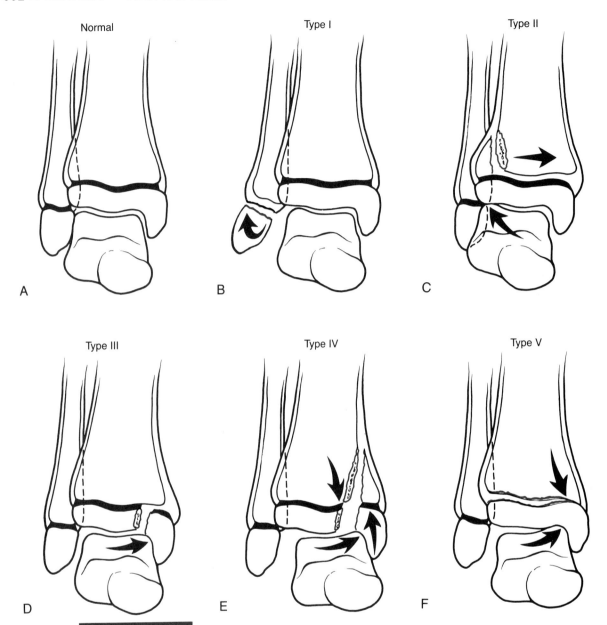

**FIGURE 9–27** ■ The Salter-Harris classification of epiphyseal plate fractures as applied to the ankle.

Fractures of the body of the calcaneus most commonly result from a large compressive force applied to the calcaneus; common mechanisms of injury are falls from ladders or roofs.

Intra-articular fractures occur in a large variety of configurations and are therefore difficult to classify for the purposes of treatment. According to Sanders et al.[101] intra-articular fractures are treated nonoperatively when (1) the fractures are nondisplaced, (2) the fractures are open, (3) early intervention is precluded, (4) soft tissue compro-mise prevents surgery, and (5) severe disease is present.

Fractures of the talus usually occur because of very large forces applied to the foot. Because 70% of the surface of the talus is covered by articular cartilage, most talar fractures are con-sidered intra-articular. In addition, the vascula-ture of the talus is tenuous and there are no muscular insertions into the talus. The talus is therefore predisposed to developing avascular necrosis after a fracture.

Fractures of the talus are classified on the basis of anatomic location and amount of displacement of the fragments and surrounding structures.[102] Talar neck fractures are classified as type I through type IV depending on the displacement of fragments and whether the subtalar joint is dislocated. Talar body fractures typically occur in the coronal and/or sagittal plane. Fractures of the lateral facet of the talus occur because of a forced dorsiflexion and external rotation of the foot. Fractures of the head of the talus are thought to be rare; when they occur, they tend to be comminuted.

Transchondral fractures of the talus are fairly common and result from forces transmitted to the articular surface and underlying subchondral bone of the talus from the adjacent joint surface. A localized area of avascular necrosis of the bone develops, followed by either repair or nonunion and separation of the fragment. The lesion is reported to occur posteromedially 57% of the time and anterolaterally 43% of the time.[103] The posteromedial lesion is thought to be caused by excessive inversion and plantar flexion and the anterolateral lesion by excessive inversion and dorsiflexion. Patients with transchondral fractures frequently report "twisting" the ankle. Transchondral fractures must be considered when examining patients with diagnoses of ankle sprains. Most experts believe transchondral fractures are due to trauma, but some cases may be attributable to atraumatic causes.[17]

Osteochondritis dissecans of the talus and transchondral fracture are separate diagnostic entities. Patients with osteochondritis dissecans typically present with bilateral lesions on their medial tali. These lesions are typically self-limiting and usually heal uneventfully.[102]

**Fractures of the Midfoot.** Isolated fractures of the midfoot are uncommon. When it occurs, the fracture is usually an avulsion of the navicular tuberosity. Treatment typically consists of cast immobilization in the supinated position for several weeks, followed by surgical repair if the immobilization is unsuccessful.[104]

**Fractures of the Forefoot.** Fractures of the forefoot can be classified as displaced or nondisplaced. Nondisplaced fractures of the second through fifth metatarsals are typically treated with tape immobilization and weight bearing as tolerated. Nondisplaced fractures of the first metatarsal are typically treated with non-weight-bearing cast immobilization for 2 weeks, followed by progressive weight bearing.[105] Displaced fractures of the metatarsals must be accurately reduced to restore normal function. Otherwise, weight-bearing forces are abnormally distributed and usually lead to altered function.[105]

Nondisplaced fractures of the fifth metatarsal are divided into those that occur at the base, the middle diaphysis, or the distal diaphysis. Fractures of the middle and distal diaphysis are treated with tape immobilization and weight bearing as tolerated. A fracture of the base of the fifth metatarsal can be either an avulsion fracture of the tuberosity or a Jones fracture.[106] Avulsion fractures are treated with simple tape immobilization and weight bearing as tolerated. Jones' fractures are located in the proximal diaphysis of the fifth metatarsal and are associated with a high incidence of delayed union and nonunion.[107]

Fractures of the phalanges are reported to be common and are most frequently caused by objects being dropped on the toes.[105] Most phalangeal fractures are treated with protected weight bearing as needed.

## Stress Fractures

Stress fractures are the result of forces that do not cause damage when applied only a few times but result in fracture when applied over many repetitions. The increased incidence of stress fractures is closely tied to the increased participation of typically sedentary people in athletic activities.[108,109] An increase in the amount of athletic activity also appears to be related to the development of stress fractures.[105]

Stress fractures are most commonly seen in the lower extremities. Much survey research has been done to determine the locations of stress fractures in large numbers of subjects. For example, Orava et al. described the characteristics of 142 patients with radiographically diagnosed stress fractures.[110] The patients participated in a variety of athletic activities. The most common location for stress fractures was the tibia. Fractures of the metatarsals were second most common.

Myerson reports that metatarsal stress fractures occur in predictable sites.[105] Stress fractures in the first metatarsal occur along its medial base. The second and third metatarsals tend to fracture along the distal diaphysis. Fourth metatarsal stress fractures tend to occur near the middle or distal diaphysis. Fifth metatarsal stress fractures tend to occur proximally near the juncture of the diaphysis and metaphysis. Knowing the most likely location for metatarsal stress fractures can be useful when examining patients with complaints of pain in the forefoot. Complaints of forefoot pain and tenderness to palpation in these areas may indicate a stress fracture.

The incidence of stress fractures of the great toe sesamoids is apparently low in sedentary populations.[110] However, athletically active patients with complaints of pain around the great toe are seen fairly commonly by some physical therapists. Stress fractures of the sesamoids are difficult to diagnose because of the frequent incidence of multipartite sesamoids. Reports in the literature suggest that approximately 10% of the population have one or more multipartite sesamoid bones in the foot.[111] The tibial (medial) sesamoid is more often found to be multipartite than the fibular (lateral) sesamoid.[112] The tibial sesamoid is also reported to be more commonly injured than the fibular sesamoid.[113,114]

Radiographic testing is required to substantiate the presence of a stress fracture. It takes up to 2 months for a stress fracture to become radiographically observable.[105] Scintigraphy (bone scanning) can be used to diagnose stress fractures before they can be identified radiographically.

Most stress fractures of the foot and ankle are nondisplaced and heal uneventfully. The treatment is usually restricted activity for 4 to 12 weeks.[105,115] Fifth metatarsal stress fractures are predisposed to delayed union or nonunion if treated incorrectly.[105] Myerson believes that stress fractures of the fifth metatarsal should be treated by immobilizing the involved foot in a non-weight-bearing cast for 6 to 8 weeks.[105] If shortened healing time is needed to allow a quick return to activity, internal fixation is the treatment of choice.

## Common Foot Deformities

*Stedman's Medical Dictionary*[116] defines deformity as "a deviation from the normal shape or size, resulting in disfigurement; may be congenital or acquired." Implicit in this definition is the assumption that we can define normal. Because normal alignment has not been clearly defined for the foot, this definition is appropriately vague. This section describes many deformities such as equinus foot that have not been typically thought of as deformities. All deformities described in this chapter have been described in the literature as "deviations from normal" that affect function.

Many deformities of the foot have been described. This chapter summarizes only the more commonly seen deformities. The references at the end of the chapter include many sources that describe thoroughly the many foot deformities not reviewed here. The classic deformities of clubfoot, pes planus, and pes cavus are described in this section. The podiatric literature has added descriptions of deformities that have only recently appeared in the physical therapy literature. These are rear foot varus, forefoot varus, forefoot valgus, and equinus foot. The operational definitions of these deformities are summarized.

Determining that a patient may have a rear foot varus, a forefoot varus, or a forefoot valgus is, at times, difficult (see examination section). The clinical presentation of a patient thought to have one or more of these deformities can also be confusing. An article by Tiberio thoroughly describes how patients with these deformities might appear clinically.[117]

### Pes Cavus

Pes cavus is a term used to describe the foot with an abnormally high arch (Figs. 9–28 to 9–30). It is similar to the term pes planus in that the definitions of these terms are not operational for clinical use. Prerequisite to distinguishing a high-arched foot (pes cavus) from a low-arched foot (pes planus) is knowing how to identify a foot with a normal arch. What constitutes a normal arch has yet to be defined.

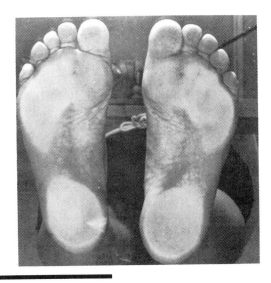

**FIGURE 9–28** ■ Plantar view of pes cavus feet while the subject was standing. Note that the middle third of the lateral longitudinal arch does not make contact with the supporting surface. (From Jahss MH, ed: Disorders of the Foot and Ankle: Medical and Surgical Management, 2nd ed, Vol 1. Philadelphia: WB Saunders, 1991, Fig. 36–1.)

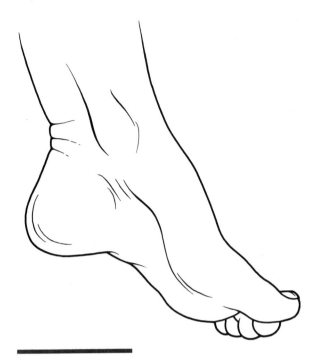

**FIGURE 9-29** ■ Medial view of a pes cavus foot in a non-weight-bearing position.

Terms used in the literature to describe a high-arched foot include calcaneocavus deformity, pes varus, and cavovarus deformity. Many authors have suggested that athletes with an excessively high arch are predisposed to overuse injuries.[118-120]

## Pes Planus

It is difficult to find a clinically useful operational definition of pes planus or flat foot in the literature. Most definitions of pes planus that are operational involve the use of radiographic measurements[121,122] (Fig. 9-31). The most commonly used and accepted definition of pes planus is a foot with an abnormally low medial longitudinal arch (Fig. 9-32). This definition is not operational—for example, it does not describe what a normal arch is or how it is measured.

Terms used in the literature to describe a foot with an abnormally low arch include pes valgus, vertical talus, calcaneal valgus, flat foot, and hypermobile pronated foot. The term pes planus appears to have little use in the clinic. It is clear from the literature, however, that feet with abnormally low medial longitudinal arches appear to present in at least two different ways.[123] The first is the foot that has what appears to be an abnormally low arch in the weight-bearing and non-weight-bearing positions. This foot has been described as a rigid pes planus foot. The second is the foot that has what appears to be a normal arch in a non-weight-bearing position but an abnormally low arch in a weight-bearing position. This foot has been described as a flexible pes planus foot (Fig. 9-33). Because these two types of pes planus feet look different in a weight-bearing versus a non-weight-bearing position, an examination of the foot in both positions appears necessary for an adequate clinical description of the low-arched foot.

## Clubfoot

Tachdjian describes two types of clubfoot deformities.[124] Postural clubfoot has the classic plantar flexed, adducted, and inverted position. The critical finding that distinguishes this type

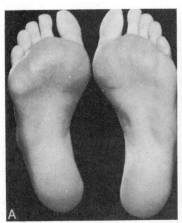
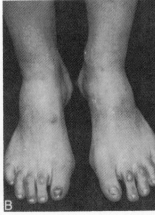
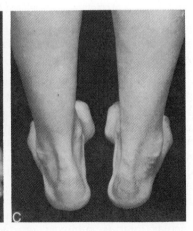

**FIGURE 9-30** ■ Plantar (A), anterior (B), and posterior (C) view of cavus feet while the subject was standing. (From Kelikian H, Kelikian AS: Disorders of the Ankle. Philadelphia: WB Saunders, 1985, Fig. 12–8A–C.)

### Pes Planus

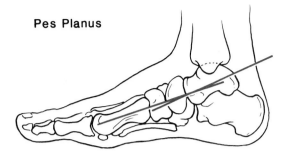

### Neutral

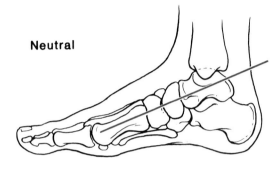

### Pes Cavus

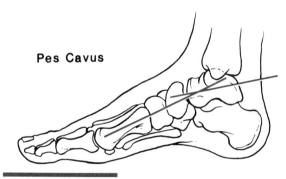

**FIGURE 9–31** ■ The talometatarsal angle used to define pes planus, neutral, and pes cavus foot types. (From Jahss MH, ed: Disorders of the Foot and Ankle: Medical and Surgical Management, 2nd ed, Vol 1. Philadelphia: WB Saunders, 1991, Fig. 5–25.)

from the more serious type of clubfoot is that the talocalcaneonavicular joint is radiographically normal. Many other clinical findings differentiate the postural clubfoot from the more serious clubfoot deformities (Table 9–9). According to Tachdjian, the cause of postural clubfoot is an abnormal intrauterine position.

Congenital talipes equinovarus is the more serious form of clubfoot because the talocalcaneonavicular joint is subluxed or dislocated.[124] The incidence of congenital talipes equinovarus

in whites is 1.2 per thousand, and it is twice as frequent in males as in females.[125] The deformity is also reported to be bilateral approximately 50% of the time.

Five theories have been proposed to explain the etiology of clubfoot. The first, proposed by Hippocrates, is that the deformity is due to mechanical factors related to the position of the fetus during development. The second theory is that clubfoot is caused by a neuromuscular defect. The third theory is based on the argument that fetal development of the foot ceases at some point, producing the deformity. Irani and Sherman proposed a fourth theory, that clubfoot is due to a germ plasm defect resulting in defective cartilage.[126] Tachdjian proposed a fifth theory, that in some cases clubfoot is caused by a ligamentous disorder.[124] The exact cause of clubfoot has not been determined and appears to be multifactorial.

The primary deformity of clubfoot is medial and plantar deviation of the head and neck of the talus.[124] The angle formed by the long axis of the head and neck of the talus with the body of the talus is normally approximately 150 degrees. In the clubfoot deformity this angle is decreased to 115 to 135 degrees.[124]

Goldner and Fitch proposed a clinical classification system with three categories for describing the severity of the clubfoot deformity[127] (Fig. 9–34). The first category consists of positional clubfoot deformities. These deformities are caused by an abnormal position of the fetus in utero. Foot size is equal and calf atrophy is not present. The hindfoot can be dorsiflexed easily to a neutral position or beyond, and the forefoot can easily be abducted to a neutral position.

Category two deformities are considered to be true clubfeet. These feet have deformities in the talonavicular and midtarsal joints. Contractures are present in the medial tendons of the foot and medial side of the joint capsules of the subtalar and midtarsal joints.

Category three deformities are considered severe. Teratologic defects, myelodysplasia, and other musculoskeletal problems are associated with category three clubfeet.

## Rear Foot Varus (Calcaneal Varus, Subtalar Varus)

The rear foot varus deformity manifests as an abnormal frontal plane relationship between the distal tibia and the calcaneus. The calcaneus is in an abnormally inverted position relative to the tibia. Normally, a line representing the bisection

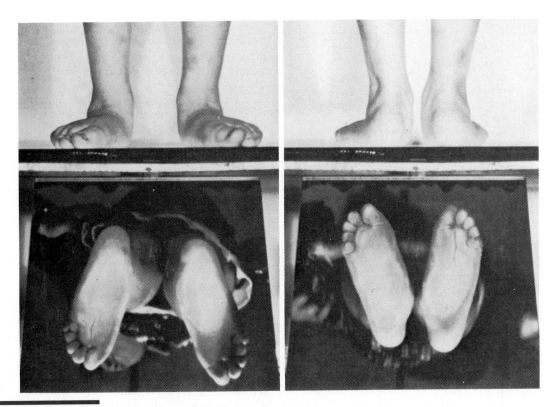

**FIGURE 9-32** ■ Anterior, posterior, and plantar views of pes planus feet in a standing subject. Note the large area of contact between the midfoot and the supporting surface. (From Jahss MH, ed: Disorders of the Foot and Ankle: Medical and Surgical Management, 2nd ed, Vol 1. Philadelphia: WB Saunders, 1991, Fig. 37-26.)

of the calcaneus should be parallel to or at an angle of approximately 3 degrees or less (slightly inverted) from a line representing the bisection of the distal third of the tibia.[128,129] A rear foot varus deformity is present when a line representing the bisection of the calcaneus is in an inverted position relative to the line representing the bisection of the tibia. This inverted position must be greater than approximately 3 degrees.

Different terms have been used in the literature to describe this abnormally inverted position of the calcaneus in relation to the tibia. For example, Tiberio[117] describes this deformity as a calcaneal varus, whereas Sgarlato[130] uses the term subtalar varus. The terms calcaneal varus and subtalar varus imply that the clinician has identified the anatomic basis for the deformity. The deformity may actually lie in the calcaneus, the talus, or the talocalcaneal joint. Because therapists typically are unable to determine the anatomic basis for this deformity, rear foot varus is probably the most appropriate term.

Some researchers have suggested that rear foot varus is caused by lack of derotation of the calcaneus or talus during development.[14] A mal-

union of the calcaneus can also result in a rear foot varus deformity. Shortening of the medial rear foot soft tissues may also cause a rear foot varus deformity. While a rear foot varus deformity is likely caused by many different factors, most clinicians and researchers agree the deformity is responsible for many types of patient complaints. Tiberio argues the rear foot varus deformity is the most common deformity of the foot.[117]

### Forefoot Varus

The forefoot varus deformity is essentially an abnormal frontal plane relationship between the plane in which the five metatarsal heads lie and the line representing the bisection of the calcaneus. Normally, the plane of the five metatarsal heads is perpendicular to the line of the calcaneal bisection when the subtalar joint is in a neutral position (Fig. 9-35). When a forefoot varus deformity is present, the line representing the plane of the five metatarsals is not perpendicular to the calcaneal bisection. The medial

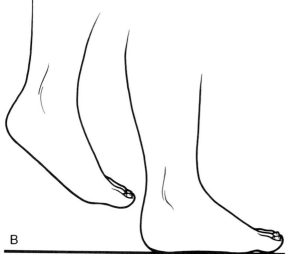

**FIGURE 9–33** ■ Tests for the difference between supple (A) and rigid (B) pes planus.

neus. Normally, the plane of the five metatarsal heads is perpendicular to the line of the calcaneal bisection (see Fig. 9–35). When a forefoot valgus deformity is present, the line representing the plane of the five metatarsals is not perpendicular to the calcaneal bisection. The lateral side of the forefoot is higher than the medial side (a valgus or everted position) when the subtalar joint is in a neutral position (see Fig. 9–35).

The cause of forefoot valgus is also thought to be abnormal development of the head and neck of the talus.[14] Root et al. hypothesized that two types of forefoot valgus exist.[131] The first is present when the plane of all five metatarsal heads is everted relative to the calcaneal bisection, the second when only the first metatarsal head is lower than the remaining metatarsal heads.

### Equinus Foot

Equinus foot is present when an abnormal sagittal plane relationship exists between the foot and the leg. The foot is in a plantar flexed position relative to the leg. Bouche and Kuwada described four types of equinus:[132] ankle equinus, in which normal dorsiflexion is limited because of an osseous block between the tibia and talus; gastrocnemius-soleus equinus, caused by an acquired or congenitally shortened triceps surae; metatarsal equinus, in which the foot is plantar flexed at the level of the tarsometatarsal joint; and forefoot equinus, in which the foot is plantar flexed at the level of the midtarsal joint.

When a metatarsal or a forefoot equinus is present, the metatarsal heads lie below the plantar aspect of the calcaneus.[132] The forefoot is in a plantar flexed position relative to the rear foot. The clinical significance of any of the equinus deformities is that the patient is thought to require more talocrural joint dorsiflexion to be able to function normally. The amount of talocrural joint dorsiflexion that is required for a normal gait is approximately 10 degrees.[133] A patient who does not have the required amount of talocrural joint dorsiflexion compensates by dorsiflexing (pronating) at the subtalar or midtarsal joint. This compensation is thought to cause symptoms in some patients.[117]

side of the forefoot is higher than its lateral side (a varus or inverted position) (see Fig. 9–35).

The cause of forefoot varus is thought to be abnormal development of the head and neck of the talus.[14] This deformity has been hypothesized to be relatively uncommon in the general population but, when present, produces significant problems.[117]

### Forefoot Valgus

The forefoot valgus deformity is essentially an abnormal frontal plane relationship between the plane in which the five metatarsal heads lie and the line representing the bisection of the calca-

## Disorders That Affect the Joints

### Ankle Sprains

The ligaments of the lateral side of the ankle are injured much more frequently than the me-

**Table 9-9.** DIFFERENTIAL DIAGNOSIS OF POSTURAL CLUBFOOT AND TALIPES EQUINOVARUS

| | Postural Clubfoot | Talipes Equinovarus |
|---|---|---|
| *Etiology* | Intrauterine malposture | Primary germ plasm defect<br>Defective cartilaginous anlage of the talus |
| *Pathologic Anatomy*<br>Head and neck of talus | Normal<br>Declination angle of talus normal 150 to 155 degrees | Medial and plantar tilt<br>Declination angle of talus decreased 115 to 135 degrees |
| Talocalcaneonavicular joint | Normal | Subluxated or dislocated medially and plantarward |
| Effect of manipulation in fetal specimens | Normal alignment of foot can be restored | Talocalcaneonavicular subluxation cannot be reduced unless ligaments connecting navicular to calcaneus, talus, and tibia are sectioned and posterior capsule and ligaments divided |
| *Clinical Features*<br>Severity of deformity<br>Heel<br>Relation between navicular and medial malleolus | Mild and flexible<br>Normal size<br>Normal space between two bones; can insert finger | Marked and rigid<br>Small, drawn up<br>Navicular abuts medial malleolus: finger cannot be inserted between two bones |
| Lateral malleolus | Normal position | Posteriorly displaced with anterior part of talus very prominent in front of it |
| Skin creases on<br>  Dorsolateral aspect of foot<br>  Medial and plantar aspects of foot<br>  Posterior aspect of ankle<br>Calf and leg atrophy | Present; normal<br>No furrowed skin<br>Normal<br>None or very minimal | Thin or absent<br>Furrowed skin<br>Deep crease<br>Moderate to marked |
| *Treatment* | Passive manipulation followed by retention by adhesive strapping, splint, or cast | Primary open reduction of talocalcaneonavicular joint often required; surgery is conservative<br>Closed methods of reduction often unsuccessful<br>Prolonged retentive apparatus essential |
| *Prognosis* | Excellent; result is normal foot | Poor with closed methods<br>Prolonged cast immobilization results in smaller foot and atrophied leg |

From Tachdjian MO: The Child's Foot. Philadelphia: WB Saunders, 1985, p 163.

dial ankle ligament. Most epidemiologic studies report that approximately 95% of all ankle sprains are lateral. Approximately 5% of ankle sprains occur on the medial side of the ankle.

Most lateral ankle sprains occur because the foot is in a plantar flexed and inverted position at the time of injury.[134] When the forces applied exceed a critical level, the lateral capsular and ligamentous structures are injured. Most medial ankle sprains occur when the foot is forcefully everted, abducted, and dorsiflexed.[135]

Many methods for classifying ankle ligament sprains have been described in the literature. This is probably because the lateral ankle ligaments function as a unit most of the time. Therefore, some classification systems are designed to grade the integrity of the entire lateral ankle ligament complex, whereas others are designed to grade individual ligaments of the complex.

There are also classification systems based on functional criteria. The first system discussed in this section is probably used most commonly for grading lateral ankle ligament injuries. Ideally, each lateral ankle ligament should be assessed and graded. However, the clinical tests available for grading these injuries probably do not allow us to make judgments about the integrity of specific ligaments on the lateral side of the ankle. Therefore, the second classification system seems to be most meaningful for grading ligament injuries of the lateral side of the ankle.

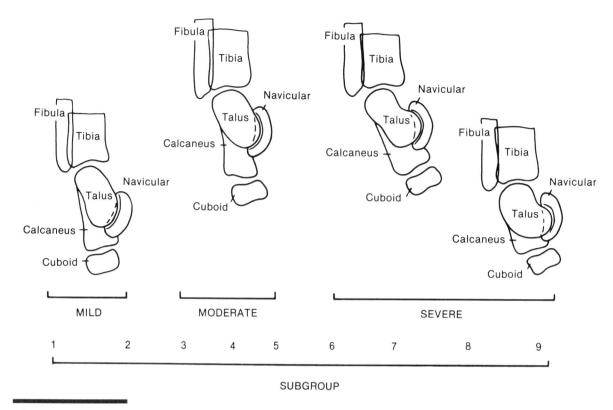

FIGURE 9–34 ■ A classification system for describing the severity of clubfoot. (From Jahss MH, ed: Disorders of the Foot and Ankle: Medical and Surgical Management, 2nd ed, Vol 1. Philadelphia: WB Saunders, 1991, Fig. 33–22A.)

The grading system described by Nicholas and Hershman is as follows:[136]

**Grade I.** Microscopic tearing of the ligament with no loss of function.
**Grade II.** Partial disruption or stretching of the ligament with some loss of function.
**Grade III.** Complete tearing of the ligament with complete loss of function.

The grading system that relies on functional criteria as well as examination findings is the system described by McConkey.[137] His classification system is as follows:

**Mild sprain (grade 1).** Minimal functional loss, little swelling, localized tenderness, and mild pain in response to stress. Pathologically, there is functional integrity with a minor ligamentous injury.
**Moderate sprain (grade 2).** Moderate functional loss, with difficulty on toe raise and walking, diffuse tenderness, and swelling. Pathologically, there is a nearly complete lateral ligament complex injury.
**Severe sprain (grade 3).** Functional disability, with marked tenderness and swelling, marked loss of range of motion, and a need for crutches. Pathologically, complete ligament rupture is indicated.

The problem with the McConkey's[137] scale is that the criteria are not defined operationally. In addition, the criteria for the grades may not be mutually exclusive. For example, a patient may have only minimal functional loss (grade 1) but marked tenderness and swelling (grade 3).

Another commonly used classification system was the scale described by Leach:[138]

**First-degree sprain.** The anterior talofibular ligament is completely ruptured.
**Second-degree sprain.** The anterior talofibular and calcaneofibular ligaments are ruptured.
**Third-degree sprain.** The ankle is dislocated and all three lateral ankle ligaments are ruptured.

The therapist must be aware that different classification systems used for grading severity of ankle ligament injuries (especially lateral ankle sprains) use the same terms (e.g., grade 2) to describe different phenomena. Some classification systems use functional criteria to determine

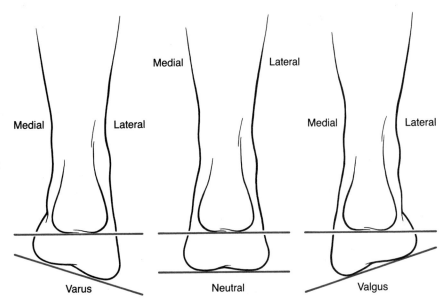

**FIGURE 9-35** ■ Forefoot varus, neutral forefoot, and forefoot valgus alignments.

the grade, whereas others attempt to identify the type and degree of pathology present. To facilitate clear communication between clinicians, the classification system used to grade ligament injuries should be defined for all clinicians treating the same patients.

### Osteoarthrosis of the Ankle

Primary osteoarthrosis (OA) of the ankle is rare. It is thought that the incidence is low for a variety of reasons. The ankle has a large surface area of contact, which minimizes the force per unit area applied to the articular cartilage during weight bearing. The innate structural stability of the ankle is also thought to help prevent primary OA. Also, the multiple joints surrounding the ankle joint help in distributing and absorbing weight-bearing forces, resulting in a decreased incidence of primary OA of the ankle.[24,77]

Secondary OA of the ankle joint is relatively common and typically results from abnormal forces applied to the ankle joint as a result of an intra-articular injury. Common causes of secondary OA of the ankle are intra-articular fractures, ligamentous instability, congenital deformity, and previous surgical treatment.

Patients with OA of the ankle report that their ankles are painful and stiff and are worse with weight-bearing activities. Patients may report locking or giving way of the ankle. Conservative treatment for these patients may include lockup ankle braces, rocker-bottom shoes with elevated heels, and ankle-foot orthoses.[139]

### Hallux Valgus Deformity

The hallux valgus deformity is commonly seen in patients with a wide variety of disorders. Often, the patient is asymptomatic but some function is significantly altered because of the deformity.

The cause of the development of hallux valgus is not completely understood. Lax ligaments, weak muscles, and abnormal bone anatomy have all been implicated as possible causes of the hallux valgus deformity.[140-142] Inman[143] and Jahss[144] have suggested that pes planus is a causative factor in the development of hallux valgus.

One factor that appears to be associated with hallux valgus deformity is the angle between the first and second metatarsal (Fig. 9-36). This angle should normally be between 3 and 9 degrees. Feet with angles of 10 degrees or more are described as having a metatarsus primus varus deformity. Abnormal angles between the first and second metatarsals are reported to vary between 10 and 20 degrees. Jahss states that metatarsus primus varus angles of 10 to 12 degrees are considered mild deformities, angles of 12 to 16 degrees moderate deformities, and angles greater than 16 degrees severe deformities.[144]

In an attempt to compensate for the medial angulation of the first ray, the hallux deviates laterally. Normally, this lateral deviation is approximately 10 degrees. Angulation beyond 10 degrees is considered to indicate a hallux valgus deformity. Kelikian has proposed a system for classifying hallux valgus deformities.[145] A defor-

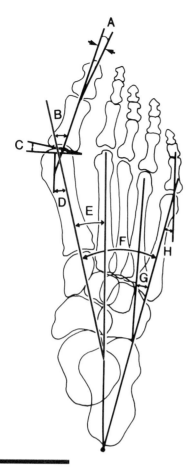

**FIGURE 9-36** ■ The first intermetatarsal angle measurement for hallux valgus deformity (angle E). (From Jahss MH, ed: Disorders of the Foot and Ankle: Medical and Surgical Management, 2nd ed, Vol 1. Philadelphia: WB Saunders, 1991, Fig. 5-9.)

mity of 20 degrees is considered to be mild, a deformity of 30 degrees moderate, and a deformity of 40 degrees or more severe.

The hallux valgus deformity is seen nine times more commonly in women than in men.[144] This greater incidence in women is thought to be due to the narrower toe boxes in most women's shoes.

Kalen and Brecher completed a retrospective study to attempt to determine whether adolescent hallux valgus deformity is associated with a flat foot deformity.[146] In addition, the authors were interested in determining whether the metatarsus primus varus angle could predict when a patient had a hallux valgus deformity.

The authors examined the radiographs of 36 adolescents with 66 hallux valgus deformities that met a set of operationally defined criteria. They found that the metatarsus primus varus angle was normal in most subjects, suggesting

that the angle between the first and second metatarsals was not predictive of who would develop a hallux valgus deformity. They also found that patients with hallux valgus deformities had a much higher incidence of pes planus deformity than would be seen in the normal population. This suggested that the hallux valgus deformity and pes planus are highly associated. The study by Kalen and Brecher[146] was retrospective and some patients did not fit all the criteria used to define pes planus, so the results should be interpreted cautiously. The study does, however, provide some basis for early intervention in young patients with pes planus deformity. Orthoses designed to allow the foot to function near its neutral position appear to be indicated. These patients appear to be predisposed to developing a hallux valgus deformity.

## Other Deformities of the Joints of the Toes

**Claw Toe.** Claw toe is present when the proximal and distal interphalangeal joints are positioned in flexion and the proximal phalanx is extended and dorsally subluxated on the metatarsal head (Fig. 9-37). The deformity may be fixed or flexible. Claw toe deformities are associated with a cavus foot type and neuromuscular

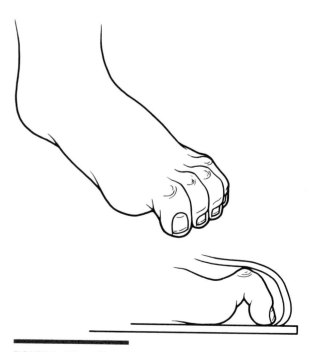

**FIGURE 9-37** ■ Claw toe deformity characterized by an extended metatarsophalangeal joint and flexed proximal and distal interphalangeal joints.

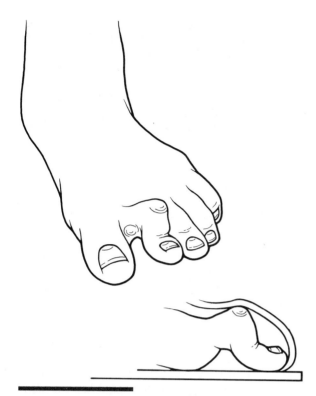

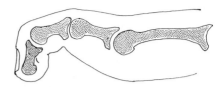

FIGURE 9-39 ■ Mallet toe deformity characterized by a flexed distal interphalangeal joint. The metatarsophalangeal and proximal interphalangeal joints are typically in a neutral position (From Jahss MH, ed. Disorders of the Foot and Ankle: Medical and Surgical Management, 2nd ed, Vol 1, Philadelphia, WB Saunders, 1991, Fig. 27-1B.)

FIGURE 9-38 ■ Hammer toe deformity characterized by an extended metatarsophalangeal joint and flexed proximal interphalangeal joint.

disorders. Often, the cause of the deformity cannot be determined. Metatarsalgia is reported to be frequently associated with the claw toe deformity.[147]

**Hammer Toe.** Hammer toe is present when the proximal interphalangeal joint is flexed and the distal interphalangeal joint and metatarsophalangeal joint are hyperextended (Fig. 9–38). The deformity may be fixed or flexible. A painful callus typically forms at the tip of the toe. The deformity may be congenital or acquired. Hammer toes are associated with cavus feet, improper footwear, hallux valgus, and muscle imbalance.[148] Brahms suggests that the shape of the cavus foot results in loss of function of the extensor digitorum brevis.[148] Because the normal relationship between the extensor and flexor muscles is altered, the hammer toe deformity develops.

**Mallet Toe.** Mallet toe is present when the distal interphalangeal joint is flexed (Fig. 9–39). The deformity may be fixed or flexible and is congenital or acquired. It becomes symptomatic when a painful callus forms on the end of the toe or the nail bed becomes inflamed.

## Disorders That Affect the Soft Tissues of the Leg

### Shin Splints

The term shin splints is a "catchall" used to describe exercise-induced posteromedial, anterolateral, or medial leg pain. Kues thoroughly reviewed the literature that examined the pathologic basis for the presence of shin splints.[149] The symptoms associated with shin splints develop gradually during repetitive weight-bearing activities. The symptoms typically decrease with rest, and the involved area may be swollen and tender to palpation.

The pain the patient reports has been attributed to many tissues. For example, the literature suggests the symptoms are due to myositis,[150] periostitis,[151] inflammation of the interosseous membrane,[152] and tendinitis.[153]

Kues argues in her review that there are data indicating that shin splints can be caused by pathology of the posteromedial cortex and periosteum of the tibia and the crural fascia in the posterior compartment.[149] More research is apparently needed to determine the role of muscle tendon and fascia in the production of shin splints.

## Disorders That Affect Neural and Vascular Structures

### Tarsal Tunnel Syndrome

The most common nerve entrapment syndrome of the ankle is reported to be tarsal tunnel syndrome.[139] Less common entrapment neuropathies of the ankle are anterior tarsal tunnel syndrome, superficial peroneal nerve entrapment, and deep peroneal nerve entrapment. The reader should review Schon and Ouzounian's review of these entrapment neuropathies.[139]

Tarsal tunnel syndrome of the foot is somewhat analogous to carpal tunnel syndrome of the wrist. It is caused by entrapment of the posterior tibial nerve or one of its branches (medial or lateral plantar nerve) within the tarsal tunnel. The tunnel is posterior to the medial malleolus and has an osseous floor covered by the flexor retinaculum. The structures passing through the tunnel are the long flexor tendons and their sheaths, the posterior tibialis tendon, and the tibial nerve, artery, and vein.

Any condition that compromises the space in the tunnel can result in the development of tarsal tunnel syndrome. Conditions reported to cause tarsal tunnel syndrome include chronic tendinitis (and the resulting fibrosis and enlargement of the tendons), old fractures, anatomic anomalies in the area, excessive pronation, venous varicosity, a ganglion, rheumatoid arthritis, and myxedema.

The patient usually reports burning dysesthesias or hypoesthesias in the plantar aspect of the foot and pain in the plantar aspect of the foot especially at night. Weight-bearing activities usually exacerbate the symptoms. These patients typically have a positive Tinel sign at the tarsal tunnel. They typically report no tenderness to palpation in the sole of the foot, which is usually the area of the pain complaint.[154] Electrodiagnostic studies of the posterior tibial nerve assist in confirming the diagnosis. Mann reports that nonsurgical methods of treatment are usually unsuccessful.[154a] However, Schon and Ouzounian report that orthoses can be beneficial in some patients with tarsal tunnel syndrome.[139] When the cause is thought to be excessive pronation, test padding to prevent excessive pronation is the treatment of choice. If it is successful, orthosis fabrication appears to be indicated.

Radin studied 14 patients with clinical evidence of tarsal tunnel syndrome and found that several of the patients responded favorably to the use of lateral heel wedges in the shoes.[154] Radin reported that these patients had varus deformities in the involved heels and splayed, pronated forefeet. The patients who responded favorably to the lateral heel wedges had varus heel deformities that could be corrected to within 5 degrees of neutral. Radin argued that rear foot inversion narrows the tarsal tunnel and therefore the patient responds favorably to treatment when placed in a position of relative pronation.

It appears from the literature that two types of patients may be predisposed to developing tarsal tunnel syndrome. The first are patients with excessive rear foot pronation with an excessive everted position of the heel during stance. The second are the patients Radin described with a heel that remains in an excessively inverted position during stance. Apparently, when a patient functions away from the neutral (vertical calcaneus) position in either an inverted or everted position, the patient may be predisposed to developing tarsal tunnel syndrome.

## Morton's Neuroma

Metatarsalgia, or pain in the area of the metatarsals, is a generic diagnosis. One of the more common causes of metatarsalgia is Morton's neuroma. Synonyms for this disease are Morton's metatarsalgia, Morton's disease, and plantar interdigital neuroma.

This disease is most commonly seen in women between the ages of 25 and 50 years. It is thought that many women's shoes predispose to this disease, although there are no data to support this theory. The disease is typically unilateral.

The symptoms reported by patients are often described as an electric shock or burning sensation. The symptoms are reported to start in the second, third, or fourth metatarsal interspace and then spread across the forefoot. Patients typically report intermittent painful symptoms associated with weight bearing or pain at night while in bed. The area of the soft tissues of the involved interspace is tender to palpation. Compression of the metatarsal heads as a unit sometimes reproduces the symptoms. In more advanced cases, a "click" may be perceived by the examiner when the metatarsals are compressed together.

Viladot states that the most common location of a Morton neuroma is the third metatarsal interspace (between the third and fourth metatarsals).[155] Mann and Reynolds studied patients with confirmed Morton's neuromas and reported an almost equal incidence of second and third interspace neuromas.[156] The fourth metatarsal space appears to be less frequently involved, and the first metatarsal space is reportedly never involved.

Viladot argues that the anatomic arrangement of the interdigital nerves predisposes the third metatarsal space to developing Morton's neuroma.[155] The medial and lateral plantar nerves anastomose at the third interspace, producing a nerve that is larger in diameter than the other digital nerves. This larger-diameter nerve may be predisposed to repetitive trauma.

Viladot states that conservative care should be attempted to allow the foot to function at or near its neutral position.[155] In addition, analgesic and anti-inflammatory medications are used. The neuroma is injected if conservative care is ineffective. Surgical treatment is used in recalcitrant cases.

### Reflex Sympathetic Dystrophy

Sympathetic nervous system dysfunction appears to play a role in some patients' pain complaints. Alexander and Johnson divide dysfunction of the sympathetic nervous system into two diagnostic classifications: reflex sympathetic dystrophy and causalgia.[157] Reflex sympathetic dystrophy is defined as a sustained burning pain combined with vasomotor dysfunction and, in later stages, trophic changes. These signs and symptoms may not be attributable to trauma. If a history of trauma is reported, the trauma may have been trivial. There is no evidence of damage to peripheral nerves. Causalgia is defined as a sustained burning pain occurring after trauma in which there is evidence of nerve damage. Vasomotor, pseudomotor, and trophic changes may be present in later stages.

### Volkmann's Ischemic Contracture

Volkmann's ischemic contracture of the foot is a result of impaired blood supply to the leg, usually caused by obstructed venous return or direct arterial injury. It is imperative to recognize the symptoms and signs of this disorder early because of the disastrous consequences, which include muscle and nerve cell necrosis. Symptoms which may indicate that a Volkmann's contracture is evolving include pain in a cast that can be confused with the initial injury and pain that is present at rest and not relieved with medication. Severe pain is usually reported by the patient during active or passive ROM testing of the involved limb. Muscle paralysis is usually present and may be the dominant symptom.

### Complications Resulting from Systemic Disease

**Systemic Diseases That Can Mimic a Foot or Ankle Disorder.** Physical therapists have found themselves in the role of primary health care providers in some states. Therapists should therefore be prepared to identify pathologies that require additional medical or surgical treatment.

Many diseases can manifest themselves in ways that suggest a primary mechanical disorder of the foot or ankle. Four of the more common systemic diseases that may mimic a local disorder of the foot or ankle are Reiter's syndrome, psoriatic arthritis, rheumatoid arthritis (RA), and gouty arthritis. These diseases are forms of inflammatory arthritis.

When taking the medical history of a patient who may have a systemic inflammatory disorder, Solomon believes the clinician must determine the pattern of joint involvement[158] and whether the disease is monoarticular or polyarticular. Because the inflammatory arthritides may present as either a monoarticular or polyarticular disease, this criterion cannot always be used with confidence to determine which type of arthritis may be present. However, patients who report a several-year history of pain in one joint are unlikely to have RA. Intermittent monoarticular disease may be suggestive of a crystal-induced disease such as gout. Persistent polyarticular disease affecting four or fewer joints is suggestive of a form of spondyloarthropathy. Spondyloarthropathies are seronegative (negative rheumatoid factor) forms of inflammatory arthritis. Psoriatic arthritis and Reiter's syndrome are considered to be spondyloarthropathies.

The clinician must also determine whether the pattern of joint involvement is symmetric or asymmetric. Patients with RA usually report symmetric joint involvement. Patients with one of the spondyloarthropathies or a crystal-induced arthritis commonly report asymmetric joint involvement.

Another issue is whether the patient reports involvement in primarily larger joints or smaller joints. RA typically involves smaller joints, whereas the spondyloarthropathies more commonly affect the larger joints. Crystal-induced arthritides affect the larger and smaller joints almost equally.

The clinician should determine whether the disease affects primarily the upper extremity joints or the lower extremity joints. Patients with RA typically report symptoms more commonly in the upper extremities. Those with crystal-induced arthritis or spondyloarthropathy report lower extremity involvement almost exclusively.

When possible, the clinician must determine whether the disease is additive (more joints becoming involved over time), migratory (different joints involved at different times), or palindromic (distinct episodes of exacerbations and remissions). RA is usually additive, but the spondyloarthropathies are either additive, migratory, or palindromic. Crystal-induced arthritides are typically palindromic.

Determining which specific joints are involved can also help in determining which of the inflammatory arthritides may be present. Proximal interphalangeal, metacarpophalangeal, and wrist joint involvement strongly suggests RA. Involvement of the sacroiliac joints, periostitis, and inflammation of tendon insertions suggest spondyloarthropathy. Involvement of the first metatarsophalangeal joint suggests gouty arthritis, although the spondyloarthropathies can also produce inflammation of the great toe.

### Reiter's Syndrome

Reiter, in 1916, described a syndrome that included a triad of pathologies: arthritis, urethritis, and conjunctivitis.[159] Reiter's syndrome affects mostly males; the cause is unknown, but it may be genetically linked.[160] Patients diagnosed with Reiter's syndrome have a negative serum rheumatoid factor.

Inflammation of connective tissue in these patients occurs at the site of attachment of ligaments, tendons, joint capsules, and fascia to the bone. The tendons and fascia of the feet are commonly involved, and this may be the patient's initial complaint. Some patients may complain of symptoms that mimic those of plantar fasciitis. Achilles tendinitis is reported to be common in these patients.[160] The patient may also report asymmetric involvement of the joints of the foot. Metatarsophalangeal joint involvement is more common than distal interphalangeal joint involvement in Reiter's syndrome.[158] Sesamoiditis is also frequently seen. New bone formation and "fluffy" periostitis are radiographic features frequently seen in the rear feet of patients with Reiter's syndrome.[158] The signs and symptoms of Reiter's syndrome reportedly can linger for months or can resolve spontaneously.[160]

Patients suspected of having Reiter's syndrome should be referred to a rheumatologist for diagnostic work-up. After adequate diagnostic testing, the physical therapist's role in the care of these patients is important. Modification of the patient's shoes to minimize the effects of the soft tissue inflammation on function is the treatment of choice in most cases.

### Psoriatic Arthritis

Patients with psoriatic arthritis typically present with asymmetric multijoint complaints and nail and joint changes, with swelling of the digits producing a characteristic sausage shape. Small joints of the hand and feet are most commonly involved. In addition to the typical musculoskeletal changes, all patients eventually have psoriatic skin lesions. Unfortunately, in 20% of the patients the musculoskeletal complaints appear before the skin lesions.[161] Spinal involvement may or may not be present.

Radiographic changes of the feet of patients with psoriatic arthritis are fairly predictable. Erosion of the proximal aspects of the terminal phalanges with periostitis is common.[160] Another characteristic radiographic deformity is the "pencil in cup" deformity, which is a narrowing of the proximal phalangeal joint surface to the degree that it has the appearance of a pencil.

Patients suspected of having psoriatic arthritis should be referred to a rheumatologist. After adequate diagnostic work-up, the conservative treatment for these patients includes medications and accommodative padding for the foot disease.

### Rheumatoid Arthritis

RA is a systemic disease that affects many systems in addition to the musculoskeletal system. Vasculitis, splenomegaly, serositis, pulmonary nodules, and inflammatory eye disease are a few of the extra-articular findings associated with RA. Women between the fourth and sixth decades are most commonly affected. The diagnosis of RA is based primarily on clinical findings. According to Arnett et al., four or more of the following criteria must be present:[162]

- Morning stiffness for at least 1 hour and present for at least 6 weeks.
- Swelling of three or more joints for at least 6 weeks.
- Swelling of the wrist, metacarpophalangeal, or proximal interphalangeal joints for 6 or more weeks.
- Symmetric joint swelling.
- Radiographic changes of the hand typical of RA, which must include erosions or unequivocal bone decalcification.
- Rheumatoid nodules.
- Serum rheumatoid factor determined by a method positive in less than 5% of normal subjects.

Patients with RA tend to report an insidious onset of pain and swelling of the small joints of the hands in a symmetric distribution. Morning stiffness that parallels the severity of the synovitis is common. The metatarsophalangeal joints and other joints of the forefoot are typically the first to become involved in the lower extremity.[158]

# TREATMENT OF SELECTED DISORDERS

This section reviews the physical therapy treatment approaches that have been proposed for four of the more common types of disorders of the foot and ankle. The treatments described for lateral ankle sprains are summarized. The treatment approaches that have been proposed for structural deformities of the forefoot and rear foot are also reviewed. Treatments for tendonopathies of the leg are described. Studies examining the efficacy of the treatment for each of these common disorders are reviewed.

References to the treatment of other ankle and foot disorders are provided at the end of the chapter. This reference list can be used to gain additional information on the treatment of disorders that are not described in this section.

## Systematic Approach to Determining Appropriate Treatment

Part one of the HOAC was described in the examination section of this chapter. Part two is used during the treatment of a patient (see Fig. 9–25). The purpose of the second part of the HOAC is to provide an organized method of reappraisal of treatment.

Therapists have often designed treatment plans that proved inadequate or only partially adequate. Part two of the HOAC provides therapists with a means of identifying when a treatment plan needs to be changed.

Therapists begin part two by asking themselves if the goals have been met. If the goals have been met, the patient is discharged. However, if they have not been met in the expected time, the therapist must determine why. The first question the therapist must answer is whether the treatment is being implemented appropriately. For example, in a patient whose functional loss is hypothesized to be due to loss of ankle joint dorsiflexion, are the active ROM (AROM) and passive ROM (PROM) exercises designed to produce increases in dorsiflexion ROM being done properly? Perhaps the patient is performing the exercise incorrectly or is not complying with the home exercise program.

If the therapist determines that a patient's treatment is not being implemented correctly, appropriate steps should be taken to ensure proper implementation. If the treatment is being implemented correctly but the goals are not being met, the therapist must determine whether the tactics (specific type of treatment) need to be modified. For example, the patient with limited dorsiflexion might benefit from a PROM exercise in which the ankle joint is positioned at the end range for a longer period of time.

If the therapist determines that the specific type of treatment is not appropriate (as in the preceding example), the tactics must be changed and then implemented. If the tactics are considered appropriate but the goals are not being met, the therapist must determine whether the treatment strategy is correct. The treatment strategy is the overall approach to the treatment. In the preceding example the overall approach centered around the use of active and passive exercises. Perhaps a better strategy would be to initiate joint mobilization procedures in addition to the ROM exercises.

If it is not possible to develop a new strategy, the therapist should seek out consultation with another clinician. When a treatment strategy is found to be inappropriate, the hypotheses generated during the examination usually require modification. Consultation with another clinician is usually required to generate new hypotheses.

## Disorders

### Lateral Ankle Sprain

Many different types of treatment regimens have been recommended for patients with lateral ankle sprains. These regimens range from conservative care in many forms to surgery, depending on the activity level of the patient and the severity of the injury.[163]

Most conservative approaches to the treatment of acute ankle sprains include the use of ice, elevation, and a compressive dressing. Some physicians use casts for patients with diagnoses of completely torn lateral ankle ligaments. In a survey study by Kay, 61% of patients diagnosed with grade III lateral ligament injuries were treated with casting.[163]

Treatment for the patient with a history of chronic or recurring lateral ankle sprains is usually different from that for the patient with an acute sprain. The patient with chronic or recurring lateral ankle sprains usually receives some type of strengthening program and proprioceptive training. Some authors believe that peroneal muscle weakness is a primary cause of lateral ankle sprains. The treatment for many of these patients, therefore, centers around the use of a peroneal muscle–strengthening program.[164]

The reason for thinking that peroneal muscle weakness contributes to ankle sprains is intuitively obvious. The peroneal muscles are in a position to prevent the motion of inversion (the motion most commonly associated with ankle sprain). However, some data suggest that the reflex response of the peroneal muscles to stretch and, secondarily, to protect the lateral ligaments is too slow to be useful.[165-167]

Freeman proposed that the functional loss attributable to an ankle sprain is due to a neuromuscular deficit and not a muscle force production deficit.[168] Specifically, Freeman argued that the functional loss was due to articular deafferentation and the resultant motor incoordination.

Tropp and colleagues undertook a series of studies to determine whether a kinesthetic deficit was present in subjects with a history of ankle sprains.[169-171] They used a device called a stabilimeter to measure postural sway. Their findings suggested that a balance deficit was present in patients with a history of ankle sprains. In a follow-up study, Tropp et al. demonstrated that, in a large group of soccer players, regular training on a simple ankle disc reduced the incidence of sprained ankles.[170] This reduced incidence was found in players with a history of recurring sprains. The frequency of sprains for the previously injured athletes was essentially the same as that for soccer players with no previous history of ankle sprains. The previously injured subjects in the study trained for approximately 10 minutes five times weekly for 10 weeks before the start of the soccer season.

Although the subjects in this study apparently were well-trained athletes, the results have significant clinical implications. Patients with recurring ankle sprains would probably benefit from similar training on a simple ankle disc.

### Forefoot and Rear Foot Disorders

Many studies have been designed to examine the effects of custom-made versus "off-the-shelf" foot orthoses on a variety of parameters. Studies have attempted to determine the effects of orthoses on the symptoms reported by patients, the effects of orthoses on the kinematics or kinetics of the foot during walking or running, and whether orthoses can enhance performance during running or bicycling.

Blake and Denton examined the affect of customized orthoses on the symptoms reported by patients with a variety of disorders of the foot and ankle.[172] The purpose of their retrospective study was to describe the results of treatment of a sample of 180 patients treated over a period of 1 year. The authors treated these patients with rigid orthoses and "physical therapy." A questionnaire was used to collect data related to symptom frequency and intensity after treatment. A total of 115 patients completed the questionnaires. Most of these patients were runners. Of the respondents, 33% reported 100% relief and 90% reported 50% relief; 78% reported feeling that their posture was improved with the use of orthoses, and 75% felt their running was improved.

Many problems are present in this study. The study was retrospective and the criteria for admission to the study were not clearly described. There was no control group, so we do not know whether the results are attributable to the treatment or simply to the passage of time. The authors did not report when the questionnaires were completed, so the time between onset of treatment and follow-up is unclear. The patients received "physical therapy" in addition to the orthotic therapy, so it is unclear which treatment accounted for the improvement reported by the subjects.

Milgrom et al. conducted a prospective study of the effect of a foot orthosis on the incidence of stress fractures in a sample of military recruits.[173] The purpose of the study was to determine whether foot orthoses designed to absorb forces would decrease the incidence of stress fractures in a sample of military recruits. A total of 295 recruits participated; half received orthoses and the other half served as a control group. The orthoses were prefabricated semirigid devices with a layer of open cell foam material added to the heel and the top. A 3-degree varus post was added to all orthoses.

The study was conducted during 14 weeks of the recruits' basic training, and the recruits were examined every 3 weeks by an orthopaedist. Subjects complaining of symptoms consistent with a stress fracture were examined radiographically and with bone scans. The bone scans indicated that 31% of the recruits had stress fractures. The incidence of femoral stress fractures in the orthosis group was significantly less than that in the control group. The incidence of tibial and metatarsal stress fractures was the same for both groups.

This study was sound but had some limitations. All subjects received the same type of orthosis. The results may have been different if the orthoses were customized. The foot type of each subject was not measured. Post hoc analyses may have revealed differences among subjects with different foot types. The benefits attributable to the shock-absorbing qualities of the orthoses may have been attributable to their shape (the 3-degree varus wedges).

Schwellnus et al. also examined the effects of orthoses designed to absorb forces on the incidence of overuse injuries.[174] The purpose of this prospective study was to examine the effect of a commercially available flat neoprene (soft) orthosis on the incidence of "tibial stress syndrome" and other overuse injuries in a sample of military recruits. The subjects were assigned to two groups, with 250 randomly assigned to the treatment group and 1151 assigned to the control group. Both groups of subjects received identical military training for 9 weeks. The severity of injuries was defined operationally in terms of the number of days the recruit was unable to train after reporting an injury. The mean incidence of overuse injuries and the incidence of tibial stress syndrome were significantly less in the experimental group. The weekly incidence of stress fractures was also less in the experimental group.

The authors did not define how tibial stress syndrome was diagnosed, so these results may not be generalizable. However, this study was well done and may be relevant to civilian populations involved in intense training programs. A weakness of the study is that the operational definition of the severity of the injury is related to the patient's ability to return to activity and not to the severity of the pathology produced.

Gardner et al. also examined the shock-absorbing qualities of foot orthoses.[175] Their prospective study was done to determine whether an orthosis designed to absorb forces (Sorbothane) could reduce the incidence of stress fractures and overuse injuries of the lower extremity to a greater degree than standard mesh inserts.

The 3025 military recruits used in this study were randomly assigned to a treatment (Sorbothane) or a control (mesh insert) group. The authors appeared to control external factors that may have affected the results. In addition, they collected much data for post hoc analysis to gain further insights into the causes of injury in this large sample. The results indicated there was no significant difference in the incidence of stress fractures or overuse injuries between the two groups. The factor that appeared to have the greatest effect on injury rate was the fitness level of the subject before military training. Subjects with low levels of perceived fitness before training had a much higher incidence of injury. A weakness of the study is that the authors reported they diagnosed some subjects as having stress fractures without radiographic evidence of a fracture.

Gross et al. conducted a retrospective study to determine whether foot orthoses reduce the symptoms reported by long-distance runners.[176] They also assessed whether certain disorders were more amenable to treatment with orthoses. A third purpose was to determine if a relationship existed between the amount of weekly running and the degree of effectiveness of the treatment.

A total of 500 questionnaires were sent to participants in running races and to members of a running club who had reported being treated with orthoses. Of the questionnaires, 347 (70%) were returned. Questions were related to the runners' diagnoses, types of orthoses used, and distance run per week. Participants were also asked how long they used their orthoses. The runners reported whether they had complete relief, great improvement, slight improvement, or no change or whether they had gotten worse as a result of use of the orthoses. Approximately 75% of the subjects reported complete relief or great improvement in their symptoms. Diagnosis or the distance run per week was not related to the degree of improvement reported.

This study suggests that orthoses may be useful in the treatment of runners with a variety of different diagnoses. However, it has several limitations. As the authors point out, the sample may have been biased. The authors chose a sample of runners who were running competitively. Therefore, they may have missed a large population of runners who were unable to run because of their symptoms but who were treated with orthoses. In addition, the authors did not collect data related to other treatments the subjects may have received. The symptomatic relief the subjects reported may have been due to other treatments. The study also does not provide any information on why the subjects responded favorably to orthoses or which types of orthoses may be most effective. Nevertheless, the data suggest that orthoses are probably useful in the treatment of runners with a variety of overuse syndromes.

Several studies have examined the effects of foot orthoses on the kinematics of the leg and foot of subjects during walking and running. Smith and colleagues investigated whether customized soft and semirigid orthoses (Foothotics) significantly altered the frontal plane kinematics of the rear foot during running.[177] The subjects were 11 runners who routinely wore orthoses and were running 30 to 70 miles per week. They were filmed with a high-speed camera at 200 frames per second. The mean maximum eversion and maximum rate of eversion were computed for three stance phases of each foot for the subjects. Each subject was filmed in random order without orthoses and with the soft and the semirigid orthoses. All subjects wore the same type of shoes. Group means were compared using *t*-tests.

The results suggest that the amounts of rear foot eversion with the soft and semirigid orthoses were not significantly different. The amount of eversion without orthoses was significantly higher than with semirigid orthoses. However, the differences in the amount of eversion between groups were approximately 1 degree, probably well within the error associated with the measurement. The velocity of eversion was significantly higher for the control group than for the soft or semirigid group. The differences in velocity of eversion between the control and treatment groups were on the order of 15%, with the treatment groups everting at a lower velocity than the control group. These may be clinically meaningful differences between groups. The reduction in the velocity of eversion may explain why orthoses are effective in reducing the symptoms of these types of patients. The authors did not examine the reliability of their measurements, which is a weakness of the study. Because reliability of the measurements was not examined and a small number of subjects were studied, further study is clearly needed.

An interesting finding reported by the authors in a post hoc analysis was that the amount of eversion measured during the control condition was poorly correlated ($r = .1$ to $.4$) with clinical measurements. These clinical measurements included the amount of subtalar inversion and eversion, subtalar neutral position, forefoot to rear foot relationship, and tibial varum. These data suggest that clinical measurements may be poor predictors of measurements taken during running.

Bates et al. examined the effects of foot orthoses on selected kinematics of running in a sample of "pronators" who had been treated successfully with orthoses.[178] Six runners who wore rigid orthoses for the previous year served as subjects. Subjects were filmed with a high-speed camera at 200 frames per second with and without the orthoses. An analysis of variance was used to determine whether group means for each variable measured were different.

No significant differences were found between the orthotic and nonorthotic conditions for measurements of maximum pronation and total time spent in pronation. Weaknesses of this study are similar to those of the study of Smith et al. Reliability was not assessed for any of the dependent measurements. The authors also did not report the clinical measurements taken for the subjects admitted to the study. The results appear to contradict those of Smith et al.[177] However, Bates et al.[178] used different types of orthoses and had a much smaller sample size.

Rodgers and Leveau examined the effects of semirigid foot orthoses on selected kinematics of running in a sample of 29 runners.[179] Each runner was filmed while running using a high-speed camera (120 frames per second) for three randomly assigned conditions: barefoot, shoes, and shoes with orthoses. The subjects were filmed while running on an outdoor track. The following variables were measured from the film: time spent in pronation, angular velocity of pronation, and maximum angular displacement in pronation.

The time spent in pronation and the total amount of pronation on the left side were significantly less (on the order of 1 degree for amount of pronation and 5% less time spent in pronation) for the orthoses condition than for the shoes-only condition. For the other dependent variables there were no differences between the orthoses condition and the shoes-only condition.

The authors attempted to reflect more accurately the natural condition of running on a track, and they allowed the runners to wear their own shoes. The authors of the two previous studies had their subjects wear a single type of shoe while running on a treadmill. This attempt to reflect the natural condition of running may have added to the variability in the measurements. For example, filming while the subject is moving away from the camera may add more error to measurements, which further emphasizes the need for reliability.

Katoh et al. examined the effect of heel cups on the ground reaction forces and center of pressure of subjects diagnosed with painful heel syndrome.[180] Painful heel syndrome was defined as a complaint of heel pain. These subjects were further divided into a plantar fasciitis group (patients complaining of pain along the plantar fascia with passive toe extension) and a painful heel group (patients with localized tenderness to palpation of only the heel). The vertical impulse (defined as the area under the ground reaction force–time curve) was measured for the forefoot, midfoot, and rear foot of the subjects with and without the heel cups. A second purpose was to compare the findings for the patients and those for a group of normal subjects. A force plate and foot switches were used to measure ground reaction forces, center of pressure, and vertical impulse.

The results suggested that the instrumentation used can differentiate between the two types of subjects tested. Using the heel cup, the patients with painful heel syndrome had a heel contact time that became equal to that of the normal group but the plantar fasciitis group continued to demonstrate abnormal heel contact times. Seven of the nine subjects with painful heel syndrome reported improvement in symptoms with the use of the heel cup, but subjects with diagnoses of plantar fasciitis reported no change in their symptoms. This method could be used to differentiate between subgroups of patients or to document changes related to treatment. However, the results of this study should be considered preliminary because of the lack of description of the two types of subjects, the small number of subjects examined, and the lack of reliability data.

Taunton et al. examined the effects of semirigid foot orthoses on selected kinematics of running in a sample of runners.[181] A triaxial electrogoniometer was used to collect data while the subjects ran on a treadmill. Variables measured were maximum eversion and time to maximum eversion. The data for the second variable are questionable because the authors did not use switches to denote where in the stance phase of gait the motion was occurring. Using an analysis of variance, the authors concluded that the total amount of eversion was significantly decreased with use of the orthoses compared to the shoes-only condition. The magnitude of the difference was on the order of 2 to 3 degrees. The time to maximum eversion was not altered with the use of orthoses.

The methodology of this study presents several major problems. The main problem concerns the use of a triaxial electrogoniometer to measure motion of the foot. The instrumentation requires that the goniometer be aligned with the axis of rotation of the joint to be measured. Many data suggest that the axis of rotation of the subtalar joint moves and would be difficult to align with a goniometer. Other problems with the use of an electrogoniometer include movement of the de-

vice on the limb and cross-talk of electrogoniometers. The many methodologic problems bring the results of this study into question.

Several studies have examined the effect of orthoses on the energy cost of locomotion. Hice et al. examined the effect of foot orthoses on heart rate and oxygen consumption during submaximal cycling.[182] Five healthy adult subjects, three of whom had never worn orthoses, served as subjects. Rigid orthoses were fabricated for each subject from a neutral position cast. Orthoses were modified until the subjects' gait patterns were "clinically improved." Toe clips were not used during the bicycle-riding tests. Subjects were tested at 10% of their maximal oxygen consumption for a total of 20 minutes. The authors did not report how maximal oxygen consumption was determined. The order of testing (orthoses or no orthoses) was randomized and retests were conducted 6 to 10 weeks apart to allow the subject to accommodate to either wearing or not wearing the orthoses. The authors did not report whether the amount of activity was controlled between the test and retest sessions.

Based on an analysis of variance, the oxygen consumption and heart rate were significantly less for the orthosis condition than for the no-orthosis condition. However, it is not clear from the results which measures of oxygen consumption or heart rate were significantly different between the two conditions. Several measures of these variables were taken during the 20-minute exercise sessions.

This study has several weaknesses. The authors did not report the methods used to measure oxygen consumption and heart rate. They provide no evidence that the orthoses enhanced the mechanics of the subjects' limb movements. The benefits measured in the study may have been due to the fact that the orthoses provided a more rigid lever during pedaling, because the subjects wore soft-soled shoes.

Berg and Sady compared the energy cost of submaximal running while wearing Sorbothane inserts and normal training flats.[183] The authors controlled many variables during the study while examining the effect of the orthoses at two different treadmill running speeds for each subject. Paired t-tests were used to compare the oxygen uptake and heart rate for the two test conditions at each speed. Results suggested that the Sorbothane insert did not significantly affect the oxygen uptake or heart rate for either test condition.

Many studies have examined the effect of

orthoses on a large number of variables, including symptoms reported by the patient, kinetic or kinematic variables, and the energy cost of locomotion. From this relatively large body of literature the following conclusions can be drawn. The symptoms reported by patients can be decreased with the use of orthoses. The extent of symptom reduction and the types of patients who can benefit most from the use of orthoses have yet to be determined. Effects of orthoses on the kinematics or kinetics of locomotion have not been adequately assessed. Orthoses appear to have little effect on the energy cost of running or bicycling.

When using orthoses to treat overuse problems related to the foot or ankle, therapists should use primarily the patients' reports of changes in symptoms as criteria for determining treatment effectiveness. The literature suggests that measurements of the kinematics or kinetics of the patient's gait pattern cannot be used to predict when a patient is responding favorably to orthoses. Some literature suggests that static measurements of foot alignment may also not be related to function.

### Tendinitis

Tendinitis of one or more of the muscles crossing the ankle joint is one of the more common pathologies seen by physical therapists. Many forms of treatment have been proposed for patients with tendinitis.[184-186] Most of these treatments, however, were not adequately defined to allow replication.

The treatment for tendinitis described by Curwin and Stanish is well defined and is used in many clinical settings.[187] The theoretic basis for the exercise program is related to the ability of the tendon to absorb and transmit forces. Curwin and Stanish argue that tendons adapt to the stresses applied to them much as bone responds to forces. If increasing forces are applied in a controlled way, the tendon essentially hypertrophies. The structural strength of the tendon is thought to increase in this process. However, when the forces applied to a tendon exceed the forces the tendon can withstand as a result of training, the tendon is disrupted. Curwin and Stanish believe that these excessive forces result in the development of tendinitis in patients.[187] The tendinitis results because the patient is performing a repetitive activity that places excessive forces on the tendon.

To treat tendinitis, Curwin and Stanish pro-pose an exercise program designed to increase the structural strength of the tendon.[187] This program has been described in a variety of sources for different types of patients.[187-189] The exercise program is based on four assumptions: (1) because most patients with tendinitis complain of pain during eccentric contractions, the exercises must produce eccentric contractions; (2) the involved muscle-tendon unit is shortened and therefore requires lengthening via a passive stretching program; (3) the load applied during the active exercise portion of the program must be gradually increased to increase the structural strength of the tendon; and (4) the speed of contraction must be gradually increased during exercise to increase the load on the tendon.

The exercise program is divided into four phases. During the first phase, the patient passively stretches the involved muscle three to five times, holding each repetition for 15 to 30 seconds. The second phase is the active exercise phase. The patient performs three sets of 10 repetitions of eccentric contractions of the involved muscle. The intensity of the exercise is such that the patient should report some pain or discomfort in the area of the involved tendon on the last set of 10 repetitions. The speed of contraction is slow the first 2 days, moderate the third to fifth days, and fast the sixth and seventh days. The patient increases the resistance after day 7 by holding weights in the hands.

No studies were found that directly support the use of Curwin and Stanish's program for patients with tendinitis of the ankle.[187] In addition, few data appear to support directly the theory Curwin and Stanish propose for the etiology of tendinitis.[187] However, based on the high frequency of clinical use and the large amount of data indirectly supporting the theory of Curwin and Stanish,[187] the method appears to be useful for some patients. More study is needed to determine whether this method is more efficacious than other methods proposed for the treatment of tendinitis.

### CASE STUDY 1

▼HISTORY

The patient was a 29-year-old woman referred for physical therapy with a chief complaint of an inability to run in local running events because of hip, knee, and ankle pain on the right side. A secondary complaint was occasional pain in the area of the right hip during low-impact aerobics that limited her ability to complete exercise sessions. The patient stated that she did not perceive pain with any other functional activities. She reported the hip pain began after running approximately 2 miles. The knee and ankle pain usually occurred shortly after the hip pain began. The patient reported no previous history of right hip pain. The patient did report that she fractured her right tibia approximately 15 years before the onset of hip pain in a gymnastics accident. The patient's goal was to be able to run in local 5-kilometer and 5-mile races without pain and to perform 1 hour of low-impact aerobics without pain.

## EXAMINATION

The patient's posture was inspected while she stood with her feet approximately a shoulder width apart. The patient's calcanei appeared to be in an inverted position bilaterally. A tibial torsion appeared to be present bilaterally because the malleoli of each leg appeared to be excessively externally rotated relative to the tibial condyles. The patellae faced medially and the right patella faced more medially than the left.

The patient's knee, foot, and ankle range of motion was assessed. She had a 10-degree rear foot varus on the right and a 5-degree rear foot varus on the left with the feet in a neutral position. In addition, she had a 9-degree forefoot varus with a flexible plantar flexed first ray on the right side and a 7-degree forefoot varus on the left side. The patient had no eversion from the neutral position on either foot. Dorsiflexion and plantar flexion of the ankle as well as flexion and extension of the knee were within normal limits actively and passively.

The lengths of the patient's lower extremities were measured by placing one end of a tape measure on the anterior superior iliac spine and the other end on the medial malleolus. The patient had a leg length discrepancy of 15 mm, with the right leg shorter than the left. With the patient standing, the right iliac crest was found to be lower than the left iliac crest.

During the gait assessment, the patient was observed to have a shorter step length on the right than the left. In addition, her right thigh was observed to rotate internally to a greater degree than the left thigh during the stance phase of gait between the foot flat and heel-off positions.

The patient's symptoms of pain were reported to be in the right hip in the area of the ischial tuberosity (posterior hip pain) and the area of the greater trochanter (lateral hip pain). The knee pain was reported to be in the area of the lateral epicondyle. The ankle pain was reported to be in the area of peroneal and extensor tendons. Palpation in the area of the ischial tuberosity reproduced the pain the patient reported in the posterior hip. Palpation in the area of the posterior aspect of the gluteus medius and the area of the deep external rotators reproduced the lateral hip pain the patient reported.

The patient was hypothesized to have inflammatory processes in the area of the proximal insertion of the hamstrings on the right side and in the area of the external rotators and gluteus medius on the right side and to have an inflammatory process in the area of the lateral epicondyle of the right knee. These inflam- matory processes appeared to be due to several mechanical problems: the rigid rear foot varus deformity and forefoot varus deformity on the right side and the leg length discrepancy, which secondarily produced the gait deviation.

## TREATMENT

The treatment was designed to address the hypothesized causes of the inflammation. The strategy was to treat the cause of the inflammation with test padding and stretching exercises and to treat the inflammation with phonophoresis and ice packs. Test padding, a method of fabricating temporary orthoses, was done to determine whether the patient would benefit from permanent orthoses. The patient was seen for a total of eight visits. The first four visits were spaced approximately 1 week apart and the last four visits approximately 2 weeks apart. This schedule was based on the type of treatment used with this patient. Because the inflammation was hypothesized to be due to mechanical factors, a significant amount of time was required between treatments to assess the effect of the test padding on the patient's functional complaints.

Initially, the patient was treated with a temporary orthosis (test padding) that consisted of a 4-degree rear foot post and a 4-degree forefoot post on the right side. The posting material was a soft felt padding enclosed with athletic tape so that the patient could use the temporary orthosis in her running shoes and aerobic shoes. The temporary orthosis was used to accommodate for the forefoot and rear foot deformities and to correct for the leg length discrepancy.

On her second visit, the patient reported that she was able to perform 1 hour of low-impact aerobics with the test pads in place without pain. She had not attempted to run since the first visit. Additional examination procedures were used at this time. The patient had a positive Ober test on the right and a straight leg raise to 55 degrees on the right before reporting a stretching sensation in her posterior thigh. The patient reported a stretching sensation in her left thigh during a straight leg raise at a position of 85 degrees. Based on these findings, the patient was instructed to begin a program of 10 sets of two repetitions per day of hamstring stretching and hip abductor stretching exercises.

The exercises were performed as follows. The patient was instructed to perform right-sided hamstring muscle lengthening exercises in seated, standing, and supine positions. The patient was therefore able to perform exercises during work and leisure times. The patient was instructed to position her hip in a neutral position on the first repetition of exercise and in an internally rotated position on the second repetition. The patient was instructed to flex at the right hip until a stretching sensation was perceived in the area of the right hamstring muscle. She was also instructed to perform right-sided hip abductor muscle stretches in a standing position. The right hip was placed in an adducted and externally rotated position. The patient was instructed to lean the pelvis to the right (producing a greater amount of right hip adduction) until a stretch was perceived in the area of the lateral hip on the right. She was instructed to hold each repetition at the end-range position (the position in which a stretching sensation was perceived in the area specified) for 10 to 15 seconds.

It appeared that the shortened hamstring muscles and abductor muscles on the right were contributing to the inflammatory processes in the hip. The patient also received phonophoresis with 10% hydrocortisone in a lotion base to the area of the ischial tuberosity and the area of the external rotator muscles of the hip. She was told to apply an ice pack to the painful areas of the involved hip twice a day to decrease the inflammation. An additional 2 degrees of felt posting was added to the test pads because they had become compressed and were no longer posting to the desired degree.

This treatment was continued during the following three visits. The original trial of test padding was modified to account for compression of the felt. By the fifth treatment the patient was running 1.5 miles three times a week with complaints of mild discomfort at the end of the runs. The test padding was changed again. A posting of 10 degrees was made for the rear foot and a posting of 9 degrees for the forefoot. The additional posting was added because excessive internal rotation during late stance was observed as described in the examination section. This excessive internal rotation was hypothesized to contribute to the inflammatory processes in the hip. The original test padding did not appear to correct the excessive internal hip rotation. With the addition of the new posting, the excessive internal hip rotation no longer appeared to be present during gait. Because of the abnormal alignment of the uninvolved limb, the patient was also given a test pad in the left shoe, which was posted at 4 degrees in the rear foot and 5 degrees in the forefoot. The leg length discrepancy was still corrected because additional felt was added to the right test pad. Because a test pad was placed in the left shoe, the right test pad had to be raised an additional amount.

The patient reported on the sixth visit that she was able to run 2 miles every other day without symptoms. On the eighth visit the patient reported running up to 4 miles without symptoms. Because the patient was now running the distance she typically ran during training and reported no symptoms, permanent orthoses were fabricated for her. The degrees of posting used in the temporary orthoses were used when fabricating the posting for the permanent orthoses.

The orthoses were fabricated using materials manufactured by Foot Tech (St. Louis, MO) and consisted of a synthetic fabric exterior with a ¼ inch layer of closed cell material designed to absorb forces. These were sealed with epoxy to a 1.1-cm layer of a rigid polyethylene-based material. The orthoses were ground to match the posting of the temporary orthoses. The patient was observed while walking and running with the permanent orthoses fitted to her running shoes. She had an equal step length and no

longer appeared to have excessive internal rotation at the right hip between the foot flat and heel-off phases of gait. In addition, she no longer had a positive Ober test. The straight leg raise test was also symmetric. The patient was discharged and instructed to continue her exercise program before and after running. The patient was also instructed to wear her orthoses whenever she ran or participated in aerobics.

The patient was seen 4 months after the fabrication of the permanent orthoses. She reported running up to 6 miles and doing a full session of low-impact aerobics without pain.

## CASE STUDY 2

### ▼ HISTORY

The patient was a 27-year-old woman referred for physical therapy with a chief complaint of pain, swelling, and loss of motion in the right ankle that made her unable to walk. The patient was playing racquetball 3 months before the initial physical therapy examination when the injury occurred. She was attempting to pivot on the right lower extremity while hitting the ball, and as the patient pivoted she felt her ankle give way.

The patient was taken to an emergency room and found to have a closed distal tibial fracture, an open distal fibular fracture, and an open talocrural joint dislocation. The patient was seen immediately by an orthopaedic surgeon. The surgeon performed a closed reduction of both the fibular fracture and the dislocation. The tibial fracture was determined to be nondisplaced and therefore did not require reduction. The patient's injured leg was then placed in a short leg cast and she was instructed to walk without weight bearing while using crutches.

Approximately 1 week later the patient was re-examined. The physician found that the fibular fracture had become displaced since the reduction. The physician then removed the cast and performed a second closed reduction, after which the patient was given another short leg cast. She was immobilized in the short leg cast for a total of 10.5 weeks until the tibial fracture healed. The physician reported that 1 week after the physical therapy examination, the patient's fibular fracture was healed.

The patient was a senior auditor who spent most of her workday in a sitting position, so she was allowed to return to work 3 weeks after the injury. The patient's goals at the time of the initial physical therapy examination were to walk and run without pain or a limp. The patient was also active in several sports and hoped to return to playing softball and racquetball.

### EXAMINATION

The patient walked to the clinic without weight bearing with crutches. An Ace wrap was positioned around the right ankle and foot. The patient was observed to have a significant amount of pitting edema of the right ankle and dorsum of the foot. A well-healed circular scar 1.5 cm in diameter was present near the talocrural joint line. The patient stated that the scar was due to the open talocrural joint dislocation.

The patient was able to dorsiflex actively to a plantar flexed position of 13 degrees. She was able to plantar flex actively to a plantar flexed position of 30 degrees. The patient's total sagittal plane motion at the talocrural joint, therefore, was 17 degrees. She had no active inversion or eversion. Passive ROM testing and talocrural joint accessory motion testing were deferred at the time of the initial examination because the fibular fracture was not healed. Accessory motion testing of the foot was deferred because the swelling was so extensive that the examiner could not assess the amount of motion present.

The causes of the patient's loss of function and pain appeared to be clear at the time of the examination. The loss of function (inability to walk without a limp and inability to participate in sports) was hypothesized to be due to the unhealed fibular fracture, the edema, and the pain produced by the inflammation that resulted from the extensive tissue damage. The inflammation and pain also appeared to result in loss of active ROM (AROM). Unfortunately, many examination procedures (e.g., accessory motion tests) could not be done because of the patient's condition. Because many procedures were not done at the time of the examination, the possibility existed that this hypothesis was incomplete and would need modification as the patient's condition improved.

TREATMENT

The treatment was designed to address the causes of loss of function, which were thought to be the swelling and inflammation that resulted from the tissue trauma. According to the physician, the fibular fracture was healed shortly after physical therapy began. The fibular fracture, therefore, was no longer considered as one of the causes of the patient's loss of function.

The treatment strategy was to use compression therapy, cryotherapy, and exercise to decrease swelling and inflammation and increase the patient's AROM. The patient was seen twice a week. The treatment was Jobst's compression therapy for 20 to 30 minutes, ice packs, pain-free non–weight-bearing active exercise into plantar flexion and dorsiflexion, and active assistive exercise into dorsiflexion and plantar flexion. The patient was instructed to use a towel looped over her foot to pull the foot into dorsiflexion and to hold the foot in an end-range dorsiflexed position for a total of 10 seconds. The end-range position was defined as the position in which the patient felt only a stretch in the ankle or calf. She was instructed to perform this exercise at least 10 times a day.

The patient's swelling decreased significantly in the first 2 weeks of therapy. In addition, her AROM improved to −4 degrees of dorsiflexion and 44 degrees of plantar flexion. However, the patient was still unable to walk without a limp. Because the physician reported that the fibular fracture was healed, the patient's passive ROM (PROM) and accessory motion of the in-

volved foot and ankle were assessed. The accessory motion of posterior and anterior glide of the talocrural joint and the accessory motion of the tarsal and tarsometatarsal joints were found to be decreased compared to those of the uninvolved side. Passive plantar flexion and dorsiflexion were also limited at this time. The end feels for all accessory motions and plantar flexion and dorsiflexion were classified as firm.

The hypothesis required modification based on the findings of decreased accessory motion and PROM, especially of the talocrural joint. The patient's functional loss appeared at this time to be due to the edema, inflammation, and resultant loss of AROM. In addition, the loss of ankle and foot (especially talocrural joint) accessory motion and PROM appeared to contribute to the patient's functional loss.

Because the hypothesis was modified, the treatment was also modified. Joint mobilization procedures were begun. Posterior glides of the talocrural joint were done. It was felt that the patient's loss of dorsiflexion was the impairment that contributed most to her abnormal gait pattern. Treatment was therefore directed at restoring normal dorsiflexion ROM and normal posterior glide. The posterior glides to the talocrural joint were done in the following way. The patient was positioned in long sitting with her involved foot off the edge of the treatment table. The examiner placed one hand over the dorsal aspect of the talus and foot while the other hand supported the involved leg. The treatment consisted of five sets of 30 posterior talar glide mobilization procedures. The mobilizations were each held at the end-range position for 1 second. The five sets were separated by a 10-second stretch into dorsiflexion. In addition, the treatment described previously that was designed to address the inflammation, edema, and decreased motion was continued.

On the seventh visit the patient was no longer using crutches. The limp was still present. The treatment approach described previously was continued except that the posterior glides were done more aggressively. Five sets of approximately 50 mobilizations were done, holding the last 10 mobilizations at the end-range position for approximately 10 seconds. The patient's AROM at this time was 7 degrees of dorsiflexion, 55 degrees of plantar flexion, 35 degrees of inversion, and 30 degrees of eversion. By the 14th treatment the patient had 9 degrees of dorsiflexion and still had her limp during gait. Specifically, the patient was observed to have a decreased stance time on the involved side with an early heel rise. It was hypothesized that the patient had a bone block into dorsiflexion that caused the limp. The physician was informed that the patient appeared to have a bone block that prevented further gains into dorsiflexion and secondarily resulted in the limp.

The patient was seen by a second orthopaedic surgeon. Radiographs were taken with the patient in an end-range position of dorsiflexion and plantar flexion (Fig. 9–40). The radiographs showed that the patient's dorsiflexion and plantar flexion were limited secondary to the talus abutting against the mortise in both end-

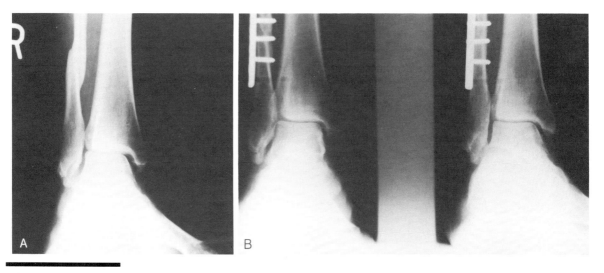

**FIGURE 9-40** ■ Radiographs of the patient's ankle before (A) and after (B) a surgical procedure designed to realign the mortise of the ankle. Note the malalignment of the ankle mortise in (A).

range positions. The physician concluded that the patient had a malunion of the fibula that resulted in an abnormally shaped ankle mortise. The ankle mortise did not permit a normal amount of talocrural joint dorsiflexion and plantar flexion.

The patient underwent a surgical procedure designed to realign the fibular malunion. She is currently receiving physical therapy in a different practice.

These case studies were chosen because they illustrate how the HOAC can be used as a format for clinical problem solving for patients with problems of the foot and ankle. The HOAC requires the therapist to hypothesize causes of the patient's functional complaints and base treatment on those hypotheses. In the first case study the therapist could adequately test the legitimacy of the hypothesis. In the second case study, the therapist hypothesized that the patient's functional deficit was due to a structural malalignment. The only way to test the legitimacy of this hypothesis was to refer the patient to an orthopaedic surgeon.

## SUMMARY

An attempt has been made to provide a scientifically based description of the anatomy, biomechanics, pathomechanics, evaluation, and treatment of the foot and ankle. Literature was reviewed where applicable to describe the usefulness of the examination and treatment approaches for patients with disorders of the foot and ankle. In addition, case studies were provided to illustrate the use of the HOAC, a theoretically sound conceptual model for use in solving patients' clinical problems.

## Acknowledgments

I would like to thank Michael Kelo, PT, for his assistance with the Case Studies.

## References

1. Manter JF: Movements of the subtalar and transverse tarsal joints. Anat Rec 80:397–410, 1941.
2. Hicks JH: The mechanics of the foot—Part 1: the joints. J Anat 87:345–357, 1953.
3. Inman VT: UC-BL dual-axis ankle-control system and UC-BL shoe insert: biomechanical considerations. Bull Prosthet Res 10:130–145, 1969.
4. Rothstein JM, Echternach JL: Hypothesis oriented algorithm for clinicians: a method for evaluation and treatment planning. Phys Ther 66:1388–1394, 1986.
5. Williams PL, Warwick R: Gray's Anatomy, 36th ed. Philadelphia: WB Saunders, 1980.
6. Inman VT: The Joints of the Ankle. Baltimore: Waverly Press, 1976.
7. Huson A: Joints and movements of the foot: Terminology and Concepts. Acta Morphol Neerl-Scand 25:117–130, 1987.
8. Lehmkulh LD, Smith LK: Brunnstrom's Clinical Kinesiology, 4th ed. Philadelphia: FA Davis, 1983, pp 6–8.
9. Steindler A: Kinesiology of the Human Body Under Normal and Pathological Conditions. Springfield, IL: Charles C Thomas, 1964.
10. Sage GH: Introduction to Motor Behavior: A Neuropsychological Approach. Reading, MA: Addison-Wesley Publishing Co., 1977, p 89.
11. Newton RA: Joint receptor contributions to reflexive and kinesthetic responses. Phys Ther 62:22–29, 1982.
12. Elveru RA, Rothstein JM, Lamb RL, et al: Methods for taking subtalar joint measurements: a clinical report. Phys Ther 68:678–682, 1988.
13. Kapandji IA: The Physiology of the Joints. New York: Churchill Livingstone, 1970.
14. Sarrafian SK: Anatomy of the Foot and Ankle. Philadelphia: JB Lippincott, 1983.

15. McMinn RMH, Hutchings RT, Logan BM: A Color Atlas of Foot and Ankle Anatomy. London: Wolfe Medical Publications, 1982.

16. Riegger CL: Anatomy of the ankle and foot. Phys Ther 68:1802–1814, 1988.

17. Kelikian H, Kelikian AS: Disorders of the Ankle. Philadelphia, WB Saunders, 1985.

18. Grant JCB: Grant's Atlas of Anatomy, 5th ed. Baltimore: Williams & Wilkins, 1962, p 356.

19. Helal B, Wilson D: The Foot. New York: Churchill Livingstone, 1988.

20. Greenfield GB: Radiology of Bone Diseases. Philadelphia: JB Lippincott, 1969.

21. Draves DJ: Anatomy of the Lower Extremity. Baltimore: Williams & Wilkins, 1986, pp 126–140.

22. Skraba JS, Greenwald AS: The role of the interosseous membrane on tibiofibular weightbearing. Foot Ankle 4:301–304, 1984.

23. Barnett CH, Napier JR: The axis of rotation of the ankle joint in man. Its influence upon the form of the talus and the mobility of the fibula. J Anat 86:1–9, 1952.

24. Greenwald AS: Ankle joint mechanics. In Ankle Injuries (Yablon IG, Segal D, Leach RE, eds). New York: Churchill-Livingstone, 1983, pp 253–264.

25. Soderberg GL: Kinesiology: Application to Pathological Motion. Baltimore: Williams & Wilkins, 1986.

26. Reference deleted.

27. Steinbach HL, Russell W: Measurement of the heel pad as an aid to diagnosis of acromegaly. Radiology 82:418–423, 1964.

28. Bojsen-Moller F, Jorgenson U: The plantar soft tissue: functional anatomy and clinical applications. In Disorders of the Foot and Ankle: Medical and Surgical Management, 2nd ed (Jahss MH, ed). Philadelphia: WB Saunders, 1991, pp 523–540.

29. Winter WG, Reiss OK: Anatomy and physiology of the heel pad. In Disorders of the Foot and Ankle: Medical and Surgical Management, 2nd ed (Jahss MH, ed). Philadelphia: WB Saunders, 1991, pp 2745–2752.

30. Kuhns JG: Changes in elastic adipose tissue. J Bone Joint Surg [Am] 31:541–547, 1949.

31. Jorgensen U: Achillodynia and loss of heel pad shock absorbency. Am J Sports Med 13:128–132, 1985.

32. Tietze A: Concerning the architectural structure of the connective tissue in the human sole. Foot Ankle 2:252–259, 1982.

33. Reference deleted.

34. Jahss MH, Kaye RA, Desai P, et al: Histology, histochemistry and biomechanics of the plantar fat pads. In Disorders of the Foot and Ankle: Medical and Surgical Management, 2nd ed (Jahss MH, ed). Philadelphia: WB Saunders, 1991, pp 2753–2762.

35. Hicks JH: The mechanics of the foot—Part 2: the plantar aponeurosis and the arch. J Anat 88:25–30, 1954.

36. Hicks JH: The foot as a support. Acta Anat 25:34–45, 1955.

37. Hicks JH: The mechanics of the foot—Part 4: the action of the muscles on the foot in standing. Acta Anat 27:180–192, 1957.

38. Hicks JH: The three weight-bearing mechanisms of the foot. In Biomechanical Studies of the Musculo-Skeletal System (Evans FG, ed). Springfield, IL: Charles C Thomas, 1961.

39. Sarrafian SK: Functional characteristics of the foot and plantar aponeurosis under tibiotalar loading. Foot Ankle 8:4–18, 1987.

40. Basmajian JV, Stecko G: The role of muscles in arch support of the foot. J Bone Joint Surg [Am] 45:1184–1190, 1963.

41. Mann RA, Inman VT: Phasic activity of intrinsic muscles of the foot. J Bone Joint Surg [Am] 66:469–481, 1964.

42. Funk DA, Cass JR, Johnson KA: Acquired adult flat foot secondary to posterior tibial tendon pathology. J Bone Joint Surg [Am] 68:95–102, 1986.

43. Mann RA, Thompson FM: Rupture of the posterior tibial tendon causing flat foot. J Bone Joint Surg [Am] 67:556–561, 1985.

44. Johnson KA: Tibialis posterior tendon rupture. Clin Orthop 177:140–147, 1983.

45. Mann RA: Acquired flatfoot in adults. Clin Orthop Relat Res 181:46–51, 1983.

46. Sutherland DH: An electromyographic study of the plantar flexors of the ankle in normal walking on the level. J Bone Joint Surg [Am] 48:66–71, 1966.

47. Reference deleted.

48. Lundberg A, Goldie I, Kalin B, et al: Kinematics of the ankle/foot complex: plantar flexion and dorsiflexion. Foot Ankle 9:194–200, 1989.

49. Lundberg A, Svensson OK, Bylund C, et al: Kinematics of the ankle/foot complex—Part 2: pronation and supination. Foot Ankle 9:248–253, 1989.

50. Lundberg A, Svensson OK, Bylund C, et al. Kinematics of the ankle/foot complex. Part 3: Influence of leg rotation. Foot Ankle 9:304–309, 1989.

51. Isman RE, Inman VT: Anthropometric studies of the human foot and ankle. Bull Prosthet Res 10–11:97–129, 1969.

52. Elftman H: The orientation of the joints of the lower extremity. Bull Hosp Jt Dis 6:139–143, 1945.

53. Soudan K, Van Audekercke R, Martens M: Methods, difficulties and inaccuracies in the study of human joint kinematics and pathokinematics by the instant axis concept. Example: the knee joint. J Biomech 12:27–33, 1979.

54. Frankel UH, Burstein AH: Orthopaedic Biomechanics. Philadelphia: Lea & Febiger, 1970.

55. Sammarco GJ, Burstein AH, Frankel VH: Biomechanics of the ankle: a kinematic study. Orthop Clinic North Am 4:75–96, 1973.

56. D'Ambrosia RD, Shoji H, Van Meter J: Rotational axis of the ankle joint: comparison of normal and pathologic states. Surg Forum 27:507–508, 1976.

57. Lundberg A, Svensson OK, Nemeth G, et al: The axis of rotation of the ankle joint. J Bone Joint Surg [Br] 71:94–99, 1989.

58. Frankel VH, Burstein AH, Brooks DB: Biomechanics of internal derangement of the knee: pathomechanics as determined by analysis of the instant centers of motion. J Bone Joint Surg [Am] 53:945–962, 1971.

59. Gardner E, Gray DJ, O'Rahilly R: Anatomy: A Regional Study of Human Structure, 3rd ed. Philadelphia: WB Saunders, 1969.

60. Crafts RC: A Textbook of Human Anatomy, 2nd ed. New York: John Wiley & Sons, 1979.

61. Reference deleted.

62. Levens AS, Inman VT, Blosser JA: Transverse rotations of the lower extremity in locomotion. J Bone Joint Surg [Am] 30:859–872, 1948.

63. Inman VT, Ralston HJ, Todd F: Human Walking. Baltimore: Williams & Wilkins, 1981.

64. Root ML, Weed JH, Sgarlato TE, et al: Axis of motion of the subtalar joint. J Am Podiatr Med Assoc 56:149–155, 1966.

65. Inman VT, Mann RA: Biomechanics of the foot and ankle. In Surgery of the Foot, 3rd ed (Inman VT, ed). St. Louis: CV Mosby, 1973.

66. Novick A: Anatomy and biomechanics. In Physical

Therapy of the Foot and Ankle (Hunt GC, ed). New York: Churchill Livingstone, 1988.

67. Van Langelaan EJ: A kinematical analysis of the tarsal joints. Acta Orthop Scand [Suppl] 204:211–239, 1983.

68. Benink RJ: The constraint mechanism of the human tarsus: a roentgenological experimental study. Acta Orthop Scand [Suppl] 215:1–135, 1985.

69. Donatelli R: The Biomechanics of the Foot. Philadelphia: WB Saunders, 1990.

70. Hallen LG, Lindahl O: The "screw home" movement in the knee joint. Acta Orthop Scand 37:97–106, 1966.

71. Tiberio D: The effect of excessive subtalar joint pronation on patellofemoral mechanics: a theoretical model. J Orthop Sports Phys Ther 9:160–165, 1987.

72. Sims DS, Cavanaugh PR: Selected foot mechanics related to the prescription of foot orthoses. In Disorders of the Foot and Ankle: Medical and Surgical Management, 2nd ed (Jahss MH, ed). Philadelphia: WB Saunders, 1991, pp 469–483.

73. Elftman H: The transverse tarsal joint and its control. Clin Orthop Relat Res 16:41–45, 1960.

74. Mann RA: Biomechanics of the foot. In American Academy of Orthopedic Surgeons' Atlas of Orthotics: Biomechanical Principles and Application. St. Louis: CV Mosby, 1975, pp 250–260.

75. Seirig A, Arvikar RJ: The prediction of muscular load sharing and joint forces in the lower extremities during walking. J Biomech 8:89–102, 1975.

76. Burdett RG: Forces predicted at the ankle during running. Med Sci Sports Exercise 14:308–316, 1982.

77. Greenwald AS, Matejczyk MB, Keppler L, et al: Preliminary observations on the weight-bearing surfaces of the human ankle joint. Surg Forum 27:505–506, 1976.

78. Wynarsky FT, Greenwald AS: Mathematical model of the human ankle joint. J Biomech 16:241–251, 1983.

79. Maitland GD: Peripheral Manipulation, 2nd ed. London: Butterworths, 1977.

80. Cyriax J: Textbook of Orthopaedic Medicine—Diagnosis of Soft Tissue Lesions, Vol 1. London: Bailliere Tindall, 1982.

81. Price DD, Harkins SW, Baker C: Sensory-affective relationships among different types of clinical and experimental pain. Pain 28(3):297–307, 1987.

82. Fromherz WA: Examination. In Physical Therapy of the Foot and Ankle (Hunt GC, ed). New York: Churchill-Livingstone, 1988.

83. Elveru RA, Rothstein JM, Lamb RL: Goniometric reliability in a clinical setting: subtalar and ankle measurements. Phys Ther 68:672–677, 1988.

84. Diamond JE, Mueller MJ, Delito A, et al: Reliability of a diabetic foot evaluation. Phys Ther 69:797–802, 1989.

85. Kaltenborn FM: Manual Mobilization of the Extremity Joints: Basic Examination and Treatment Techniques, 4th ed. Oslo: Olaf Norlis Bokhandel, 1989.

86. Lamb RL: Manual muscle testing. In Measurement in Physical Therapy (Rothstein JM, ed). New York: Churchill Livingstone, 1985.

87. Perry J, Ireland ML, Gronley J, et al: Predictive value of manual muscle testing and gait analysis in normal ankles by dynamic electromyography. Foot Ankle 6:254–259, 1986.

88. Rothstein JM, Lamb RL, Mayhew TP: Clinical uses of isokinetic measurements. Phys Ther 67:1840–1945, 1987.

89. Rasmussen O, Tovborg-Jensen I: Anterolateral rotational instability in the ankle joint. Acta Orthop Scand 52:99–102, 1981.

90. Cedell CA: Supination-outward rotation injuries of the ankle. Acta Orthop Scand [Suppl] 110:1–148, 1967.

91. Thompson TC, Doherty JH: Spontaneous rupture of tendon of Achilles: a new clinical diagnostic test. J Trauma 2:126–129, 1962.

92. Subotnik SI: Leg length of the lower extremity. J Orthop Sports Phys Ther 3:11–16, 1981.

92a. Anderson WV: Modern Trends in Orthopaedics. New York: Appleton-Century-Crofts, 1972.

93. Beattie P, Isaacson K, Riddle DL, et al: Validity and reliability of measurements of leg length differences obtained with a tape measure. Phys Ther 70:150–157, 1990.

94. Shrout PE, Fleiss JL: Intraclass correlations: uses in assessing rater reliability. Psychol Bull 86:420–428, 1979.

95. Salter RB: Textbook of Disorders and Injuries of the Musculoskeletal System, 2nd ed. Baltimore: Williams & Wilkins, 1983.

96. Pankovich AM: Trauma to the ankle. In Disorders of the Foot and Ankle: Medical and Surgical Management, 2nd ed (Jahss MH, ed)., Vol 3. Philadelphia: WB Saunders, 1991, pp 2361–2414.

97. Lauge-Hansen N: Fractures of the ankle. II. Combined experimental-surgical and experimental-roentgenological investigation. Arch Surg 60:957–972, 1950.

98. Salter RB, Harris WR: Injuries involving the epiphyseal plate. J Bone Joint Surg [Am] 45:587, 1963.

99. Siffert RS, Weiner LS, Feldman DJ: Trauma to the child's foot and ankle, including growth-plate and epiphyseal injuries. In Disorders of the Foot and Ankle: Medical and Surgical Management, 2nd ed (Jahss MH, ed). Philadelphia: WB Saunders, 1991, pp 2514–2546.

100. Kling TF, Bright RW, Hensinger RN: Distal tibial physeal fractures in children that may require open reduction. J Bone Joint Surg [Am] 66:647, 1984.

101. Sanders R, Hansen ST, McReynolds IS: Trauma to the calcaneus and its tendon. In Disorders of the Foot and Ankle: Medical and Surgical Management, 2nd ed (Jahss MH, ed). Philadelphia: WB Saunders, 1991, pp 2326–2354.

102. King RE, Powell DF: Injury to the talus. In Disorders of the Foot and Ankle: Medical and Surgical Management, 2nd ed (Jahss MH, ed). Philadelphia: WB Saunders, 1991, pp 2293–2325.

103. Canale ST, Belding RH: Osteochondral lesions of the talus. J Bone Joint Surg 62A:97–102, 1980.

104. Coker TP: Sports injuries to the foot and ankle. In Disorders of the Foot and Ankle: Medical and Surgical Management, 2nd ed (Jahss MH, ed). Philadelphia: WB Saunders, 1991, pp 2415–2445.

105. Myerson MS: Injuries to the forefoot and toes. In Disorders of the Foot and Ankle: Medical and Surgical Management, 2nd ed (Jahss MH, ed)., Vol 3. Philadelphia: WB Saunders, 1991, pp 2233–2273.

106. Zelko RR, Torg JS, Rachun A: Proximal diaphyseal fractures of the fifth metatarsal—treatment of the fractures and their complications in athletes. Am J Sports Med 7:95, 1979.

107. Kavanaugh JH, Brower TD, Mann RV: The Jones fracture revisited. J Bone Joint Surg [Am] 60:776, 1978.

108. McBride AM: Stress fractures in athletes. Am J Sports Med 3:212, 1975.

109. Drez D, Young JC, Johnston RD, et al: Metatarsal stress fractures. Am J Sports Med 8:123, 1980.

110. Orava S, Puranen J, Ala-Ketola L: Stress fractures caused by physical exercise. Acta Orthop Scand 49:19, 1978.

111. Inge GL, Ferguson AB: Surgery of the sesamoid bones of the great toe. Arch Surg 21:456, 1933.

112. Jaffe WL, Gannon PF, Laitman JT: Paleontology, embryology and anatomy of the foot. In Disorders of the

Foot and Ankle: Medical and Surgical Management, 2nd ed. (Jahss MH, ed). Philadelphia: WB Saunders, 1991, pp 3–34.

113. Hobart MH: Fracture of the sesamoid bones of the foot. J Bone Joint Surg 27:298–302, 1929.

114. Van Hal ME, Keene JS, Lange TA, et al: Stress fractures of the great toe sesamoids. Am J Sports Med 10:122–128, 1982.

115. Clement DB: Stress fractures of the foot and ankle. In Foot and Ankle in Sport and Exercise (Shephard RJ, Taunton JE, eds). New York: Karger, 1987, pp 56–70.

116. Stedman's Medical Dictionary, 25th ed. Baltimore: Williams & Wilkins, 1990.

117. Tiberio D: Pathomechanics of structural foot deformities. Phys Ther 68:1840–1849, 1988.

118. Lutter LD: Cavus foot in runners. Foot Ankle 1:225–228, 1981.

119. Subotnik SI: The cavus foot. Physician Sports Med 8:53–55, 1980.

120. O'Donoghue DH: Treatment of Injuries to Athletes. Philadelphia: WB Saunders, 1976.

121. Bleck EE, Berzins UJ: Conservative management of pes valgus with plantar flexed talus, flexible. Clin Orthop Relat Res 122:85–94, 1977.

122. Bordelon RL: Correction of hypermobile flatfoot in children by molded insert. Foot Ankle 1:143–150, 1980.

123. Duckworth T: The hindfoot and its relation to rotational deformities of the forefoot. Clin Orthop Relat Res 177:39–48, 1983.

124. Tachdjian MT: The Child's Foot. Philadelphia: WB Saunders, 1985.

125. Wynne-Davies R: Family studies and cause of congenital clubfoot. J Bone Joint Surg [Br] 46:445–463, 1964.

126. Irani RN, Sherman MS: The pathological anatomy of idiopathic clubfoot. Clin Orthop Relat Res 84:14–20, 1972.

127. Goldner JL, Fitch RD: Idiopathic congenital taliper equinovarus (clubfoot). In Disorders of the Foot and Ankle: Medical and Surgical Management, 2nd ed (Jahss MH, ed). Philadelphia: WB Saunders, 1991, p 793.

128. Bernhardt DB: Prenatal and postnatal growth and development of the foot and ankle. Phys Ther 68:1831–1839, 1988.

129. Tax H: Podopediatrics. Baltimore: Williams & Wilkins, 1980, pp 14–20.

130. Sgarlato TE: A Compendium of Podiatric Biomechanics. San Francisco: California College of Podiatric Medicine, 1971.

131. Root ML, Orien WP, Weed JH: Biomechanical Examination of the Foot, Vol 1. Los Angeles: Clinical Biomechanics, 1971.

132. Bouche RT, Kuwada GT: Equinus deformity in the athlete. Physician Sports Med 12:81–91, 1984.

133. Inman VT, Ralston HJ, Todd F: Human Walking. Baltimore: Williams & Wilkins, 1981.

134. Gould N, Seligson D: Early and late repair of the lateral ligament of the ankle. Foot Ankle 1:84–89, 1980.

135. Pankovich AM, Shivaram MS: Anatomical basis of variability in injuries of the medial malleolus and the deltoid ligament. Acta Orthop Scand 50:225–236, 1979.

136. Nicholas J, Hershman EB: The Lower Extremity and Spine in Sports Medicine. St. Louis: CV Mosby, 1986.

137. McConkey JP: Ankle sprains, consequences and mimics. In Foot and Ankle in Sport and Exercise (Shephard RJ, Taunton JE, eds). New York: Karger, 1987, pp 39–55.

138. Leach RE: Acute ankle sprains: Vigorous treatment for best results. J Musculoskel Med 1:68–76, 1983.

139. Schon LC, Ouzounian TJ: The ankle. In Disorders of the Foot and Ankle: Medical and Surgical Management, 2nd

ed (Jahss MH, ed). Philadelphia: WB Saunders, 1991, 1417–1460.

140. Cholmeley JA: Hallux valgus in adolescants. Proc R Soc Med 51:903–906, 1958.

141. Scranton PE, Zuckerman JD: Bunions surgery in adolescents: results of surgical treatment. J Pediatr Orthop 4:39–43, 1984.

142. Goldner JL: Hallux valgus and hallux flexus associated with cerebral palsy: analysis and treatment. Clin Orthop Rel Res 157:98–104, 1981.

143. Inman VT: Hallux valgus: A review of etiologic factors. Ortho Clin North Am 5:59–66, 1974.

144. Jahss MH: Disorders of the hallux and the first ray. In Disorders of the Foot and Ankle: Medical and Surgical Management, 2nd ed (Jahss MH, ed). Philadelphia: WB Saunders, 1991, 945–971.

145. Kelikian H: Hallux Valgus, Allied Deformities of the Forefoot and Metatarsalgia. Philadelphia: WB Saunders, 1965, pp 213–225.

146. Kalen V, Brecher A: Relationship between adolescent bunions and flatfeet. Foot Ankle 8:331–336, 1988.

147. Mann RA, Coughlin MJ: Lesser toe deformities. In Disorders of the Foot and Ankle: Medical and Surgical Management, 2nd ed (Jahss MH, ed). Philadelphia: WB Saunders, 1991, pp 1205–1288.

148. Brahms MA: The small toes: Corns and deformities of the small toes. In Disorders of the Foot and Ankle: Medical and Surgical Management, 2nd ed (Jahss MH, ed). Philadelphia: WB Saunders, 1991, pp 1175–1197.

149. Kues J: The pathology of shin splints. J Orthop Sports Phys Ther 12:115–122, 1990.

150. DeLacerda FG: Iontophoresis for treatment of shin splints. J Orthop Sports Phys Ther 3:183–185, 1982.

151. D'Ambrosia RD, Zelis RF, Chuinard RO, et al: Interstitial pressure measurements in the anterior and posterior compartment in athletes with shin splints. Am J Sports Med 5:127–131, 1977.

152. O'Donoghue DH: Treatment of Injuries to Athletes. Philadelphia: WB Saunders, 1976.

153. Scheuch PA: Tibialis posterior shin splint: diagnosis and treatment. Athletic Training 19:271–274, 1984.

154. Radin EL: Tarsal tunnel syndrome. Clin Orthop Relat Res 181:167–170, 1983.

154a. Mann RA: Diseases of the nerves of the foot. In Surgery of the Foot, 5th ed (Mann RA, ed). St. Louis: CV Mosby, 1986, pp 205–207.

155. Viladot A: The metatarsals. In Disorders of the Foot and Ankle: Medical and Surgical Management, 2nd ed (Jahss MH, ed). Philadelphia: WB Saunders, 1991, pp 1229–1268.

156. Mann RA, Reynolds JD: Interdigital neuroma: a critical analysis. Foot Ankle 3:238, 1983.

157. Alexander IJ, Johnson KA: Reflex sympathetic dystrophy syndrome. In Disorders of the Foot and Ankle: Medical and Surgical Management, 2nd ed (Jahss MH, ed). Philadelphia: WB Saunders, 1991, pp 2187–2191.

158. Solomon G: Inflammatory arthritis. In Disorders of the Foot and Ankle: Medical and Surgical Management, 2nd ed (Jahss MH, ed). Philadelphia: WB Saunders, 1991.

159. Reiter H: As described by Solomon G in The Foot in Systemic and Acquired Disorders. In Disorders of the Foot and Ankle: Medical and Surgical Management, 2nd ed (Jahss MH, ed). Philadelphia: WB Saunders, 1991.

160. Rana NA: Rheumatoid arthritis, other collagen diseases, and psoriasis of the foot. In Disorders of the Foot and Ankle: Medical and Surgical Management, 2nd ed (Jahss MH, ed)., Vol 3. Philadelphia: WB Saunders, 1991, pp 1719–1751.

161. Scarpa R, Oriente P, Pucino A, et al: Psoriatic arthritis in psoriatic patients. Br J Rheumatol 23:246, 1984.

162. Arnett FC, Edworthy S, Bloch DA, et al: The American Rheumatism Association 1987 revised criteria for the classification of rheumatoid arthritis. Arthritis Rheum 31:315–324, 1988.

163. Kay DB: The sprained ankle: current therapy. Foot Ankle 6:22–27, 1985.

164. Smith RW, Reischl SF: Treatment of ankle sprains in young athletes. Am J Sports Med 14:465–471, 1986.

165. Pope MH, Johnson RJ, Brown DW, et al: The role of the musculature in injuries to the medial collateral ligament. J Bone Joint Surg [Am] 61:398–402, 1979.

166. Jones GM, Watt DGD: Observations on the control of stepping and hopping movements in man. J Physiol (Lond) 219:709–727, 1971.

167. Jones GM, Watt DGD: Muscular control of landing from unexpected falls in man. J Physiol (Lond) 219:729–737, 1971.

168. Freeman MAR: Instability of the foot after injuries to the lateral ligament of the foot. J Bone Joint Surg [Br] 47:669–677, 1965.

169. Tropp H, Ekstrand J, Gillquist J: Factors affecting stabilometry recordings of single limb stance. Am J Sports Med 12:185–188, 1984.

170. Tropp H, Ekstrand J, Gillquist J: Stabilometry in functional instability of the ankle and its value in predicting injury. Med Sci Sport Exercise 16:64–66, 1984.

171. Tropp H, Askling C, Gillquist J: Prevention of ankle sprains. Am J Sports Med 13:259–262, 1985.

172. Blake RL, Denton JA: Functional foot orthoses for athletic injuries. J Am Podiatr Med Assoc 75:359–362, 1985.

173. Milgrom C, Giladi M, Kashdan H, et al: A prospective study of the effect of a shock-absorbing orthotic device on the incidence of stress fractures in military recruits. Foot Ankle 6:101–104, 1985.

174. Schwellnus MP, Jordaan G, Noakes TD: Prevention of common overuse injuries by the use of shock absorbing insoles. Am J Sports Med 18:636–641, 1990.

175. Gardner LI, Dziados JE, Jones BH, et al: Prevention of lower extremity stress fractures: a controlled trial of a shock absorbing insole. Am J Public Health 78:1563–1567, 1988.

176. Gross ML, Davlin LB, Evanski PM: Effectiveness of orthotic shoe inserts in the long-distance runner. Am J Sports Med 19:409–412, 1991.

177. Smith LS, Clarke TE, Hamill CL, et al: The effects of soft and semi-rigid orthoses upon rearfoot movement in running. J Am Podiatr Med Assoc 76:227–233, 1986.

178. Bates BT, Osternig LR, Mason B, et al: Foot orthotic devices to modify selected aspects of lower extremity mechanics. Am J Sports Med 7:338–342, 1979.

179. Rodgers MM, Leveau BF: Effectiveness of foot orthotic devices used to modify pronation in runners. J Orthop Sports Phys Ther 4:86–93, 1982.

180. Katoh Y, Chao EYS, Morrey BF, et al: Objective technique for evaluating painful heel syndrome and its treatment. Foot Ankle 3:227–237, 1983.

181. Taunton JE, Clement DB, Smart GW, et al: A triplanar electrogoniometer investigation of running mechanics in runners with compensatory over pronation. Can J Appl Sports Sci 10:104–115, 1985.

182. Hice GA, Kendrick Z, Weeber K, et al: The effect of foot orthoses on oxygen consumption while cycling. J Am Podiatr Med Assoc 75:513–516, 1985.

183. Berg K, Sady S: Oxygen cost of running at submaximal speeds while wearing shoe inserts. Res Q Exerc Sport 56:86–89, 1985.

184. Clancy WG: Tendinitis and plantar fascitis in runners. In Prevention and Treatment of Running Injuries (D'Ambrosia R, Drez D, eds). Thorofare, NJ: Charles B. Slack, 1982, pp 77–78.

185. Fox JM, Blazina ME, Jobe FW, et al: Degeneration and rupture of the achilles tendon. Clin Orthop Relat Res 107:201–204, 1975.

186. Smart GW, Taunton JE, Clement DB: Achilles tendon disorders in runners—a review. Med Sci Sport Exercise 12:231–243, 1980.

187. Curwin S, Stanish WD: Tendinitis: its etiology and treatment. Lexington, MA: Callamore Press, 1984.

188. Stanish WD, Rubinovich RM, Curwin S: Eccentric exercise in chronic tendinitis. Clin Orthop Relat Res 208:65–68, 1986.

189. Stanish WD, Curwin S, Rubinovich RM: Tendinitis: The analysis and treatment for running. Clin Sports Med 4:593–609, 1985.

## Bibliography

Allard P, Duhaime M, Labelle H, et al: Spatial reconstruction technique and kinematic modeling of the ankle. Transaction on Biomedical Engineering 6:31–36, 1987.

Anderson WV: Modern Trends in Orthopaedics. New York: Appleton-Century-Crofts, 1972.

Bailey DS, Perillo JT, Forman M: Subtalar joint neutral: a study using tomography. J Am Podiatr Med Assoc 74:59–64, 1984.

Benas D, Jokl P: Shin splints. Am J Corrective Ther 32:53–57, 1976.

Bernstein A, Stone JR: March fracture: a report of three hundred and seven cases, and a new method of treatment. J Bone Joint Surg 26:743, 1944.

Bosien WR, Staples OS, Russell SW, et al: Residual disability following acute ankle sprains. J Bone Joint Surg [Am] 37:1237–1243, 1955.

Brand PW: The insensitive limb (special issue). Phys Ther 59:8–33, 1979.

Brenner MA, ed: Management of the Diabetic Foot. Baltimore: Williams & Wilkins, 1987.

Brody DM: Running Injuries. Ciba Clin Symp 32:1–36, 1980.

Chusid JG, ed: Correlative Neuroanatomy and Functional Neurology. Los Altos, CA: Lange, 1979.

Ciccone CD: Pharmacology in Rehabilitation. Philadelphia: FA Davis, 1990.

Close JR, Inman VT, Poor PM, et al: The function of the subtalar joint. Clin Orthop 50:159–179, 1967.

Cox JS, Brand RL: Evaluation and treatment of lateral sprains. Phys Sports Med 5:51–55, 1977.

Engh CA, Robinson RA, Milgram J: Stress fractures in children. J Trauma 10:532–541, 1970.

Engsberg JR: A biomechanical analysis of the talocalcaneal joint—in vitro. J Biomech 20:429–442, 1987.

Frankel VH, Burstein AH: Orthopaedic Biomechanics. Philadelphia: Lea & Febiger, 1979.

Freeman MAR, Dean MRE, Hanham IWF: The etiology and prevention of functional instability of the foot. J Bone Joint Surg [Br] 47:678–685, 1965.

Freeman MAR, Wyke B: Articular reflexes at the ankle joint: an electromyographic study of normal and abnormal influences of ankle joint mechanoreceptors upon reflex activity in the leg muscles. Br J Surg 54:990–1000, 1967.

Freer DH: The treatment and evaluation of ankle sprains. J Am Podiatr Assoc 73:337–343, 1983.

Frost HM, Hanson CA: Techniques for testing the drawer

sign in the ankle. Clin Orthop Relat Res 123:49–51, 1977.

Green DR, Whitney AK, Walters P: Subtalar joint motion: a simplified view. J Am Podiatr Assoc 69:83–91, 1979.

Greenwald AS, Matejczyk MB, Keppler L, et al: Preliminary observations on the weight-bearing surfaces of the human ankle joint. Surg Forum 27:505–506, 1976.

Greenwald AS: Ankle joint mechanics. In Ankle Injuries (Yablon IG, Segal D, Leach RE, eds). New York: Churchill-Livingstone, 1983, pp 253–264.

Hicks JH: The mechanics of the foot—Part 2: the plantar aponeurosis and the arch. J Anat 88:25–30, 1954.

Hill JJ, Cutting PJ: Heel pain and body weight. Foot Ankle 9:254–255, 1989.

Hlavac HF: The Foot Book. Mountain View, CA: World Publications, 1977.

Horstman JK, Kantor GS, Samuelson KM, et al: Investigation of lateral ankle ligament reconstruction. Foot Ankle 1:338–342, 1981.

Hunt GC, ed: Physical Therapy of the Foot and Ankle. New York: Churchill-Livingstone, 1988.

Hunt GC: Examination of lower extremity dysfunction. In Orthopaedic and Sports Physical Therapy (Gould JA III, Davies GJ, eds), Vol 2. St. Louis: CV Mosby, 1985, pp 408–436.

Hurwitz S: Surgical overview. In Physical Therapy of the Foot and Ankle (Hunt GC, ed). New York: Churchill-Livingstone, 1988, pp 315–330.

Inman VT, ed: DuVries' Surgery of the Foot. St. Louis: CV Mosby, 1973.

Inman VT, Mann RA: Biomechanics of the foot and ankle. In DuVries' Surgery of the Foot (Inman VT, ed). St. Louis: CV Mosby, 1978, pp 3–21.

James SL, Bates BT, Osternig LR: Injuries to runners. Am J Sports Med 6:40–49, 1978.

Johnson EE, Markolf KL: The contribution of the anterior talofibular ligament to ankle laxity. J Bone Joint Surg 65:81–88, 1983.

Jordon RP, Coupe M, Schuster RO: Ankle dorsiflexion at the heel off phase of gait. J Am Podiatr Med Assoc 69:40–43, 1979.

Kapandji IA: The Physiology of the Joints, Vol 2, Lower Limb. New York: Churchill-Livingstone, 1983.

Kelikian H, Kelikian AS: Osteocartilaginous bodies in and around the ankle joint. In Disorders of the Ankle (Kelikian H, Kelikian AS, eds). Philadelphia: WB Saunders, 1985, pp 725–758.

Kellgren JH, Samuel EP: The sensitivity and innervation of the articular capsule. J Bone Joint Surg [Br] 32:84–91, 1950.

Kessler RM, Hertling D: Management of Common Musculoskeletal Disorders, 2nd ed. New York: Harper & Row, 1990.

Kimura IF, Nawoczenski, DA, Epler M, et al: Effect of the air stirrup in controlling ankle inversion stress. J Orthop Sports Phys Ther 9:190–193, 1987.

Kirby KA: Methods of determination of positional variations in the subtalar and transverse tarsal joints. Anat Rec 80:397–410, 1947.

Lane JM, ed: Fracture Healing. New York, Churchill-Livingstone, 1987.

Lautin CA, Quellet R, St. Jacques R: Talar and subtalar tilt: an experimental investigation. Can J Surg 11:270–279, 1968.

Lehmkuhl LD, Smith LK, eds: Brunnstrom's Clinical Kinesiology, 4th ed. Philadelphia: FA Davis, 1983.

Lundberg A: Kinematics of the ankle and foot. In vivo roentgen stereophotogrammetry. Acta Orthop Scand [Suppl] 233:1–24, 1989.

MacConnaill MA, Basmajian JV: Muscles and Movements: A Basis for Human Kinesiology. Baltimore: Williams & Wilkins, 1969.

Mack RP, ed: American Academy of Orthopaedic Surgeons Symposium on the Foot and Leg in Running Sports. St. Louis: CV Mosby, 1982.

Magee DJ: Orthopedic Physical Assessment. Philadelphia: WB Saunders, 1987.

Maitland GD: Vertebral Manipulation. London: Butterworths, 1986.

Matheson GO, Clement DB, McKenzie DC, et al: Stress fractures in athletes: a study of 320 cases. Am J Sports Med,15:46–58, 1987.

Mann RA: Surgical implications of biomechanics of the foot and ankle. Clin Orthop Relat Res 146:111–118, 1980.

Mann RA, Baxter DE, Lutter LD: Running symposium. Foot Ankle 1:190–224, 1981.

Mann RA, Hagy JL, Simon SR: Biomechanics of gait: a critical visual analysis. Gait Analysis Laboratory, Shriners Hospital for Crippled Children, San Francisco, 1975.

Marti B, Vader JP, Minder CE, et al: On the epidemiology of running injuries: the 1984 Bern Grand Prix study. Am J Sports Med 16:285–293, 1988.

McMinn RM, Hutchings RT: Color Atlas of Human Anatomy. Chicago: Year Book Medical, 1983.

McPoil TG, Brocato RS: The foot and ankle: biomechanical evaluation and treatment. In Orthopaedic and Sports Physical Therapy, 2nd ed (Gould JA III, Davies GJ, eds). St. Louis: CV Mosby, 1990, pp 293–322.

Mennell JM: Joint Pain—Diagnosis and Treatment Using Manipulative Techniques. Boston: Little, Brown, 1964.

Michael RH, Holder LE: The soleus syndrome: a cause of medial tibial stress (shin splints). Am J Sports Med 13:87–94, 1985.

Mittleman G: Transverse plane abnormalities of the lower extremities: intoe and outtoe gait. J Am Podiatr Med Assoc 61:1–7, 1971.

Munro CF, Miller DI: Ground reaction forces in running: a reexamination. J Biomech 20:147–155, 1987.

Murray MP, Kory RC, Clarkson BH: Comparison of free and fast speed walking patterns of normal men. Am J Phys Med 45:8–15, 1966.

Newell SG, Miller SJ: Conservative treatment of plantar fascial strain. Physician Sports Med 5:68–73, 1977.

Nisell R, Mizrahi J: Knee and ankle joint forces during steps and jumps down from two different heights. Clin Biomech 3:92–100, 1988.

Parlasca R, Shoji H, D'Ambrosia RD: Effects of ligamentous injury on ankle and subtalar joints: a kinematic study. Clin Orthop Relat Res 140:266–272, 1979.

Perry J: Anatomy and biomechanics of the hindfoot. Clin Orthop Relat Res 177:9–15, 1983.

Physical Therapy. Special issue published on the foot and ankle. December 1988.

Procter P, Paul JP: Ankle joint biomechanics. J Biomech 15:627–634, 1982.

Quiles M, Requena F, Gomez L, et al: Functional anatomy of the medial collateral ligament of the ankle joint. Foot Ankle 4:73–82, 1983.

Rastegar J, Miller N, Barmada R: An apparatus for measuring the load-displacement and load-dependent kinematic characteristics of articulating joints—application to the human ankle. J Biomech Eng 102:208–213, 1980.

Regnauld B: The Foot: Pathology, Aetiology, Semiology, Clinical Investigation and Therapy. New York: Springer-Verlag, 1986.

Riddle DL, Freeman DB: Management of a patient with a diagnosis of bilateral plantar fasciitis and Achilles tendinitis: a case report. Phys Ther 68:1913–1916, 1988.

Rijke AM, Jones B, Vierhout PA: Injury to the lateral ankle ligaments of athletes: a posttraumatic followup. Am J Sports Med 16:256–259, 1988.

Root ML, Orien WP, Weed JH: Clinical Biomechanics: Normal and Abnormal Function of the Foot, Vol 2. Los Angeles: Clinical Biomechanics, 1971.

Ryerson SD: The foot in hemiplegia. In Physical Therapy of the Foot and Ankle (Hunt GC, ed). New York: Churchill-Livingstone, 1988.

Sanner WH, Page JC, Tolbol HR, et al: A study of ankle joint height changes with subtalar joint motion. J Am Podiatr Med Assoc 71:158–161, 1981.

Shephard E: Tarsal movements. J Bone Joint Surg [Br] 33:258–263, 1951.

Shephard RJ, Taunton JE, eds: Foot and Ankle in Sport and Exercise. New York: Karger, 1987.

Stauffer RN, Chao EYS, Brewster RC: Force and motion analysis of the normal, diseased and prosthetic ankle joint. Clin Orthop Relat Res 127:189, 1977.

Stormont DM, Morrey BF, An K, et al: Stability of the loaded ankle. Am J Sports Med 13:295–300, 1985.

St. Pierre R, Allman F, Bassett FH, et al: A review of lateral ankle ligamentous reconstructions. Foot Ankle 3:114–123, 1982.

St. Pierre RK, Rosen J, Whitesides PE, et al: The tensile strength of the anterior talofibular ligament. Foot Ankle 4:83–85, 1983.

Subotnick SI, ed: Podiatric Sports Medicine. New York: Futura, 1975.

Thompson JP, Loomer RL: Osteochondral lesions of the talus in a sports medicine clinic. Am J Sports Med 12:460–463, 1984.

Tropp H, Askling C: Effects of ankle disc training on muscular strength and postural control. Clin Biomech 3:88–91, 1988.

Turek SL: Orthopaedics: Principles and Their Application, 4th ed. Philadelphia: JB Lippincott, 1984.

Wallenstein SL: Scaling clinical pain and pain relief. In Pain Measurement in Man (Bromm B, ed). New York: Elsevier, pp 389–396, 1984.

Wright DG, Desai SM, Henderson WH: Action of the subtalar and ankle joint complex during the stance phase of walking. J Bone Joint Surg [Am] 46:361–182, 1964.

Wu KK: Surgery of the Foot. Philadelphia: Lea & Febiger, 1986.

Yablon IG, Segal D, Leach RE: Ankle Injuries. New York: Churchill-Livingstone, 1983.

Zohn DA, Mennell JM: Musculoskeletal Pain—Diagnosis and Physical Treatment. Boston: Little, Brown, 1976.

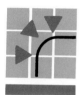

# CHAPTER *Ten*

## The Posture-Movement Dynamic

### *DAVID L. McKINNIS*

## INTRODUCTION

Movement is perhaps the most critical aspect of the human experience. Movement enhances perception and fosters exploration of an individual's environment. The more functional the movement, the greater the individual's ability to manipulate and control the environment. Higher performance levels may result in more meaningful interaction and better understanding. The significance of movement to the individual's continued development makes the human body the basic tool for life.

Each human being's working definition of life depends greatly on the performance level of movement experience. Fetal movement and successful passage through the postnatal developmental sequence begin to define not only physi-

cal but also intellectual, emotional, and social parameters for exploring life. Through each succeeding decade the capacity for efficient and pain-free movement remains central to an individual's life-enhancing experiences.

Postural reactions form the basis of movement and posture remains inextricably intertwined with movement. Motor performance continues to improve only when movement strategies evolve around postures that cope effectively with gravity. Even highly skilled motor performances that depend on learning have their origin in the functional development of the posture-movement dynamic. Posture may be viewed as the arrangement of body segments at any point or focus of points during movement. This arrangement may be loosely considered as performance enhancing or performance detracting. A performance-enhancing posture offers the positive potentials of movement. A performance-detracting posture offers the negative potentials of movement. Performance-detracting postures that are not appropriately utilized as feedback to movement strategies may tend to persist and become life detracting or even life threatening.

The conception of a human being initiates a life force seeking the highest human potential. To this end, posture is genetically safeguarded not only by reflexes but also by nonlearned predetermined responses once considered reflexes and now viewed as inherited subprograms. These subprograms translate into an innate urge for movement that triggers the central nervous system (CNS) and its feedback mechanisms. The progressive integration of reflexes, reactions, subprograms, and sensory-motor feedback leads the human organism through the developmental sequence and toward increasingly complex motor activity. The process continues to superimpose more sophisticated neuromuscular control on the musculoskeletal force-leverage system. The skeleton attempts to develop and maintain itself as a structure well suited to a range of forces from gravity to the stress and strain imposed by voluntary movement. During growth and development stages and also throughout life, the CNS attempts to integrate information to keep the orientation of the eyes and head, and the trunk and limbs, in an efficient response mode to gravity. This neurologically based posture-movement dynamic remains capable of pursuing the positive potentials of movement unless disrupted by disease, trauma, abuse, or disuse.

# NEUROLOGIC BASIS OF THE POSTURE-MOVEMENT DYNAMIC: AN OVERVIEW

## The Motor Hierarchy

The posture-movement dynamic is controlled by a four-level CNS hierarchy. Each level is a separate neural circuit, and all four levels are organized for hierarchical interdependence and also parallel independence. The levels are

■ Spinal cord
■ Brain stem
■ Brodmann's area 4 of the cortex
■ Motor planning area

Each level receives sensory information and can use its sensory information to modify descending

motor commands. Each progressive level has an increased ability to control selectively the ascending sensory information that reaches it. Each level has specific command responsibilities but no level works in isolation. The hierarchy monitors, analyzes, and adapts its actions using two fundamental routes of information feedback. Sensory feedback from proprioceptors and exteroceptors is supplemented with reference copies of outgoing motor commands. These reference copies are known as corollary discharges, efferent copies, or re-efference. Sensory feedback and reference copy feedback form a basis of comparison between intended motor outcomes and actual results. The continuous integrative sensory-motor processing in the motor hierarchy focuses on the motor neuron, the final common pathway of the motor system.

## Spinal Cord

The first level of the motor hierarchy is the spinal cord. It is responsible for organizing reflex behavior. The basic unit of the spinal cord is the reflex arc consisting of a sensory neuron and its sense organ, an interneuron located in the spinal cord, and a motor neuron with its effector, a muscle or a gland.

The stretch reflex or myotatic reflex is the fundamental reflexive base of the posture-movement dynamic. The proprioceptor or sense organ of the stretch reflex is the muscle spindle. This specialized receptor consists of an encapsulated group of fibers called intrafusal fibers. Intrafusal fibers are arranged in parallel with the extrafusal or large skeletal muscle fibers. The stretch reflex has a phasic component of short duration but strong force. This phasic component is best observed in deep tendon reflexes. The stretch reflex also has a tonic component that lasts longer but is weaker and responds to the continued stretch of muscles. The tonic component appears to be most important in postural stability and postural adjustment, but it requires integrative control by the brain stem.

The stretch reflex receives sensory input from the intrafused fibers of the muscle spindle. This sensory input concerns the muscle length and the rate of muscle length change. The stretch reflex sends motor commands to regulate the length of the same muscle. Some motor commands are sent to extrafusal fibers via alpha motor neurons for the purpose of increasing muscle tension. Other motor commands are sent to intrafusal fibers via gamma motor neurons to help the muscle spindle maintain and regulate its sensitivity to muscle length status.

The stretch reflex is aided by the Golgi tendon organs, which sense muscle tension levels. The Golgi tendon organs are able to sense muscle tension because each organ is placed in series with a bundle of extrafusal skeletal muscle fibers. Together, the stretch-sensitive muscle spindles and the contraction-sensitive Golgi tendon organs reflexively monitor and control the muscular length-tension relationship. The stretch reflex control of the length-tension relationship is dominant in the physiologic extension muscles —the flexor or extensor muscles whose main function is to oppose gravity.

The presence of interneurons in the spinal cord permits the stretch reflex to operate in more ways than simple autogenic excitation, which permits only the innervation of the same muscle. Coordination through interneurons provides the foundation of such important muscular control mechanisms as synergistic innervation, reciprocal inhibition, recurrent inhibition, disinhibition, and cocontraction. Interneurons also connect motor neuron pools into segmental networks that are in turn connected to other spinal segments via the propriospinal tract. The result is spinal cord–mediated segmental control of reflex activity. When ascending input and descending control signals from higher levels of the motor hierarchy are superimposed on the spinal cord's segmental network, a highly efficient negative feedback servomechanism controls postural stability and postural adjustment (Fig. 10–1).

## Brain Stem

The second level of the motor hierarchy is the brain stem. The brain stem processes ascending information from the spinal cord and integrates descending motor commands from higher levels. The cranial nerve nuclei located in the brain stem process related cranial nerve and special sensory information including visual, auditory, and vestibular inputs. Without the integrative control of the brain stem the stretch reflex would be mediated only by the spinal cord and would produce phasic rather than tonic activity.

Except for the corticospinal and corticobulbar tracts, all descending motor pathways begin in the brain stem. The two systems of pathways that descend from the brain stem are the ventromedial pathways and the dorsolateral pathways. The ventromedial pathways control proximal muscles. The dorsolateral pathways control distal muscles. The two combine to bring equilibrium and balance, stability, force, speed, coordination, directionality, targeting, and manipulation to the posture-movement dynamic (Fig. 10–2).

## Brodmann's Area 4 of the Cortex

The third level of the motor hierarchy is Brodmann's area 4 of the cortex. This level is more

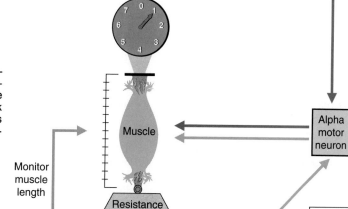

**FIGURE 10–1** ■ Simple representation of the postural length–tension control mechanism. The red loop shows tension feedback (tendons). The pink loop shows length change feedback (muscles).

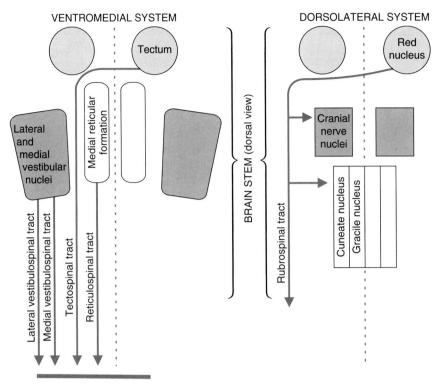

FIGURE 10-2 ■ The descending motor pathways originating in the brain stem.

commonly known simply as the motor cortex. The motor cortex contains a somatotopic map of the body's muscles. In response to sensory, cognitive, affective, and motor planning inputs, the motor cortex can carry out voluntary movement. The motor cortex can mediate commands for muscle selection, force regulation and application, and the sequence of action. These motor commands descend by way of the corticospinal or pyramidal pathways and corticobulbar pathways. The lateral corticospinal tract controls distal limb muscles, and the ventromedial corticospinal tract controls axial and proximal muscles. The corticobulbar tract controls the head and facial muscles. Although the motor cortex plays an important role in voluntary control, it is primarily the highest level in the automatic sensory-motor integrative control of the posture-movement dynamic. For this reason it is also important to view the sensory cortex as a vital part of this hierarchical level (Fig. 10-3).

## Motor Planning Area

The fourth level of the motor hierarchy is the motor planning area. This area includes the premotor cortex, the supplemental motor cortex of the frontal lobe, and the posterior parietal cortex. The premotor cortex seems to coordinate sensory and motor messages to stabilize proximal muscles, guide limb movement, direct the arm toward a target, and regulate the intent of movement. The supplemental motor areas seem to play important roles in programming complex motor behavior as well as controlling both proximal and distal muscles to orient the body. The posterior parietal cortex seems to utilize sensory information from the environment to devise targeting and timing strategies for movement (Fig. 10-4).

The motor planning area is responsible for the formation of strategies that initiate and direct the voluntary aspect of the posture-movement dynamic. However, the motor planning area must share the top level of the motor hierarchy with the limbic system. The limbic system includes the cingulate gyrus, the hippocampus, the fornix, the parahippocampal gyrus, the amygdala, the caudate, the putamen, and other structures. The limbic system is a vast network of intercortical connections and is critically linked to the hypothalamus. The limbic system blends emotions, memories, drives, and survival needs with hypothalamic inputs concerning vital signs into a

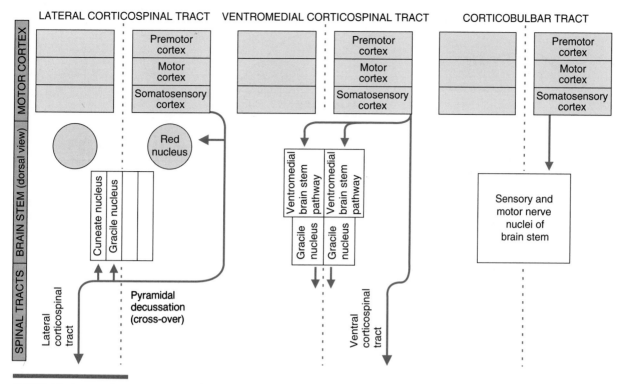

**FIGURE 10–3** ■ (Left) Lateral corticospinal tract. Originates in the motor cortex, the premotor cortex, and the somatosensory cortex and controls spinal segmental motor neuron pools that innervate distal limb muscle. (Center) Ventromedial corticospinal tract. Originates in the motor cortex, the premotor cortex, and the somatosensory cortex and controls spinal segmental neuron pools that innervate axial and proximal muscles. (Right) Corticobulbar tract. Originates in the motor cortex, the premotor cortex, and the somatosensory cortex; terminates in the sensory and motor cranial nerve nuclei of the brain stem; and controls the muscles of the face and head.

global association of experiences. This global association appears to be important in mediating experience-referenced learning.

The entire motor hierarchy plus the limbic system is still insufficient to explain the brain's control of the posture-movement dynamic. The roles of the cerebellum, the basal ganglia, and the thalamus cannot be disregarded.

The cerebellum controls the posture-movement dynamic by regulating descending motor commands. The cerebellum can perform this regulation because it receives and compares information concerning sensation, motor planning, and motor execution. By comparing information from the periphery, the brain stem, the motor cortex, and the motor planning area, the cerebellum is involved in balance, equilibrium, posture adjustment, eye movements, muscle tone, motor planning, motor initiation, and motor learning.

The basal ganglia include the caudate, the putamen, the globus pallidus, and the subthalamic nuclei as well as the substantia nigra. The role of the basal ganglia in controlling the posture-

movement dynamic includes spatial-temporal cognition, muscle tone regulation, postural reflex modulation, coordination, speed and rhythm, motor planning, and volition.

The thalamus serves the posture-movement dynamic as an extensive relay center linking both sensory and motor information from the motor cortex and motor planning areas, the basal ganglia, the cerebellum, the brain stem, and the spinal cord (Fig. 10–5).

## Primitive Reflexes, Genetic Subprograms, Integration, and Postural Reactions

Primitive reflexes appear from the time of fetal development until the time of birth. By the age of 6 months most primitive reflexes, except those that remain unchanged and persist throughout life, are assimilated into more complex movements. Once assimilated, primitive reflexes do

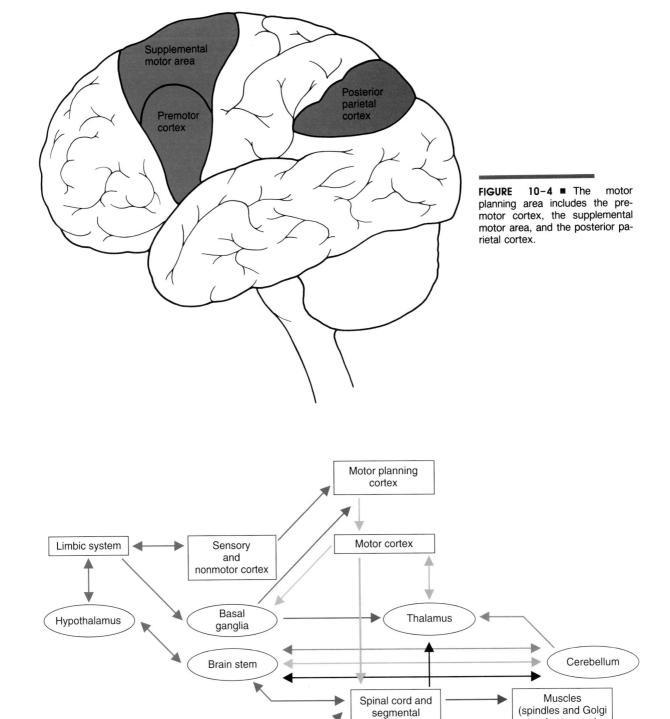

**FIGURE 10-4 ■** The motor planning area includes the premotor cortex, the supplemental motor area, and the posterior parietal cortex.

**FIGURE 10-5 ■** Simplified representation of control of the posture-movement dynamic by the motor hierarchy.

not reappear except in response to extreme stress or effort or to CNS damage.

Genetic subprograms contain nonlearned automatic stereotyped predetermined responses. Once triggered, these genetic subprograms generate a cascade of coordinated actions to produce their motor patterns. The stimulus for a genetic subprogram may range from simple maturation of neuronal networks to activation of either a primitive or highly integrated reflex. An activated genetic subprogram can sequentially stabilize limb joints in time frames far less than required for reflex arc activity. It can also produce a specific and repeatable automatic motor pattern composed of independent elements not responsive to the initial stimulus.

Integration is an organizational process that the brain stem and higher levels can apply to modulation and assimilation of primitive reflexes and genetic subprograms to attain coordinated motor control. With sensory feedback and reference copy feedback, appropriate facilitation or inhibition can modify motor commands and eventually produce more complex motor responses that supersede the primitive reflexes and genetic subprograms.

As integration progresses, complex movement appears and the primitive reflexes and genetic subpatterns are relegated to indistinguishable parts of the whole motor performance. Integration of primitive reflexes and genetic subprograms usually occurs between 1 and 12 months of age.

Although the ultimate level of integration occurs with the voluntary control of highly skilled movement, integration can also be temporarily or permanently fixated at lower levels to produce postural reactions. Postural reactions are critical to the posture-movement dynamic. Temporary postural reactions appear from birth through approximately the first 21 months of childhood. Some temporary postural reactions are integrated as early as the first 1 to 2 months of life; others are integrated as late as 7 years of age. Permanent postural reactions appear as early as 3 months and persist throughout life.

### Primitive Reflexes and Genetic Subprograms

The following list of stimulus-generated responses includes behaviors that have traditionally been considered primitive reflexes. Some of these behaviors may in fact be true primitive reflexes, whereas others may represent genetic subprograms. Precise delineation is lacking, con-flicting research definitions abound, and the term "reflexes" not only persists but dominates the professional literature. The important consideration is that these behaviors are the early foundation of the posture-movement dynamic.

**Deep tendon reflexes.** Deep tendon reflexes are present from birth but require much skill to elicit, observe, and classify. Best responses appear to be in the biceps tendon, the patellar tendon, and the calcaneal tendon. Deep tendon reflexes persist throughout life (Fig. 10–6).

**Babinski's response.** When the plantar surface of the foot is stimulated from heel to toe following a path along the lateral border, the great toe extends and the other toes fan out (Fig. 10–7). This primitive withdrawal response is integrated in 5 to 7 months. It does not reappear except in individuals with upper motor neuron lesions.

**Superficial reflexes.** This group of reflexes includes mucous membrane reflexes such as the corneal reflex, the nasal reflex, the phalangeal reflex, and the uvular reflex. The group also includes skin reflexes such as the upper and lower abdominal reflexes and the anal reflex (Fig. 10–8). These reflexes persist throughout life.

**Visceral reflexes.** This group of reflexes includes pupillary reflexes, blink reflexes, the oculocardiac reflex, the carotid sinus reflex, and various bladder and rectal reflexes. These reflexes persist throughout life (Fig. 10–9).

**Rooting or search reflex.** This reflex enables

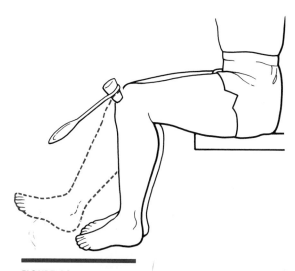

FIGURE 10–6 ■ Deep tendon reflex of the quadriceps.

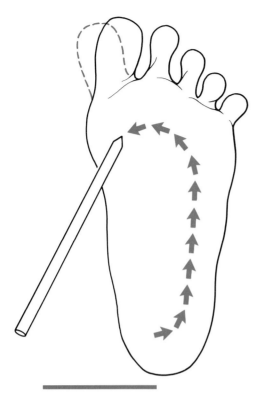

**FIGURE 10–7** ■ Babinski's response.

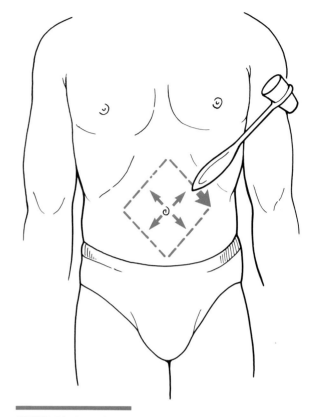

**FIGURE 10–8** ■ Superficial abdominal reflex. Umbilicus deviates to side of stimulus.

the infant to locate mother's milk without being directed to the nipple. Head, lips, tongue, and mandible respond to light touch by moving toward the point of stimulation. Integration of the rooting reflex occurs at approximately 3 months (Fig. 10–10).

**Sucking and swallowing reflexes.** These reflexes enable the infant to obtain food. The stimulus is the placement of the nipple into the infant's mouth. The response is closing the lips, rhythmic sucking, and swallowing. The sucking and swallowing reflexes are integrated at approximately 3 months (Fig. 10–11).

**Eye reflexes.** Derived from both the superficial and visceral categories, the eye reflexes are designed to protect the eyes. The eye reflexes include the following:

Cochleal-palpebral reflex
Visuopalpebral reflex (Fig. 10–12)
Nasopalpebral reflex
Cutaneopalpebral reflex
Ciliary reflex
Corneal reflex
Peiper's optic reflex
McCarthy's reflex

Additional eye reflexes include the pupillary reflex, the photic-sneeze reflex, and the resistance to passive opening of the eyes. Some eye reflexes such as the ''doll's eye'' reflex are integrated as early as 10 days after birth. Others persist throughout life.

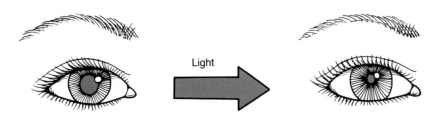

Light

**FIGURE 10–9** ■ Visual reflex. The pupil constricts in reaction to illumination.

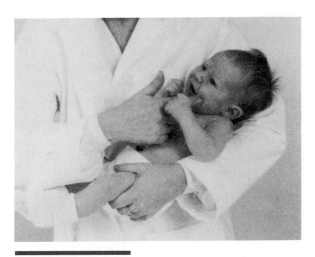

**FIGURE 10-10** ■ Rooting reflex. Baby begins to suck as finger, bottle, or nipple touches his mouth. (From Jarvis C: Physical Examination and Health Assessment. Philadelphia: WB Saunders, 1992, p 767.)

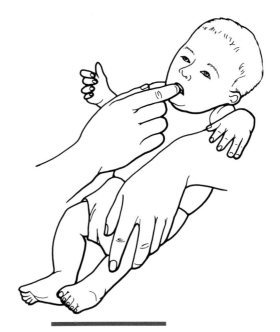

**FIGURE 10-11** ■ Suck-swallow reflex.

**Moro's reflex.** This behavioral pattern may be a primitive protective or equilibrium response. With the infant supine and the head held in flexion, a sudden extension of the cervical region simulating loss of head support triggers a twofold response. Extension and abduction of the upper extremities, opening of the hands, and extension of the neck and trunk appear first. These movements are followed by flexion and adduction of the upper extremities (Fig. 10-13). This pattern is usually accompanied by crying and some movements of the lower extremities. Moro's reflex is usually integrated at 5 to 6 months.

**Startle reflex.** This reflex is protective in nature. It is elicited by a loud noise, a tap on the sternum, or a quick change in head position from flexion to extension. The response is immediate bilateral elbow flexion with hands remaining closed (Fig. 10-14). Elements of the startle reflex parallel those of Moro's reflex and are integrated in the same

time frame. With severe stimuli, certain aspects of the startle reflex may reappear throughout life.

**Traction reflex and the grasp reflexes.** The traction reflex is a flexor response of the extremities when a gently pulling force is applied to them. In the upper extremities, application of stretch to the adductors and flexors via a gentle pull on the forearms of the infant elicits the traction reflex. The traction reflex is integrated as early as 2 months or as late as 5 months. The grasp reflexes appear in both the hands and the feet. They are integrated only after integration of the traction reflex (Fig. 10-15).

**Crossed extension reflex.** This behavior may be a form of protection or withdrawal. While the examiner holds one of the infant's legs in extension, pressure is applied to the

**FIGURE 10-12** ■ Protective corneal reflex.

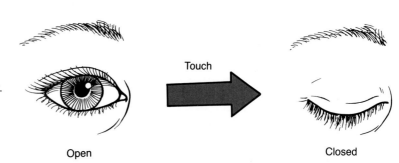

Touch

Open                                        Closed

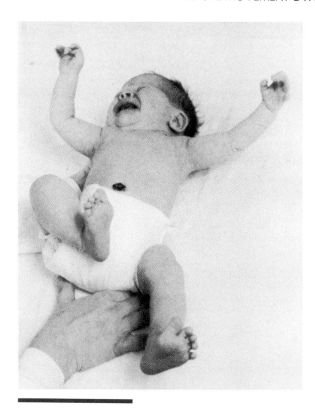

**FIGURE 10–13** ■ Moro's reflex (From Jarvis C: Physical Examination and Health Assessment. Philadelphia: WB Saunders, 1992, p 770.)

plantar surface of the ipsilateral foot. The response involves the free leg in what appears to be an attempt to push away the stimulus. The crossed extension reflex is integrated at 2 months but may reappear throughout life as a protective response to noxious stimuli (Fig. 10–16).

**Withdrawal reflex.** This protective reflex results in quick flexion of the limb in response to a noxious stimulus to the foot (Fig. 10–17). The withdrawal reflex is integrated at 2 months but its protective function remains throughout life.

**Galant's reflex.** This reflex appears to be the basis for lateral trunk flexion. With the infant in a prone position, a gentle stimulus is applied along the thoracolumbar paravertebral line. The response is an incurving of flexion of the trunk toward the stimulated side (Fig. 10–18). The Galant reflex integrates by 2 months.

**Neck-on-body righting reflex.** This response seems to guarantee head-body rotational components of movement necessary for supine to side lying. The examiner turns the infant's head to one side and the infant's trunkal unit log rolls to side lying on the same side (Fig. 10–19). The neck-on-body reflex is integrated at 4 to 5 months.

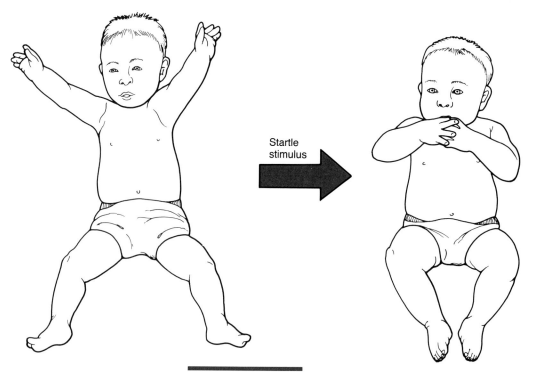

Startle stimulus

**FIGURE 10–14** ■ Startle reflex.

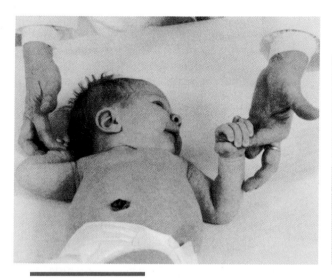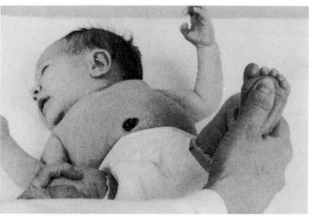

**FIGURE 10–15** ■ (Left) Palmar grasp. (Right) Plantar grasp. (From Jarvis C: Physical Examination and Health Assessment. Philadelphia: WB Saunders, 1992, p 768.)

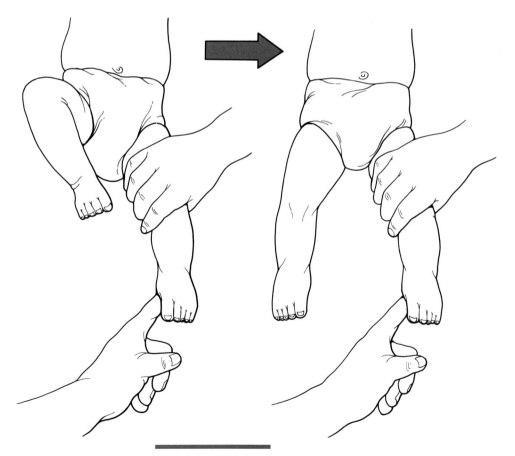

**FIGURE 10–16** ■ Crossed extension reflex.

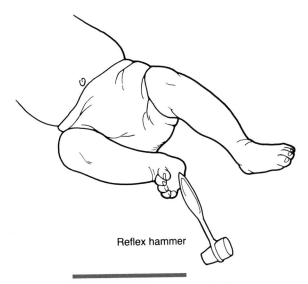

**FIGURE 10-17 ■** Withdrawal reflex.

**Body-on-body righting reflex.** With the infant supine, the trunkal segment of the body is stimulated to turn to side lying. The response is for the infant's trunkal unit to log roll to side lying (Fig. 10-20). This log-rolling reaction precedes development of segmental rolling. Integration of the body-on-body righting reflex occurs at 4 to 5 months.

**Placing reflexes.** Certain tactile or proprioceptive stimuli result in a positional placement of the hands or feet (Fig. 10-21). The motor patterns of the placing reflexes are integrated at 2 months.

**Positive support reflex.** When the infant is held vertically with feet on a surface, the response is partial weight bearing with hips and knees remaining flexed (Fig. 10-22). This behavior is integrated at 2 months.

**Automatic walking reflex.** When the infant is held vertically with feet touching a surface, a coordinated and rhythmic heel-toe walking pattern follows the support reflex (Fig. 10-23). This behavior is integrated at 2 months.

**Tonic labyrinthine reflex.** With the body supine and the head in neutral position, extensor patterns are facilitated and flexor patterns are inhibited (Fig. 10-24). With the body prone and the head in neutral position, flexor patterns are facilitated and extensor patterns are inhibited. This behavior is integrated by 6 months; however, integration of the tonic labyrinthine responses appears to have more to do with suppression, maturation, and motor learning than simple assimilation. The tonic labyrinthine reflex is closely related to other otolithic-based responses such as the acceleration reflex and the positional reflex.

**Asymmetric tonic neck reflex.** With the infant supine, turning of the head to one side stimulates proprioceptors in the neck and produces a postural response. The typical response pattern of an asymmetric tonic neck reflex with head turned right includes right upper and lower extremity extension, right upper extremity abduction of approximately 90 degrees, left upper and lower extremity flexion, and left upper extremity ab-

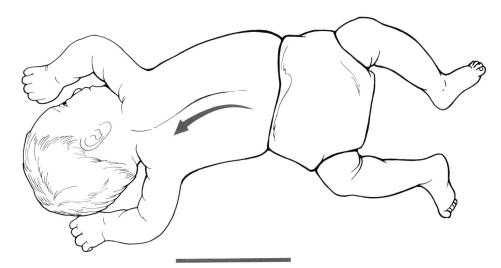

**FIGURE 10-18 ■** Galant's reflex.

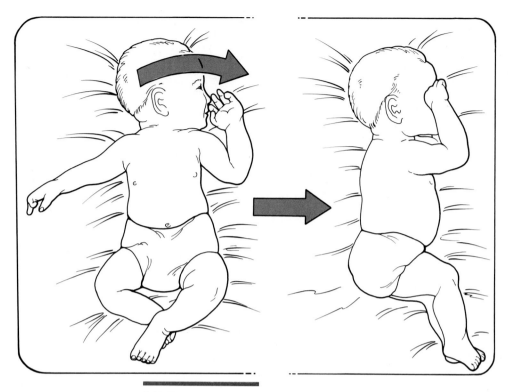

**FIGURE 10–19** ■ Neck-on-body righting reflex.

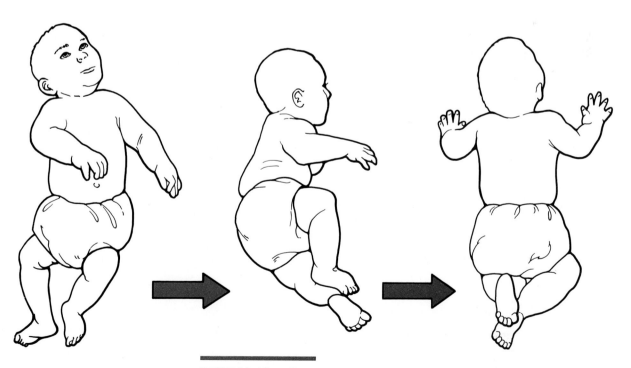

**FIGURE 10–20** ■ Body-on-body righting reflex.

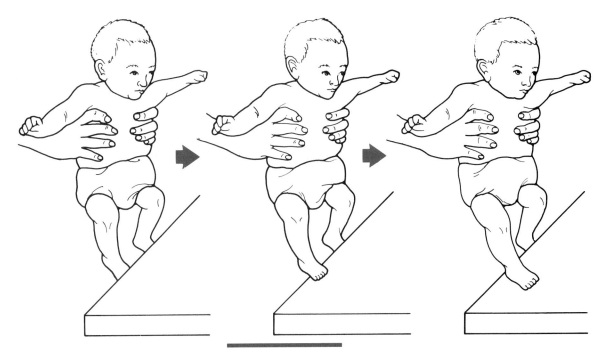

**FIGURE 10–21** ■ Placing reflex.

duction (Fig. 10–25). The involvement of the lower extremities is often minimal. The flexion pattern of the response is often stronger than the extension pattern. The asymmetric tonic neck reflex is integrated at 4 to 6 months. Without integration, neck righting reactions do not appear, posture is not symmetric, and motor milestones are not reached.

**Symmetric tonic neck reflex.** The symmetric tonic neck reflex does not appear until 4 to 6 months. The basic stimuli for the reflex are head flexion and head extension. When the head is flexed or extended, proprioceptors in the neck are stimulated. The response to head flexion is flexion of the upper extremities and extension of the lower extremities (Fig. 10–26, left). The response to head ex-

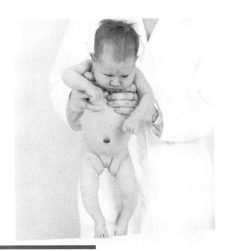

**FIGURE 10–22** ■ Positive support reflex. (From Jarvis C: Physical Examination and Health Assessment. Philadelphia: WB Saunders, 1992, p 771.)

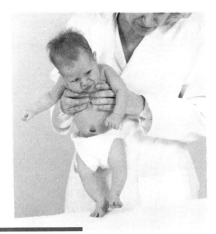

**FIGURE 10–23** ■ Automatic walking reflex. (From Jarvis C: Physical Examination and Health Assessment. Philadelphia: WB Saunders, 1992, p 771.)

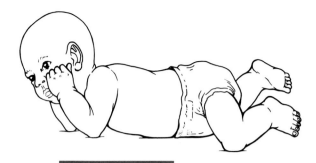

**FIGURE 10–24** ■ Tonic labyrinthine reflex.

tension is upper extremity extension and lower extremity flexion (Fig. 10–26, right). The symmetric tonic neck reflex is integrated between 8 and 12 months.

### Postural Reactions

The following list of stimulus-generated responses represents behaviors still considered permanent reflexes. Growing evidence suggests that, like many of the primitive reflexes, these behaviors might be better considered as genetic subprograms existing at various levels of integration. Many of these postural reactions are global events with a programmed series of reactions that proceed much faster than reflex activity. Whether these behaviors are reflexes or subprograms, postural reactions remain as lifelong influences on the posture-movement dynamic.

**Avoidance and grasp reactions.** These reactions enable the infant and developing child to build coordinated movement patterns for manipulation of the environment by the hand (Fig. 10–27). The eventual capability for voluntary control of individual muscles independently of each other, a capacity known as fractionation of movement, allows the infant access to the unique human prehensile skills. Avoidance reactions appear at birth and are integrated at 6 years. Grasp reactions appear between 4 and 11 months and remain throughout life.

**Body-orienting righting reactions.** These righting reactions function to orient the body in relation to gravity. They permit transitions from one position to another. They maintain eye, head, trunk, and segmental postural relationships to each other as well as to the ground and the horizon. In the labyrinthine head-righting reactions, otolithic organs respond to gravity by keeping the head level (Fig. 10–28). The optical righting reactions respond to visual cues to keep the head upright and the visual field horizontal. The body-on-head righting reactions respond to exteroceptor information to keep the head upright. The body-on-body righting reactions respond to exteroceptor information to right the body even if the head remains in a less than upright attitude. The neck-on-body righting reactions respond to neck muscle spindle information to right the thorax, the shoulders, and the pelvis. These reactions appear between birth and 6 months and persist until 5 years, except for the labyrin-

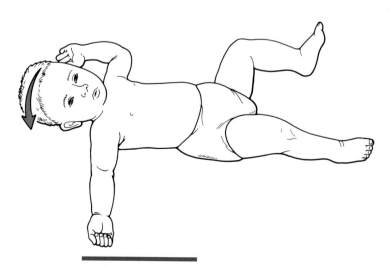

**FIGURE 10–25** ■ Asymmetric tonic neck reflex.

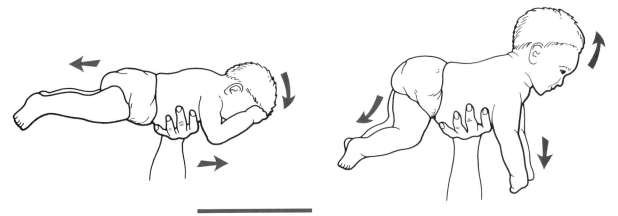

**FIGURE 10-26** ■ Symmetric tonic neck reflex.

thine and optical righting reactions, which are lifelong.

**Ventral suspension behaviors.** The Landau reflex causes an infant held in ventral suspension to move from head, spine, and leg extension to flexion of the hips, knees, and elbows when the head is depressed. This reflex appears at 3 months and is integrated at 6 months. The parachute reaction occurs when the child is held in ventral suspension and quickly lowered. The child responds by extending the arms to protect against falling (Fig. 10–29). The parachute reaction appears at 6 months and persists throughout life. The Landau and the parachute behaviors

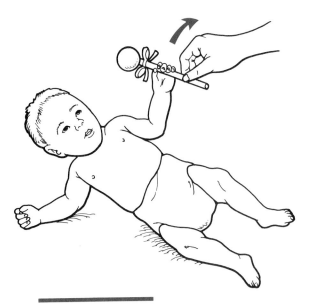

**FIGURE 10-27** ■ Avoidance and grasp reactions.

are foundations of protective, support, and righting reactions.

**Positive supporting reactions.** These reactions promote weight bearing through the extremities. The first positive supporting reaction of the upper extremities appears at 3 months, permits prone-on-elbow weight bearing, and persists throughout life (Fig. 10–30). The second positive supporting reaction of the upper extremities appears at 4 to 6 months, permits weight bearing on the hands, and persists throughout life. The positive supporting reaction of the lower extremities appears at 6 to 9 months, permits weight bearing for eventual stance and ambulation, and persists throughout life.

**Equilibrium reactions.** The equalization of opposing forces to maintain balance is attained by visual, vestibular, and other kinesthetic inputs (Fig. 10–31). Visual equilibrium reactions of the upper extremities appear at 3 months and those of the lower extremities at 4 months. These visual equilibrium reactions aid in placing, orientation, and motion compensation. The visual equilibrium reactions persist throughout life. Protective equilibrium reactions appear between 4 and 18 months and persist throughout life. Protective equilibrium reactions respond to multiple sensory inputs and especially to vestibular stimuli. Downward protective extension appears at 4 months; forward protective extension appears at 6 months; sideward protective extension appears at 7 months; backward protective extension appears at 9 months. Protective staggering and shifting reactions appear at 15 to 18 months. Tilting equilibrium reactions appear between 6 and 21 months and persist throughout life. Tilt-

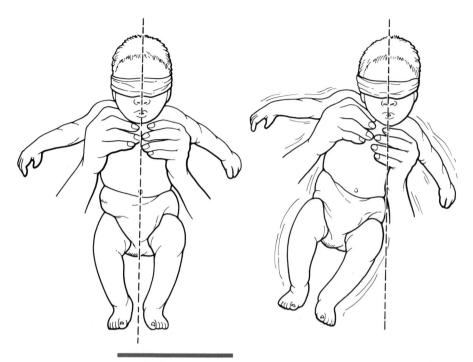

**FIGURE 10–28** ■ Body-orienting righting reaction.

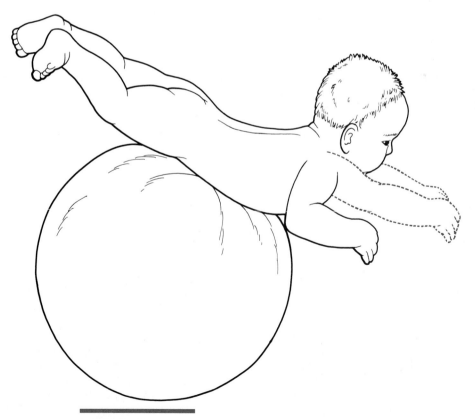

**FIGURE 10–29** ■ Ventral suspension reaction (parachute reaction).

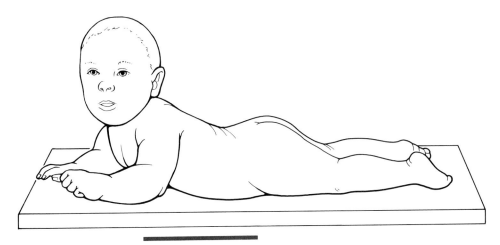

FIGURE 10-30 ■ Positive supporting reaction.

ing equilibrium reactions can be elicited by visual or kinesthetic inputs, but they are primarily a response to vestibular stimuli. Prone tilting reactions appear at 6 months, supine tilting reactions at 7 months, sitting tilting reactions at 8 months, quadruped tilting reactions at 10 months, and standing tilting reactions some time after 12 months. Postural stabilizing equilibrium reactions appear between 6 and 21 months and persist throughout life. Postural stabilization occurs in response to visual and vestibular stimuli, but kinesthetic feedback is essential. Postural stabilization reactions begin proximally and progress distally. Postural stabilization equilibrium reactions mirror tilting equilibrium reactions in their times of appearance.

## THE DEVELOPMENTAL SEQUENCE

The posture-movement dynamic is a sensory-motor growth, maturation, and maintenance process that occurs in a relatively constant progression called the developmental sequence. Certain principles govern the developmental sequence. Reflex activities predominate for prescribed time frames and then become integrated at higher levels until cortical control permits voluntary movement. Motor reflex expression appears in the body first and then the neck and head. Motor control, however, begins with neck and facial muscles and proceeds cephalocaudally. Upper trunk control precedes lower trunk control. Upper extremity control precedes lower extremity control. Motor control also develops proximal to distal, with shoulder control preced-

ing arm control and pelvic and hip development preceding leg development. Muscular activation progresses from physiologic extension to flexion dominating extension, extension equalizing flexion, reciprocal inhibition, cocontraction, and synergistic innervation. Movement develops from whole body responses to segmental dissociation to fractionalized and isolated small muscle actions. Motor control develops progressively by incremental adjustments in the mobility-stability-mobility (MSM) loop. Reflex-based MSM loops progress to integratively modulated MSM loops and ultimately to learned MSM skills.

The developmental sequence is marked by accomplishment of motor milestones that follow CNS maturation and movement experience. The developmental sequence is composed of parallel formations of posture-movement improvements in the areas of head control, prone and supine progressions, rolling, sitting, standing, and walking progressions (Fig. 10-32).

### First-Year Milestones

#### Milestones of Head Control

1. At 12 weeks the baby can maintain the head-up position while the body is held in ventral suspension.
2. At 3 months the baby can hold the head vertically while in a prone and forearm support position.
3. At 6 months the baby can lift the head independently when the body is pulled to sit.
4. At 12 months most righting and equilibrium reactions are well integrated except in the standing position.

fied or full plantigrade position and can creep on hands and feet.

### Milestones of the Supine Progression

1. At 4 months the baby is able to hyperextend the neck and roll from supine to side while in a hands-to-knees posture.
2. At 5 months the baby is able to roll from supine and assume a full side-lying position.
3. At 6 months the baby is able to roll from supine to prone.
4. At 7 months the baby dislikes the supine position and rolls out of it.

### Milestones of the Rolling Progression

1. At 4 months the baby is able to log roll from prone or supine to side lying in a hands-to-knees position.
2. At 6 months the baby is able to roll segmentally from supine to prone and prone to supine.
3. At 7 months the baby rolls to full side lying and plays in side lying.

### Milestones of the Sitting Progression

1. At 3 months the baby displays a slight head lag when pulled to sit.
2. At 5 months the baby has no head lag when pulled to sit.
3. At 7 months the baby can move from quadruped to sitting.
4. At 7 months the baby can move from sitting to quadruped.
5. At 11 months the baby can long sit (sit with the weight distributed on both hips and legs) and side sit (sit with the weight on one hip and leg).

### Milestones of the Standing Progression

1. At 3 months the baby displays minimum weight bearing while held in trunkal support.
2. At 6 months the baby displays full weight bearing while held by the hands.
3. At 7 months the baby can pull itself to stand.
4. At 11 months the baby can stand alone.

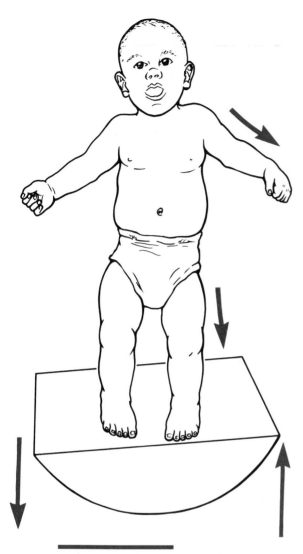

**FIGURE 10–31** ■ Equilibrium reaction.

### Milestones of the Prone Progression

1. At 3 months the baby can maintain a prone and forearm position.
2. At 4 months the baby can roll from prone to side while in a hands-to-knees posture.
3. At 5 months the baby can roll from prone to supine.
4. At 6 months the baby can maintain a prone and extended arm position.
5. At 7 months the baby can assume a quadruped position and begin to crawl.
6. At 8 months the baby begins creeping on hands and knees.
7. At 10 months the baby can assume a modi-

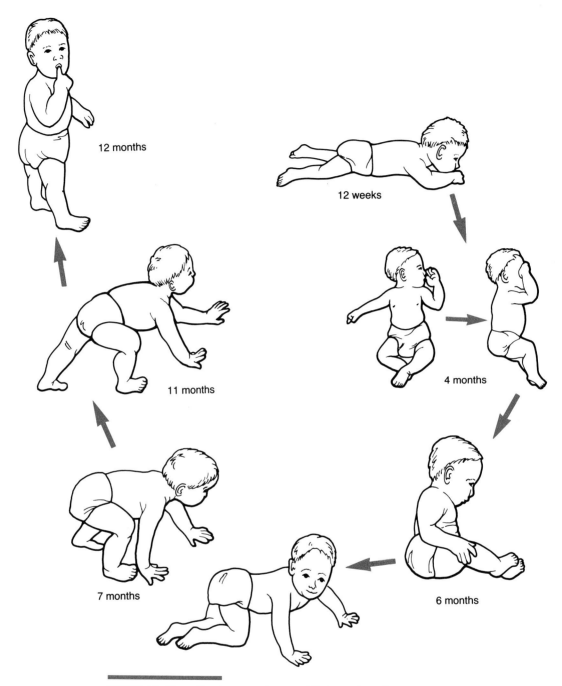

**FIGURE 10–32** ■ Development of motor skills in the first 12 months of life.

5. At 12 months the baby can shift its weight and lift one leg.

### Milestones of the Walking Progression

1. At 1 month the baby may display the automatic walking reflex.

2. At 2 months the baby displays astasia-abasia.

3. At 8 months the baby can perform a steppage gait when held by the hands.

4. At 9 months the baby can walk when held by the hands.

5. At 11 months the baby can cruise while holding onto furniture.

6. At 12 months the baby attempts walking with a high guard and a wide base of support.

## Motor Milestones Beyond the First Year

1. At 15 months the child can sit in a chair with independent entry and exit.
2. At 13 months the child can walk alone with a high guard and a wide base of support.
3. At 15 months the child can stand up without help.
4. At 2 years the child can run, walk backward, and pick an object up from the floor.
5. At 2 years the child can go upstairs with a step-to pattern and at 3 years with an alternate pattern up but a step-to pattern down.
6. At 4 years the child climbs and descends stairs with a normal alternating pattern.
7. At 5 years the child can hop on one foot, hop with both feet together, gallop, slide, and run backward slowly.
8. At 6 years the child can skip, jump in horizontal and vertical patterns, and display elemental throwing, kicking, striking, and catching skills.

Although the developmental sequence is normally associated with motor milestones attained in a child's period of growth and development, it might easily be viewed as much more. The posture-movement dynamic does not come to a halt just because motor milestones have been reached. The posture-movement dynamic instead becomes a mechanism for coping with and adapting to the demands of a new, more random and loosely structured developmental sequence —aging through the decades of life. The motor milestones of youth give way to somatoemotional, somatosocial, somatocultural, somatointellectual, and somatoenvironmental interactions that may result in performance-enhancing or performance-detracting postures. The positive potentials of movement available through the aging process offer the new, albeit abstract developmental sequence. Superimposed on the existing feedback systems of youth are the new and demanding feedback requirements of aging: conscious awareness and intelligent care and use of one's posture-movement dynamic and appropriate medical and therapeutic care of injury, disease, developmental deficits, and disuse-abuse problems. Maintenance of the posture-movement dynamic throughout life permits the human body to perform its function as the basic tool for life.

## MOTOR LEARNING

The goal of each individual's posture-movement dynamic is to pursue and maximize the positive potentials of movement. The highest level of this pursuit is motor learning. The significance of motor learning tends to be lost in the stereotypic view of motor learning as progressive skill development for the purpose of athletic performance. Motor learning is of much greater importance because it organizes interactive responses with the environment, refines perception, and builds temporal-spatial references on which abstract concepts may be developed.

Learning itself should be viewed as not simply a change in behavior but rather an advancement in thought processes yielding greater insight, inductive and deductive reasoning, problem solving, and creativity. Learning may proceed to metaphysical levels but it is firmly rooted in the reflex integration–motor learning continuum. An individual's interpretation of physical reality via sensory-motor experience is at the least a springboard to that person's working definition of life and the learning derived from it.

Motor learning begins as adaptations of randomized movements to gain more functional responses. Motor learning progresses to task-oriented behavior that can be refined through repeated performance (Fig. 10–33). The motor learning process attempts to integrate a retained motor pattern that efficiently accomplishes a desired task despite extraneous interference and yet remains malleable. The highest-level skills retain the capacity for creative change.

The posture-movement dynamic gives the CNS its primary reason to integrate visual, auditory, vestibular, tactile, kinesthetic, and proprioceptive information. That reason is perception. Both motor learning and cortical learning depend on perception. Perception is the combination of sensation and interpretation. Perceptual changes result in changes in comprehension. All learning, in effect, becomes a function of perception within the dimension of time.

Motor learning begins to develop a body image on the basis of a movement gestalt. The developmental sequence integrates important conceptual images including midline attention; midline crossing; laterality; rotation; weight shifting; rolling; stabilization; mobility; segmentalization; prone, supine, and vertical orientation; flexion; extension; hand-eye relationships; weight bearing; and many more. Two-dimensional conceptual grids form around principles such as fig-

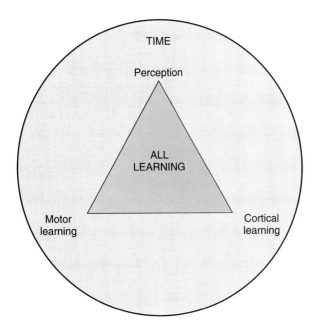

**FIGURE 10-33** ■ Theoretical model relating motor learning, cortical learning, perception, and time.

ure and ground, proximity, similarity, and closure. Three-dimensional conceptual grids form around principles such as linear perspective, color intensities and tonalities, interpositions of objects, texture, and feedback-established relationships. Temporal references form around elapsed time, event intervals, and event durations. Both gross and fine movement concepts of body image form from a spectrum of principles including

■ Tension or load
■ Force of movement
■ Velocity of movement
■ Amplitude of movement
■ Direction of movement
■ Balance, stability, and mobility
■ Variability in comparison
■ Opposition
■ Perceptual detail
■ Inhibition
■ Impulsiveness, compulsiveness, or contradiction
■ Initiation of judgment
■ Finality of judgment
■ Perseverance
■ Extinction

Body image enhances, and is itself enhanced by, development of communication skills. The random movements, tactile responses, visual tracking and fixations, vocal sounds, and crying of the infant eventually become communication techniques such as eye contact, recognition, body language, and speech. Successful communication enables the individual to progress from self-centeredness to recognition and acceptance of others. The sensory-motor roots of movement and communication produce a body image that fosters both self-confidence and socialization.

Motor learning joins the cognitive and affective aspects of learning to play a continual role in forming and re-forming an individual's behavior. As reflexive and random movements become integrated, the baby uses movement to aid its search for primary needs. The search for these primary needs results in pleasure from satisfaction, pain from unfulfillment, or conflict or irritability from mixed signals. These sensations may be loosely associated with the development of primary emotions: pleasure with love, pain with fear, and conflict or irritability with anger. The limbic system begins to blend all these sensations and behaviors into a global association of experiences, and an emotionally based link is established. The limbic system is a future source of motivations for motor learning.

As the child develops, primary needs seldom take the forefront and primary emotions begin to blend and blur. Secondary needs like cognizance, affiliation, dominance, and aggression begin to appear and secondary emotions, which often remain nameless, ambiguous, and confusing for much of life, begin to dominate. Motor learning and cortical learning are often inhibited, misdirected, or sometimes fixated by distorted limbic and cognitive inputs based on secondary needs and secondary emotions.

When tertiary needs present themselves, motor learning and cortical learning can focus on goal-directed activity. Goal attainment functions as both reward and motivation for new goals. Limbic and cortical inputs find degrees of effective modulation for motivational inputs and learning proceeds in a more orderly fashion. The motor learning–cortical learning relationship gains because perception is enhanced, body and self-image concepts improve, socialization improves, and the individual is ready to learn.

Motor learning does not stop with goal-oriented activity. Instead, motor learning parallels cortical learning through the highest developmental levels of self-realization, self-actualization, autonomy, and creativity. At these levels motor learning reaches the apex of the neurologic basis of the posture-movement dynamic. Cognitive, affective, and psychomotor dimensions unite to produce the highest learning and behavioral responses available through the various decades of life.

## DISRUPTIONS OF THE POSTURE-MOVEMENT DYNAMIC

Disruptions of the posture-movement dynamic are the result of neuromuscular pathologies, musculoskeletal disorders, and posture-movement abuse and disuse syndromes. Neuromuscular pathologies have their origin in an extensive categorization of disorders and diseases (see Neuromuscular Pathologies chart).

Neuromuscular pathologies result in acute, chronic, or permanent destruction of nerve cell function, loss of normal motor inhibitory control, or pain-initiated hyperactivity of nervous tissue. Upper motor neuron lesions of the pyramidal system cause the following (Fig. 10–34):

- Paresis of voluntary movement patterns
- Increased muscle tone with related spasticity
- Hyperactive stretch reflex
- Hyperactive deep tendon reflexes and clonus
- Babinski's response

Upper motor neuron lesions of the extrapyramidal system cause (Fig. 10–35):

- Increased muscle tone and related characteristics
- Athetosis, tremor, and other involuntary movements
- Rigidity and poverty of movement

Cerebellar lesions decrease muscle tone and produce balance and coordination deficits (Fig. 10–36). Lower motor neuron lesions cause the following (Fig. 10–37):

- Flaccid paralysis
- Absence of muscle tone and related characteristics
- Muscular atrophy
- Sensory loss

Spinal cord lesions produce a combination of upper and lower motor neuron deficits, including various forms of paralysis.

Musculoskeletal disorders are generally the result of bone deformities, joint deformities, and muscle function restraints. Bone deformities may

# NEUROMUSCULAR PATHOLOGIES

| | |
|---|---|
| Malformation of the CNS | Spina bifida, other dysraphisms |
| Hereditary diseases | Huntington's chorea, Friedreich's ataxia, familial amyotrophic lateral sclerosis, Charcot-Marie-Tooth disease |
| Chromosomal anomalies | Down's syndrome |
| CNS metabolic diseases | Phenylketonuria, Hurler's disease |
| CNS infectious diseases | Meningitis, poliomyelitis |
| Perinatal and postnatal trauma | Cerebral palsy, subdural hematoma |
| Motor unit diseases | Infantile muscular atrophy, myasthenia gravis, muscular dystrophy |
| Paroxysmal disorders | Epilepsy, familial paroxysmal choreoathetosis |
| CNS tumors | Astrocytomas, blastomas, gliomas |
| Autoimmune disease | Rheumatoid arthritis, multiple sclerosis |
| Toxic disorders | Neonatal drug addiction |
| Mental development disorders | Autism, speech and language disorders |

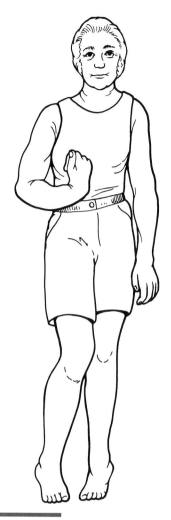

strains, tears, and ruptures; and local anomalies such as pain-spasm cycles (Fig. 10–40).

Posture-movement abuse and disuse syndromes are products of occupation and lifestyle. Long-duration static postures, repetitive skills, poor body mechanics, heavy lifting, and many other stressors are the core of the occupational posture-movement abuse syndrome (Fig. 10–41). These factors all tend to be repeated in some form in home, avocational, and leisure activities, reinforcing the abuse syndrome. A global decrease in movement variety to exercise coupled with muscle weakness, muscle imbalance, a sed-

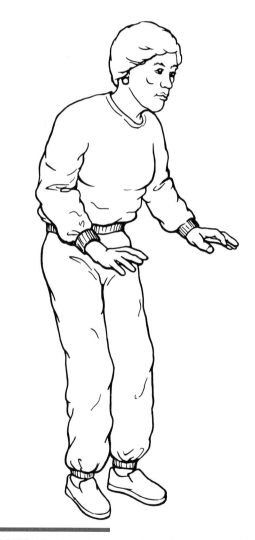

**FIGURE 10–34** ■ Typical posture of person with right-side hemiplegia, the residual deficit of a cerebrovascular accident producing upper motor neuron lesions of the pyramidal system. Asymmetric head and trunk position, unequal weight bearing in the lower extremities, and increased muscle tone or spasticity in the right hemibody predominate.

result from congenital or developmental abnormalities, epiphyseal growth plate disturbance, bone disease, nutritional deficits, fractures, and problems in healing (Fig. 10–38). They include variations in length, circumference, shape, and alignment. Joint deformities may result from congenital or developmental abnormalities, pathologic or traumatic instability, articular incongruity, internal derangements, adhesions and scarring, and idiopathic origins (Fig. 10–39). Muscle function restraints, other than those of neuromuscular origin, include muscle imbalances with such causes as excessive and isolated atrophy or hypertrophy; protective responses to contusions,

**FIGURE 10–35** ■ Typical posture of a person with Parkinson's disease, an upper motor neuron disease of the extrapyramidal system. Rigidity of the neck, trunk, and extremity muscles characterizes the more advanced stages of the disease. Resultant loss of freedom of motion produces postural instability and poverty of movement.

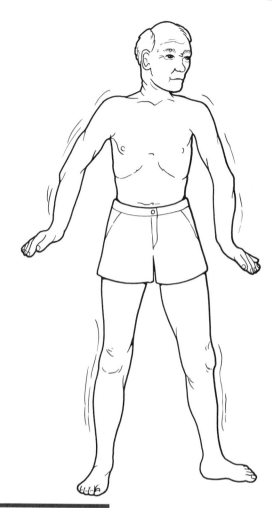

**FIGURE 10–36** ■ Lesions of the cerebellum cause decreases in muscle tone, coordination, and balance. Gait is often described as ataxic. Typical posture of ataxic person is a wide base of support with extraneous movements of trunk and extremities in efforts to maintain upright position.

entary lifestyle, and related weight gain adds to the abuse syndrome. The posture-movement dynamic is de-emphasized, sensory-motor perception is minimized, learning often levels off or even regresses, and emotional stability may decrease by degrees. The posture-movement dynamic tries to adapt to this destructive cycle but breakdowns inevitably occur sooner or later, resulting in a variety of conditions including

■ Carpal tunnel syndrome
■ Mechanical cervical and lumbar dysfunction and pain
■ Rotator cuff tendinitis
■ Muscular strain
■ Muscular spasms

■ Osteoarthritis
■ Temporomandibular joint dysfunction
■ Bulging discs
■ Peripheral neuropathies

When the abuse syndrome becomes the disuse syndrome, further complications develop, such as

■ Muscle disuse atrophy
■ Bone disuse atrophy in the form of disuse osteoporosis
■ Increased arthritic and degenerative changes
■ Diffuse or nonspecific somatic pain increases
■ Protective responses that promote guarding re-

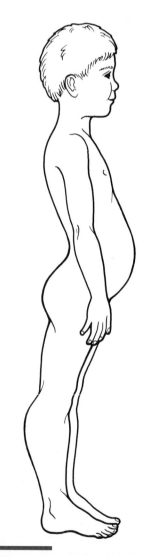

**FIGURE 10–37** ■ Typical posture of child with muscular dystrophy, a lower motor neuron disease producing progressive muscle atrophy. Predominant weakness of spinal and gluteal muscles causes the postural compensation of increased lumbar lordosis.

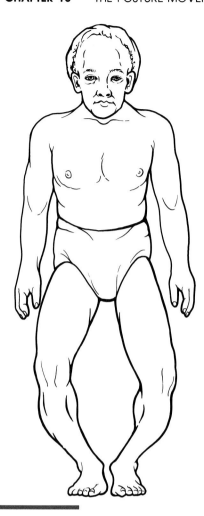

**FIGURE 10-38** ■ Bone deformities resulting from Paget's disease, or osteitis deformans. The disease is characterized by disorganized skeletal remodeling producing enlargement of the cranium, kyphosis of the spine, and bowing of the lower extremities.

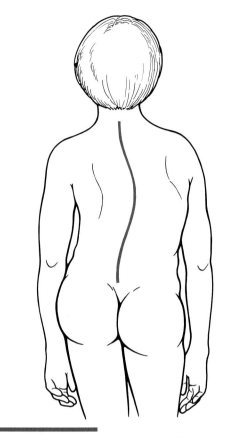

**FIGURE 10-39** ■ Postural deformity of kyphorotoscoliosis secondary to developmental joint abnormalities.

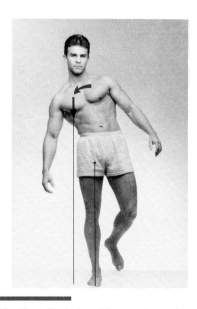

**FIGURE 10-40** ■ Typical walking posture of person with weakness of the right gluteus medius muscles. Insufficient stabilization of the right hip joint during stance phase produces the postural compensation of right lateral trunk bending at stance phase. This asymmetric compensation is often described as the gluteus medius "lurch."

actions that decrease range of motion (ROM) and result in inflammation, capsulitis, and contractures

The drastic changes in the limbic and cortical roles in motivation further negate any restoration of the posture-movement dynamic. Disintegration proceeds in any available direction.

Neuromuscular pathologies, musculoskeletal disorders, and posture-movement abuse and disuse syndromes all lead directly or indirectly to dysfunction and deformity. The observable bases for such dysfunctions and deformities are usually muscular imbalances, muscular atrophy, muscular contractures and fibrosis, connective tissue scarring, and deficits in osteogenesis and formation of bone architecture.

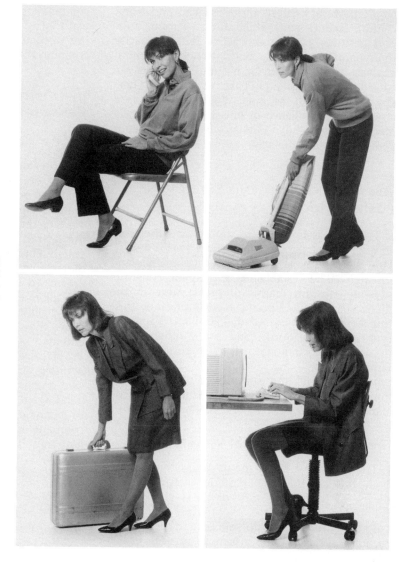

**FIGURE 10–41** ■ Examples of typical postural abuse and disuse habits common to modern lifestyles. Note sustained or repetitive thoracic and lumbar flexion combined with forward head position.

## POSTURAL ANALYSIS

The concept of the posture-movement dynamic is founded on several considerations:

■ Posture is the arrangement of body segments at any point or locus of points during movement.
■ A performing-enhancing posture offers the positive potentials of movement.
■ The positive potentials of movement are a key to the lifelong process of self-discovery.
■ A performance-detracting posture offers the negative potentials of movement.
■ The negative potentials of movement have a disintegrative effect on perception, development and maintenance, emotions, learning, socialization, and self-actualization.

■ The temporal summation of performance-detracting postures alters biomechanics, produces pain, dysfunction and deformity, and emphasizes the negative potentials of movement.

Problems of the posture-movement dynamic, whether orthopaedic or neurologic in nature, can often be reduced or even corrected. An assessment of the patient's present status may be compared to accepted norms of structural relationships and biomechanics. The results may then be used to formulate a plan to restore part or all of the posture-movement dynamic.

The assessment of present status should include both static and dynamic postural analysis. Static postural analysis includes comparison of the patient's standing posture to a biomechanically accepted ideal or standard posture. Dynamic postural analysis includes head and trunk control, balance and equilibrium in various support postures, passive and active ROM, capacity for voluntary control, and strength. Postural analysis and correction of postural problems are considered the essential basis of physical therapy. Proper body segment alignment, balanced strength and resilience of muscles, efficient body mechanics, and full ROM are usually the major goals of physical therapy.

## The Ideal or Standard Static Posture Model

The body is in continual motion and therefore in the strictest sense static posture does not exist. However, the work of experienced clinicians and researchers has established a theoretic construct of static posture that is of great value to the physical therapist. Specific models of static posture as theorized by Kendall, Cailliet, Kapandji, Brunnstrom, McMorris, and many others differ in details and rationale. It is important to be familiar with the wealth of information presented in all these works. What follows is intended only as a generalized distillation of the standard posture model (Figs. 10–42 to 10–46).

### The Head and Cervical Vertebrae

The line of reference should bisect the head in both the anterior and posterior coronal plane views. In the lateral view of the sagittal plane the line of gravity passes slightly posterior to the coronal suture, through the external auditory meatus, through the odontoid process, and through or slightly posterior to the axis of rotation of the cervical vertebrae. When the line of gravity does not pass directly through the flexion-extension axis, gravitational moments of force promote the more likely of the two directions. The relationship of the line of gravity to the cervical vertebral axis of flexion-extension causes an extension response to gravity. The relationship of the line of gravity to the head's axis of flexion-extension causes a flexion response to gravity. Ligamentous structures alone cannot counter gravity; the neck and spinal muscles must assist. In the erect positions, regardless of alignment problems, there is a constant effort to maintain visual reference to the horizon.

Typical problems of head and neck alignment include lateral tilts, excessive flexion or extension at the atlanto-occipital joint or throughout the cervical vertebrae, and side bending–rotation combinations that occur to the same side. A forward head with related adaptive shortening of the neck extensor muscles is one of the most common disorders of the area (Fig. 10–47).

### The Thorax and Thoracic Vertebrae

The line of reference for the anterior coronal plane should bisect the thoracic vertebral bodies and the sternum. The anterior view of the thorax should be symmetric. The line of reference for the posterior coronal plane should fall on the thoracic spinous processes, and the posterior view of the thorax should also be symmetric. In the lateral view of the sagittal plane the line of gravity should pass anterior to the bodies of the thoracic vertebrae. The relationship of the line of gravity to the thoracic vertebral axis of flexion-extension causes a flexion response to gravity. The ligamentous structures require much help from the spinal extensor muscles to counter gravity.

Typical problems of thoracic alignment include kyphosis or excessive flexion, verticality or excessive extension, and scoliosis or abnormal side bending–rotation combinations (Fig. 10–48). Problems of thoracic vertebral alignment are accompanied by adaptive changes in the rib cage and the shoulder complex. Focal points of specific dysfunction also tend to appear at the C-7 to T-3 and T-11 to L-1 transition areas.

### The Pelvis and Lumbosacral Vertebrae

The line of reference for the anterior coronal plane should bisect the lumbosacral vertebral bodies and pass through the pubic symphysis. The anterior view of the pelvis should be symmetric and landmarks should be level. The line of reference for the posterior coronal plane should fall on the lumbar spinous processes and bisect the sacrum, and the posterior view of the pelvis should be symmetric with level landmarks. In the lateral view of the sagittal plane the line of gravity passes through or slightly posterior to the axis of rotation of the lumbar vertebrae and close to the axis of rotation of the lumbosacral joint. A line connecting the anterior superior iliac spines and posterior superior iliac spines should be horizontal. The lumbosacral angle formed by the inclination of the superior plateau of the first sacral vertebra should be approximately 30 degrees. The line of gravity also passes slightly an-

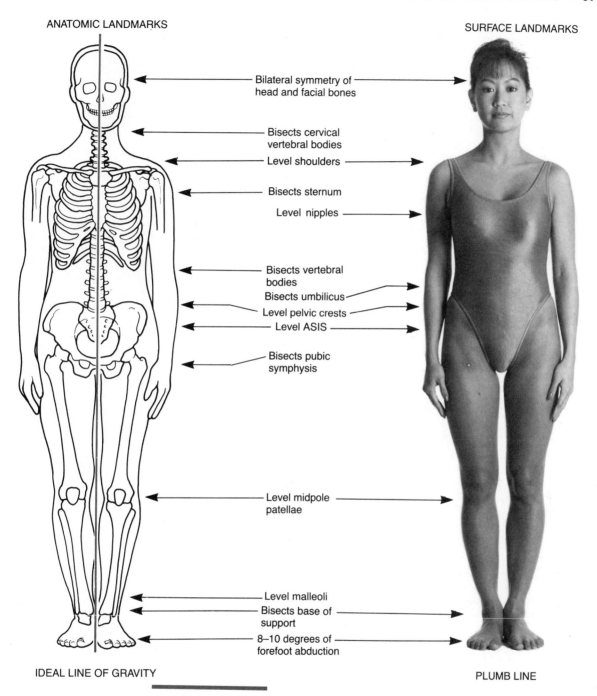

ANATOMIC LANDMARKS

SURFACE LANDMARKS

Bilateral symmetry of head and facial bones

Bisects cervical vertebral bodies

Level shoulders

Bisects sternum

Level nipples

Bisects vertebral bodies

Bisects umbilicus

Level pelvic crests

Level ASIS

Bisects pubic symphysis

Level midpole patellae

Level malleoli

Bisects base of support

8–10 degrees of forefoot abduction

IDEAL LINE OF GRAVITY

PLUMB LINE

**FIGURE 10–42** ■ Ideal posture. Anterior view of coronal plane.

terior to the sacroiliac joints. The relationship of the line of gravity to the lumbar vertebral axis of flexion-extension causes an extension response to gravity. The relationship of the line of gravity to the sacroiliac joint causes a flexion or anterior-to-inferior response to gravity by the superior portion of the sacrum. Ligamentous structures stabilize the sacrum but the iliopsoas and other muscles must counter the lumbar extension moment.

Typical problems of lumbosacral and pelvic alignment include the following (Fig. 10–49):

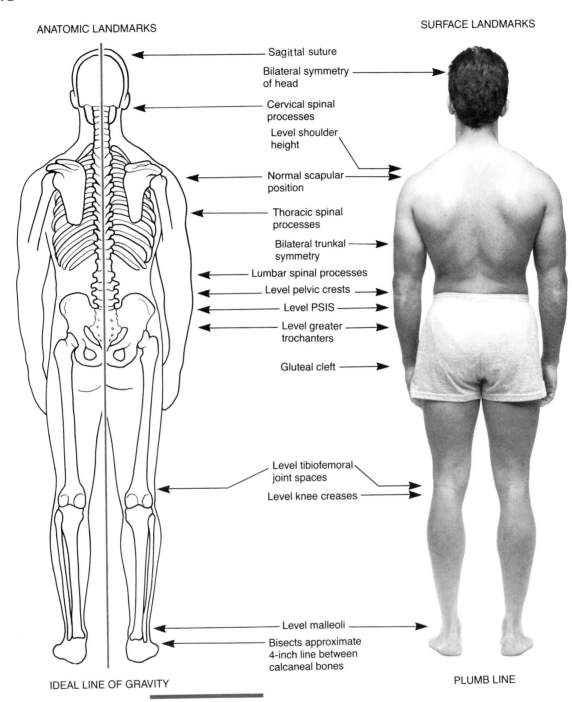

ANATOMIC LANDMARKS

SURFACE LANDMARKS

- Sagittal suture
- Bilateral symmetry of head
- Cervical spinal processes
- Level shoulder height
- Normal scapular position
- Thoracic spinal processes
- Bilateral trunkal symmetry
- Lumbar spinal processes
- Level pelvic crests
- Level PSIS
- Level greater trochanters
- Gluteal cleft
- Level tibiofemoral joint spaces
- Level knee creases
- Level malleoli
- Bisects approximate 4-inch line between calcaneal bones

IDEAL LINE OF GRAVITY

PLUMB LINE

**FIGURE 10–43** ■ Ideal posture. Posterior view of coronal plane.

- Excessive lumbar lordosis
- Flat back or loss of lumbar lordosis
- Lumbar scoliosis
- Anterior or posterior pelvic tilts
- Disturbed iliosacral positioning

## The Lower Extremities

The line of reference for both the anterior and posterior views of the coronal plane should bisect the body and reveal symmetry and equal

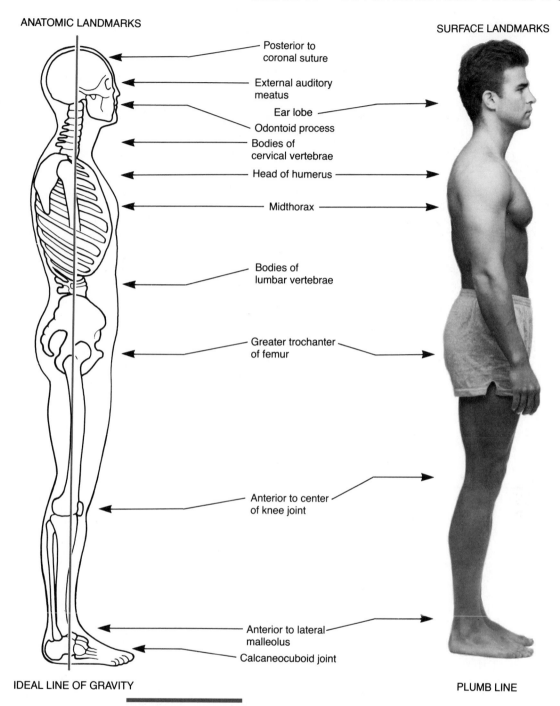

ANATOMIC LANDMARKS

SURFACE LANDMARKS

Posterior to
coronal suture

External auditory
meatus

Ear lobe

Odontoid process

Bodies of
cervical vertebrae

Head of humerus

Midthorax

Bodies of
lumbar vertebrae

Greater trochanter
of femur

Anterior to center
of knee joint

Anterior to lateral
malleolus

Calcaneocuboid joint

IDEAL LINE OF GRAVITY

PLUMB LINE

**FIGURE 10–44** ■ Ideal posture. Lateral view of sagittal plane.

weight distribution. The anterior view should be supplemented with the mechanical axis for each lower extremity. The mechanical axis should form a straight line connecting the center of the head of the femur, the center of the patella, and the center of the head of the talus. In the lateral view of the sagittal plane the line of gravity should pass slightly posterior to the center of the hip joint, slightly anterior to the center of the knee joint, and through the calcaneocuboid joint. The relationship of the line of gravity to the hip and knee joints causes a flexion response to

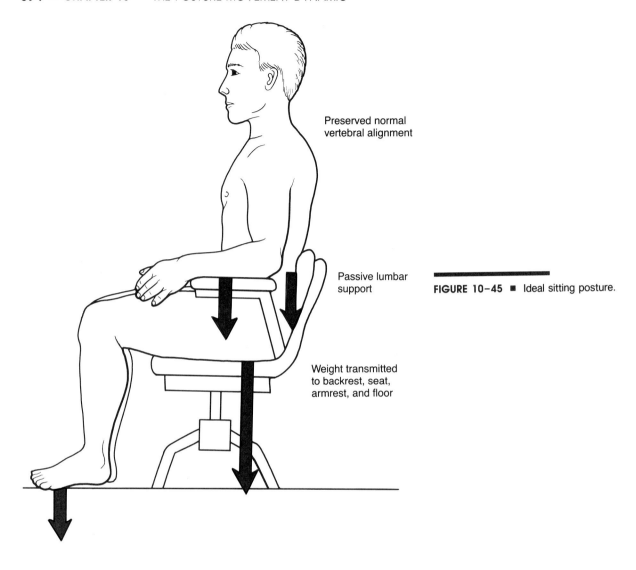

Preserved normal
vertebral alignment

Passive lumbar
support

**FIGURE 10–45** ■ Ideal sitting posture.

Weight transmitted
to backrest, seat,
armrest, and floor

gravity at each. The relationship of the line of gravity to the ankle joint causes a dorsiflexion response to gravity. Ligamentous structures stabilize the hip and knee joints without any muscular help. No ligamentous stability is present in the ankle to stabilize the dorsiflexion moment, so the counterforce is provided by the soleus muscle.

Typical problems of alignment in the lower extremities include

■ Excessive joint flexion or extension
■ Excessive abduction or adduction
■ Excessive internal or external rotation

Pathologic problems (Fig. 10–50) include

■ Coxa varus and coxa valgus retroversion and anteversion
■ Genu varum and genu valgus
■ Tibial torsion

## The Foot

Kendall's version of standard posture, the barefoot position, has the heels about 3 inches apart and each forefoot abducted 8 to 10 degrees. Weight is distributed equally on each foot. In this position, the line of gravity should pass through the calcaneocuboid joint and the mechanical axis of the lower extremity should pass through the center of the head of the talus. A posterior view in the coronal plane should reveal a straight calcaneus and calcaneal tendon. A medial view in the sagittal plane should reveal a straight Feiss line—the line drawn from the medial malleolus to the navicular tuberosity to the head of the first metatarsal.

Typical problems of the foot (Fig. 10–51) include

■ Excessive plantar flexion or dorsiflexion

| POSTURE EVALUATION | | |
|---|---|---|
| NAME:             AGE:      SEX:      HEIGHT:        WEIGHT:        DATE: | | |

Body type: Ectomorph / Mesomorph / Endomorph / Slight Build / Medium Build / Heavy Build

| ANTERIOR VIEW | Comments: | |
|---|---|---|
| Head (aligned, forward, flexed, extended) | | |
| Mandible (resting position, retracted) | | |
| Shoulders (level, uneven) | | |
| Rib cage (symmetric, asymmetric) | | |
| Pelvis (level, anterior/posterior tilt) | | |
| Hips (coxa varus, coxa valgus, anteversion, retroversion) | | |
| Femurs (alignment) | | |
| Knees (level, genu varus, genu valgus) | | |
| Tibias (alignment, torsions) | | |
| Ankles (inversion, eversion) | | |
| Feet (pes cavus, pes planus, supination/pronation) | | |
| Toes (alignment, deformities) | | |
| **LATERAL VIEW** | | |
| Head (forward, flexed/extended) | | |
| Mandible (resting, protracted/retracted) | | |
| Scapulae (winging, elevation/depression) | | |
| Thoracic kyphosis (increased/decreased) | | |
| Lumbar lordosis (increased/decreased) | | |
| Pelvis (anterior/posterior tilt) | | |
| Knees (hyperextension/flexion) | | |
| Feet (longitudinal arch) | | |
| **POSTERIOR VIEW** | | |
| Head (alignment, tilt) | | |
| Shoulders (level) | | |
| Scapulae (bilateral symmetry) | | |
| Spine C-1 to sacrum (rotations, deviations) | | |
| Pelvis (level, tilt) | | |
| Sacrum (level at base and inferior lateral angles) | | |
| Hips (level, uneven) | | |
| Knees (creases level/uneven) | | |
| Ankles (inversion/eversion) | | |
| Calcaneal position (inverted/everted) | | |

Pertinent Medical History:

Pertinent Radiographic Findings / Other Tests:

**FIGURE 10–46** ■ Example of posture evaluation form. Information is obtained by visual observation and palpation.

■ Excessive abduction or adduction
■ Excessive pronation and supination

Pathologic problems include

■ Rigid pes planus or pes cavus
■ Calcaneal varus or valgus
■ Hallux valgus

■ Claw toes
■ Hammer toes

## The Shoulder Complex

The line of reference for both anterior and posterior views of the coronal plane should bi-

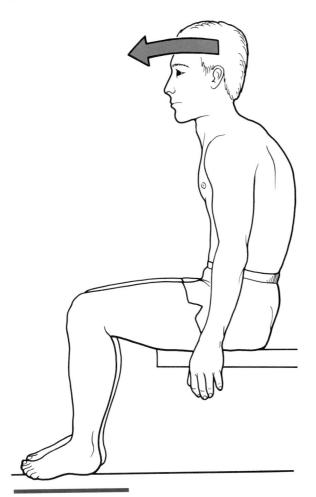

**FIGURE 10-47** ■ The common postural fault of the forward head position is usually associated with related increases in thoracic kyphosis and decreases in lumbar lordosis. These positional deficits may begin early in life but cause the most devastating effects later in life.

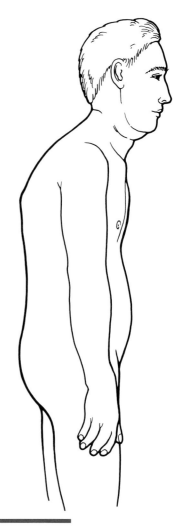

**FIGURE 10-48** ■ Excessive thoracic kyphosis often begins in adolescence as "slouching" posture. Habitual thoracic flexion can lead to associated cervical and lumbar compensations, abducted scapulae, dysfunctional shoulder girdle mechanics, overstretched and weak posterior trunk musculature, and shortened anterior trunk musculature. The hypomobile kyphotic spine in osteoporotic elderly persons is susceptible to anterior wedge compression fractures of the vertebral bodies.

sect the body and reveal symmetry and level landmarks. In the posterior view the scapulae should rest congruously against the thoracic cage between the second and seventh ribs with the vertebral borders approximately parallel and about 2 inches from midline. In the lateral view of the sagittal plane the line of gravity passes through the center of the shoulder joint. In this instance the line of gravity serves only as a line of reference to help locate the proper position of the shoulder complex. The force of gravity on the glenohumeral joint is observed better in the coronal plane, where an adduction response to gravity becomes apparent. This adduction moment is countered by abduction forces supplied by the superior joint capsule and the coracohumeral ligament. In ideal posture the upper ex-

tremity can hang at the side of the body without requiring active muscular assistance.

Typical problems of the shoulder complex posture (Fig. 10-52) include

■ Scapular winging
■ Scapular protraction or retraction
■ Scapular elevation or depression

Problems of the shoulder complex may also originate with the sternum and the clavicle. Any al-

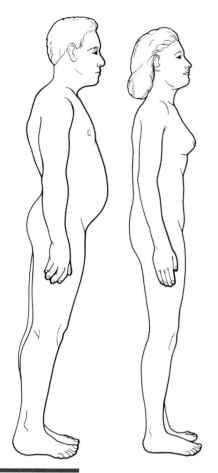

**FIGURE 10–49** ■ Typical postural dysfunctions of the lumbosacral-pelvic complex. (Left) Increased lumbar lordosis is often associated with hypermobile lumbar joints, excessive shear stresses at L-4 to L-5 and L-5 to S-1, and anterior pelvic tilt. Abdominal musculature is generally weak and overstretched; posterior lumbar muscles and hip flexors tend to be shortened. (Right) Decreased lumbar lordosis is often associated with posterior pelvic tilt, loss of lumbar joint mobility, and tight hamstrings. In either of these examples, related cervical and thoracic compensations exist, as do compensations in the distal kinetic chain of the lower extremities.

teration in the standard postural position of the glenohumeral joint is a potentially serious postural problem.

## The Dynamic Posture Model

The ideal model for dynamic posture is based on full integration of reflexes, reactions, sensation, motor milestones, and volitional movement. Head and trunk control, trunk rotation, bilateral and unilateral contractions against gravity-related elongation of reciprocally inhibited antagonist,

positional stability and equilibrium, segmental control, mobility, and fine motor coordination are some of the many characteristics of the dynamic posture model. Analysis of dynamic posture ranges from the singular measurements of goniometry to the complexities of anthropometry and kinesiology. Dynamic posture is not a theoretic construct for plumb line and posture grid comparison but is instead the individual's expression of neuromusculoskeletal development.

The true model for dynamic posture is individualized and describes the individual's potential for

■ ROM-strength-endurance expression
■ Righting-equilibrium-protective reaction expression
■ Mobility-stability-mobility (MSM) loop expression
■ Motor control–motor planning–motor execution expression
■ Integrated cognitive-affective-psychomotor expression

### Range of Motion–Strength–Endurance Expression

Range of motion is the movement permitted at an articulation by the bone structure, soft tissue elasticity, and contraction of muscles crossing that joint (Fig. 10–53). Strength is the force generated by muscle contraction. Endurance is the capacity to sustain force over a period of time. Individually, each of these areas can present special problems. An articulation may be hypomobile or hypermobile. Strength may be trace or absent, permitting only passive ROM. Endurance may have no practical value until a position or movement can be sustained. However, when an individual displays maximum positive expression of all three, freedom of motion, delicate and/or powerful motion, and sustained motion blend into skilled and creative movement patterns.

The clinical assessment of ROM-strength-endurance expression may begin with goniometry, manual muscle testing, and isokinetic repetitions. Meaningful analysis, however, must examine the individual's expression of function, performance, and potential.

### Righting-Equilibrium-Protective Reaction Expression

Righting reactions utilize visual, vestibular, and proprioceptive information to orient the head and body to the ground, the horizon, and the

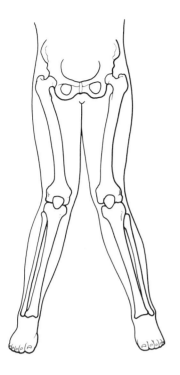 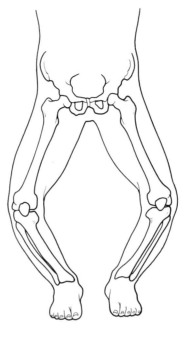

**FIGURE 10–50** ■ Alignment dysfunctions of the lower extremities may originate developmentally or in response to injury or disease. A mechanical problem existing at one weight-bearing joint always has some compensatory effect on the joints proximal and distal to it in the kinetic chain. Also, postural problems that are observed to be unilateral have some degree of compensatory effect on the contralateral extremity.

force of gravity. Equilibrium reactions utilize visual, vestibular, and proprioceptive information to maintain balance when the center of gravity is disturbed. Protective reactions are specialized equilibrium reactions that rely heavily on vestibular information to detect loss of balance and initiate extremity responses to stop or catch the fall. The combination of the three reaction types provides the foundation for balance and orientation in the upright positions (Fig. 10–54). They eventually produce weight shifting, ambulation, manipulation, and movement strategies.

Clinical assessment may begin with rolling activities, seated balance and weight shifting, and

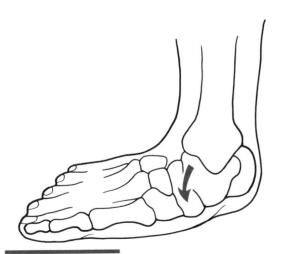 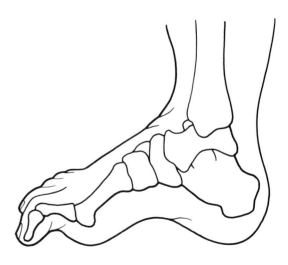

**FIGURE 10–51** ■ Common postural dysfunctions at the foot. (Left) Pes planus or flat foot. This postural dysfunction is often associated with calcaneal eversion, subtalar joint pronation, and ligamentous laxity. Proximal extremity malalignments may include knee valgus that shifts the line of weight bearing medially. A flexible flat foot describes the foot whose longitudinal arch is restored upon non–weight bearing. A rigid flat foot exhibits no preservation of the longitudinal arch. (Right) Pes cavus or high longitudinal arch. This type of foot is usually associated with an inflexible forefoot, extensor ligamentous shortening with resultant dorsiflexion of the proximal phalanges, and excessive weight-bearing stresses at the metatarsal heads.

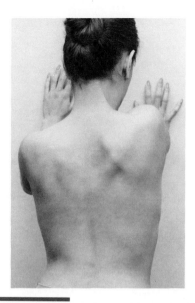

**FIGURE 10–52** ■ Weakness of the serratus anterior muscles causes "winging" of the scapula during this wall push-up test. Altered position of the scapula caused by isolated muscle weakness leads to a cascade of soft tissue lesions in the shoulder complex secondary to dysfunctional joint mechanics. Muscles, tendons, bursae, and neurovascular structures are susceptible to strain, compression, and friction during abnormal scapuloglenohumeral rhythm.

simple perturbations of the center of gravity. Advanced analysis may include performance tests on balance beams, rocker boards, stairs, uneven surfaces, and large balls. When an individual displays maximum positive expression of all three, a dynamic skill base already exists and potential for more creative movement is available.

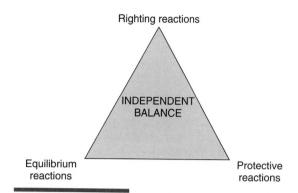

**FIGURE 10–54** ■ Righting-equilibrium-protective reaction expression. An individual's posture-movement dynamic progresses in direct relation to development of balance and orientation skills. Independent balance might well be viewed as a perceptual skill critical to learning.

## Mobility-Stability-MSM Loop Expression

Mobility is movement, whether random or voluntary. Stability is a sustained pattern of muscular contraction or cocontraction that produces weight bearing, support, and fixation of body segments. MSM loop is a term of convenience used to describe patterns of mobility-stability integration pre-existing within or progressively developed by the motor hierarchy for the purpose of automatic and voluntary control (Fig. 10–55). MSM loops use all the resources available in the motor hierarchy to build head, neck, trunk, and proximal control skills that lead to and enhance locomotor and manipulative skills of the extremities.

Clinical assessment of stability may begin with

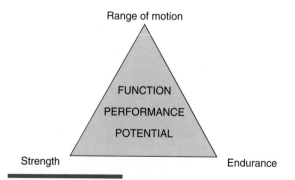

**FIGURE 10–53** ■ ROM-strength-endurance expression. An individual's potential for performance of motor activity requires not only an intact neuromuscular system but also a blend of freedom of movement, application of force to leverage systems, and the physiologic capacity for sustained effort.

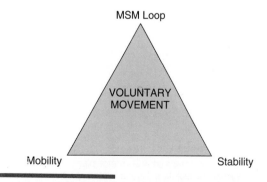

**FIGURE 10–55** ■ Mobility-stability-MSM loop expression. MSM loops are movement patterns skills, and established movement strategies built step by step from oscillations over the stability-mobility continuum until a desired measure of control is obtained.

an evaluation of muscle tone, the capacity for contraction and cocontraction, and weight bearing. Clinical assessment of mobility may add ROM to the neuromuscular evaluation. Clinical assessment of MSM loop development may begin with analysis of movements from the developmental sequence. Advanced analysis includes the level of locomotor and manipulative skills that the individual has available to express mobility-stability integration.

## Motor Control–Motor Planning–Motor Execution Expression

Motor control is ultimately the development of skilled locomotion and manipulation (Fig. 10–56). Motor planning is the selection of an appropriate motor response. Motor execution is actual performance of the selected response. Clinical assessment may find all three facets well developed in controlled situations, yet the patient's abilities disintegrate when the controls are removed. Sensory overload, stimulus generalization, emotions, experience, and timing are among many factors that may interfere with performance.

Motor control–motor planning–motor execution expression shows the critical link between dynamic posture and higher learning. Abilities developed outside the environment in which they must be used often prove ineffective. An individual's motor expression of learning should be rooted in the individual's real world of behavioral experiences.

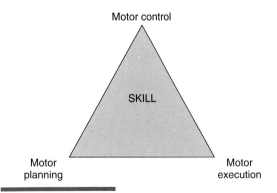

**FIGURE 10–56 ■** Motor control–motor planning–motor execution expression. Skill is initially a motor act linking perception and cortical activity to performance of a task. Higher learning builds concepts from the enhanced perceptions attained not only by skills but also by the planning-control-execution aspect of the posture-movement dynamic.

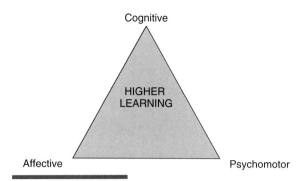

**FIGURE 10–57 ■** Cortical learning and motor learning may finally be considered as two separate functions, but motor learning's critical role in perception and its contributions to cognitive and affective centers form the basis for an individual's learning.

## Integrated Cognitive-Affective-Psychomotor Expression

Cognition is the use of perception, memory, and thought to enhance observation and experience, gain understanding through association, and develop a reasoning process to use and create knowledge. Affective behavior is the blending of sensation, emotions, memories, survival needs, pain, and vital signs of physiologic function into motivations. Psychomotor behavior is intended here to represent predominantly the voluntary aspect of motor control. Knowledge, emotions, memories, drives, attitudes, opinions, values, inhibitions, will power, self-control, initiative, and voluntary movement are all interrelated. Clinical assessment of dynamic posture cannot be only one-dimensional. An individual's cognitive-affective-psychomotor expression of dynamic posture is an expression of the entire personality (Fig. 10–57).

## SUMMARY

Movement is perhaps the most critical aspect of human experience. Movement enhances perception and fosters exploration and manipulation of an individual's environment. Each human being's working definition of life depends greatly on the performance level of movement experience. Through each decade of life the capacity for efficient and pain-free movement remains central to an individual's life-enhancing experiences. The posture-movement dynamic is a sensory-motor system controlled by the motor hierarchy, constructed on a foundation of integrated reflexes, subprograms, and reactions, developed in a sequence of motor milestones, and actualized through motor learning. The posture-movement dynamic pursues the positive potentials of movement unless disrupted by disease, trauma, abuse, or disuse. Problems of the posture-movement dynamic can often be reduced or even corrected. Assessment of static posture is a present-status comparison to a theoretic construct known as the ideal or standard posture model. Assessment of dynamic posture is a view of the individual's expression of neuromusculoskeletal development ranging from motor milestone achievements to cognitive, affective, and psychomotor integration of personality. The posture-movement dynamic enables the human body to function as the basic tool for life.

## Bibliography

Barnes MR, Crutchfield CA, Heriza CB: The Neurophysiological Basis of Patient Treatment, Vol II. Morgantown, WV: Stokesville Publishing, 1979.

Bly L: The Components of Normal Movement During the First Year of Life and Abnormal Motor Development. Oak Park, IL: The Neuro-Developmental Treatment Association, 1983.

Bobath B: Adult Hemiplegia: Evaluation and Treatment, 2nd ed. London: William Heinemann Medical Books, 1979.

Bobath B: Abnormal Postural Reflex Activity Caused by Brain Lesions, 3rd ed. Rockville, MD: Aspen Systems, 1986.

Bouchard C, Shephard RJ, Stephens T, et al: Exercise, Fitness, and Health: A Consensus of Current Knowledge. Champaign, IL: Human Kinetics, 1990.

Brooks VB: The Neural Basis of Motor Control. New York: Oxford University Press, 1986.

Brunnstrom S: Movement Therapy in Hemiplegia. Philadelphia: Harper & Row, 1970.

Carr JH, Shepherd RB: A Motor Relearning Programme for Stroke. Rockville, MD: Aspen Systems, 1984.

Carpenter MB: Core Text of Neuroanatomy, 3rd ed. Baltimore: Williams & Wilkins, 1985.

Chaffin DB, Andersson GBJ: Occupational Biomechanics, 2nd ed. New York: John Wiley & Sons, 1991.

Chusid JG: Correlative Neuroanatomy and Functional Neurology, 19th ed. Los Altos, CA: Lange Medical Publications, 1985.

Connor FP, Williamson GG, Siepp JM: Program Guide for Infants and Toddlers with Neuromotor and Other Developmental Disabilities. New York: Teachers College Press, 1978.

Cratty BJ: Movement Behavior and Motor Learning. Philadelphia: Lea & Febiger, 1964.

Crutchfield CA, Barnes MR: The Neurophysiological Basis of Patient Treatment, 2nd ed. Morgantown, WV: Stokesville Publishing, 1972.

Davies PM: Steps to Follow—a Guide to the Treatment of Adult Hemiplegia. Berlin: Springer-Verlag, 1985.

Duesterhaus Minor MA, Duesterhaus Minor S: Patient Care Skills. Reston, VA: Reston Publishing, 1984.

Duesterhaus Minor MA, Duesterhaus Minor S: Patient Evaluation Methods for the Health Professional. Reston, VA: Reston Publishing, 1985.

Heiniger MC, Randolph SL: Neurophysiological Concepts in Human Behavior. St. Louis: Mosby Year Book, 1981.

Hoppenfeld S: Physical Examination of the Spine and Extremities. New York: Appleton-Century-Crofts, 1976.

Hughes C: Postural assessment. Unpublished manuscript, 1985. (Available from C. Hughes, Slippery Rock University, Slippery Rock, PA.)

Illingworth RS: The Development of the Infant and Young Child, 8th ed. Edinburgh: Churchill-Livingstone, 1985.

Kandel ER, Schwartz JH: Principles of Neural Science, 2nd ed. New York: Elsevier, 1985.

Kendall HO, Kendall FP, Boynton DA: Posture and Pain. Malabar, FL: Robert E. Krieger Publishing, 1981.

Kendall HO, Kendall FP, Wadsworth GE: Muscles, Testing and Function, 2nd ed. Baltimore: Williams & Wilkins, 1971.

Kisner C, Colby LA: Therapeutic Exercise. Philadelphia: FA Davis, 1985.

Lawther JD: The Learning and Performance of Physical Skills, 2nd ed. Englewood Cliffs, NJ: Prentice-Hall, 1977.

Magee DJ: Orthopedic Physical Assessment. Philadelphia: WB Saunders, 1987.

Menkes JH: Textbook of Child Neurology. Philadelphia: Lea & Febiger, 1974.

Nixon V: Spinal Cord Injury. Rockville, MD: Aspen Systems, 1985.

Nordin M, Frankel VH: Basic Biomechanics of the Musculoskeletal System, 2nd ed. Philadelphia: Lea & Febiger, 1989.

Norkin C, Levangie P: Joint Structure and Function. Philadelphia: FA Davis, 1985.

Rasch PJ, Burke RK: Kinesiology and Applied Anatomy, 6th ed. Philadelphia: Lea & Febiger, 1977.

Salter RB: Textbook of Disorders and Injuries of the Musculoskeletal System, 2nd ed. Baltimore: Williams & Wilkins, 1983.

Saunders HD: Evaluation, Treatment and Prevention of Musculoskeletal Disorders. Minneapolis: Anderberg-Lund Printing, 1985.

Soderberg GL: Kinesiology. Baltimore: Williams & Wilkins, 1986.

Sullivan PE, Markos PD, Minor MAD: An Integrated Approach to Therapeutic Exercise. Reston, VA: Reston Publishing, 1982.

Uram P, McKinnis DL: Refining Human Movement. Butler, PA: Thoma Printing, 1968.

Watson RR, Eisinger M: Exercise and Disease. Boca Raton: CRC Press, 1992.

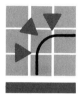

# CHAPTER *Eleven*

## Gait

*MARCIA EPLER*

## INTRODUCTION

The evaluation of patients is based on a number of factors, including diagnosis, diagnostic testing results, medical history, subjective information provided by the patient and/or family, and physical examination. The physical examination sometimes includes an assessment of a localized body area or segment but most often requires the clinician to approach the individual as a total entity. The examination process not only detects problems of the musculoskeletal, neurologic, and cardiovascular systems but also provides information about how abnormalities in these systems contribute to deviations in posture and gait. Any disorder of such magnitude as to affect an individual's overall posture and/or gait can be expected to be manifest in the individual's difficulties in performing activities of daily living and level of function.

Human walking can be defined as the process of locomotion in which the erect moving body is supported first by one leg and then the other. Many animals travel on all fours, but the human has evolved to a level of moving from one location to another by means of a bipedal gait. Although there are countless variations of styles of gait that would be considered normal, virtually all individuals exhibit certain characteristics common to all gait and from which deviations from normal can be detected. It is crucial that all clinicians involved in the rehabilitation process have a thorough understanding of the biomechanics of normal gait. Equally important is the ability to recognize deviations in gait resulting from disease, trauma, postural abnormalities, and age. The clinician's ability to visualize and assess gait abnormalities is essential to the formulation of appropriate treatment programs aimed at normalizing structure and function.

In order to fully appreciate and comprehend human locomotion, an understanding of basic definitions and concepts used in the description of gait is necessary. The following terminology provides the framework for a detailed description of gait analysis.

## BASIC CONCEPTS OF GAIT

**Base of Support.** Base of support in gait refers to the distance between an individual's feet while in a weight-bearing position. The base of support helps provide both the stability and balance necessary to maintain an upright posture. A normal base of support is considered to be between 5 and 10 cm. Naturally, the larger the base of support, the greater the stability provided. Conversely, balance and stability are progressively compromised as the base of support becomes smaller. Clinically, larger than normal bases of support are observed in individuals who have muscular imbalances of the lower limbs and trunk as well as those who have problems with overall static and dynamic balance.

**Center of Gravity.** The center of gravity refers to the point of an object at which all mass tends to be concentrated and the point at which the force of gravity acts. In the human body, the center of gravity lies approximately 5 cm anterior to the second sacral vertebra. The center of gravity shifts both horizontally and vertically during gait.

**Toe-out.** Toe-out is defined by the angle formed by the intersection of the foot's line of progression and the line extending from the center of the heel through the second metatarsal. The normal toe-out angle is approximately 7 degrees. The amount of toe-out typically decreases as the speed of gait increases.

**Step Length.** Step length is the linear distance between the point of contact of one heel or toe with the ground and the point of contact of the contralateral heel or toe with the ground. Some individuals, such as those diagnosed with cerebral palsy, typically do not exhibit heel contact with the ground. For those individuals, step length is measured from the point of contact of the toe with the ground. Step length is always discussed in relation to the limb moving forward. For example, the step length on the left would be measured as the distance from the point of contact of the right heel with the ground to the point of contact of the left heel with the ground. Step lengths are equal in gait that is observed to be symmetric. Asymmetric gait patterns demonstrate inequality in step lengths (Fig. 11–1).

**Step Duration.** Step duration is the amount of time spent during a single step. Therefore, it is measured as the time between contact of the heel of one foot with the floor and contact of the heel of the contralateral foot with the floor.

**Cadence.** Cadence is defined as the number of steps per minute. Normal values for cadence fall between 90 and 120 steps per minute.

**Stride Length.** Stride length refers to the sequence of motions that occur between two consecutive repetitions of a body part and is also commonly referred to as the basic *gait cycle.* Stride length is determined by measuring the distance from the point of heel contact or toe contact of one lower limb to the subsequent point of heel contact or toe contact with the same lower limb. A stride length contains both a left and a right step and is directly affected by leg length. Obviously, individuals with greater leg lengths have larger stride lengths. Decreases in stride length occur commonly with aging. Also, as the velocity of gait increases, accompanying increases in stride length and number of strides become evident. Normal values for stride length range from 70 to 82 cm.

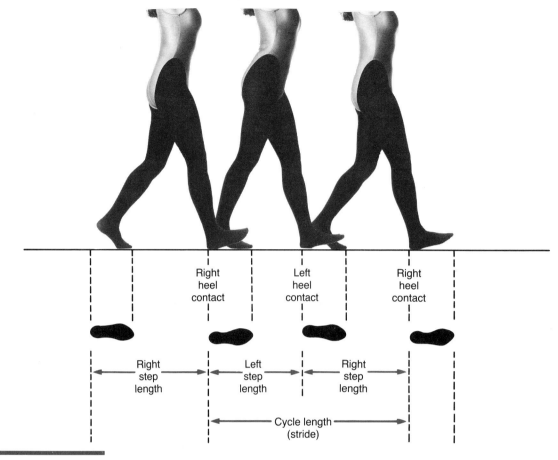

**FIGURE 11–1** ■ Measurement of step and stride lengths throughout the gait cycle. (Modified from Inman VT, Ralston HJ, Todd F: Human Walking. Baltimore: Williams & Wilkins, 1991.)

**Stride Duration.** Stride duration refers to the amount of time required to accomplish one stride. Knowledge of stride length and stride duration allows computation of walking speed: walking speed = stride distance/stride duration and is expressed as cm/sec or m/sec.

**Stance.** Stance is the phase in the gait cycle when the foot is in contact with the ground in preparation for weight bearing and propulsion of the body in a forward direction. The stance phase of gait occupies approximately 60% of the walking gait cycle (Fig. 11–2).

**Swing.** Swing is defined as the phase of the gait cycle in which the lower limb is non–weight bearing and moving forward. The swing phase occupies 40% of the walking gait cycle.

**Double Support.** Double support refers to the period of time when the feet of both lower limbs are simultaneously in contact with the ground and weight is being transferred from one foot to the other. In normal gait, the period of double support constitutes approximately 25% of the gait cycle. The time of double support is inversely proportional to the speed of walking. Therefore, as the speed of walking decreases, the period of double support increases. Conversely, as the speed of walking increases the period of double support decreases, and when running there may be no phase of double support.

## GENERAL BODY DISPLACEMENTS DURING GAIT

This section deals with the major displacements that occur in the body during the normal walking process. These vertical and lateral oscillations are a result of the harmonious movement of all body segments during ambulation.

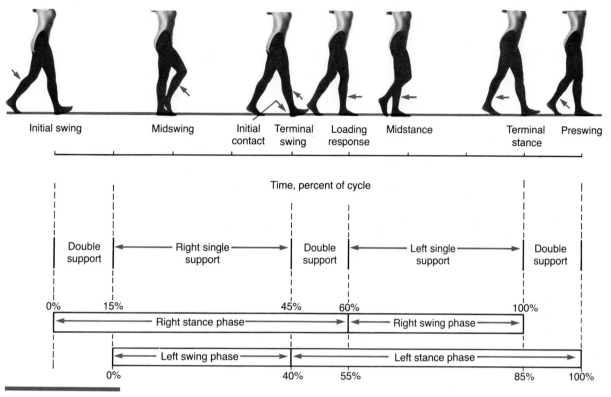

**FIGURE 11-2** ■ Percentage of time spent in each phase of the gait cycle. (Modified from Inman VT, Ralston HJ, Todd F: Human Walking. Baltimore: Williams & Wilkins, 1991.)

## Center of Mass

The center of mass of the human body lies midline in the frontal plane and slightly anterior to the second sacral vertebra in the sagittal plane. During normal ambulation, the center of mass continues to remain within the pelvis, although it displaces both vertically and laterally. A tracing of the center of mass in the sagittal plane is a sinusoidal curve as the body moves forward in its line of progression, with the amount of vertical displacement or oscillation totaling approximately 5 cm (Fig. 11–3). The peak of vertical displacement occurs at midstance of the weight-bearing phase and midswing of the opposite limb. The low point of vertical displacement is observed at the phase of double support. The lateral displacement of the center of mass also moves in a sinusoidal manner, alternating between the left and the right support phase.

Maximal displacement occurs just after midstance as the body weight is shifted over the stance limb, and the total amount of lateral displacement is approximately 4 to 5 cm.

## INDIVIDUAL FACTORS CONTRIBUTING TO NORMAL GAIT

Certain individual body movements, in combination, contribute to the process of normal gait. Deviations from or absences of these movements undoubtedly result in gait disturbances of various magnitudes. These gait disturbances may be manifest in abnormalities of the stance and swing phases, alteration of the velocity of gait, and increased energy cost of walking. This section provides a breakdown of these essential individual movements, along with the contribution that each makes to the gait cycle. The elements of pelvic rotation, pelvic list, knee flexion during

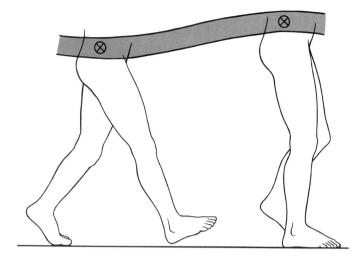

**FIGURE 11-3** ■ Sinusoidal waveform resulting from the vertical displacement of the center of gravity during gait. (Redrawn from Norkin C, Levangie P: Joint Structure and Function—A Comprehensive Analysis, 2nd ed. Philadelphia: FA Davis, 1991.)

stance, and foot attachment to the distal segment all contribute to a vertical displacement during gait. Pelvic rotation also results in a lateral displacement of the body, along with rotation of the thorax and shoulders, motion of the thigh and leg, and motion of the ankle and foot.

## Pelvic Rotation (Transverse Plane)

The pelvis rotates left and right about a vertical axis in the transverse plane (Fig. 11-4). The total pelvic rotation is approximately 8 degrees, 4 degrees to the left and 4 degrees to the right. The pelvic rotation effectively lengthens the femur from the phase of terminal swing through initial contact, thereby allowing the foot to make contact with the floor with minimal vertical displacement of the trunk.

## Pelvic Rotation (Frontal Plane)

The pelvis rotates or "lists" downward approximately 5 degrees in the frontal plane on the contralateral side of the stance limb (Fig. 11-5). This listing creates a relative adduction of the weight-bearing limb and a relative abduction of the non–weight-bearing limb. The relative adduction of the stance limb increases the efficiency of the hip abductor mechanism. Weakness of the abductor musculature, particularly the gluteus medius muscle, causes a situation of pelvic instability depicted in a Trendelenburg sign both statically and dynamically. A positive Trendelenburg sign exists when the pelvis drops toward the non–weight-bearing side during sin-

gle limb support. This often results from inability of the gluteus medius to stabilize the pelvis by pulling effectively from its distal attachment.

## Knee Flexion During Stance

Knee flexion during the swing phase must occur so that the body is able to advance forward during the gait cycle with minimal vertical displacement of the center of gravity. Typically, knee flexion is at its maximum at midstance, when the body is passing over the weight-bearing limb.

## Foot Attachment to Distal Segment

The concept of a mobile foot attached to a distal segment may help to explain the minimal deviations of the knee from the horizontal plane during stance. This is achieved by talocrural plantar flexion and dorsiflexion as well as subtalar joint pronation and supination, which provide relative shortening and lengthening of the supporting limb throughout the stance phase. Dorsiflexion and pronation effectively shorten the limb, and plantar flexion and supination lengthen it.

## Thorax and Shoulders

The shoulders and trunk rotate out of phase with each other during the gait cycle to ensure stability and balance.

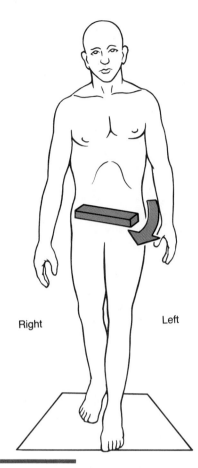

Right

Left

**FIGURE 11–4** ■ Pelvic rotation during the gait cycle. (Redrawn from Norkin C, Levangie P: Joint Structure and Function—A Comprehensive Analysis, 2nd ed. Philadelphia: FA Davis, 1991.)

## Thigh and Leg (Shank)

The movements of the thigh and leg occur in conjunction with rotation of the pelvis. Normally, the pelvis, thigh, and leg rotate toward the weight-bearing limb at the beginning of the swing phase of the reference extremity. Rotation continues until single-limb support, when the thigh and leg reverse direction and move into external rotation.

## Ankle and Foot

At the beginning of the stance phase, the ankle is dorsiflexed and the subtalar joint supinated. After heel contact, plantar flexion occurs at the talocrural joint and pronation at the subtalar joint. The rapid subtalar joint pronation results in a flexible foot, enabling accommodation

to the terrain. By the end of the midstance period, maximum dorsiflexion occurs at the talocrural joint and the subtalar joint begins to supinate. Supination of the subtalar joint continues throughout the remainder of the stance period as the foot functions as a rigid lever during push-off. Plantar flexion occurs at the ankle joint until toe-off, at which point a change toward dorsiflexion takes place, which continues throughout swing.

## PHASES OF GAIT

The two primary phases of gait, stance and swing, can be further subdivided into distinct components that are discussed in this section. As the study of gait biomechanics can be difficult, the following section has been organized by identifying each specific phase of the gait pattern along with the kinematics and kinetics that occur during that particular phase.

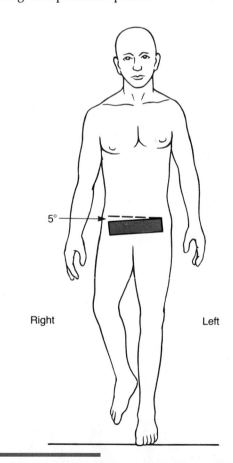

5°

Right

Left

**FIGURE 11–5** ■ Pelvic listing during the gait cycle. (Redrawn from Norkin C, Levangie P: Joint Structure and Function—A Comprehensive Analysis, 2nd ed. Philadelphia: FA Davis, 1991.)

## Stance Phase

As previously mentioned, the stance phase of gait occupies approximately 60% of the gait cycle. Stance may be further broken down into the following five categories (Fig. 11–6):

- Initial contact (heel strike)
- Loading response (foot flat)
- Midstance (single-leg support)
- Terminal stance (heel-off)
- Preswing (toe-off)

### Initial Contact

Initial contact occurs at the instant at which the heel (midfoot or toe in some cases) of the leading lower limb strikes the ground. It is this phase of stance that prepares the forward moving limb for weight bearing as the trailing limb prepares to leave the ground. Because portions of both feet are in contact with the ground during this phase, it represents a period of double support.

**Kinematics of Initial Contact.** During initial contact, the trunk remains erect and neutral. The pelvis is level and in a position of forward rotation. The hip joint is in a position of 30 degrees of flexion, neutral or slight abduction, and neutral rotation. The knee is close to full extension, the tibia externally rotated, and the knee abducted 5 to 10 degrees. The ankle is maintained in a neutral position and the toes are neither flexed nor extended.

**Kinetics of Initial Contact.** A flexion moment is created at the hip as the ground reaction force falls anterior to the joint. Eccentric contraction of the gluteus maximus is necessary to assist in deceleration of the forward-moving limb. The contractile capability of the gluteus maximus is enhanced by the elongated position of the muscle resulting from the posture of hip flexion. At the knee, the quadriceps are contracting eccentrically to control knee flexion during weight acceptance.

At the ankle, the ground reaction force falls posterior to the talocrural joint, creating a plantar flexion moment. Eccentric activity of the tibialis anterior and the long toe extensors is important in maintaining the ankle in a neutral position. The ground reaction force also lies lateral to the axis of the subtalar joint at initial contact, creating an eversion moment of the calcaneus.

### Loading Response

The loading response occurs immediately after initial contact and is the point in the gait cycle at which the foot is fully in contact with the floor. Forefoot loading usually occurs within the first 20% of the stance phase.

**Kinematics of Loading Response.** During the loading response, the trunk continues to remain erect and level while the pelvis is positioned level and inclined forward approximately 5 degrees. The hip maintains its posture of approximately 30 degrees of flexion with slight adduction. The knee moves into increased flexion of approximately 15 to 20 degrees with accompanying internal rotation of the tibia. The ankle plantar flexes to 15 degrees from the neutral position observed during initial contact and the subtalar joint is pronated. The toes are neither flexed nor extended.

**Kinetics of Loading Response.** The pelvis, during the loading response, is stabilized in the frontal plane by the gluteus medius, gluteus minimis, and tensor fasciae latae muscles. The posture of the hip remains flexed in accordance with the ground reaction force falling anterior to the hip joint. The flexion motion of the hip is countered by the eccentric contraction of the gluteus maximus early in weight acceptance to control hip flexion and to assist in controlling forward thigh rotation and thus the amount of knee flexion. The hip flexion moment is also countered in part by the adductor magnus and gracilis. A flexion moment exists at the knee and is controlled by the eccentric contraction of the

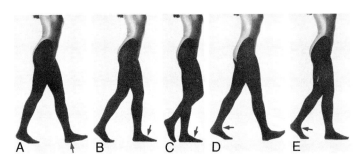

**FIGURE 11–6** ■ Subcategories of the stance phase of gait. (A) Initial contact. (B) Loading response. (C) Midstance. (D) Terminal stance. (E) Preswing.

quadriceps musculature, particularly in the first 10% of the stance period. At the ankle, the rapid plantar flexion moment requires that the anterior leg muscles, especially the tibialis anterior, contract eccentrically in order to control the lowering of the foot to the floor.

## Midstance

Midstance is the point in the stance phase at which the body weight passes directly over the supporting limb. Midstance is also a period of single-limb support in which the body is propelled forward over the fixed foot.

**Kinematics of Midstance.** The trunk remains erect and neutral throughout midstance and the pelvis also remains level with neutral rotation. The hip extends from the flexed posture observed in the previous phase to a neutral position and continues to remain in slight adduction and internal rotation. The knee moves from a position of approximately 20 degrees of flexion to a position of full extension. The ankle moves from the plantar flexed position found in the loading response to that of approximately 10 degrees of dorsiflexion. The 10 degrees of dorsiflexion during midstance is essential for the smooth progression of the limb over the supporting surface. The toes remain neutral.

**Kinetics of Midstance.** The pelvis is stabilized in the frontal plane by the hip abductor group, namely the gluteus medius, which acts to prevent dropping of the pelvis on the contralateral side. Pelvic stability is also assisted by the slightly adducted posture of the weight-bearing stance femur. The hip extension to neutral, with accompanying pelvic rotation to neutral, is obtained in part by the momentum of the contralateral swing limb. An extension moment at the hip exists together with activity of the hip flexors and/or tensor fasciae latae muscle. A mild adduction torque, along with the extension torque, continues throughout the period of single-limb support. The location of the ground reaction force and the transfer of weight over the supporting limb, partially assisted by the swing of the contralateral limb, result in minimal contribution from the quadriceps muscles during this phase. As the ankle is dorsiflexed 10 degrees, the plantar flexors are in a position of optimal stretch for concentric contraction and power generation in terminal stance to provide an explosive push-off. A dorsiflexion moment is present at the ankle. The tibialis anterior may play a minor role in contracting concentrically to pull the tibia forward over the foot. As the leg rotates over the foot, the gastrocnemius and soleus muscles eccentrically contract to decelerate and control the motion of the tibia over the foot.

## Terminal Stance

Terminal stance is the point at which the heel of the weight-bearing limb leaves the ground. During this phase, the weight-bearing limb begins to unload in preparation for preswing and the swing phase. Like the initial contact phase of stance, this phase is also characterized by a period of double support.

**Kinematics of Terminal Stance.** The trunk remains erect and neutral. The pelvis continues to be level with posterior rotation of 5 degrees. The hip joint remains essentially neutral but gives the appearance of being in 10 degrees of extension beyond neutral. This apparent hip extension is a result of the 5 degrees of posterior rotation at the pelvis and backward bending of the lumbar spine. The hip also remains in mild internal rotation and abduction. The knee achieves a position of full extension along with tibia external rotation. The ankle moves from a position of dorsiflexion at midstance to rapid plantar flexion at push-off. The heel of the foot at this point is off the floor in preparation for swing. The metatarsophalangeal joints are extended 30 degrees with the interphalangeal joints remaining neutral.

**Kinetics of Terminal Stance.** During terminal stance, the trunk continues to remain level and erect. The neutral position of the hip joint is maintained by essentially the same muscular activity found in midstance with the addition of the iliacus, which contracts to protect the joint capsule. The elongation of the iliacus as well as other hip flexors in this phase enhances the muscles' contraction concentrically to initiate flexion during the subsequent swing phase. Anterior fibers of the tensor muscle also contract late in this phase. The weight line continues to lie posterior to the hip joint, resulting in an extension moment of 40 foot-pounds of force. At the knee, eccentric contraction of the hamstring group and gastrocnemius muscle provide control of hyperextension. This counters the extension moment resulting from the ground reaction force causing the weight line to fall anterior to the knee joint axis. Eccentric contraction of the gastrocnemius and soleus muscles also plays a role in controlling the forward motion of the body. During push-off, the gastrocnemius and soleus muscles shorten, causing the foot to plantar flex actively and generate an explosive push-off. Activity then drops off rapidly until toe-off.

## Swing Phase

The swing phase, constituting 40% of the gait cycle, can be further subdivided into four categories (Fig. 11–7):

- Preswing (acceleration)
- Initial swing
- Midswing
- Terminal swing (deceleration)

### Preswing

Although preswing is actually a period of double support, it is considered part of swing because the events in this phase must occur in preparation for the limb to move into the swing phase.

**Kinematics of Preswing.** During preswing, the trunk continues to be erect and neutral. The pelvis remains in its position of backward rotation of 5 degrees and level. The hip remains in neutral extension and slight internal rotation. Knee flexion occurs passively to 30 to 35 degrees in response to active plantar flexion at the ankle of approximately 20 degrees. The metatarsophalangeal joints continue to extend to 60 degrees while the interphalangeal joints remain neutral.

**Kinetics of Preswing.** The backward rotation of the pelvis and neutral extension of the hip are both passive events due to the momentum generated by push-off. At the hip, the weight line now comes to lie anterior to the joint, creating a flexion moment. The hip is now in a position to accelerate forward into flexion by concentric contractions of the iliacus and rectus femoris. A flexion moment at the knee results in knee flexion to 30 to 35 degrees, which is mostly passive in nature, although low levels of activity are seen

in the gastrocnemius muscle, presumably to ensure adequate knee flexion before swing-through. Low levels of quadricep activity are also noted: at the hip to assist in hip flexion to bring the swinging limb forward and at the knee to decelerate the backward-swinging leg and foot. At the time of toe-off, the strong plantar flexion moment generated by the plantar flexors at heel-off ceases and minimal muscle activity is seen.

### Initial Swing

Initial swing begins the moment the toes of the weight-bearing limb leave the ground and continues until midswing (the point at which the extremity passes directly beneath the body). During this phase, acceleration of the swinging limb, created by the ankle plantar flexors during late stance and the burst of hip flexor activity, is critical to adequate toe clearance and forward advancement of the limb.

**Kinematics of Initial Swing.** The trunk during this phase remains erect and level. Although the pelvis remains backwardly rotated and level, it begins to move into forward rotation accompanying the motion of flexion at the hip. The hip flexes to 20 degrees and rotates externally. The knee continues to flex to a position of 60 degrees and abducts to neutral throughout swing. The tibia rotates externally until midswing. The ankle position begins to change from approximately 10 degrees of plantar flexion to a neutral position.

**Kinetics of Initial Swing.** A hip extension moment exists because of the tendency of gravity to pull the limb downward. This is countered by concentric contractions of the iliacus, adductor longus, iliopsoas, gracilis, tensor fasciae latae, rectus femoris, and sartorius muscles. As the knee flexes, the quadriceps initially contract eccentrically to decelerate the backward-swinging leg. This is followed by a concentric contraction of the quadriceps muscles to assist in swinging the leg forward. Little activity of the knee extensors is required to swing the limb forward at natural cadences. Most of the energy used to swing the limb forward comes from a pendulum action and moments that provide an appropriate couple at the knee joint. Gravity acts on the ankle and foot, causing a plantar flexion moment in its attempt to pull the foot downward.

### Midswing

Midswing occurs as the limb passes directly beneath the body, aligned with the opposite limb, which is in a position of midstance.

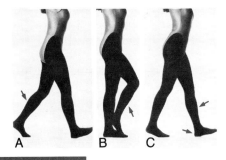

**FIGURE 11–7** ■ Subcategories of the swing phase of gait. (A) Initial swing. (B) Midswing. (C) Terminal swing.

**Kinematics of Midswing.** The trunk continues to be erect and level and the pelvis is now in a position of neutral rotation. Hip flexion is observed to be 20 to 30 degrees with minimal external rotation. The knee moves toward extension from its previous position of 60 degrees to that of 30 degrees. The tibia also remains in a position of external rotation throughout midswing. The ankle and toes are observed to be neutral.

**Kinetics of Midswing.** An extension moment continues to exist at the hip as a result of the influence of gravity. Concentric contractions of the hip flexors and adductors are present, although the adductor longus and iliacus are inactive. A minimal extension moment is present at the knee with the quadriceps group contracting eccentrically when the tibia moves beyond the perpendicular to the ground. The ankle is maintained in neutral by the counterbalancing effects of a plantar flexion moment with static contraction of the anterior leg muscles, notably the tibialis anterior.

### Terminal Swing

Terminal swing, characterized by deceleration of the limb, occurs after midswing when the tibia passes beyond perpendicular in relation to the foot and the knee is extending in preparation for initial contact.

**Kinematics of Terminal Swing.** The trunk continues to be erect and neutral with the pelvis level and in forward rotation of 5 degrees. Hip flexion continues at 30 degrees with a position of mild external rotation, which changes to internal rotation just before initial contact. The knee continues to extend, approaching full extension before heel contact. The tibia also moves into a position of internal rotation. The ankle and toes are in neutral positions.

**Kinetics of Terminal Swing.** The gracilis is the only muscle during terminal swing that continues to function as a hip flexor and is assisted by a flexion moment. The quadriceps contract concentrically to provide knee extension. The hamstring group functions eccentrically to assist in deceleration of the limb in preparation for initial contact. The ankle continues to remain in a neutral position as a result of the combination of the plantar flexion moment and the isometric control of the anterior leg muscles. The tibialis anterior muscle, in particular, begins its major activity at the end of swing and peaks at heel contact.

Certain components of the gait cycle are more easily explained when discussed by individual segment analysis. Among these components are the activity of the trunk, the contribution of the subtalar joint, and movement of the upper limbs.

## BIOMECHANICS OF GAIT

### Trunk Biomechanics

As seen in the previous sections on the phases of gait, the trunk remains erect and level throughout the entire gait cycle, helping to keep the body positioned over the base of support. The trunk acts in rhythm with the pelvis: when the pelvis is rotating in one direction, the trunk rotates in the opposite direction. For example, as the right limb advances forward during its swing phase, the pelvis rotates to the left. Simultaneously, the trunk moves in the direction of right rotation. This relationship between the trunk and the pelvis contributes to the overall smoothness and stability of gait. As the stance limb is being loaded, the deep back extensor muscles on the contralateral side contract eccentrically to assist in maintenance of the erect trunk posture. This occurs in harmony with a concentric contraction of the ipsilateral deep back muscles. In approaching the terminal phase of stance, the ipsilateral deep trunk extensors contract eccentrically and the contralateral deep back extensors contract concentrically to assist in providing the stability necessary for the transfer of weight from one limb to the other.

The role of the abdominal muscles, namely the rectus abdominis and the internal and external obliques, appears to be minimal, if they are active at all during the gait cycle. Electromyographic activity indicates that the internal and external oblique muscles are active throughout the cycle but the rectus is active in only 50% of individuals. In any event, the functioning of the abdominal group appears to be of little consequence for the function of normal gait.

### Subtalar Biomechanics

The biomechanics of the subtalar joint and its relationship to the function of the midtarsal joint and the lower limb are complex but important to the understanding of the gait cycle during open and closed chain events.

A brief overview of subtalar joint function

shows that at the moment of initial contact, the calcaneus is in a position of inversion relative to the lower limb. Immediately, as loading occurs, the calcaneus everts, resulting in subtalar joint pronation and "unlocking" of the midtarsal area. This results in a flexible foot that adapts readily to changes in the terrain. By the middle of mid-stance and continuing into terminal stance, the subtalar joint moves toward supination and the calcaneus again inverts, causing the midtarsal joint to "lock up." This results in a stable foot so that propulsion can occur.

It is suggested that the reader seek other sources that describe the biomechanics of the foot and ankle in detail, so that these principles can be applied to the movements that occur normally and abnormally during gait.

## Motion of the Upper Limbs

Although movement of the upper limbs is not essential for gait to occur, it assists in providing stability and smoothness to the gait cycle. Normally, there is a reciprocal relationship between motions of the upper limbs and the lower limbs: as one lower limb advances, the opposite upper limb moves forward. Therefore, as the right lower limb advances in swing, the left upper limb is also moving forward.

## VELOCITY OF GAIT

Individuals walk at various speeds in accordance with the demands imposed on them at any given time. Velocity is measured as the product of cadence and step length. If the step length is increased with the cadence remaining constant, there is a resultant increase in the velocity of gait. Also, if the cadence is increased with the step length remaining constant, an increase in velocity is seen. Natural cadences reported in the literature range from 101 to 122 steps per minute. Natural cadence in females has been found to be 6 to 9 steps higher than that in males. As changes in the velocity of gait occur, accompanying changes in all aspects of the gait cycle are noted. Higher speeds of walking are characterized by a decrease in the amount of time spent in stance and an increase in the time spent in swing. The angular displacement and rate of acceleration and deceleration of the joints of the lower limb, along with motion of the trunk and upper limbs, also increase with higher speeds of walking. With lower speeds of walking, there is a noticeable increase in the amount of time spent in the stance phase with a simultaneous decrease in the amount of time spent in swing. In addition, angular displacements and rates of acceleration and deceleration of the upper limbs, trunk, and lower limbs are found to be diminished.

Speed of gait is also a function of age, with the elderly typically exhibiting a lower speed of walking. This slowing down of gait is often the result of loss of flexibility of the joints of the lower limb, an increased energy cost of gait, and in some individuals problems with balance and coordination. In an attempt to walk faster, an elderly person increases the frequency of steps rather than increasing the stride length. Increasing the stride length decreases the stability of the individual and is usually avoided in this population. Difficulties in ambulation begin to occur in some individuals around the age of 60. However, more severe gait abnormalities do not appear until about 75 to 80 years.

Energy cost is another factor that affects the speed of walking. Energy cost during ambulation is measured by determining the oxygen consumption over a set distance traveled. The energy cost is lowest at a cadence of 75 to 100 steps per minute or approximately 3 miles per hour and is dependent on stride length as well as the rate of walking. An optimal gait pattern is one in which there is a minimal amount of energy expenditure. Individuals naturally adapt their walking speed to ensure that the energy expenditure remains minimal. Both higher and lower rates of walking, as well as the use of an assistive device, result in an increase in the energy cost.

## CLINICAL GAIT ANALYSIS

To perform gait analysis, the clinician must be able to apply the principles of the biomechanics of walking to the patient who presents with deviations from normal as a result of age, disease, postural abnormalities, or trauma. Before observing an individual walk, the clinician should have knowledge and understanding of the limitations of the individual that may be related to a particular pathology. Much of this information can be gathered during the initial evaluation and re-evaluations throughout the rehabilitation process. The clinician should have an idea how the abnormalities may be manifested throughout the gait cycle. Obviously, a patient who has marked restrictions in the range of motion of knee flexion would be expected to have difficulty achieving a normal swing-through with the affected limb. Also, patients with muscle weakness, balance difficulties, and coordination problems have problems with normal gait, in both stance and swing phases.

Gait analysis should begin with a gross, total body analysis looking at overall posture, cadence, stride length, step length, arm swing, and the general velocity of ambulation. The presence of abnormalities requires that the clinician next determine the cause of the abnormality, in terms of identifying the segment or segments involved and the phases of gait that are affected. In order to achieve this, the examiner must closely observe all body segments that play a role in normal gait and understand how those segments interact with one another. Usually, the examination proceeds with the clinician observing the individual from head to toe, then reversing and looking from toe to head. Each individual segment is observed for the appropriate angular displacement and expected velocity throughout the swing and stance phases. If deviations are detected for a particular segment, attention must be paid to the effect on other body segments that contribute to the gait cycle. If there are deviations from normal in any segment or segments, there are accompanying compensations by other body parts so that the individual remains able to walk. It is critical that the examiner be able to differentiate between deviations resulting from the original pathology and those that may be present for compensation. The rehabilitation program should be directed to correcting the abnormal physical findings resulting from the pathology. It is important to remember that gait training is an adjunct to the total rehabilitation process and that the optimal effect of "normalizing gait" is achieved by various forms of therapeutic exercise, gait training, and evaluation of appropriate orthotic and assistive devices.

Examples of gait evaluation forms are provided in Figures 11–8 to 11–12. Generally, visual gait analysis should be performed from lateral, posterior, and anterior views. Examination from different points of view ensures that all components of gait are observed accurately. Some components of gait can be assessed in more than one position, although one position usually provides the best information. Gait should be analyzed with the patient both with and without footwear. In addition, the footwear should be closely examined for patterns of wear. The information provided in the following should be observed relative to its expected occurrence within the gait cycle and any deviations from normal should be noted.

## Lateral View

The lateral view allows the examiner to assess the following:

■ Reciprocal arm swing
■ Rotation of shoulders and thorax
■ Pelvic rotation
■ Hip flexion and extension
■ Knee flexion and extension
■ Ankle dorsiflexion and plantar flexion
■ Step length
■ Stride length
■ Heel rise
■ Preswing
■ Cadence

## Anterior View

The anterior view allows the following examination:

■ Reciprocal arm swing
■ Rotation of shoulders and thorax
■ Pelvic rotation
■ Pelvic list
■ Hip rotation and abduction-adduction
■ Knee rotation and abduction-adduction
■ Degree of toe-out
■ Base of support measurement

## Posterior View

The posterior view allows assessment of the following:

■ Reciprocal arm swing
■ Rotation of the shoulders and thorax
■ Pelvic rotation
■ Pelvic list
■ Hip rotation and abduction-adduction
■ Knee rotation and abduction-adduction
■ Subtalar movement
■ Heel rise
■ Preswing
■ Base of support

## ABNORMALITIES IN GAIT

This section deals with common clinical abnormalities encountered in gait (Tables 11–1 and 11–2). Emphasis is directed to areas of musculoskeletal and related neurologic pathology, al-

Instructions for Gait Analysis: Total Body
1. Perform gait analysis with the least possible bracing and support.
2. Place a check in the appropriate box. With bilateral involvement, use (R) or (L) instead of a check.

| | | WEIGHT ACCEPTANCE | | SINGLE LIMB STABILITY | | SWING LIMB ADVANCEMENT | | | | LIST MAJOR PROBLEMS: |
|---|---|---|---|---|---|---|---|---|---|---|
| | | IC | LR | MSt | TSt | PS | IS | MSw | TSw | |
| TRUNK | Backward lean | | | | | | | | | Weight acceptance |
| | Forward lean | | | | | | | | | |
| | Lateral lean R/L | | | | | | | | | |
| | Rotates backward | | | | | | | | | |
| | Rotates forward | | | | | | | | | |
| PELVIS | Hikes | | | | | | | | | |
| | Posterior tilt | | | | | | | | | |
| | Anterior tilt | | | | | | | | | |
| | Lacks forw. rotation | | | | | | | | | |
| | Lacks backw. rotation | | | | | | | | | |
| | Excess forw. rotation | | | | | | | | | Single limb stability |
| | Excess backw. rotation | | | | | | | | | |
| | Ipsilateral drop | | | | | | | | | |
| | Contralateral drop | | | | | | | | | |
| HIP | Flexion: Limited | | | | | | | | | |
| | Absent | | | | | | | | | |
| | Excess | | | | | | | | | |
| | Inadequate extension | | | | | | | | | |
| | Past retracts | | | | | | | | | |
| | External rotation | | | | | | | | | |
| | Internal rotation | | | | | | | | | |
| | Abduction | | | | | | | | | Swing limb advancement |
| | Adduction | | | | | | | | | |
| KNEE | Flexion: Limited | | | | | | | | | |
| | Absent | | | | | | | | | |
| | Excess | | | | | | | | | |
| | Inadequate extension | | | | | | | | | |
| | Wobbles | | | | | | | | | |
| | Hyperextends | | | | | | | | | |
| | Extension thrust | | | | | | | | | |
| | Varus | | | | | | | | | |
| | Valgus | | | | | | | | | Excessive U.E. weight bearing |
| | Excess contra. flexion | | | | | | | | | |
| ANKLE AND FOOT | Forefoot contact | | | | | | | | | |
| | Foot flat contact | | | | | | | | | |
| | Foot slap | | | | | | | | | |
| | Excess plantar flexion | | | | | | | | | |
| | Excess dorsiflexion | | | | | | | | | |
| | Excess varus | | | | | | | | | |
| | Excess valgus | | | | | | | | | |
| | Heel off | | | | | | | | | |
| | No heel off | | | | | | | | | |
| | Drag | | | | | | | | | |
| | Contralateral vaulting | | | | | | | | | |
| TOES | Up | | | | | | | | | |
| | Inadequate extension | | | | | | | | | |
| | Clawed | | | | | | | | | |

**FIGURE 11-8** ■ Recording form for full body gait analysis. Dark squares: need not consider whether deviation occurs during this phase. White squares: subphase during which gait deviation is most pronounced. Light squares: subphase during which gait deviation is less pronounced. IC, initial contact; LR, loading response; MSt, midstance; TSt, terminal stance; PS, preswing; IS, initial swing; MSw, midswing; TSw, terminal swing. (Modified from Scully RM, Barnes MR: Physical Therapy. Philadelphia: JB Lippincott, 1989. Adapted by permission of Ranchos Los Amigos Medical Center, Pathokinesiology and Physical Therapy Department.)

Instructions for Gait Analysis: Trunk and Pelvis
1. Perform gait analysis with the least possible bracing and support.
2. Place a check in the appropriate box.  With bilateral involvement, use (R) or (L) instead of a check.

| | | WEIGHT ACCEPTANCE | | SINGLE LIMB STABILITY | | SWING LIMB ADVANCEMENT | | | | LIST MAJOR PROBLEMS: |
|---|---|---|---|---|---|---|---|---|---|---|
| | | IC | LR | MSt | TSt | PS | IS | MSw | TSw | |
| TRUNK | Backward lean | | | | | | | | | Weight acceptance |
| | Forward lean | | | | | | | | | |
| | Lateral lean R/L | | | | | | | | | |
| | Rotates backward | | | | | | | | | |
| | Rotates forward | | | | | | | | | Single limb stability |
| PELVIS | Hikes | | | | | | | | | |
| | Posterior tilt | | | | | | | | | |
| | Anterior tilt | | | | | | | | | |
| | Lacks forw. rotation | | | | | | | | | |
| | Lacks backw. rotation | | | | | | | | | Swing limb advancement |
| | Excess forw. rotation | | | | | | | | | |
| | Excess backw. rotation | | | | | | | | | |
| | Ipsilateral drop | | | | | | | | | |
| | Contralateral drop | | | | | | | | | |

**FIGURE 11–9** ■ Recording form for gait analysis of the trunk and pelvis. See Figure 11–8 for explanation. (Modified from Scully RM, Barnes MR: Physical Therapy. Philadelphia: JB Lippincott, 1989. Adapted by permission of Ranchos Los Amigos Medical Center, Pathokinesiology and Physical Therapy Department.)

Instructions for Gait Analysis: Hip
1. Perform gait analysis with the least possible bracing and support.
2. Place a check in the appropriate box.  With bilateral involvement, use (R) or (L) instead of a check.

| | | WEIGHT ACCEPTANCE | | SINGLE LIMB STABILITY | | SWING LIMB ADVANCEMENT | | | | LIST MAJOR PROBLEMS: |
|---|---|---|---|---|---|---|---|---|---|---|
| | | IC | LR | MSt | TSt | PS | IS | MSw | TSw | |
| HIP | Flexion: Limited | | | | | | | | | Weight acceptance |
| | Absent | | | | | | | | | |
| | Excess | | | | | | | | | |
| | Inadequate extension | | | | | | | | | Single limb stability |
| | Past retracts | | | | | | | | | |
| | External rotation | | | | | | | | | Swing limb advancement |
| | Internal rotation | | | | | | | | | |
| | Abduction | | | | | | | | | |
| | Adduction | | | | | | | | | |

MOTIONS REFERRED FROM OTHER JOINTS:

Excessive pelvic motion ☐

Excessive trunk motion ☐

**FIGURE 11–10** ■ Recording form for gait analysis of the hip. See Figure 11–8 for explanation. (Modified from Scully RM, Barnes MR: Physical Therapy. Philadelphia: JB Lippincott, 1989. Adapted by permission of Ranchos Los Amigos Medical Center, Pathokinesiology and Physical Therapy Department.)

Instructions for Gait Analysis: Knee
1. Perform gait analysis with the least possible bracing and support.
2. Place a check in the appropriate box. With bilateral involvement, use (R) or (L) instead of a check.

| | | WEIGHT ACCEPTANCE | | SINGLE LIMB STABILITY | | SWING LIMB ADVANCEMENT | | | | LIST MAJOR PROBLEMS: |
|---|---|---|---|---|---|---|---|---|---|---|
| | | IC | LR | MSt | TSt | PS | IS | MSw | TSw | |
| KNEE | Flexion: Limited | | | | | | | | | Weight acceptance |
| | Absent | | | | | | | | | |
| | Excess | | | | | | | | | |
| | Inadequate extension | | | | | | | | | Single limb stability |
| | Wobbles | | | | | | | | | |
| | Hyperextends | | | | | | | | | |
| | Extension thrust | | | | | | | | | Swing limb advancement |
| | Varus | | | | | | | | | |
| | Valgus | | | | | | | | | |
| | Excess contra. flexion | | | | | | | | | |

MOTIONS REFERRED FROM OTHER JOINTS:

External rotation ☐
Internal rotation ☐
Abduction ☐
Adduction ☐

**FIGURE 11-11** ■ Recording form for gait analysis of the knee. See Figure 11-8 for explanation. (Modified from Scully RM, Barnes MR: Physical Therapy. Philadelphia: JB Lippincott, 1989. Adapted by permission of Ranchos Los Amigos Medical Center, Pathokinesiology and Physical Therapy Department.)

though these areas are by no means covered in their entirety.

## Antalgic Gait

Any physical disability resulting in pain in the lower limb and/or pelvic region may result in an antalgic gait pattern. The characteristics of this type of gait pattern include a decrease in the duration of stance of the affected limb, usually in response to reluctance and/or inability of the individual to bear weight through the painful limb. Accordingly, there is a noticeable lack of weight shift laterally over the stance limb, also in an attempt to keep weight off the involved limb. The result of a decreased stance phase on the affected side is a decrease in the swing phase of the uninvolved limb, creating a shorter step length on the uninvolved side, a decreased cadence, and an overall decrease in the velocity of walking. In addition, pain specifically located in the joints of the lower limb or pelvis with accompanying decreases in range of motion and/or strength may result in other deviations in both the stance and swing phases.

## Leg Length Discrepancy

Patients who have both true and apparent leg length discrepancies demonstrate deviations from the normal gait cycle. On the side of the shorter limb, as the foot prepares to make initial contact with the ground, the pelvis drops laterally in an attempt to lengthen the limb. Visually and in frontal plane view, the gross appearance is that of the individual limping. In addition, the individual may supinate the foot on the short side to effectively lengthen the limb. The joints of the unaffected, longer limb commonly demonstrate exaggerated flexion in order to achieve swing-through. Alternative compensations to allow swing-through of the longer leg include vaulting on the short limb side and hip hiking and circumduction of the long limb side.

## Muscle Weakness or Paralysis

### Weakness of Gluteus Medius

An individual with gluteus medius weakness demonstrates a classic Trendelenburg gait pattern

Instructions for Gait Analysis: Ankle, Foot, and Toes
1. Perform gait analysis with the least possible bracing and support.
2. Place a check in the appropriate box. With bilateral involvement, use (R) or (L) instead of a check.

| | | WEIGHT ACCEPTANCE | | SINGLE LIMB STABILITY | | SWING LIMB ADVANCEMENT | | | | LIST MAJOR PROBLEMS: |
|---|---|---|---|---|---|---|---|---|---|---|
| | | IC | LR | MSt | TSt | PS | IS | MSw | TSw | |
| ANKLE AND FOOT | Forefoot contact | | | | | | | | | Weight acceptance |
| | Foot flat contact | | | | | | | | | |
| | Foot slap | | | | | | | | | |
| | Excess plantar flexion | | | | | | | | | |
| | Excess dorsiflexion | | | | | | | | | |
| | Excess varus | | | | | | | | | Single limb stability |
| | Excess valgus | | | | | | | | | |
| | Heel off | | | | | | | | | |
| | No heel off | | | | | | | | | |
| | Drag | | | | | | | | | |
| | Contralateral vaulting | | | | | | | | | Swing limb advancement |
| TOES | Up | | | | | | | | | |
| | Inadequate extension | | | | | | | | | |
| | Clawed | | | | | | | | | |

MOTIONS REFERRED FROM OTHER JOINTS:

External rotation ☐
Internal rotation ☐
Abduction ☐
Adduction ☐

**FIGURE 11-12** ■ Recording form for gait analysis of the ankle, foot, and toes. See Figure 11-8 for explanation. (Modified from Scully RM, Barnes MR: Physical Therapy. Philadelphia: JB Lippincott, 1989. Adapted by permission of Ranchos Los Amigos Medical Center, Pathokinesiology and Physical Therapy Department.)

in which the pelvis drops on the unaffected side during single-limb support of the side of weakness. This dropping of the pelvis is due to the inability of the gluteus medius to pull from its distal attachment on the femur and stabilize the pelvis in a level position in the frontal plane. Accompanying the pelvis drop on the unaffected side is a relative adduction of the femur of the stance limb. Another deviation, sometimes termed the "gluteus medius lurch," involves the individual laterally flexing the trunk over the affected limb during single-limb support in order to maintain the center of gravity over the base of support. This minimizes the torque due to body weight and hence the gluteus medius force required to stabilize the pelvis.

## Weakness of Psoas

Weakness of the psoas muscle is reflected in the patient's difficulty initiating swing-through. In order to compensate for the psoas weakness, the individual rotates the limb externally at the hip and uses the hip adductors to achieve swing-through. The individual may also demonstrate exaggerated trunk and pelvis motion in order to compensate for the weakness in the hip flexion movement.

## Paralysis or Weakness of the Gluteus Maximus

Paralysis or weakness of the gluteus maximus results in inability to counter the flexion moment at the hip at the moment of initial contact. The individual must compensate by quickly moving the trunk posteriorly at initial contact so that the weight of the trunk can oppose the flexion moment present. This compensation allows the individual to maintain an upright posture during the gait cycle.

■■■■■■ **Table 11-1.** PRIMARY DEVIATIONS AFFECTING WEIGHT ACCEPTANCE AND SINGLE-LIMB SUPPORT

| Deviations | Causes | Penalties |
| --- | --- | --- |
| Hip adduction | Increased adductor muscle activity<br>Inadequate strength of abductors<br>Decreased proprioception | Narrow base of support leading to loss of balance |
| Contralateral pelvic drop | Weakness or inadequate control of hip abductors | Decreased stance stability<br>Potential loss of balance |
| Inadequate hip extension | Inadequate hip extension strength or control<br>Hip flexion contracture<br>Increased muscle activity of hip flexors<br>Painful joint<br>Decreased proprioception<br>Secondary to excessive knee flexion posture | Increased energy demand<br>Decreased forward progression; decreased velocity |
| Inadequate knee extension | Inadequate quadriceps strength or control<br>Knee flexion contracture<br>Increased hamstring muscle activity<br>Increased gastrocnemius muscle activity<br>Secondary to inadequate hip extension or excessive dorsiflexion<br>Painful joint<br>Decreased proprioception | Increased energy demand<br>Decreased stance stability leading to decreased stance time<br>Decreased forward progression and velocity |
| Knee extension thrust | Inadequate quadriceps control<br>Increased quadriceps muscle activity<br>Secondary to primary ankle instability<br>Increased plantar flexion muscle activity<br>Plantar flexion contracture<br>Decreased proprioception<br>Painful knee (avoids flexion) | Loss of loading response at knee<br>Decreased forward progression and velocity<br>May result in joint problems, pain |
| Excessive plantar flexion | Increased plantar flexion muscle activity<br>Inadequate plantar flexion strength and control<br>Plantar flexion contracture<br>Decreased proprioception | Decreased forward progression and velocity<br>Need for compensatory postures<br>Increased energy demand<br>Shortened stance time |
| Excessive dorsiflexion | Accommodation for knee flexion contracture<br>Inadequate plantar flexion strength<br>Decreased proprioception<br>Dorsiflexion contracture (rare) | Stance instability with resultant decreased stance time<br>Compensatory hip and knee flexion resulting in increased energy<br>Decreased forward progression and velocity |
| No heel-off | Inadequate plantar flexion strength and control<br>Painful ankle-foot-metatarsal heads<br>Restricted ankle or midfoot or metatarsal phalangeal motion | Decreased preswing knee flexion<br>Decreased forward progression and velocity |
| Excess varus | Increased invertor muscle activity<br>Decreased proprioception | Unstable base of support with potential for falling and injury<br>Decreased forward progression and velocity |
| Claw toes | Increased toe flexor muscle activity<br>Muscle imbalance with weak intrinsics<br>Exaggerated response to compensate for poor balance<br>Toe flexion contracture | Pain resulting from skin pressure and from weight bearing on distal end of toes<br>Decreased forward progression and velocity |

From Scully RM, Barnes MR: Physical Therapy. Philadelphia: JB Lippincott, 1989, p 693.

## Inability of Quadriceps to Contract

Inability of the quadriceps to contract effectively results in varying degrees of compensation depending on the integrity of other muscles, namely the hip extensors and ankle plantar flexors. Assuming that those muscles have good contractile capabilities, compensation occurs by forward bending of the trunk combined with rapid plantar flexion of the ankle. These compensations are effective because they create an extension moment at the knee with resulting hyperextension, negating the need for quadriceps muscle activity to provide support. If the hip extensors and ankle plantar flexors are also

**Table 11–2.** PRIMARY DEVIATIONS AFFECTING LIMB ADVANCEMENT

| Deviations | Causes | Penalties |
|---|---|---|
| Limited or absent flexion | | |
|   Hip | Increased extensor muscle activity or posturing expecially at knee and ankle | Decreased forward progression and velocity |
| | Inadequate strength or control of hip flexors | Decreased step length |
| | Painful joint | Compensatory deviations leading to increased energy demands |
| | Decreased proprioception | |
|   Knee | Inadequate preswing knee flexion | Toe drag at initial swing |
| | Increased knee extensor muscle activity | |
| | Painful joint | |
| | Restricted knee flexion range | |
| | Decreased hamstring muscle strength | |
| | Decreased proprioception | |
| Inadequate knee extension, terminal swing | Knee flexion contracture | Decreased step length |
| | Synergy dependent; unable to extend the knee selectively with hip flexion | Decreased forward progression and velocity |
| | Increased knee flexor muscle activity | |
| | Dominated by flexor withdrawal response | |
| Hip adduction | Increased adductor muscle activity | Swing limb touches stance limb resulting in potential for fall, decreased forward progression |
| | Excessive flexor or extensor synergy | |
| | Decreased proprioception | Limb placement in front of the stance limb resulting in a narrow base of support |
| Excessive plantar flexion, midswing, terminal swing | Inadequate dorsiflexion strength | Toe drag, midswing |
| | Ankle plantar flexion contracture | Inadequate preparation for initial contact resulting in foot flat or toes first, initial contact; leads to loss of loading response at ankle |
| | Increased plantar flexor muscle activity | |
| | Excessive extensor synergy | |
| | Decreased proprioception | |

From Scully RM, Barnes MR: Physical Therapy. Philadelphia: JB Lippincott, 1989, p 694.

weak, compensation occurs by the patient manually pushing the knee into extension at initial contact.

### Steppage Gait

Involvement of the muscles necessary for ankle dorsiflexion results in what is universally known as a steppage gait, because the individual's swing phase on the involved side is said to resemble the high steppage gait of a horse. The excessive hip and knee flexion compensates for the dropfoot and allows swing-through of the affected limb to occur without scuffing or dragging the toes on the floor. Initial contact occurs at the forefoot rather than normally at the heel, and a characteristic "slap" can be heard at the moment of contact. This slapping is the result of inability of the dorsiflexors to decelerate and control contact of the foot with the floor.

### Weakness or Paralysis of the Ankle Plantar Flexors

A calcaneal gait pattern is typical in individuals who have weakness or paralysis of the ankle plantar flexors. The abnormalities in this gait are seen during the phase of single support because the tibia and knee are not well stabilized. In addition, there is no real propulsion because of the plantar flexion weakness. Consequently, the amount of time spent in the stance phase is diminished, accounting for the smaller step length on the unaffected side.

## Joint Hypomobility

Hypomobility of hip or knee flexion results in a need for the individual to lengthen the uninvolved limb to achieve swing-through of the involved limb. Compensations in the uninvolved limb may include plantar flexion of the ankle during stance or vaulting, hip hiking, or circumduction. These compensations may present individually or in combination.

## Muscular Contracture

### Hip Flexion Contracture

Hip flexion contractures result in a need for compensation to counteract the flexion moment at the hip at the moment of initial contact. Increasing the lumbar lordosis and backward bending of the trunk are typical compensations. Simultaneous knee flexion may also be observed. An assistive device to support the trunk may be necessary depending on the severity of the hip flexion contracture and/or the ability to compensate at the lumbar spine, trunk, and knee.

### Knee Flexion Contracture

An individual with a knee flexion contracture demonstrates excessive dorsiflexion of the ankle from late swing phase to early stance of the uninvolved limb. The involved limb exhibits early heel rise in terminal stance.

### Plantar Flexion Contracture

A plantar flexion contracture results in early heel rise during terminal stance and possibly during midstance in the case of a more severe contracture. Knee hyperextension is also apparent at midstance, and forward bending of the trunk with accompanying hip flexion is noted during midstance to terminal stance.

## Fractures

The trend in fracture care is for early mobilization to minimize the detrimental effects of immobility. It is important that this early mobilization occur without interfering with the healing requirements of bone. In accordance with Wolff's law that form follows function, healthy formed bone is laid down in response to the stresses imposed on it. Bone repair is best facilitated by placing loading stresses on the bone and not by forces that are tensile in nature. Early weight-bearing and gait activities are important to provide those loading stresses to the fracture site. It is, however, critical that sufficient healing of bone occur before these compressive types of stresses are imposed. Patients walking with a partial weight-bearing gait when the bone is not fully healed may benefit most by using a foot flat posture during the stance phase of the gait cycle. This allows more compressive types of loading rather than the bending moments of force that are present when using a normal heel-to-toe pattern. It has been noted that heel-to-toe weight-bearing gait during the early phase of

bone repair may result in a fatigue fracture in which "conversion of soft fiber bone to fibrous tissue" occurs.[1]

## GAIT TRAINING WITH ASSISTIVE DEVICES

Despite aggressive rehabilitation, many patients still require assistive devices in order to walk safely and independently. The selection of the appropriate assistive device to use with a patient is often difficult because factors such as age, balance coordination, muscle weakness, cardiopulmonary status, level of function, supportive personnel, and environmental conditions must be considered. Safety must be the primary consideration in choosing an assistive device and subsequent training with that device.

This section discusses gait patterns associated with the use of common assistive devices, from the device that offers the greatest stability to that which offers the least stability. The following description of devices is not complete.

Education of the patient is an important consideration in gait training. In many instances, education and training of family members are also indicated to ensure optimal safety of the patient after discharge. Instruction should include periodic checking and subsequent replacement of crutch tips, hand grips, and axillary pads when signs of wear are present. The patient should bear weight on the hands only and not on the axillary pads, because weight bearing on the axilla may result in radial nerve damage. Wet floors, ice, and snow should be avoided because of the risk of slips and falls. Care must be taken when walking on or near throw rugs to avoid tripping over an edge of the carpet or having the carpet shift. Finally, individuals who use axillary crutches should learn to hug them against the lateral chest wall to prevent the crutches from slipping out from under the axilla.

Patients should be instructed in moving the assistive device a comfortable reach from them during walking. Moving the assistive device too far forward results in loss of balance and an increased risk of falling. On the other hand, if the device is not advanced far enough, gait may be impeded by the device and the base of support may be too small, which compromises balance. In using unilateral and bilateral supports, the patient must also be instructed to keep the device by the side rather than in front of the foot, where it can be tripped over.

## Fitting the Patient with an Assistive Device

The fitting of assistive devices varies depending on the type of device used. Fitting of walkers is accomplished by adjusting the height of the walker to the level of the greater trochanter of the patient's hip. The same measurement principle is involved in fitting hemi-walking canes, quadripod canes, and standard canes. Measurement of axillary crutches is done keeping in mind that the crutch tip should be vertical to the ground at an approximate distance of 6 inches lateral and 6 inches anterior to the foot. The handgrips of axillary crutches should be adjusted to the level of the greater trochanter. There should be a two- to three-finger space between the tops of the axillary pads and the patient's axilla to prevent pressure on the area of the brachial plexus. Forearm or Lofstrand crutches should be fitted with the handgrip at the level of the greater trochanter and the top of the forearm cuff just distal to the elbow. With a proper fit, the degree of elbow flexion allows depression of the shoulder girdle to facilitate the advancement of the body and lower limbs during the gait cycle. The fit of platform walkers should include location of the platform height at a level in which the individual can stand comfortably with good posture, the arms relatively at the sides, and the shoulder girdle slightly elevated. This elevated position of the shoulder girdle allows the patient to push down on the platform and elevate the body, thereby allowing progression of the lower limbs during walking. The distance to the handgrip should be a comfortable reach with the forearm resting on the platform. It is important that any selected assistive device be fitted correctly to allow safe, independent gait with minimal energy expenditure. The energy cost of ambulation increases with use of an assistive device; therefore a gait pattern as close to normal as possible is desired to keep the energy cost down.

## Four-Point Gait Pattern

A four-point gait pattern (Fig. 11–13) is one in which there are four points of contact with the floor, the feet accounting for two and the assistive device for two. This gait pattern is typical in training patients with bilateral assistive devices, such as two axillary or forearm crutches. The pattern sequence is that one crutch advances, followed by the contralateral lower limb, followed by the other crutch and finally the re-

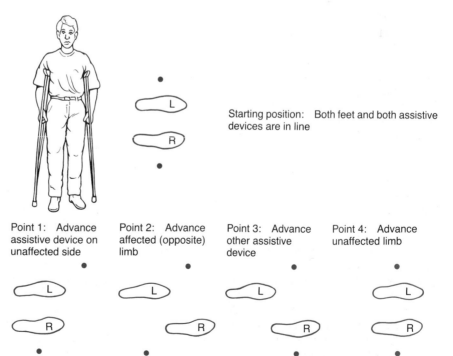

**FIGURE 11–13** ■ Four-point gait pattern.

Starting position: Both feet and both assistive devices are in line

Point 1: Advance assistive device on unaffected side

Point 2: Advance affected (opposite) limb

Point 3: Advance other assistive device

Point 4: Advance unaffected limb

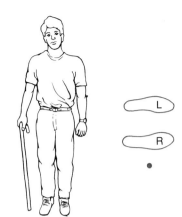

Starting position:   Both feet and unilateral assistive device are in line

FIGURE 11–14  ■  Three-point gait pattern.

Point 1:   Advance assistive device on unaffected side

Point 2:   Advance affected limb

Point 3:   Advance unaffected limb

FIGURE 11–15  ■  Two-point gait pattern.

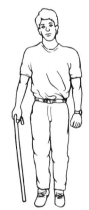

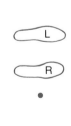

Starting position: Both feet and unilateral assistive device are in line

Point 1:   Advance assistive device and affected limb simultaneously

Point 2:   Advanced unaffected limb

maining lower limb. For example, the right crutch advances, followed by the left lower limb, advancement of the left crutch, and finally the right lower limb. This gait pattern is designed to break down and simulate the reciprocal motion that occurs between the upper and lower limbs during normal gait. A progression of this gait pattern is to have the upper limb with the assistive device and the opposite lower limb move forward simultaneously, resulting in a two-point gait pattern.

## Three-Point Gait Pattern

The three-point pattern (Fig. 11–14) is represented by the contact of the individual's feet (two points) and the assistive device (one point) with the floor.

A unilateral assistive device is typically held on the side opposite the involved lower limb. Initially, the assistive device is advanced forward, followed by the involved lower limb and lastly the uninvolved lower limb. Three-point gait with a unilateral assistive device may be used for individuals who have no medical weight-bearing restrictions but for various reasons exhibit only partial weight bearing of the affected limb.

This gait pattern can also be taught with use of a walker in which the walker is advanced, followed by the involved lower limb and finally the uninvolved lower limb. This gait pattern with a walker is often used by individuals with a partial weight-bearing orthopaedic status.

## Two-Point Gait Pattern

A two-point gait pattern (Fig. 11–15) is one in which the assistive device and involved lower limb move forward simultaneously (one point), followed by the uninvolved lower limb (one point).

Gait training with a walker may involve a two-point gait in which the four legs of the

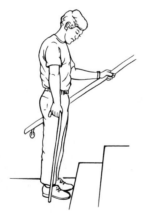

Starting position:  Both feet and unilateral assistive device are on same step; hand is on railing

**FIGURE 11–16** ■ Ascending stairs.

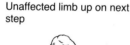
Unaffected limb up on next step

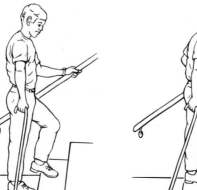
Affected limb up on next step

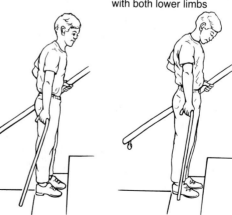
Assistive device up to step with both lower limbs

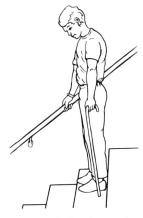

Starting position: Both feet and unilateral assistive device are on same step; hand is on railing

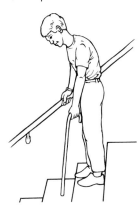

Assistive device down onto next step

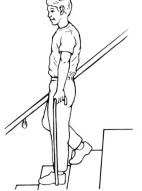

Affected limb down onto next step

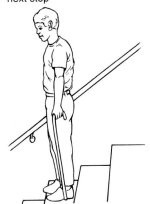

Unaffected limb down onto next step

**FIGURE 11-17** ■ Descending stairs.

walker make contact with the floor simultaneously (one point), followed by the uninvolved lower limb making contact with the floor (second point). The involved lower limb has a restriction of non-weight bearing.

When a unilateral device is used, the device and involved lower limb advance together as one point followed by the uninvolved lower limb. This is a high-level gait pattern in which normal reciprocal movement occurs between the upper and lower limbs. Individuals trained with this gait pattern usually require the assistive device only for minimal support of balance.

## Stair Climbing with Assistive Devices

In teaching stair-climbing gait, the patient's safety should be the primary consideration. In any situation in which the patient and/or assisting family members are at risk of injury, alternatives to stair climbing should be explored. These alternatives may include building ramps if architecturally feasible and arrangements for the patient to live and perform activities of daily living on a single level of the home.

A basic principle of instruction in stair climbing (Fig. 11-16) is that the patient should always use a handrail if one is available. Handrails provide a fixed and stable support for the patient in case of loss of balance. Another principle of stair-climbing gait is that the uninvolved leg advances up to the next step before the involved leg in ascending the stairs. In descending stairs (Fig. 11-17), the involved leg moves to the step below before the uninvolved leg is lowered.

Using walkers, even stair-climbing walkers, can be unsafe on stairs. Therefore, patients who use walkers may best be served by making alternative arrangements to managing steps.

In stair climbing, bilateral assistive devices, such as axillary and forearm crutches, are held by the upper limb opposite the railing. The order of progression in ascending the stairs is that the uninvolved lower limb advances to the next step, followed by the involved leg and assistive devices. In descending stairs, the assistive devices are first lowered, followed by the involved limb and finally the uninvolved limb. The patient walking with a unilateral assistive device also follows this stair-climbing sequence.

In climbing stairs without railings, as well as in managing curbs, the patient should follow the sequence just described. Obviously, the decreased support and balance on steps that do not have railings requires closer attention and guarding of patients in this situation.

## SUMMARY

The study of gait analysis is an ongoing process that is mastered only by years of clinical experience coupled with a strong didactic background. In this chapter we have attempted to provide the reader with a solid foundation in the biomechanics of gait and gait analysis that can readily be applied to the clinical environment for rehabilitation as well as research purposes. The study of gait is dynamic, with ongoing clinical research providing even more information to enhance the understanding of the factors involved in the walking process and how these factors are affected by disease or trauma. It is the responsibility of the clinician to keep up with this new information in order to provide the best possible clinical care.

## Reference

1. Barrett JB: Plantar pressure measurements: rational shoe wear in patients with rheumatoid arthritis. JAMA 235:1138, 1976.

## Bibliography

Bampton S: A Guide to the Visual Examination of Pathological Gait. Philadelphia: Temple University Rehabilitation Research and Training Center, 1979.

Basmajian JV: Muscles Alive, 5th ed. Baltimore: Williams & Wilkins, 1985.

Finley FR, Cody KA: Locomotive characteristics of urban pedestrians. Arch Phys Med Rehabil 51:423, 1970.

Grieve DW: Gait patterns and the speed of walking. Biomed Engineering 3:119, 1968.

Inman VT, Ralsyon HJ, Todd F: Human Walking. Baltimore: Williams & Wilkins, 1981.

Lehmkuhl LD, Smith LK: Brunnstrom's Clinical Kinesiology, 5th ed. Philadelphia: FA Davis, 1992.

Magee DJ: Orthopedic Physical Assessment. Philadelphia: WB Saunders, 1992.

Morrison JB: The mechanics of muscle function in locomotion. J Biomech 3:431–451, 1970.

Murray MP: Gait as a total pattern of movement. Am J Phys Med 46:290–333, 1967.

Murray MP, Brought AB, Kory RC: Walking patterns of normal men. J Bone Joint Surg [Am] 46:335, 1964.

Norkin C, Levangie P: Joint Structure and Function—A Comprehensive Analysis, 2nd ed. Philadelphia: FA Davis, 1991.

Root ML, Arien WP, Weed JH: Normal and Abnormal Function of the Foot. Clinical Biomechanics, Vol 11. Los Angeles: Clinical Biomechanics, 1975.

Scully RM, Barnes MR: Physical Therapy. Philadelphia: JB Lippincott, 1989.

Smidt GL: Hip motion and related factors in walking. Phys Ther 51:9–21, 1971.

Smidt GL, ed: Gait in Rehabilitation. New York: Churchill-Livingstone, 1990.

Soderberg GL: Kinesiology—Application to Pathological Motion. Baltimore: Williams & Wilkins, 1986.

Sutherland DH, Cooper L, Daniel D: The role of the ankle plantarflexors in normal walking. J Bone Joint Surg [Am] 62:354–363, 1980.

Winter DA: Biomechanics of Human Movement. New York: John Wiley & Sons, 1979.

Winter DA: The Biomechanics and Motor Control of Human Gait. Waterloo, IA: University of Waterloo Press, 1988.

# *Twelve*

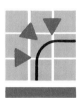

# Fundamentals of Radiology for Physical Therapists

*LYNN NOWICKI McKINNIS*

## INTRODUCTION

In traditional undergraduate physical therapy programs, radiology has not been taught in any formal manner to physical therapists. This is unfortunate because plain film radiography is the *first-order* diagnostic or screening procedure for virtually every patient in the clinic. In graduate programs, radiology is a fundamental course.

Plain film radiography denotes taking simple x-ray films without use of contrast medium (Fig. 12–1). The results of plain film radiography correlated with the clinical evaluation dictate any further diagnostic studies to be done. They also form the basis for treatment or nontreatment and possible referrals.

This chapter provides a fundamental understanding of the science of radiology and an interpretation of the language of the written radiology report. This basic knowledge should assist physical therapists in gaining a comprehensive understanding of musculoskeletal disease and dysfunction, augment education of patients, and enhance communication with physicians.

## THE ART AND SCIENCE OF RADIOLOGY

Radiologic technicians combine 2 years of academic and clinical training to master the art of photography, the physics of technology, and anatomy. Radiologists are medical doctors who specialize in reading radiographs and interpreting their findings for the referring physicians.

X-radiation is a form of electromagnetic vibrations of short wavelength, 1/10,000 the wavelength of visible light rays (Fig. 12–2). X-rays can penetrate dense substances and ionize matter, and their ionization of silver atoms on film produces the gray images of the radiograph. The use of x-rays in diagnostic radiology depends on the various densities inherent in the human body and their attenuation of x-rays.

Briefly, the process begins when a high-voltage

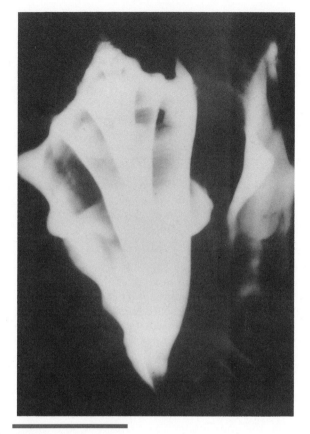

FIGURE 12–1 ■ Plain film radiograph of a conch shell. (Courtesy of Sarah A. Hample, RTR, North Hills Passavant Hospital, Pittsburgh, PA.)

electric current is passed through an x-ray tube containing positive (anode) and negative (cathode) electrodes. Electrons are driven from the cathode and strike the anode, where an energy conversion takes place. The sudden deceleration of electrons converts energy to x-rays, which are beamed through a series of lead shutters and then travel in divergent lines to the patient (Fig. 12–3). X-rays passing through the patient are attenuated in amounts that depend on the thickness, density, and composition of body structures. Radiation that is not attenuated continues

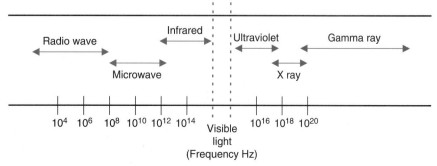

FIGURE 12–2 ■ The electromagnetic spectrum.

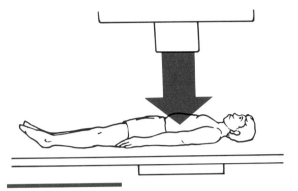

**FIGURE 12–3** ■ Diagram of basic tools required in conventional plain film radiography: an x-ray source, an object (the patient), and a recording medium (film).

out of the patient to the film. The silver emulsion on the film undergoes chemical ionization when exposed to radiation. This reaction creates blackness in areas exposed to more radiation and whiteness in areas of less radiation, so that the radiograph is an accurate representation of the radiographic densities of the structures the x-ray beam has encountered. Developed films (similar to photographic negatives) are then sent to the radiologist for reading. Films become a permanent part of a patient's medical record, along with the radiologist's typewritten report. Scrap film and older discarded film are recycled or sold to recover the silver and plastic base. Radiographs, or films, are often incorrectly referred to as "x-rays," but they are actually developed *films.*

## GENERAL POSITIONING FOR RADIOGRAPHS

The most common radiograph, the chest film, is routinely taken as a posterior-anterior (PA) projection. That is, the patient stands with the anterior chest pressed to the film cassette, and the x-ray tube is behind the patient (Fig. 12–4). The x-ray beam is projected in a posterior-to-anterior direction through the patient and finally onto the film. This position is used because the lungs are more anterior in the chest cavity and structures closer to the film are more sharply defined. The farther structures are from the film plate, the more magnification and distortion of the image take place. A distorted image of a structure is also obtained if the structure is outside the central focal ray of the x-ray beam. The farther a structure is from the central ray, the more geometric distortion of the image takes

place. For example, if a patient's hands were x-rayed together on one film plate, the central ray would fall between the hands. The sharpest image would be of the thumbs, and the remainder of the hands would be increasingly distorted out toward the periphery of the fifth digits.

Standard radiographs of the skeletal system are usually anterior-posterior (AP) projections with lateral projection taken at a right angle to the AP plane. Right and left oblique projections are standard projections at the spine, pelvis, and some extremity joints. The obliques are named in reference to either the AP or PA position (Fig. 12–5). Internal rotation (IR) or external rotation (ER) of a limb before the AP projection is often used when evaluating the hip or shoulder joint in order to visualize more of the circumference of the spherical heads and tubular shafts.

## IDENTIFYING RIGHT AND LEFT ON RADIOGRAPHS

Films are labeled with a registration plate stating the patient's name and case number, the date, and the facility where the radiographs were taken. Films are also usually labeled with identifying markers to discern right (R) and left (L) limbs or halves of the body and whether the patient was erect (ERECT) or weight bearing (WTB). The R and L markers can be confusing because they are usually upside down and backward. They are usually placed on the film at the time the patient is being positioned. An "R" or "Я" or "Я" or " Я" is still a right limb or the right side of the body. Do not attempt to orient the film to correctly position the "R" or "L".

The standard projection is AP, and the film should be positioned as if the patient is facing

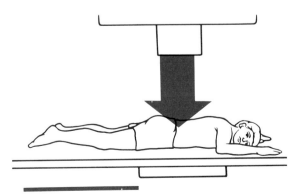

**FIGURE 12–4** ■ Posterior-anterior chest film position.

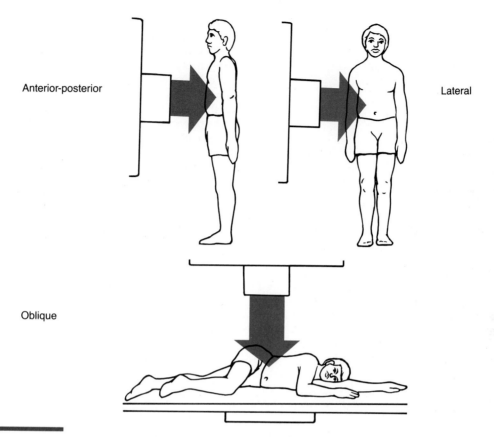

FIGURE 12–5 ■ Standard anatomic projections are frontal (AP or PA), lateral, and oblique projections. Many radiographers in the United States name obliques in reference to the side of the patient closest to the film—for example, left anterior oblique (LAO). This terminology is noted in parentheses.

the individual reading the film. The R or L marker, somewhere on the film, indicates a right or left leg. If it is a right lower extremity, the film should be oriented so that the fibula is to the reader's left (Fig. 12–6). When viewing an AP projection of the lumbar spine, the R marker on one side of the spine denotes the patient's right side. The film should be positioned so that the right side is on the reader's left-hand side of the film.

Many special positions for radiographs exist, and these are requested by the radiologist who is seeking some specific pathology. In general, physical therapists review radiographs with standard projections: AP, PA, LAT, OBLIQUE, ERECT, WTB, or AP combined with IR or ER.

## SEEING RADIOGRAPHIC DETAIL

Interpreting radiographic detail is a skill that must be taught. Three dimensions are flattened,

layers become a "composite shadowgram," and curves in bone throw visual curves. Two fundamental concepts are prerequisite to developing a knowledge of radiographic detail: an understanding of radiographic density and an appreciation of form and thickness and the shadows they produce.

## Radiographic Density

When x-rays reach the silver emulsion on film, the chemical reaction renders the image black. When x-rays are totally absorbed by an object, no radiation reaches the film and the corresponding area on the film is white. When an object partially attenuates x-rays, the remaining radiation reaches the film and a gray image is produced. Thus the principle of medical radiology is dependent on the human body's various densities and thus its various attenuation properties.

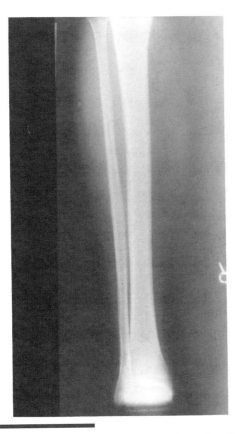

FIGURE 12–6 ■ AP projection of right lower leg. Do not orient the film to correctly position the R marker. (Courtesy of Tri-Rivers Surgical Associates, Inc., Pittsburgh, PA.)

The term radiolucent refers to the transparency of an object to x-radiation. Radiopaque refers to an object's lack of transparency to x-radiation. Radiolucency and radiopaqueness are both degrees of radiodensity. Objects are described as more or less radiodense than each other. Decreased radiodensity, or radiolucency, denotes a blacker shadow on the film; increased radiodensity, or radiopacity, denotes a whiter shadow on film. Radiographic contrast refers to the density difference between two areas in a radiograph. The greater the difference in densities, the higher the contrast and the easier it is to identify structures.

Radiographically, the human body contains four different densities, produced by air, fat, water, and bone. Air is present in the lungs, stomach, and intestines. It is the most radiolucent of the four, and its image is blackest. Fat is more radiodense than air and is found subcutaneously, around organs, and along muscle sheaths. Water has approximately the same density and attenuation properties as most soft tissues of the body, including muscle, blood, viscera, cartilage, tendons, ligaments, nerves, and skin. Water and these like structures are somewhat more radiodense than fat. Bone is the most radiodense of the inherent body structures and so casts the whitest shadow of the four. Dentin of the teeth is the most radiodense bone tissue and appears very white in radiographs.

Two inorganic substances are commonly seen in medical radiography. Contrast media, such as the barium used in upper and lower gastrointestinal studies, are radiopaque and cast a bright white outline. Heavy metals used in prosthetic appliances, such as total joint replacements, or internal fixation devices, such as wires, pins, or compression screws, are the most radiopaque or radiodense materials and appear solid white on film (Fig. 12–7).

Another explanation of relative radiodensity is based on the composition or atomic weight of structures. The greater the atomic weight of a substance, the greater its attenuation of x-rays. Lead has an atomic number of 82 and attenuates so completely that it is used as a radiation shield. Barium has an atomic number of 56, so its attenuation is less than that of lead but much more than that of the calcium of bone (atomic number 20). Thus, barium attenuates more x-rays than bone and appears much whiter on film than bone (Fig. 12–8).

## Form and Thickness

Radiodensity depends on the composition of the materials of a structure and is also a function of thickness. For example, if several blocks of homogeneous composition were lined up in a row and each block was 1 inch thicker than its predecessor, the radiographic shadows produced

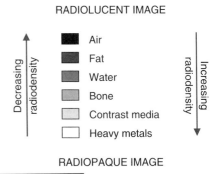

FIGURE 12–7 ■ Relative radiodensities of the human body, commonly used contrast media, and heavy metals.

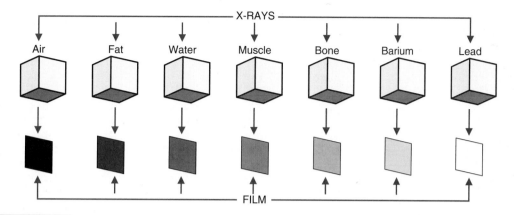

**FIGURE 12–8** ■ Radiodensity as a function of composition of matter. (Reprinted by permission of the publishers from Fundamentals of Radiology by Lucy Frank Squire and Robert A. Novelline, Cambridge, Mass.: Harvard University Press, Copyright © 1975, 1982, 1988 by the President and Fellows of Harvard College.)

would be progressively whiter (Fig. 12–9). This is simply a rule of summation: the thicker the structure, the more relative radiodensity it possesses.

Because of the great variety of bone shapes in the body, it is necessary to think of thickness as a function of form. Figure 12–10 depicts the form of a wedge projected from three of its sides. Assume that the wedge has uniform composition. In example A, the wedge is projected through its triangular flat side and casts a triangular radiographic image. In example B, the wedge is placed upright on its base. The projection from above now casts a rectangular image with a denser center line. The image in example B is analogous to the image created by a prominent bone ridge. That is, the top ridge of the wedge appears more white or radiodense than the rest of the wedge. Because the wedge is uniform, the increased radiodensity is due to the

increased amount of wedge through which the x-rays have traveled. The greater the thickness, the more attenuated the x-rays and the whiter the image. Compare this ridge of the wedge to the radiodense lines of real ridges of the proximal femur (Fig. 12–11). Example C in Figure 12–10A shows that the thicker end of the side-lying wedge casts a whiter image than its thinner edge. These different radiographic images of the same wedge show that density is a function of thickness. The effect of the angle of projection on the radiographic image is also well demonstrated in this example.

The effects of form and thickness combined with different angles of projection are now illustrated for curved surfaces. Figure 12–12A and B show a hollow cylinder projected from two different angles. Stood on its end, the cylinder casts the image of a hollow circle (see Fig. 12–12A). With the cylinder viewed from its side, the image

**FIGURE 12–9** ■ Radiodensity as a function of thickness of an object. (Reprinted by permission of the publishers from Fundamentals of Radiology by Lucy Frank Squire and Robert A. Novelline, Cambridge, Mass.: Harvard University Press, Copyright © 1975, 1982, 1988 by the President and Fellows of Harvard College.)

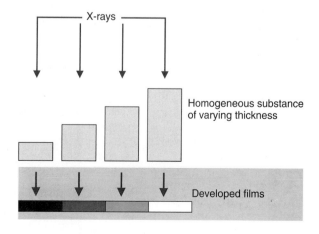

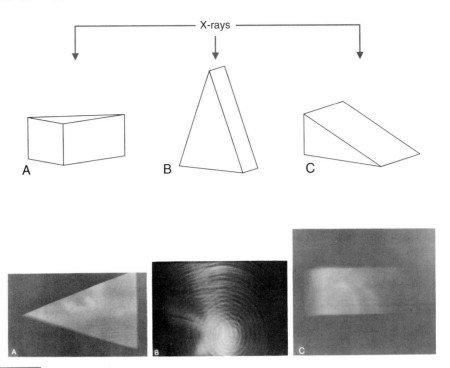

**FIGURE 12-10** ■ (A, B, and C) Radiodensity as a function of thickness and form. The three different angles of projection produced three different images of the same wedge of wood. (Courtesy of Sarah A. Hample, RTR, North Hills Passavant Hospital, Pittsburgh, PA.)

**FIGURE 12-11** ■ Bone landmarks of the proximal femur. (Courtesy of Tri-Rivers Surgical Associates, Inc., Pittsburgh, PA.)

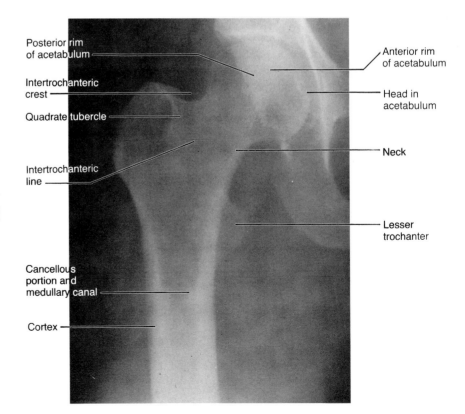

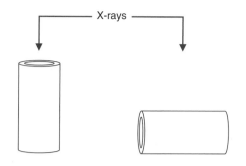

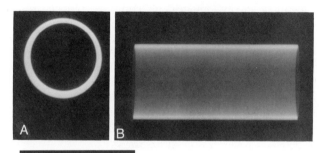

**FIGURE 12–12** ■ (A and B) Two projections of a hollow plastic cylinder. (Courtesy of Sarah A. Hample, RTR, North Hills Passavant Hospital, Pittsburgh, PA.)

is of two dense parallel lines, representing the margins of the cylinder (see Fig. 12–12B). But if the cylinder is of uniform composition, why are the margins imaged as lines? If a beam of sunshine traversed the side-lying cylinder flatly across its side, the shadow would be rectangular. The answer again lies in the rule of summation. X-rays that pass directly through the center of the side-lying hollow cylinder traverse a thickness equal to the sum of two sides of the cylinder. X-rays that pass through the long side margins of the hollow cylinder traverse curved planes of much greater cumulative thickness than the sum of the two sides. Thus, the margins are radiographed tangentially and, by the rule of summation, produce a whiter, more radiodense image than the rest of the cylinder. Human long bones are somewhat tubular in form and have an outer cortex of strong, dense bone and a core of spongy trabecular bone and marrow. Again, because the margins of long bones are curved planes, they are radiographed tangentially and produce whiter, denser images. See the example of the femur in Figure 12–11 and compare it with the image of the cylinder in Figure 12–12B.

Another way to understand curved surfaces is to remember that parts of structures are either approximately parallel to the x-ray film or relatively perpendicular to the film (Fig. 12–13).

Clearly, an x-ray beam travels through much more thickness in a perpendicular structure than a flat parallel structure. Curved planes can be visualized by seeing them as a transition from a parallel plane to a perpendicular plane then to a parallel plane again. It is obvious that a basic understanding of radiology requires knowledge of anatomy and its forms and structures.

## A Composite Shadowgram

Radiodensity is understood to be a function of a structure's material composition, thickness, and form. The angle of projection determines the plane in which the beam traverses the object and so defines the outline of the image. X-ray films are simply images produced by the densities through which the x-ray beam has traveled. Squire, in her text *Fundamentals of Radiology,* described x-ray films not as pictures but as "composite shadowgrams" representing the sum of the densities interposed between beam sources and film.

Keeping this description in mind, it is necessary to think three-dimensionally while looking at the two-dimensional films. The viewer must mentally "add" and "subtract" the radiographic shadows that are superimposed on one another.

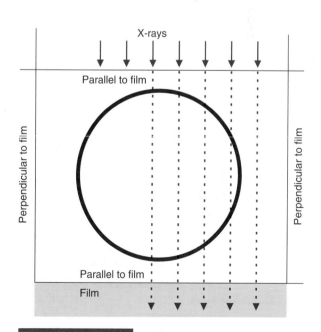

**FIGURE 12–13** ■ X-rays travel through a greater thickness of material in structures perpendicular to the film than in structures parallel to the film.

In this way the anatomic layers are sorted out and their contribution to the composite shadow-gram accounted for.

For example, the AP view of the lumbar spine in Figure 12–14 was obtained by the x-rays traversing, in anterior-to-posterior-order, skin, fat, abdominal muscles, intestines containing fecal matter and gas, deeper muscles of the spine such as the psoas, the spine itself with related cartilage and disc spaces, more muscles of the erector spinae and posterior back, fat, and finally skin again. If the lumbar vertebrae are of interest, the viewer mentally subtracts the images of gray superimposed anterior to them. That is, the outlines of fat, muscle, and intestine are identified and then ignored. Then the cortical outlines of the vertebral body are recognized and outlines of the pedicle lamina, facet articulations, transverse processes, and spinous processes are added, all positioned posterior to the vertebral body. The

relative radiolucency of the soft tissues anterior to the vertebrae makes it possible to "see through" to the more radiodense bone structures. Vertebral structures are considered in more detail later.

## A Rose Is a Rose

The radiographic principles related to composition, form, thickness, and angles of projection can be summarized and interpreted by applying them to a familiar object. Squire illustrates the logic of x-ray images of complex objects by presenting x-ray films of three roses, as shown in Figure 12–15.

By gross form, roses, leaves, and stems are recognized. It is easily seen that one rose is unopened, another is in bloom, another is about finished blooming. Thickness principles are evi-

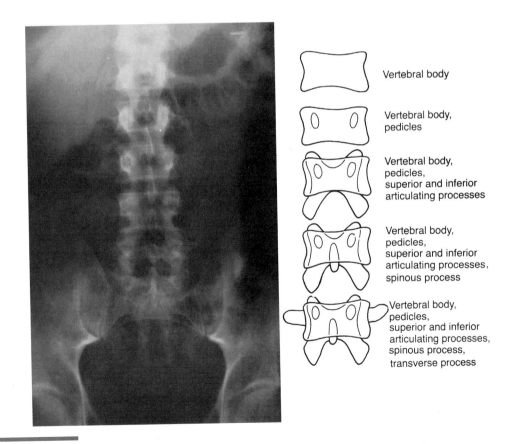

**FIGURE 12–14** ■ (A) AP view of the lumbar spine. Note the different densities of air and bone and the various shades of gray representing muscles and organs. (B) Use the schematic to understand the outlines of the vertebrae. (Reprinted by permission of the publishers from Fundamentals of Radiology by Lucy Frank Squire and Robert A. Novelline, Cambridge, Mass.: Harvard University Press, Copyright © 1975, 1982, 1988 by the President and Fellows of Harvard College.)

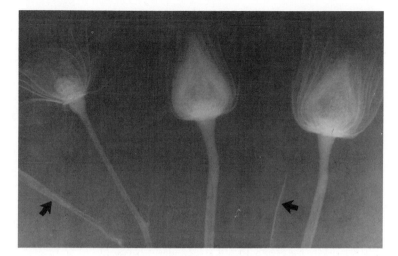

**FIGURE 12–15** ■ Radiograph of roses. Arrows point to leaves positioned perpendicular to film. Leaves parallel to the film were too radiolucent to produce an image. (Courtesy of Sarah A. Hample, RTR, North Hills Passavant Hospital, Pittsburgh, PA.)

dent in the delicate transparency and radiolucency of one rose petal compared to the increased density of the closed rose, whose several petals overlap in a tight bud. Some information about the composition of the stems and veins of the leaves can be discerned. They appear denser than the flat surfaces of the leaves because of their stronger cell structure and the fact that they are fluid filled. The various parallel and perpendicular planes in which the petals and leaves lie are revealed by various white density changes. The leaf that is perpendicular on the film is easily seen, as opposed to leaves lying flat on the film. The rose petals illustrate numerous curved planes. By understanding angles of projection, it can be deduced that the stems are tubular, as the denser white parallel margins of the stems represent curved planes filmed tangentially.

## HOW TO EVALUATE RADIOGRAPHS

In studying a plain film, it is important to see musculoskeletal structures grossly and then in detail. Bone must be considered as both an anatomic framework and a portion of a large, sensitive physiologic organ. A working knowledge of pathology and disease states is needed to appreciate how the musculoskeletal system adapts or fails to adapt. Basic radiographic assessment of the musculoskeletal system should include examination of

- General body architecture
- General contour of bone
- General density of bone
- Local density of bone

- Articulating relationships between bones
- Cortical outline of bones
- Periosteum of bones
- Articular cartilage and potential space
- Subchondral bone
- Joint capsules
- Epiphyses and epiphyseal plates
- Medulla of bone
- Soft tissues

## General Body Architecture

First, look at the overall film. Radiographic images are approximately 30% larger than life size. Assess gross normal appearance of form. Note whether any bones are missing because of congenital absence or amputation. Also note whether any "extra" bones are present, such as a cervical rib, a "sixth" lumbar vertebra, or an extra navicular among the tarsals. Note the general size of the bones. Do they appear normal? Are there gross enlargements such as in Paget's disease?

## General Contour of Bone

The normal shape of each bone should be apparent. Note any internal or external irregularities. Observe any congenital, developmental, or pathologic deformities.

## General Density of Bone

Normal contrasting radiodensities between soft tissues and bone should be seen. Note any overall increase in bone density typical of an osteosclerotic disease or any overall decrease in bone density typical of osteoporosis. Trabecular patterns should be distinct. These should be looked for in areas of weight bearing, particularly the head and neck of the femur, distal femur, proximal tibia, and calcaneus.

## Local Density of Bone

Localized osteoarthritis causes sclerotic changes that are seen as increased density on film. Sclerotic areas should be sought on weight-bearing surfaces of joints. These areas are usually associated with loss of articular cartilage and degenerative joint disease. Sclerotic areas also represent areas of bone healing following fracture, infection, or local bone death.

## Articular Relationships Between Bones

Assess the normal congruity between articulating joint surfaces, and note any dislocations or subluxations. Subluxations involve less displacement then dislocations, and the joint remains partially articulating. Dislocations are usually caused by direct trauma. Subluxations may be caused by direct trauma that causes tearing or laxity of ligaments or joint capsules. Subluxations may also result from inflammatory diseases that erode supporting structures.

## Cortical Outline of Bone

Trace the outline of each bone. The cortex should be smooth and continuous. Sharp angles along curved shafts may indicate impaction fractures. Breaks in continuity are fractures. Healthy cortex should appear denser than the remainder of bone. Loss of cortical density indicates loss of bone density. The best example of such bone loss is osteoporosis.

## Periosteum of Bone

Healthy periosteum is indistinct in plain film radiography. The appearance of callus at a fracture site usually suggests a functional periosteum. A thickened periosteum that appears elevated or lifted away from the cortex is characteristic of osteomyelitis, a bone infection that has formed a subperiosteal abscess.

## Articular Cartilage and Potential Space

Cartilage is not readily seen in plain films, but its presence is made known by the potential joint spaces. Absence of the space indicates loss of articular cartilage. Observe each joint for well-preserved joint space. Decreased joint space associated with sclerotic subchondral bone indicates osteoarthritis. Generalized loss of joint spaces, even to the degree that bone appears to be articulating directly with bone, is indicative of painful inflammatory diseases such as rheumatoid arthritis. Remember that some joints progress with age into synostoses. In a synostosis, the joint space is obliterated by fibrous union.

## Subchondral Bone

Loss of hyaline cartilage causes synovial joints to lose their optimal articulating congruity. With the cartilage thinned, the unprotected and malaligned surfaces mechanically stress the subchondral bone. As deterioration progresses, joint biomechanics become more severely altered. In accordance with Wolff's law,[1] subchondral bone reacts to increased stress by increasing its density, which presents as sclerosis. Osteochondritis dissecans, or detachment of necrotic subchondral bone, is a complication of osteochondral fracture. In contrast, the osteolytic lesions of gouty arthritis or systemic processes like rheumatoid arthritis cause erosion of subchondral bone that presents as radiolucent areas on film.

## Joint Capsules

Normal joint capsules are not seen radiographically. Effusion, hemorrhage, or hemarthrosis distends the capsule, and its outline is clearly discerned. Effusion of the capsule may also displace fat pads that are not normally detectable. The "fat pad" sign of the elbow or the pronator fat pad of the palmar side of the distal radius, when made obvious by joint effusion, is a clue to joint trauma or possible occult (hidden) fracture.

## Epiphyses and Epiphyseal Plates

The epiphyses should be recognized as normal in size in terms of general skeletal maturity and chronologic age. Disruptions of the epiphyseal plate, as described by the Salter-Harris classification,[2] can be difficult to diagnose and contralateral films may be needed for comparison.

## Medulla of Bone

A sharply defined interface should be seen between the cortex and the medullary cavity. Note any radiolucent areas that could represent tumors.

## Soft Tissues

Normal soft tissues are not readily detected by plain film radiography. Trauma to soft tissues, however, produces abnormal images. Joint capsules are distended by effusion, hemorrhage, or hemarthrosis. Films of patients with inflammatory joint diseases reveal evidence of periarticular swelling. Calcium deposits in soft tissues are abnormal and can easily be seen in calcific bursitis or myositis ossificans. Edema or abscesses may be present in conditions such as cellulitis or may be secondary to osteomyelitis.

## GENERAL CHARACTERISTICS OF NORMAL BONES AND JOINTS

In viewing films of joints and bones, an understanding of normal structure is needed to serve as a base for understanding the abnormal characteristics of fracture and disease.

Normal bone grows in width by the process of intramembranous ossification and grows in length by endochondral ossification. Primary centers of ossification are in the diaphyses. Ossification progresses out toward the epiphyses. Secondary centers of ossification develop in the cartilaginous epiphyses at various ages after birth. The zones of the epiphyseal plate progressively calcify cartilage into bone (Fig. 12–16). The process of ossification continues from the embryo to approximately 25 years of age. Thereafter, local growth is possible, as in healing of fractures.

Remodeling of bone occurs continuously during longitudinal growth. As the epiphysis moves continually away from the shaft, the metaphysis is remodeled by osteoblastic cell deposition of bone on one surface and osteoclastic cell resorption on the opposite surface. Total bone deposition exceeds bone resorption during normal growth years, resulting in positive bone balance. In the last decades of life, bone deposition cannot keep up with bone resorption, resulting in negative bone balance or senile osteoporosis.

Of paramount importance to physical therapists is the remodeling of bone in response to physical stress. Wolff's law, formulated by Julius Wolff in 1969, states that "every change in the form and function of bones or in their function alone is followed by certain definite changes in their internal architecture, and equally definite changes in their external conformation, in accordance with mathematical laws."[1] Simply speaking, bone is deposited in sites subjected to stress. Wolff's law also works in reverse; that is, bone is resorbed from sites deprived of stress. Physical therapists must be aware of this phenomenon and its clinical implications. Disuse atrophy of a limb affects not only the muscle tissue but also bone tissue. Lack of weight bearing or lack of muscle pulling on bone over a prolonged period leads to disuse osteoporosis or a decrease in total bone mass. Loss of bone mass appears on radiographs as loss of density of the bone image relative to the soft tissue image.

Joints are simply articulations between two or more bones. Joints are generally classified into five types:

**Syndesmosis.** Two bones are bound by fibrous connective tissue. An example may be found at the distal tibiofibular joint.

**Synchondrosis.** Two bones are bound together by cartilage. An example is the temporary epiphyseal plate.

**Synostosis.** The joint has been obliterated by bone union across the joint space. All synchondroses of growing bones eventually fuse, as do some syndesmoses.

**Symphysis.** Two bones with articulating hyaline cartilage are bound tightly by dense fibrous connective tissue. The best example is the pubic symphysis.

**Synovial.** Two bones with articulating hyaline cartilage are supported nutritionally by synovial fluid and encased peripherally by the joint capsule. The inner layer of the capsule specializes into the synovial membrane; the

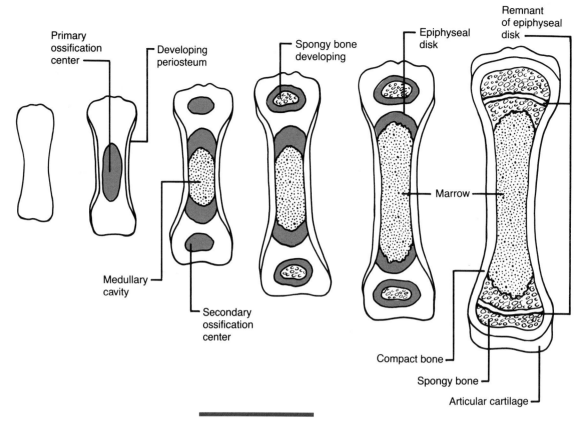

**FIGURE 12-16 ■** Development of bone.

outer layer differentiates into fibrous tissue that blends with stabilizing ligaments and anchors to bone.

Articular cartilage, or hyaline cartilage of synovial joints, depends on synovial fluid for nourishment. Distribution, circulation, and recycling of synovial fluid depend on joint motion and normal compression forces to aid diffusion of the fluid to the cartilage matrix. Prolonged immobilization, after fracture, for example, inhibits this crucial process and leads to disuse atrophy of the cartilage. Figure 12-17 of the shoulder illustrates glenohumeral degenerative joint disease secondary to an old humeral impaction fracture. The decreased joint space and sclerotic joint surfaces indicate abnormally thin and damaged articular cartilage. These degenerative changes are unusual for a non-weight-bearing joint.

This x-ray film is a good example of why physical therapists need to see films. With this visual information, physical therapists can be properly vigilant for the detrimental effects of immobilization. Physical therapists can then design appropriate exercise programs to prevent

this synovial stasis when possible and, of equal importance, guard against aggressive rehabilitation in the presence of cartilaginous atrophy. Normal arthrokinematics (joint play or normal roll, spin, and glide) are reduced as a result of immobilization. Forced osteokinematics, or range of motion, without the prerequisite normal arthrokinematics compresses the already weakened and rigid articular cartilage. The results are delayed gains in range of motion, continued pain, abnormal biomechanics, and a contribution to degenerative osteoarthritis of the joint.

## COMMON DISORDERS OF BONES AND JOINTS

Bone is both an anatomic structure that provides the body's rigid framework and leverage system and a systemic physiologic living organ that reacts in ways that mirror organic disease. Bone manifestations of disease are often detected by radiographs. Bone is a common site for metastatic tumors from primary cancerous organ sites.

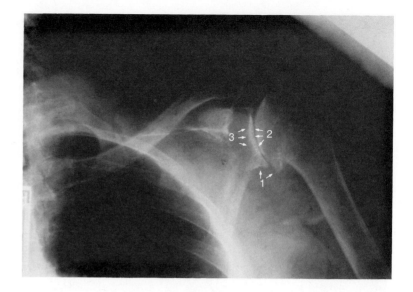

**FIGURE 12–17** ■ Degenerative osteoarthritis of the glenohumeral joint. Note decreased joint space, sclerotic subchondral bone, and osteophyte formation at joint margins. (1) Spurs; (2) narrow joint; (3) whitish bone. (Courtesy of Slippery Rock University School of Physical Therapy, Slippery Rock, PA.)

Osteomyelitis, or bone infection, and septic arthritis, or joint infection, may be caused by extension of adjacent soft tissue infection, by external contamination of punctures or open fractures, or by hematogenous routes.

Disorders of bone may have their etiology in genetic abnormalities, metabolic or dietary abnormalities, endocrine abnormalities, or many unknown sources.

Bone has a limited number of reactions to a wide variety of abnormal physiologic conditions. In general, bone reacts to abnormal conditions in one of three ways:

■ Altered bone deposition
■ Altered bone resorption
■ Local bone death

## Osteoporosis

When bone deposition is less than bone resorption, there is a generalized decrease in bone mass. Radiologically, bone appears less dense and the cortex thinner. A radiologic term for thin bone is osteopenia. It is a descriptive term rather than a clinical diagnosis. Rarefaction also refers to the radiologic appearance of an abnormal loss of bone mass. Osteoporosis, or porous bone, was already mentioned as a clinical diagnosis of decreased total bone mass. Disuse atrophy was cited as a causative factor, as was the negative bone balance of the elderly (more than 65 years of age). Prolonged steroid therapy and some disease processes result in osteoporotic bone. Post-

menopausal osteoporosis is related to estrogen deficiency in females. A similar condition can occur in amenorrheic teenage girls, who should normally be laying down the bulk of their total bone mass. Both the elderly and teenage osteoporotics are at risk for pathologic fractures secondary to acquired structural weaknesses or fractures caused by relatively minor trauma. Elderly women frequently suffer fractures of the distal radius when reaching out to catch themselves in a fall. Fractures of the neck of the femur have the same high incidence as distal radius fractures and may cause a fall or happen as a result of a fall. The neck of the humerus is also weakened by osteoporosis, and humeral neck fractures occur as often as wrist and hip fractures (Fig. 12–18). Compression fracture, or collapse of the vertebral body with anterior wedging and resultant progressive thoracic kyphosis (Fig. 12–19), is also common among the elderly. Particularly common in the teenage group are chronic stress fractures and delayed union of fractures.

It has been estimated that osteoporosis is seen radiographically in more than half of patients over age 65. Osteoporosis cannot be detected radiographically until more than 30% of total bone mass has been lost. Thus, physical therapists should anticipate some degree of osteoporosis in all persons over 65 and especially in postmenopausal women, who, in effect, have the double risk of postmenopausal plus senile osteoporosis. Considering the added factor of disuse osteoporosis, the aging population could well benefit from appropriate preventive and postural instruction. When reading radiologic reports, it

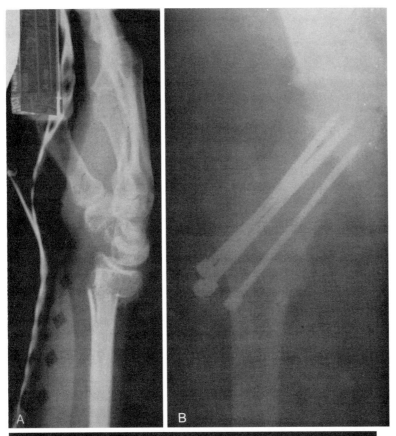

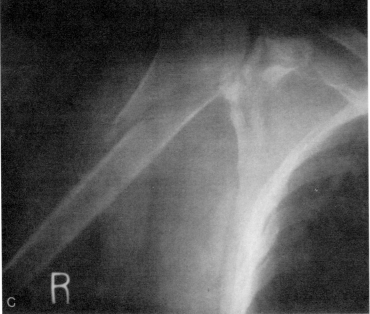

**FIGURE 12–18** ■ (A) Fracture of the distal radius with a volar apex of fracture and dorsal angulation of the fracture fragment. (B) Intertrochanteric fracture of the femur after reduction and internal fixation with Steimann pins. (C) Spiral fracture of the humoral neck. The highest incidence of these fractures is in the elderly female population. (Courtesy of Slippery Rock University School of Physical Therapy, Slippery Rock, PA.)

should be remembered that osteoporosis is a clinical diagnosis, not a description of the radiologic image of bone. Bone mass is decreased in osteoporosis because of a reduction in bone deposition activity. Bone mass may also be decreased by diseases, such as hyperparathyroidism, that cause gross bone destruction. These two diverse metabolic processes result in radiologic similarities. Cortex appears thinner and bone appears more radiolucent. The radiologist describes decrease in bone mass as osteopenia or as demineralization of bone.

## Osteomalacia

Osteomalacia, also known as adult rickets, is a disorder caused by hypocalcification and characterized by loss of bone mass. The body continues to make bone but is not able to calcify the matrix. Thus, there is an appearance of wide but thin bone with no visible cortex (Fig. 12–20). Bowing of the long bones and compression of vertebral bodies often occur. Osteomalacia is related to vitamin deficiencies or renal disorders.

## Osteosclerosis

In conditions in which bone deposition is greater than bone resorption, there is a general increase in bone mass. Osteosclerosis is a category of some rare skeletal diseases such as acromegaly, osteopetrosis, and osteopoikilosis, which involve increases in total body bone mass. However, osteosclerosis is also a common orthopaedic term describing localized areas of increased density. Sclerotic refers to more density, secondary to increased mechanical stress or prior healing.

Degenerative osteoarthritis, or degenerative joint disease, is a condition in which articular cartilage has been worn down so that subchondral bone takes on more stress than normal and becomes sclerotic. Degenerative osteoarthritis is discussed in more detail later.

Hypertrophy of bone is also due primarily to increased stresses, in accordance with Wolff's law. The classic example is the rigid foot with varus or supinated-like deformity. The fifth metatarsal bears excessive weight in stance, instead of the weight being properly transmitted across the forefoot. The result is a hypertrophic fifth ray appearing denser or whiter on film.

Exostoses, sometimes called spurs, bunions, or osteophytes, are local bone protuberances formed by excessive friction, stress, or muscle tension.

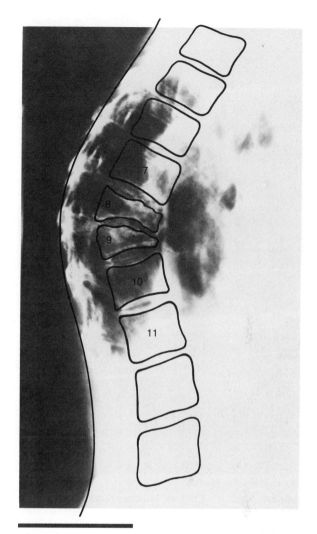

**FIGURE 12–19** ■ Thoracic kyphosis resulting from generalized osteoporosis. (Courtesy of Slippery Rock University School of Physical Therapy, Slippery Rock, PA.)

Figure 12–21 shows a common heel spur, possibly secondary to abnormal plantar fascia tension. Figure 12–22 shows a spur on the acetabular rim of the hip joint. Clinically, hip range of motion would be mechanically limited by this protuberance. Passive rotations of the hip joint would probably produce hard end feels.

The neuropathic foot in Figure 12–23 has lost a great deal of normal bone architecture and appears sclerotic. In cases of diabetes or syphilis or diseases in which there is loss of autonomic sensation, the feet are often subjected to bumps, cuts, or bruises unnoticed by the patient. Over the years there are constant episodes of trauma and/or infection, and thus attempts at healing constantly take place. The resultant radiographic

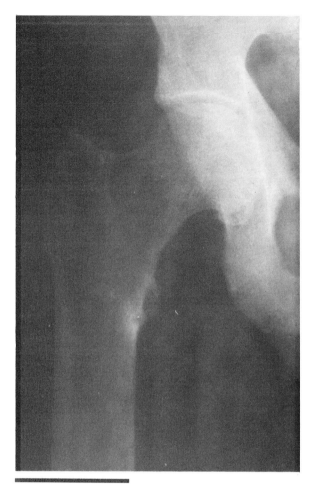

**FIGURE 12-20** ■ Osteomalacia of the femur. Note the loss of sharp interface between cortical bone and cancellous bone caused by demineralization of the cortex. (Courtesy of North Hills Passavant Hospital, Pittsburgh, PA.)

appearance is whitish because of the multiple sclerotic layers deposited in this chronic condition. The total bone mass of the foot, however, may be demineralized and brittle.

## Paget's Disease (Osteitis Deformans)

Paget's disease is a progressive bone disease that affects 3% of the population over 40 years of age. Its etiology remains unknown. The disease is characterized by random proliferation with both osteoblast formation and osteoclast resorption. The result is thickened, deformed, and eventually porous bone. Paget's disease usually affects the skull, the vertebral bodies, the pelvis,

the femur, and the tibia. Figure 12-24 is a radiograph of a skull showing cranial enlargement and uneven density caused by Paget's disease.

Figure 12-25 is a film of the pelvis of the same patient. The sacroiliac joints have been obliterated by bone proliferation across the joint space. These radiographs represent first-order diagnostic tests that reveal the present extent of the damage caused by the disease. Figure 12-26 shows that a more in-depth test—a bone scan—can overcome the limits of the plain radiograph by revealing areas where the disease process continues to develop. In bone scanning, radioactive isotopes are used to illuminate areas of increased bone activity. The black patches on the bone scan represent these areas of increased activity.

## Slipped Femoral Capital Epiphysis

Epiphyseal slippage of the femoral head is a developmental abnormality of the hip that occurs more frequently in males than females and appears between 9 and 16 years of age. The etiology is theorized to be a hormonal imbalance that weakens epiphyseal plates. Because the head of the femur is subjected to strong shear forces, this plate is most vulnerable to displacement. Figure 12-27 shows the characteristic "jockey cap" deformity caused by the downward and backward slippage of the epiphysis. This image of the hip in wide abduction and external rotation provides a better view of the relationship of the epiphysis to the femoral neck in this instance. Internal fixation is required in more severe cases of displacement, and avascular necrosis of the femoral head is a serious complication.

## Myositis Ossificans

Abnormal calcification within muscle is a painful condition known as myositis ossificans. Hemorrhage within a muscle belly, most commonly caused by direct trauma, may result in abnormal blood coagulation and calcification into bone-like substance. Figure 12-28A is a film of the humerus of a young man who had recently injured his biceps during weight lifting. The biceps was tender to palpation. The film at this time is negative. Figure 12-28B is a film of the same man 6 weeks later. By this time, calcifica-

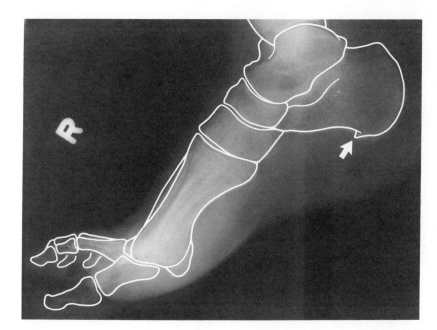

**FIGURE 12–21** ■ Heel spur located at anteromedial plantar surface of the calcaneus (arrow). (Courtesy of North Hills Passavant Hospital, Pittsburgh, PA.)

**FIGURE 12–22** ■ Osteophyte protruding from the superior rim of the acetabulum. Other degenerative changes include decreased joint space and sclerotic subchondral bone at the articulating surfaces. The arch of white shadow at the top half of the film is adipose tissue. Arrow points to bone spur. (Courtesy of North Hills Passavant Hospital, Pittsburgh, PA.)

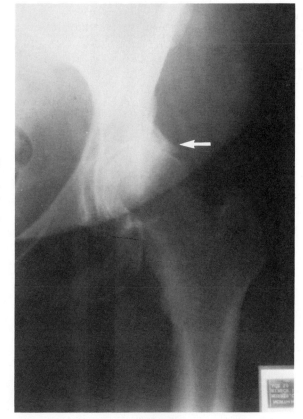

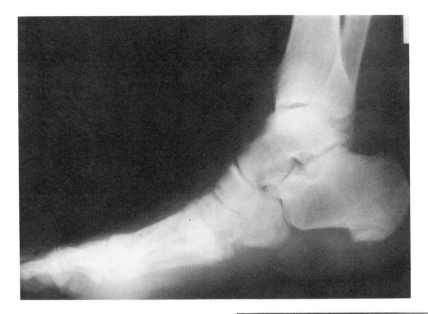

FIGURE 12-23 ■ Neuropathic foot. Note the loss of normal bone arches and abnormal density changes. (Courtesy of North Hills Passavant Hospital, Pittsburgh, PA.)

FIGURE 12-24 ■ Paget's disease manifested at the cranium. The radiopaque image at the mouth was produced by metallic dental work. (Courtesy of North Hills Passavant Hospital, Pittsburgh, PA.)

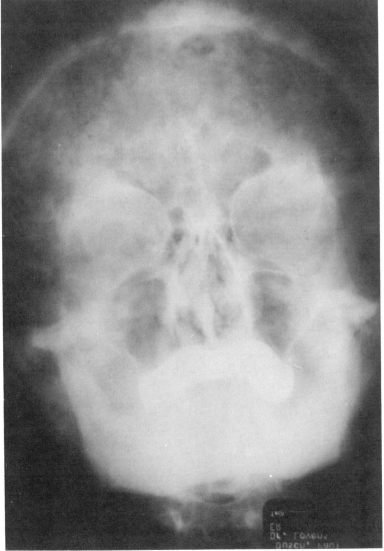

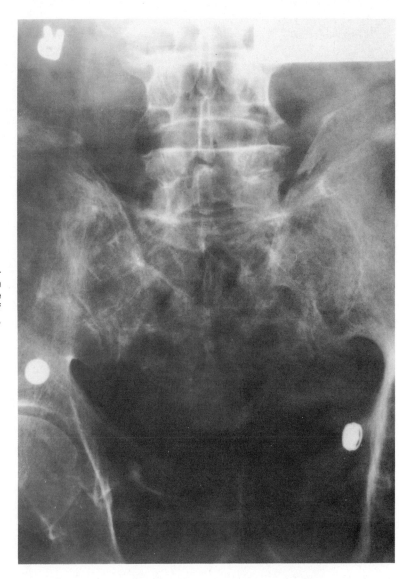

**FIGURE 12–25** ■ Paget's disease manifested at the pelvis. Note bone obliteration of sacroiliac joint spaces. Radiopaque circle images are clothing snaps. (Courtesy of North Hills Passavant Hospital, Pittsburgh, PA.)

tion had progressed to the extent of radiopacity. The biceps had become extremely painful to active contraction, and palpation revealed a bone-like mass within the muscle belly. Myositis ossificans can also be caused by repetitive microtrauma. Such microtrauma may even be induced by the physical therapist performing aggressive passive stretching of a contracted muscle. An example is microhemorrhage in the brachioradialis muscle during passive stretching of an elbow joint contracture. Heterotrophic ossification is a similar calcification that can occur insidiously along myofascial planes. It is usually secondary to neurologic damage in patients suffering some form of paralysis but may occur after total joint replacements or even after minor trauma.

## Degenerative Osteoarthritis

Degenerative osteoarthritis is a noninflammatory chronic arthritis of middle and late age. It affects weight-bearing joints primarily and is characterized by thinning of articular cartilage, sclerosis of subchondral bone, and bone overgrowth at joint margins. The term *degenerative joint disease* is used interchangeably with degenerative osteoarthritis.

Primary osteoarthritis refers to degenerative changes without antecedent trauma. It has been described by Salter as an exaggeration of the normal aging process of joints.[1] The specific etiology is unknown, although genetics may be a

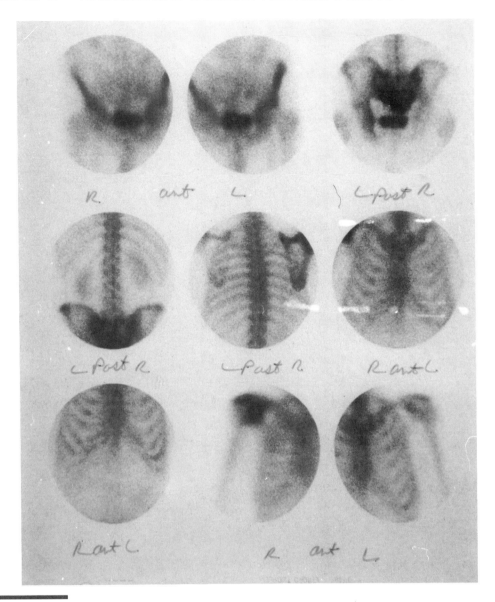

**FIGURE 12-26 ■** Early detection of Paget's disease via bone scanning. The right humerus and scapula demonstrate increased bone activity indicated by increased uptake of the radioactive isotope that renders a blacker image than that of surrounding normal bone. (Courtesy of North Hills Passavant Hospital, Pittsburgh, PA.)

factor. Overuse and, in the case of weight-bearing joints, obesity are aggravating factors. Figure 12–29 illustrates severe osteoarthritis of the first carpometacarpal joint. This painful condition is exacerbated by using the thumb in forceful opposition to the rest of the digits. Adaptive devices for normal activities of daily living can lessen overuse of this joint. Figure 12–30 of the hand reveals a common sign of osteoarthritis at the distal interphalangeal joints. Heberden's nodes are particles of joint debris engulfed by

synovial tissue that subsequently enlarge and deform the small joints. Figure 12–31 of the spine shows an example of bone overgrowth at joint margins. Osteophyte formation (also called bone lipping or spur development) is another characteristic of osteoarthritis. Osteophytes can break off into the synovial joints and cause mechanical blocking and local inflammation.

Secondary osteoarthritis refers to degenerative changes precipitated by some trauma. The trauma may have been fracture, torn menisci,

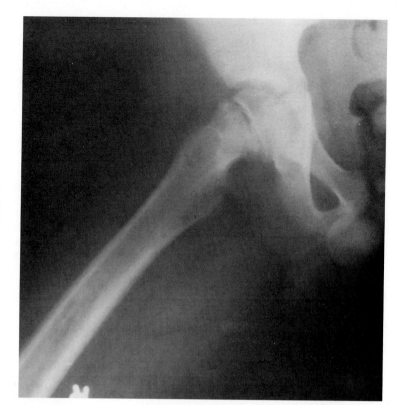

**FIGURE 12-27** ■ Slipped femoral capital epiphysis in a 10-year-old boy. Dashed line indicates proper alignment. (Courtesy of North Hills Passavant Hospital, Pittsburgh, PA.)

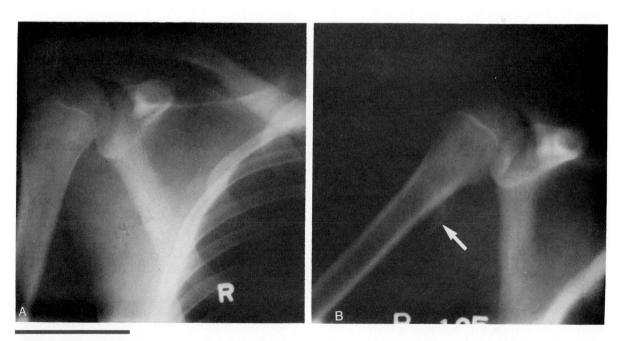

**FIGURE 12-28** ■ (A) Right bicep of a 28-year-old male injured during weight lifting. X-ray film is negative at this time. (B) Myositis ossificans of the biceps of the same patient 6 weeks later. By this time the hemorrhage in the muscle had calcified and was radiodense (arrow). (Courtesy of North Hills Passavant Hospital, Pittsburgh, PA.)

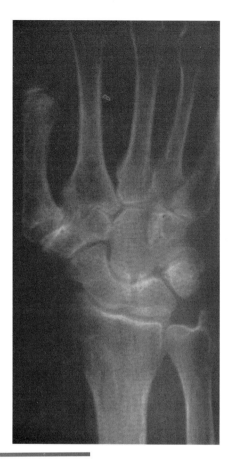

**FIGURE 12–29** ■ Degenerative osteoarthritis of the first car-pometacarpal joint. (Courtesy of Slippery Rock University School of Physical Therapy, Slippery Rock, PA.)

dense, according to Wolff's law. This whiter, denser localized area of bone is radiologically described as sclerotic.

The patient in Figure 12–32 was a 40-year-old male. Compare this mild degree of degenerative osteoarthritis with that shown in Figure 12–33, for an 80-year-old female with severe degenerative arthritis of the medial knee joint. Note the loss of joint space and sclerotic subchondral bone. Also note the valgus deformity of the knee joint resulting from loss of joint congruity and medial ligamentous laxity. These changes occur progressively over years and are synchronous with the loss of articular cartilage. Periarticular swelling of the soft tissues is evident over the medial joint area. Loss of knee function, decreased ability to walk, and increased joint pain made this patient an appropriate candidate for a total knee arthroplasty. Figures 12–34 and 12–35 are postoperative films of the same patient after joint replacement.

infection, microtrauma from occupational or athletic stresses, or maladaptive congruity of joints secondary to ligamentous laxity or congenital deformities. Many other conditions can contribute to degenerative joint disease. Post-traumatic arthritis is a term commonly used to describe the osteoarthritis that develops after fracture. The fracture may have been intra-articular, extending to the articular joint surface. A fracture may also have resulted in malunion deformity, altering joint congruity and normal joint mechanics.

The medial joint surface of the knee in Figure 12–32 illustrates degenerative osteoarthritis. Note the decreased joint space of the medial side compared to the lateral side of the joint. This indicates that articular cartilage has been abnormally worn thin on the medial side of the joint. The white reactive subchondral bone of the medial tibial plateau has responded to the thinning of the articular cartilage and has become more

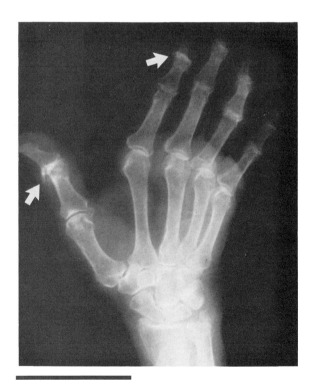

**FIGURE 12–30** ■ Degenerative changes at all distal interphalangeal joints. Osteophytes, decreased joint spaces, and sclerotic articulating surfaces are present. Herberden's nodes (arrows) are more obvious on clinical examination on the dorsum of the joints. Note also a fracture at the base of the fourth phalanx. (Courtesy of Slippery Rock University School of Physical Therapy, Slippery Rock, PA.)

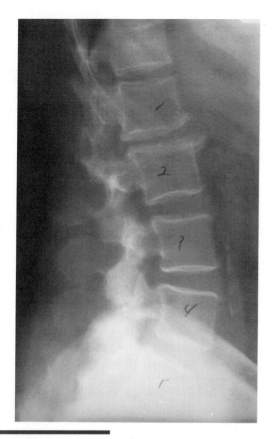

**FIGURE 12–31** ■ Osteophytic spur development at sites of attachment of the anterior longitudinal ligament. These spurs are theorized to be traction spurs related to the pull of the ligament. (Courtesy of Slippery Rock University School of Physical Therapy, Slippery Rock, PA.)

## Gouty Arthritis

Gout is a hereditary metabolic abnormality characterized by an elevated serum uric acid level. Gouty arthritis is a clinical manifestation of the disease presenting as monoarticular pain and inflammation. This disease affects men predominantly and occurs most often at the first metatarsophalangeal joint and other small joints of the feet and hands. Attacks of gouty arthritis are intermittent and are precipitated by sudden deposition of sodium monourate crystals in the synovial membrane. The body attempts to phagocytose the crystals, and lysosomal enzymes are released as by-products of this process. These enzymes are responsible for the local inflammatory process. Early attacks of gouty arthritis are often completely resolved and the joint returns to normal. Successive attacks can cause chronic

degenerative joint changes with deformities. Tophi are nodule deposits of urate crystals that form within or outside the joint. Erosions of bone near the joint can be seen as radiolucent lesions representing areas of urate deposits. Figure 12–36 is a classic example of the degenerative changes of gouty arthritis at the first metatarsophalangeal joint.

## Rheumatoid Arthritis

Rheumatoid arthritis is a progressive connective tissue disease estimated to affect almost 3% of populations in countries with a temperate climate. Women are affected three times more frequently than men, and onset is most common in young adulthood.

Early stages of the disease are characterized by exacerbations and remissions of synovial membrane inflammation. The smaller joints of the hands and feet, primarily the proximal interphalangeal joints, usually exhibit symptoms first. Repeated joint capsule distention promotes laxity of supporting structures and contributes to subse-

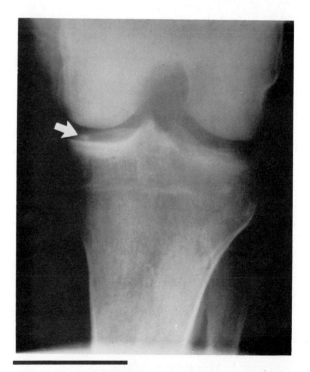

**FIGURE 12–32** ■ Mild degenerative changes at the medial knee joint: slightly decreased joint space, sclerosis of medial tibial plateau, and loose body (arrows) within the medial joint. (Courtesy of Slippery Rock University School of Physical Therapy, Slippery Rock, PA.)

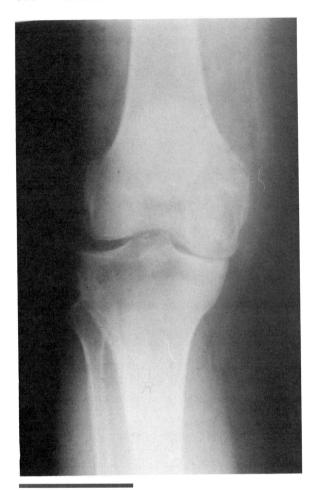

FIGURE 12-33 ■ Advanced degenerative osteoarthritis at the medial knee joint with associated valgus deformity and soft tissue swelling. This film was taken before a total joint replacement. (Courtesy of Tri-State Orthopaedics, Ltd., Pittsburgh, PA.)

teolytic bone areas. Rarefaction, or localized demineralization, gradually becomes evident. Articular cartilage spaces progressively decrease. Later, joint subluxations and dislocations are seen, most commonly at the hands and feet. Bony ankyloses at the wrists and ankles are manifestations of advanced rheumatoid arthritis. Figures 12–37 and 12–38 illustrate early soft tissue changes and the later progressively deforming characteristics of rheumatoid arthritis.

## Avascular Necrosis

Avascular necrosis is also referred to as ischemic necrosis or aseptic necrosis. This pathologic condition is characterized by interruption of circulation to bone, subsequent bone death, and eventual bone growth and replacement of dead bone.

Avascular necrosis appears idiopathically in many epiphyseal disorders of children. Legg-Calvé-Perthes disease, Köhler's disease, and Freiberg's disease are eponyms for avascular necrosis of the femoral head, tarsal navicular bone, and metatarsal head, respectively. Idiopathic avascu-

quent joint subluxations and dislocations. Later stages of the disease are characterized by formation of granulation tissue into a pannus that covers and erodes articular cartilage. In response, reparative fibrous scars form and lead to joint contractures and deformities. Eventually, fibrous and bony ankylosis within the joint causes further disability. Flexion contractures are common because the patient usually rests the swollen joints in this position of maximum capsular volume. Muscle contractures also result from fibrosis within muscle tissue. Ruptured tendons further contribute to progressive deformities.

Radiographs show periarticular swelling and joint capsule distention in the early stages of the disease. Radiolucent cysts may eventually be seen at the subchondral bone, representing os-

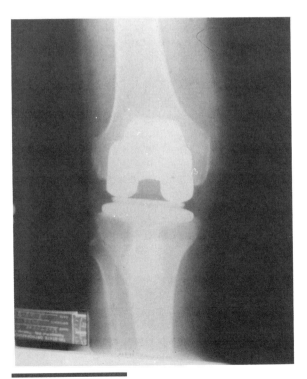

FIGURE 12-34 ■ Postoperative AP projection of total joint replacement. (Courtesy of Tri-State Orthopaedics, Ltd., Pittsburgh, PA.)

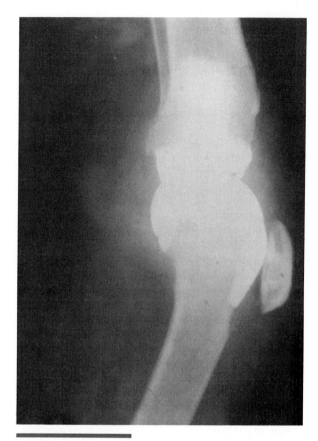

**FIGURE 12-35** ■ Lateral projection of total joint replacement. (Courtesy of Tri-State Orthopaedics, Ltd., Pittsburgh, PA.)

lar necrosis also appears in young adults at the carpals. Kienböck's disease and Preiser's disease refer to necrotic changes of the lunate and scaphoid bones, respectively. The entire course of the disease, from initial avascularity through revascularization, bone growth, and remodeling, may take several years if not arrested at any stage. The remodeling attempts are often compromised and residual deformity is common.

Post-traumatic avascular necrosis results from interruption of blood supply to bone after injury, fracture, or dislocation. The disruption of circulation may have been caused by direct tearing of vessels or sustained compression of the vessels. In adults, the femoral neck fractures may be complicated by associated tearing of retinacular vessels. The proximal pole of the scaphoid bone is susceptible to necrosis after fracture.

Alcoholism, prolonged steroid use, sickle-cell disease, systemic lupus erythematosus, and renal disorders are examples of pre-existing conditions that favor the development of avascular necrosis.

Radiologic evidence varies depending on the stage of the disease. Regions of early avascular necrosis and bone death may appear normal on plain films. Weight-bearing bones, such as the femoral head, may collapse in later stages, and loss of bone contour and joint congruity is then evident radiographically (Fig. 12–39). At end stages of the disease, areas of new bone growth and repair appear sclerotic in images. Deformity may be present.

## FORCES THAT FORM FRACTURES

Most musculoskeletal injuries occur in predictable patterns determined by a structure's inherent properties and the characteristics of the external forces. Fractures, likewise, occur in predictable patterns determined by the viscoelastic properties of bone and the biomechanics of load.

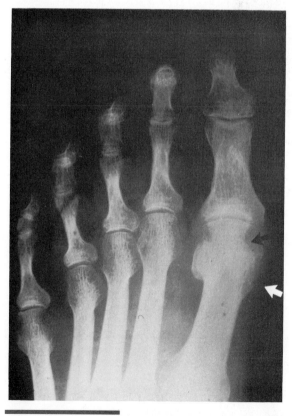

**FIGURE 12-36** ■ Dorsoplantar projection demonstrating soft tissue swelling (white arrow) at the first metatarsophalangeal joint and erosion of adjacent bone margins (black arrow). These changes characterize the later stages of gouty arthritis. (Reprinted from the Clinical Slide Collection on the Rheumatic Diseases, copyright 1991. Used by permission of the American College of Rheumatology)

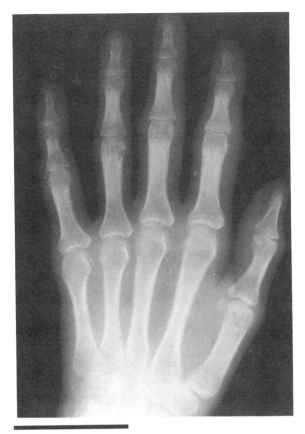

FIGURE 12-37 ■ Characteristics of early stage of rheumatoid arthritis. Note soft tissue swelling of the proximal interphalangeal and metacarpophalangeal joints and thinning of the radial cortices of the metacarpal heads. Osteopenia is present in cancellous bone, primarily periarticularly. These are pre-erosive changes common in rheumatoid arthritis. (Reprinted from the Clinical Slide Collection on the Rheumatic Diseases, copyright 1991. Used by permission of the American College of Rheumatology.)

Load is defined as an application of force. Bone can be loaded by the forces of tension, compression, bending, and torsion. Gozna and Harrington describe five basic patterns of injury resulting from these forces or combinations of them.[3] These patterns are diaphyseal impaction, transverse fracture, oblique-transverse (or butterfly) fracture, spiral fracture, and oblique fracture. These fractures and their corresponding precipitating loads are summarized in Figure 12-40.

Note that tension is absent as a causative force load in the five basic bone injury patterns. Bone withstands pure tension forces quite well. Joints and ligaments are most vulnerable to tension forces, and injury occurs in these structures primarily as sprains or degrees of tearing. Tension forces may also cause an avulsion fracture, or a disruption of bone at the site of ligamentous or musculotendinous attachment. Figures 12-41 and 12-42 show examples of avulsion fractures at the patella and the ulnar styloid.

External forces may render a fracture displaced or undisplaced. Displaced fragments may be overriding one another, lateral to each other, extremely distracted from one another, angulated, or rotated out of alignment (Fig. 12-43). Displaced fractures may be open fractures with a fragment breaking through the skin, which exposes the fracture site to the external environment and increases the risk of infection. Closed fractures denote intact skin (Fig. 12-44).

Occult fractures are so named because they are subtle, hidden fractures, not readily detectable on plain films, especially in areas of irregular bone shape. Areas of irregular bone shape often sus-

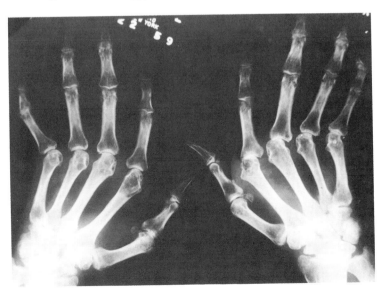

FIGURE 12-38 ■ Characteristics of advanced rheumatoid arthritis. The metacarpophalangeal joints demonstrate marked narrowing with subluxation and ulnar deviation. Demineralization is present in periarticular areas adjacent to the metacarpal and proximal interphalangeal joints. The ulnar styloid processes and carpal bones also reveal erosions. (Reprinted from the Clinical Slide Collection on the Rheumatic Diseases, copyright 1991. Used by permission of the American College of Rheumatology.)

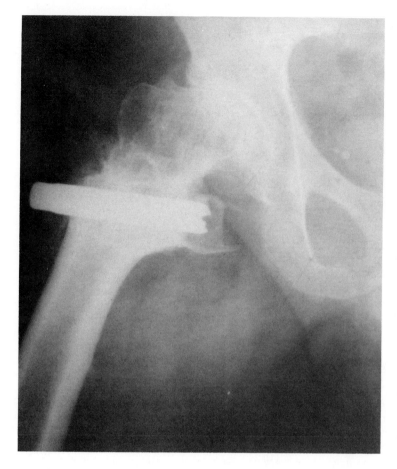

**FIGURE 12-39** ■ This patient originally sustained a femoral neck fracture and underwent open reduction and internal fixation with hip nailing. The patient subsequently developed avascular necrosis of the femoral head. Over time, the femoral head collapsed and joint congruity was lost. Ambulation became increasingly painful and the patient elected to have a total joint replacement. (Courtesy of Tri-State Orthopaedics, Ltd., Pittsburgh, PA.)

tain fractures secondary to compressive forces, and further diagnostic studies are done to define the limits of the fracture.

## FRACTURE HEALING

After a fracture has occurred, repair cells from the periosteum and endosteum proliferate and form a callus. Radiodense lines may be seen bridging the fracture gap. After a few weeks, the callus unites the fracture site, which is termed clinical union. At this point there is no movement at the fracture site but the repair lacks normal strength. (Some bone fragments, if perfectly aligned, forgo callus formation, and trabecular bone patterns are seen crossing the fracture site. This is called primary bone union.) As the callus is gradually resorbed, trabecular patterns appear across the fracture site, a stage called early union. Established union is the next stage of healing, evidenced by appearance of cortical structure and remodeling changes. Remodeling continues as trabeculae are organized along lines of stress according to Wolff's law. Fibrous union denotes a clinically stable, pain-free fracture site without any radiologic evidence of the fracture line remaining. The time frame of these stages depends on the age of the patient, site and configuration of the fracture, blood supply to the fragments, and amount of displacement of the fragments. Figures 12–45, 12–46, and 12–47 illustrate the stages of successful fracture healing.

## Complications

Failure of bone fragments to unite is termed nonunion. Unwanted movement at a healing fracture site is the most common cause of nonunion. Autogenous bone grafting may be a solution.

Healing of a fracture, but with significant deformity, is termed malunion. If the degree of deformity is enough to cause marked cosmetic problems, loss of function, or potential for de-

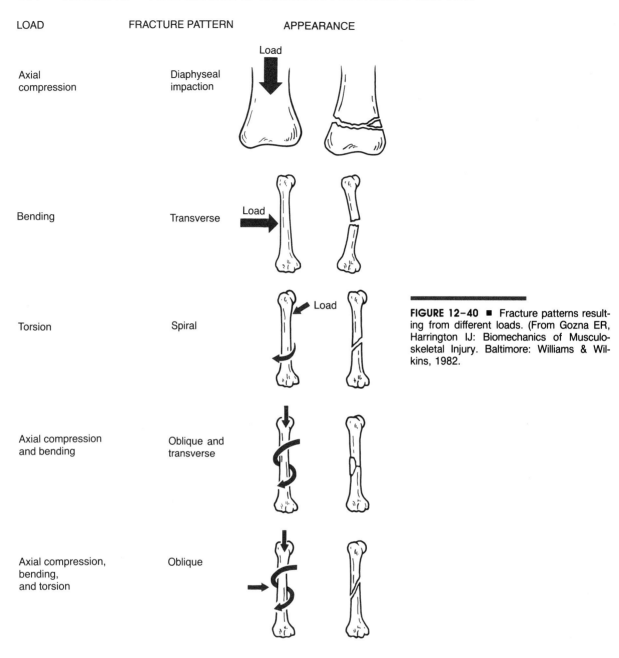

| LOAD | FRACTURE PATTERN | APPEARANCE |
|------|------------------|------------|
| Axial compression | Diaphyseal impaction | |
| Bending | Transverse | |
| Torsion | Spiral | |
| Axial compression and bending | Oblique and transverse | |
| Axial compression, bending, and torsion | Oblique | |

**FIGURE 12-40** ■ Fracture patterns resulting from different loads. (From Gozna ER, Harrington IJ: Biomechanics of Musculoskeletal Injury. Baltimore: Williams & Wilkins, 1982.

generative joint disease, corrective surgery is warranted. Delayed union describes healing at a fracture site that progresses much too slowly compared to norms. The solution is often patience, but occasionally autogenous bone grafting is necessary.

Post-traumatic osteoarthritis describes osteoarthritis that is accelerated after intra-articular fracture or as a result of malunion deformities that alter joint mechanics. It was discussed in more detail earlier.

## FRACTURE CLASSIFICATION

In the early 1980s, the Orthopedic Trauma Association and the American Academy of Orthopedic Surgeons devised a system of fracture classification. Their goal was to unify the descriptive language used for fracture configurations to adapt to computer technology and an international data base. The result was a Trauma Registry consisting of a coding system for all

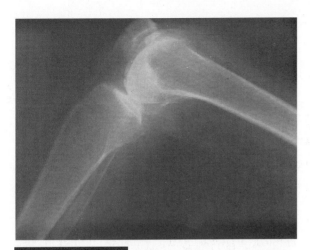

**FIGURE 12–41** ■ Avulsion fracture through the midpole of the patella. (Courtesy of Slippery Rock University School of Physical Therapy, Slippery Rock, PA.)

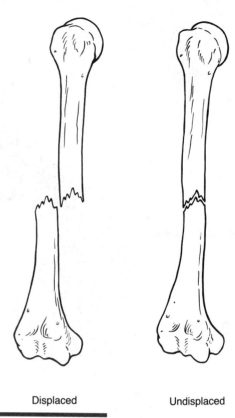

Displaced                    Undisplaced

**FIGURE 12–43** ■ Displaced and undisplaced fractures.

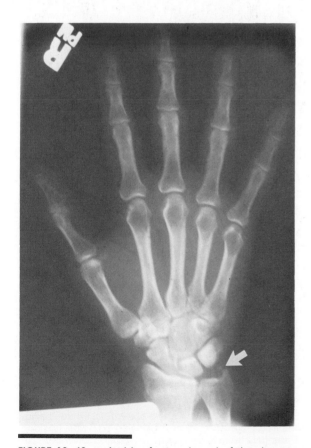

**FIGURE 12–42** ■ Avulsion fracture (arrow) of the ulnar styloid. (Courtesy of Slippery Rock University School of Physical Therapy, Slippery Rock, PA.)

fractures and complications. *The Fracture Classification Manual,* by Gustilo, provides an outline of the basic concepts of this standardized fracture classification system.[4]

Bones are broadly classified as long bones or flat bones. Long bones include the humerus, phalanges, and tibia. Flat bones include the scapula, vertebrae, and carpals.

Long bones are divided into

1. The intra-articular portion
2. The extra-articular portion consisting of
   a. Proximal end metaphysis and neck
   b. Distal end metaphyseal portion
   c. Shaft divided into proximal, middle, and distal thirds

Flat bones are divided into

1. The articular portion
2. The body or extra-articular portion (Fig. 12–48)

Fracture configuration is categorized based on shaft fractures or articular fractures.

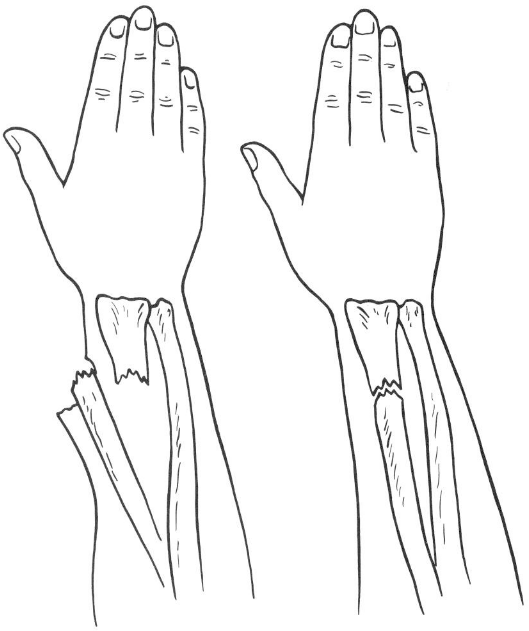

Open          Closed

**FIGURE 12–44** ■ Older terminology referred to simple fracture and compound fracture. Closed and open are the preferred terms currently.

Shaft fractures may be one of four types, each with its subtypes:

1. Linear
   a. Transverse
   b. Oblique
   c. Spiral
2. Comminuted
   a. Butterfly fragments less than 50% of shaft diameter
   b. Butterfly fragments 50% or more of shaft diameter
   c. Comminuted less than 50% of shaft diameter
   d. Comminuted 50% or more of shaft diameter
3. Segmental
   a. Two levels
   b. Three or more levels
   c. Intramedullary fragment split
   d. Intramedullary fragment comminuted
4. Bone Loss
   a. Less than 50% of shaft diameter
   b. More than 50% of shaft diameter
   c. Segmental loss (Fig. 12–49)

Articular fractures may be one of four types:

1. Linear
2. Comminuted
3. Impacted
4. Bone loss (Fig. 12–50)

The traditional naming of fractures after the activity that caused the fracture, or after the physician who first documented the fracture pattern, predates the discovery of x-rays in 1895. Common usage of these familiar fracture names through the decades has firmly entrenched them among health professionals and laypeople. "Baseball" finger, Colles' fracture, "Little League" elbow, and "greenstick" fracture are examples of well-known fracture terms in use today. The radiologist, however, avoids using common but inexact language in the appraisal of radiographs. Fracture patterns are described in anatomic, directional, and standardized terms.

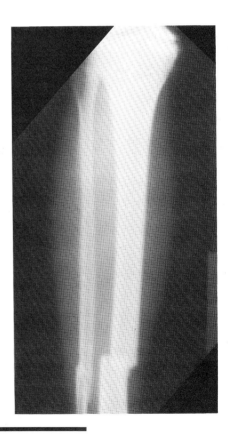

**FIGURE 12–45** ■ Shaft fracture of the distal third of the fibia and fibula sustained by a 10-year-old boy while sledding. These films taken in the emergency room demonstrated complete transverse fractures with overriding of fracture fragments. (Courtesy of Tri-Rivers Surgical Associates, Inc., Pittsburgh, PA.)

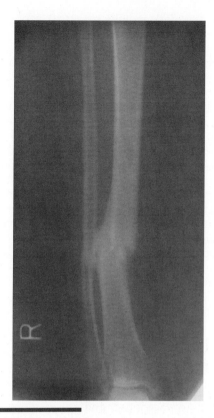

**FIGURE 12–46** ■ In the patient in Figure 12–45, good callus formation is noted at both fracture sites 4 months after injury. (Courtesy of Tri-Rivers Surgical Associates, Inc., Pittsburgh, PA.)

Some well-founded, well-documented, older systems of fracture classification have been incorporated in the Trauma Registry. For example, the Salter-Harris classification of epiphyseal plate injuries should be understood by physical therapists.

## SALTER-HARRIS CLASSIFICATION

This classification of children's epiphyseal fractures is widely known and accepted. In the growing child, epiphyseal plates are structurally weaker than surrounding bone, capsule, muscles, ligaments, and tendons. Thus, an ankle sprain that might stretch or tear a collateral ligament in an adult can damage the epiphyseal plate in a child. A disrupted epiphyseal plate may lead to early fusion of the epiphysis and result in deformity or a short leg. Salter and Harris[2] outlined the possible types of epiphyseal plate injuries and described prognosis and treatment of each

type (Fig. 12–51). The film in Figure 12–52 is an example of the most common type of epiphyseal plate injury—Salter-Harris type II. This injury involves separation of the epiphyseal plate of the distal tibia with a large triangular metaphyseal fragment. Treatment is usually by closed reduction and the prognosis is good.

The thick periosteum of bones in children is loosely attached to the shafts and is rarely torn completely across during fracture. The intact periosteum helps in maintaining reduction of the underlying fractured cortex and accelerates fracture healing. Constant remodeling of growing bone also acts via Wolff's law on moderate deformity after fracture, and subsequent bone growth often leaves no trace of the earlier deformity. Adult periosteum, in contrast, is thin and firmly attached to bone. Fractures often tear and separate the periosteum, rendering bone union less certain. This periosteal interruption makes

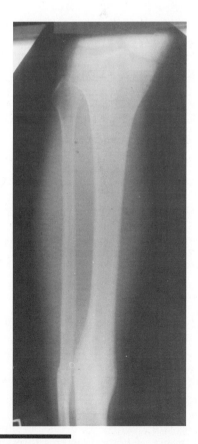

**FIGURE 12–47** ■ In the patient in Figure 12–45, successful fracture healing with remodeling is demonstrated 10 months after injury. (Courtesy of Tri-Rivers Surgical Associates, Inc., Pittsburgh, PA.)

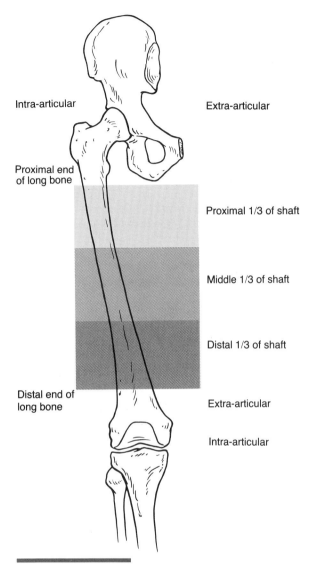

Intra-articular

Extra-articular

Proximal end
of long bone

Proximal 1/3 of shaft

Middle 1/3 of shaft

Distal 1/3 of shaft

Distal end of
long bone

Extra-articular

Intra-articular

**FIGURE 12–48** ■ Shaft division. (From Gustilo RB: The Fracture Classification Manual. St. Louis: Mosby-Year Book, 1991.)

adult fractures slower to heal than the fractures of childhood.

## RECOGNIZING FRACTURES ON RADIOGRAPHS

Fractures are defined as breaks in the structural continuity of bone. Fractures through cortical bone are seen on film as disruptions in the smooth margins of the cortex. Associated hemorrhage and soft tissue swelling may increase the gap between fracture fragments. This gap is imaged as a dark radiolucent streak representing the extent of the fracture (Fig. 12–53).

It is necessary to distinguish between the radiolucent streaks characteristic of both cartilaginous epiphyseal growth plates and fractures. The radiolucent spaces of growth plates show smoothly curved cortical margins, in contrast to the abrupt discontinuity of cortical bone fracture. The epiphyseal plate is also bounded by a smooth radiodense line representing the increased bone activity related to growth (Fig. 12–54).

Fractures of spongy bone may be impacted. In this instance, trabeculae become enmeshed and override adjacent trabeculae. Impaction fractures are imaged as areas of increased bone density and appear as whiter patches of bone (Fig. 12–55).

Avulsion fractures should be looked for in areas of musculotendinous or ligamentous attachment (Fig. 12–56).

## VIEWING RADIOGRAPHS

The radiographs in this section show some fractures, dislocations, and disease processes common to the patients treated by physical therapists. Normal radiographs are presented for comparison. This selection is by no means comprehensive but should provide a foundation for viewing the films of patients.

### Radiographs of the Spine

Figure 12–57 is a normal film of the pelvis and hips. Bone architecture varies from individual to individual. Anomalies, or deviations from the usual, occur with some frequency. "Normal" is used in a general context to denote absence of pathology, deformity, fracture, or dislocation. Note that Figures 12–58 and 12–59 are also normal images of the pelvis and hips but appear quite different from Figure 12–57.

Figure 12–58 illustrates a transitional lumbar vertebra. The fifth lumbar vertebra articulates through its transverse processes directly with the sacrum. This anomaly is not pathologic, and its presence was an incidental finding. Patients may need to be reassured of this. A unilateral articulation may, however, promote asymmetric and possibly maladaptive biomechanics throughout the proximal and distal kinetic chain.

Figure 12–59 is a film of an elderly patient.

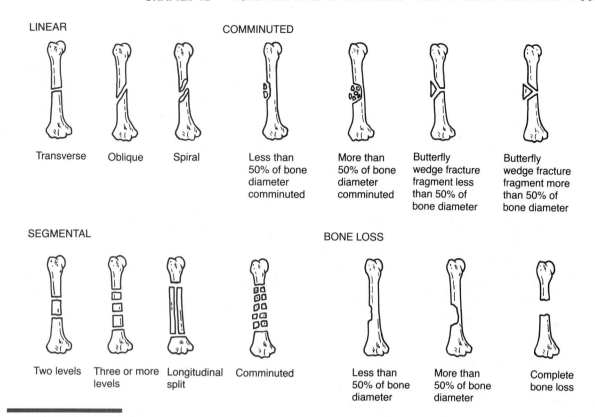

**FIGURE 12–49** ■ Classification of long bone fractures. (From Gustilo RB: The Fracture Classification Manual. St. Louis: Mosby-Year Book, 1991.)

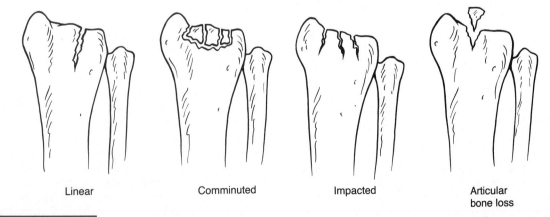

**FIGURE 12–50** ■ Classification of intra-articular fractures. (From Gustilo RB: The Fracture Classification Manual. St. Louis: Mosby-Year Book, 1991.)

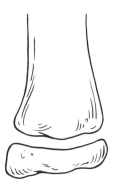

Type I
Separation of
epiphyseal plate

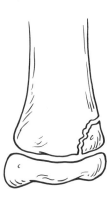

Type II
Separation of
epiphyseal plate
plus metaphyseal
wedge fracture

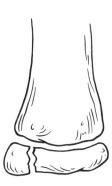

Type III
Separation of
epiphyseal plate
plus epiphyseal
wedge fracture

**FIGURE 12–51** ■ Salter-Harris classification of epiphyseal plate injuries.

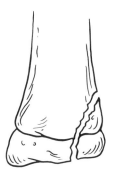

Type IV
Metaphyseal and
epiphyseal
fracture fragment

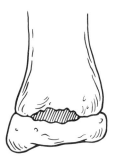

Type V
Impaction fracture
of epiphyseal plate
and adjacent surfaces

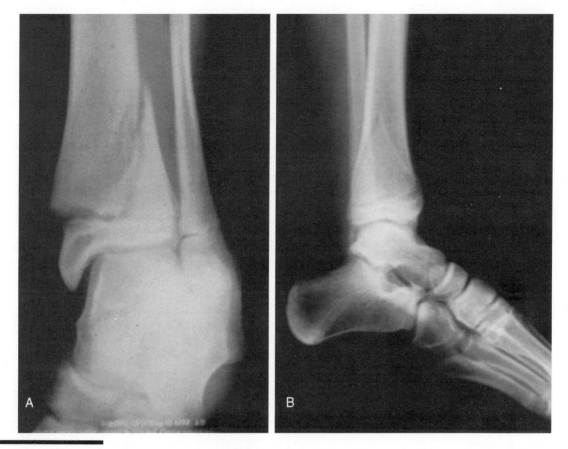

**FIGURE 12–52** ■ (A) AP projection of Salter-Harris type II epiphyseal plate injury. Note triangular metaphyseal fragment and separation of tibial epiphyseal plate. (B) Lateral projection of Salter-Harris type II injury. The metaphyseal fragment is not seen to be displaced when viewed from this angle. Compare this view to the radiograph in (A). It is necessary to view at least two projections at right angles to each other when evaluating the musculoskeletal system. (Courtesy of Slippery Rock University School of Physical Therapy, Slippery Rock, PA.)

The bilateral sacroiliac joints have narrowed with age.

Figure 12–60 is an oblique film of the lumbar spine. This projection provides the best view of the lumbar facet joints. The appearance of a "Scotty dog" outline indicates that the facet joints have been well demonstrated. Right and left oblique films are obtained to view both right and left facet joints. The obliques may be projected from an AP or PA direction. Note a fracture of the pars articularis at L-5.

Figure 12–61 is a lateral view of the lumbosacral joint, demonstrating a decreased joint space at L-5 to S-1 compared to L4-5.

Figure 12–62 demonstrates rib articulations of the thoracic spine. The first three lumbar vertebrae are differentiated from the lower thoracic vertebrae because they lack rib articulations.

Figure 12–63 is a typical chest x-ray film with a radiopaque metal object located at the upper spine. Without a lateral view of this patient, there would be no way to know where this metal object is located in the anatomy. This might be a bullet lodged in the sternum, the trachea, or the spinal cord. Fortunately, this object was a medallion on a necklace resting harmlessly on the skin.

Figure 12–64 is a lateral projection of the cervical spine. This angle is best for viewing cervical facet joint articulations. Intervertebral joint spaces, or disc spaces, are also well defined. Although disc spaces appear normal in this film, there is marked narrowing of facet joint spaces at all levels. Facet joint margins are clearly sclerosed. These findings represent degenerative osteoarthritis of the cervical spine.

Figure 12–65 is a cervical film representative of cervical spondylosis, the formation of osteo-

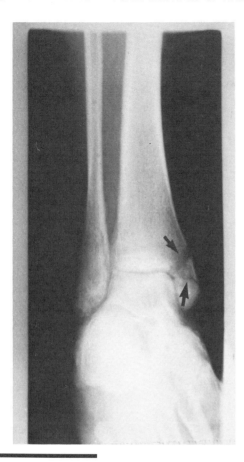

FIGURE 12-53 ■ Butterfly fracture fragment (arrows) at the medial malleoli of the tibia. (Courtesy of Slippery Rock University School of Physical Therapy, Slippery Rock, PA.)

to become a source of compression of the neurovascular bundle as it crosses the thoracic outlet.

Figure 12–68 demonstrates the relationship between the first and second cervical vertebrae. This AP projection is made through the patient's wide-open mouth. This view is standard after cervical sprain to rule out fracture or ligamentous disruption of these segments.

Figure 12–69 is a film of a 14-year-old girl with idiopathic scoliosis. Scoliosis is a rotational deformity of the spine and ribs. The curves that result are measured on radiographs most commonly by the Cobb method. Horizontal lines are drawn at the superior border of the superior end vertebrae and at the inferior border of the inferior end vertebrae. Perpendicular lines are then drawn through these horizontal lines and the re-

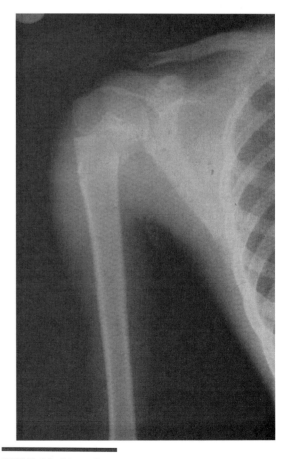

FIGURE 12-54 ■ Greenstick fracture. Note the epiphyseal plates at the humeral head and distal humeral condyles. There is an incomplete transverse fracture at the humeral neck. Compare the radiolucent lines defining the epiphyseal plate to the radiolucent line of the fracture. (Courtesy of Slippery Rock University School of Physical Therapy, Slippery Rock, PA.)

phytes in response to degenerative disc disease. This lateral projection demonstrates narrowing of the disc space at C5-6 with osteophytes arising from both the anterior and posterior vertebral bodies.

Figure 12–66 is an oblique projection of a cervical spine with spondylosis. Encroachment on the intervertebral foramina is best viewed in this projection. Osteophytes from the posterior vertebral bodies have protruded into the intervertebral foramina at multiple levels. This can cause nerve root irritation or compression resulting in radicular symptoms. This patient also has degenerative disc disease at C5-6 and C6-7.

Figure 12–67 demonstrates another kind of anomaly. Vestiges of ribs project from the transverse processes of C-7. The rib on the right side is larger and has formed an articulation with the angle of the first thoracic rib. This condition in itself is not pathologic. It does have the potential

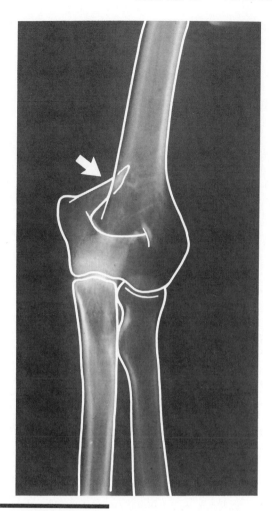

**FIGURE 12–55** ■ The fragments of this supracondylar humeral fracture are partly impacted (arrow), producing an area of increased density. (Courtesy of Slippery Rock University School of Physical Therapy, Slippery Rock, PA.)

sulting intersecting angle is measured. This patient is noted to have a 25-degree curve. The amount of vertebral rotation is measured by the distance the radiographic image of the pedicle has rotated toward midline. It is reported as increasing plus numbers as in 1+, 2+, 3+, or 4+ rotation.

## Radiographs of the Lower Extremity

Figures 12–70, 12–71, and 12–72 demonstrate three types of fractures common at the hip. Figure 12–70 is a film of an intertrochanteric fracture repaired with a side plate and compres-

sion screws. This fracture is common to osteoporotic, elderly females. Figure 12–71 demonstrates an impaction fracture of the inferior femoral head and the inferior acetabular rim. The fracture is difficult to see, and comparison with the contralateral hip is helpful. This fracture occurs commonly in automobile accidents when the knee strikes the dashboard and the femur is driven into the acetabulum. The mechanism of the fracture in Figure 12–72 is the same, although in this case only the posterior acetabular rim has fractured. The acetabulum was repaired with two compression screws.

Figure 12–73 demonstrates changes in the femoral head caused by avascular necrosis. Note

*Text continued on page 668.*

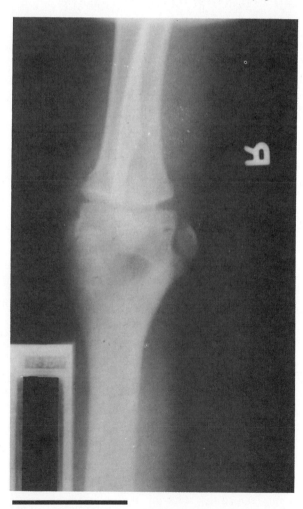

**FIGURE 12–56** ■ Avulsion fracture at the medial epicondyle of the humerus secondary to forceful contraction of the flexor muscle group of the forearm. This fracture has earned the nickname "Little League" elbow. The patient was a 12-year-old boy injured pitching baseball. (Courtesy of North Hills Passavant Hospital, Pittsburgh, PA.)

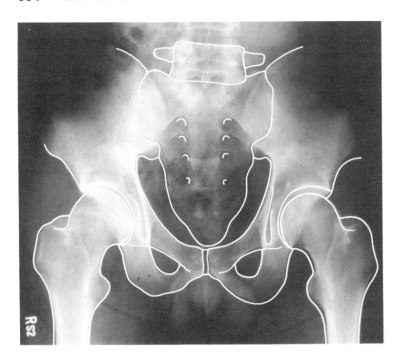

**FIGURE 12-57** ■ Normal radiograph of the pelvis and hips. Note the radiographic "teardrop." This normal image medial to the acetabulum comprises the cortical surfaces of the pubic bone and ischium, forming the anteroinferior aspect of the acetabular fossa. (Courtesy of Slippery Rock University School of Physical Therapy, Slippery Rock, PA.)

**FIGURE 12-58** ■ Transitional lumbar vertebrae. The transverse processes of the fifth lumbar vertebra have formed articulations with the sacrum and the iliac bones. (Courtesy of Slippery Rock University School of Physical Therapy, Slippery Rock, PA.)

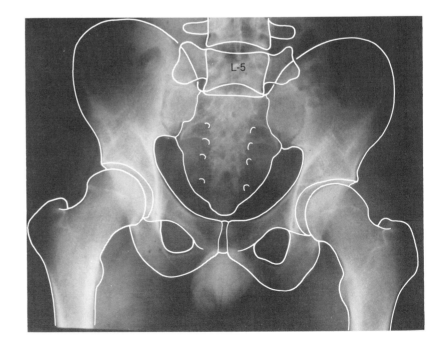

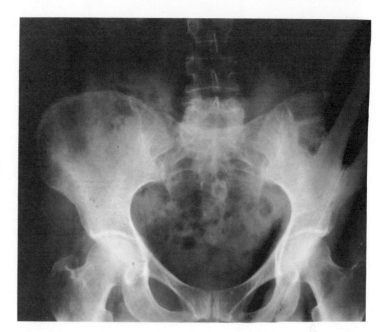

**FIGURE 12-59** ■ Normal pelvis in an elderly adult. (Courtesy of Slippery Rock University School of Physical Therapy, Slippery Rock, PA.)

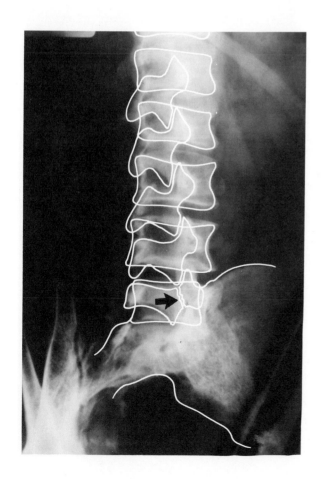

**FIGURE 12-60** ■ Note the "collar" of the Scotty dog at L-5 (arrow). The appearance of a collar indicates a fracture of the pars interarticularis. Although this defect can be demonstrated in approximately 10% of adults, its etiology remains unclear. It is theorized to be a developmental defect, a stress fracture caused by repetitive trauma, or a fracture from a single injury. The defect is called spondylolysis and occurs primarily at L-5. It may be unilateral or bilateral. (Courtesy of Slippery Rock University School of Physical Therapy, Slippery Rock, PA.)

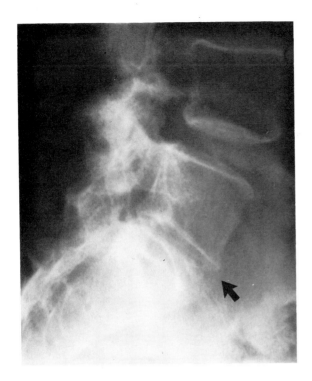

FIGURE 12-61 ■ Lateral projection of the lumbosacral joint demonstrating decreased joint space at L-5 to S-1 (arrow), indicative of a degenerative disc at that level. (Courtesy of Slippery Rock University School of Physical Therapy, Slippery Rock, PA.)

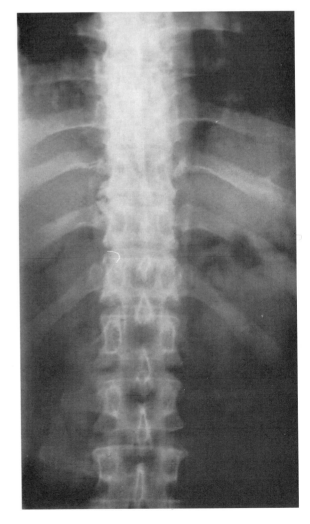

FIGURE 12-62 ■ AP projection of normal lower thoracic and lumbar spine. (Courtesy of Slippery Rock University School of Physical Therapy, Slippery Rock, PA.)

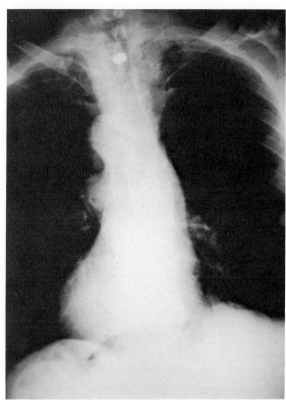

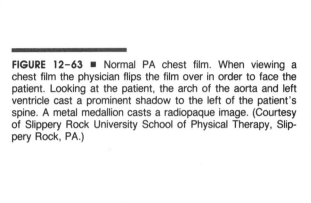

**FIGURE 12-63** ■ Normal PA chest film. When viewing a chest film the physician flips the film over in order to face the patient. Looking at the patient, the arch of the aorta and left ventricle cast a prominent shadow to the left of the patient's spine. A metal medallion casts a radiopaque image. (Courtesy of Slippery Rock University School of Physical Therapy, Slippery Rock, PA.)

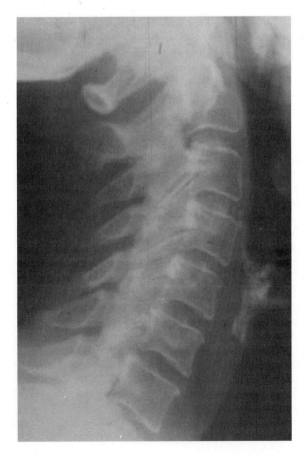

**FIGURE 12-64** ■ Degenerative osteoarthritis of the cervical spine. (Reprinted from the Clinical Slide Collection on the Rheumatic Diseases, copyright 1991. Used by permission of the American College of Rheumatology.)

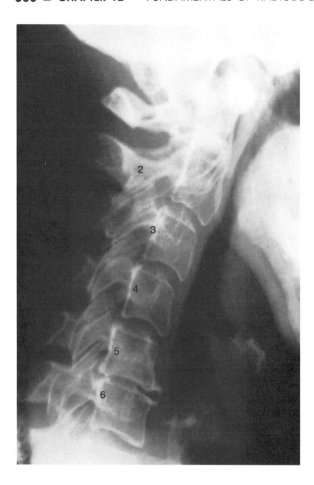

**FIGURE 12-65** ■ Cervical spondylosis. (Reprinted from the Clinical Slide Collection on the Rheumatic Diseases, copyright 1991. Used by permission of the American College of Rheumatology.)

the web-like pattern of sclerosis throughout the head that defines the reparative stage of the disease. Compare this film with the normal film of Figure 12–11. Also, compare the stage of avascular necrosis in Figure 12–73 with the later stage of this condition in Figure 12–39.

Figure 12–74 is a postoperative film of a total hip prosthesis. Total joints are indicated when loss of articular cartilage or loss of joint congruity causes severe pain and loss of function. This patient had suffered collapse of the femoral head as a result of avascular necrosis. The preoperative film was shown in Figure 12–39.

Figure 12–75 demonstrates severe rheumatoid arthritic changes at the hips. There is complete loss of articular cartilage, and the heads of femurs appear to be in direct contact with the acetabular roofs. This patient would experience severe pain, loss of motion, and impaired function. This patient is also a candidate for joint replacement.

Figure 12–76 is an AP projection of a normal knee. Figure 12–77 is a view of the patellofemoral joint referred to as a tangential patella. The purpose of this view is to visualize the articulating relationship of the patella to the femur, the surfaces of the femoral condyles, the articulating surfaces of the joint, and the soft tissues interposed at the joint. This film shows some mild sclerosis at the lateral joint surfaces.

Figure 12–78 is a lateral view of the knee in Figure 12–76. Note mild osteoarthritic changes at the articular surface of the patella. The tangential view helped define the more specific lateral location of the osteoarthritis.

Figures 12–79 and 12–80 show films of a bilateral shaft fracture of the lower leg at evaluation and after casting. A great deal of bone detail is lost when x-raying through a cast. This immediate postcasting film is made to verify good alignment of fracture fragments. Later x-ray studies that are done to assess progress in heal-

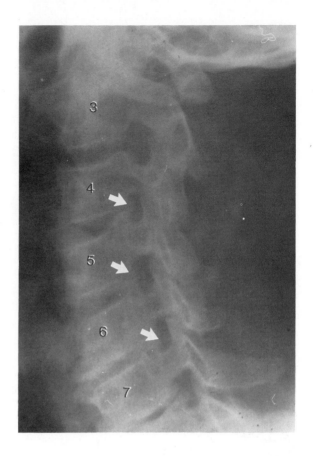

FIGURE 12-66 ■ Oblique projection of cervical spondylosis with foraminal encroachment (arrows). (Reprinted from the Clinical Slide Collection on the Rheumatic Diseases, copyright 1991. Used by permission of the American College of Rheumatology.)

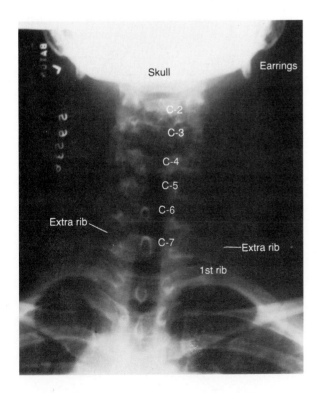

FIGURE 12-67 ■ Cervical rib present at C-7. (Courtesy of Slippery Rock University School of Physical Therapy, Slippery Rock, PA.)

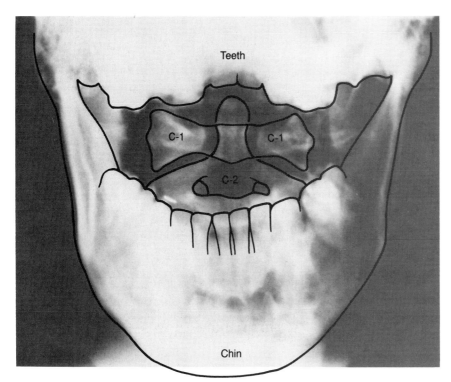

Teeth

C-1    C-1

C-2

Chin

**FIGURE 12-68** ■ Open mouth AP projection of C-1 and C-2. (Courtesy of Slippery Rock University School of Physical Therapy, Slippery Rock, PA.)

**FIGURE 12-69** ■ Right lumbar major curve scoliosis measured at 25 degrees. (Courtesy of Tri-Rivers Surgical Associates, Inc., Pittsburgh, PA.)

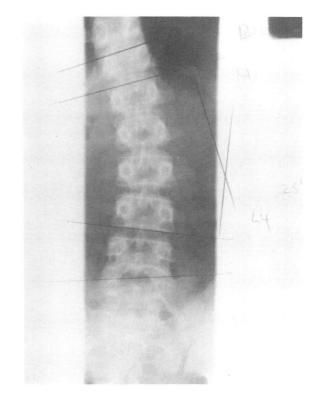

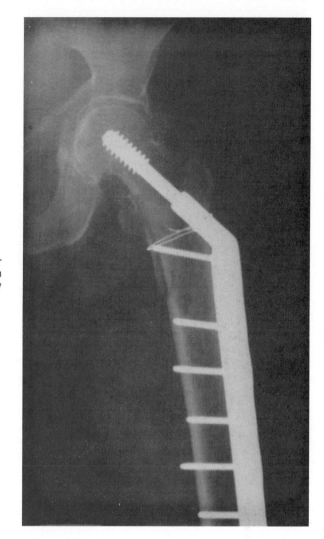

FIGURE 12-70 ■ Intertrochanteric fracture of the femur after open reduction and internal fixation with compression screws and side plate. (Courtesy of Slippery Rock University School of Physical Therapy, Slippery Rock, PA.)

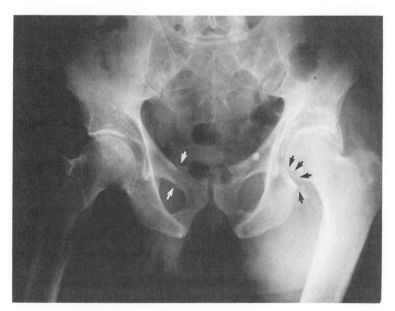

FIGURE 12-71 ■ Impaction fracture of the inferior femoral head and inferior acetabular rim. Black arrows point to the fracture area. Note the bone fragment at the inferior acetabular rim. There is a transverse fracture of the superior ramus of the pubis on the patient's right side (white arrows).

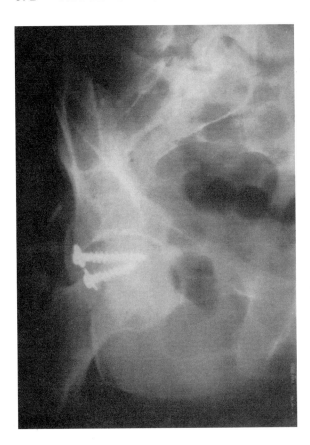

**FIGURE 12-72** ■ Posterior acetabular rim fracture fixated with compression screws.

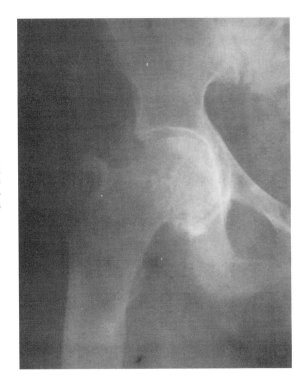

**FIGURE 12-73** ■ Avascular necrosis of the femoral head. Revascularization and healing have occurred, evidenced by a pattern of sclerosis extending from the articular surface to the femoral neck. The articular cartilage is thinned. Weight-bearing surfaces may eventually collapse. (Courtesy of North Hills Passavant Hospital, Pittsburgh, PA.)

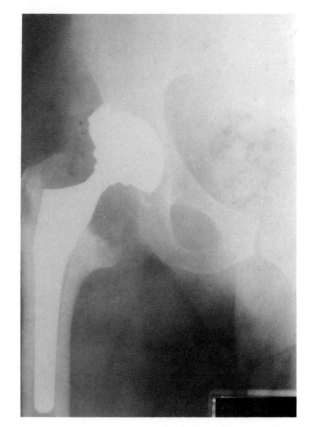

**FIGURE 12–74** ■ Total hip arthroplasty. This surgery was done to salvage the hip joint damaged by avascular necrosis seen in Figure 12–39. (Courtesy of Tri-State Orthopaedics, Ltd., Pittsburgh, PA.)

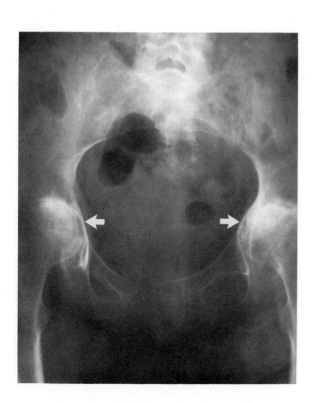

**FIGURE 12–75** ■ Rheumatoid arthritis of the hips. Note the loss of articular cartilage (arrows) and bone density changes periarticularly. Rheumatoid arthritis commonly affects joints bilaterally. (Courtesy of North Hills Passavant Hospital, Pittsburgh, PA.)

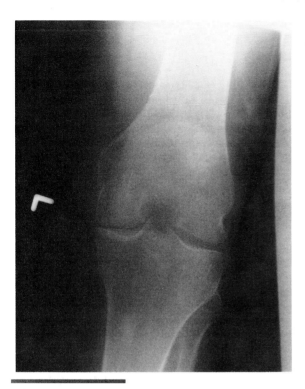

**FIGURE 12–76** ■ Normal radiographic appearance of the knee. (Courtesy of North Hills Passavant Hospital, Pittsburgh, PA.)

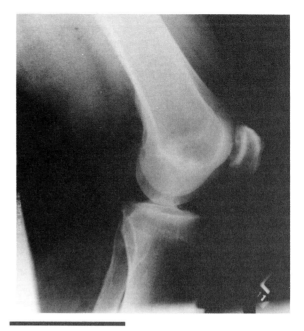

**FIGURE 12–78** ■ Lateral projection of patellofemoral and tibiofemoral joints. (Courtesy of Slippery Rock University School of Physical Therapy, Slippery Rock, PA.)

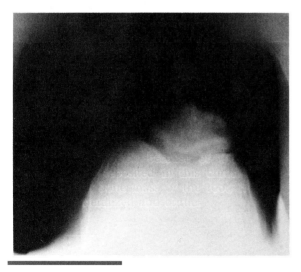

**FIGURE 12–77** ■ Tangential or "skyline" projection of the patellofemoral joint. This radiograph was made with the patient supine, the lower extremity flexed approximately 60 degrees at the hip and 110 degrees at the knee, and the foot flat on the table. The x-ray beam is projected through the knee in a caudal-cephalic direction. Looking at this left knee as the x-ray beam traveled puts the medial joint on our left and the lateral joint on our right. There are mild degenerative changes at the lateral patellofemoral joint. (Courtesy of Slippery Rock University School of Physical Therapy, Slippery Rock, PA.)

ing are usually done with the limb out of plaster, between cast changes.

Figure 12–81 is a dorsal view of the foot seen in Figure 12–23. This second projection, taken at a right angle to the first, reveals information not available on the lateral view alone. Note the subluxations and dislocations at the tarsometatarsal joints. Note also the amputation of the fifth metatarsal bone.

The necessity of viewing at least two right-angle radiographic projections when evaluating the musculoskeletal system should be well understood at this point.

## Radiographs of the Upper Extremity

Figure 12–82 shows a film of a traumatically dislocated glenohumeral joint. Most glenohumeral dislocations occur in an anterior direction as a result of forced external rotation combined with abduction and extension of the shoulder. An axillary projection is often obtained to define the exact relationship of the humeral head to the glenoid fossa in this condition. Recurrent dislocations are common, especially in athletes and physically active young adults. A radiologic finding in recurrent dislocations is a bone defect or

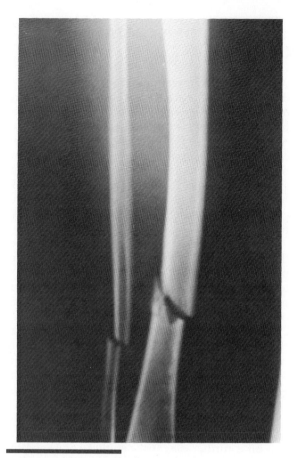

**FIGURE 12-79** ■ Bilateral shaft fracture of the lower leg. The fracture lines are described as oblique at the fibula and spiral with comminution at the tibia. (Courtesy of Slippery Rock University School of Physical Therapy, Slippery Rock, PA.)

verse fractures of the radial and ulnar shafts in AP and lateral views through cast material. The amount of displacement is more evident on the lateral view.

Figure 12–89 shows a distal radial fracture. The fracture extends intra-articularly. The radio-carpal joint is susceptible to post-traumatic osteoarthritis. Distal radial fractures are often combined with ulnar styloid fractures. The common name for this fracture pattern is a Colles fracture.

Figure 12–90 is called a navicular projection. The hand is positioned palm down on the film plate and deviated ulnarly. This produces a gap on the radial side of the wrist joint and provides the best view of the scaphoid (navicular) bone. The standard hand projection is PA, as is this navicular projection. This patient was being evaluated for a possible scaphoid fracture. The radiographic findings are normal.

Figure 12–91 shows a normal hand in a PA

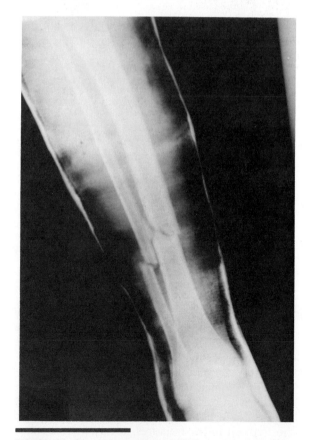

**FIGURE 12-80** ■ Postcasting radiograph done to confirm acceptable reduction of fracture fragments. Apposition of fracture fragments is necessary for successful fracture healing without residual deformity. (Courtesy of Slippery Rock University School of Physical Therapy, Slippery Rock, PA.)

"dent" of the posterolateral humeral head. This defect is actually a compression or impaction fracture sustained during each episode of dislocation when the humeral head strikes the glenoid rim. It is commonly called the Hill-Sachs lesion. It can be viewed radiographically if the humerus is rotated internally at least 60 degrees. Figure 12–83 shows a postoperative film of the relocated and repaired joint.

Figures 12–84, 12–85, and 12–86 show normal elbow joints of subjects in three different age groups. Figure 12–84 shows the elbow of a 5-year-old child. Note the size of the epiphysis and growth plates. Figure 12–85 shows the elbow of a 10-year-old child. Compare the developmental growth changes between these two children. Figure 12–86 is the elbow of a 30-year-old adult.

Figures 12–87 and 12–88 demonstrate trans-

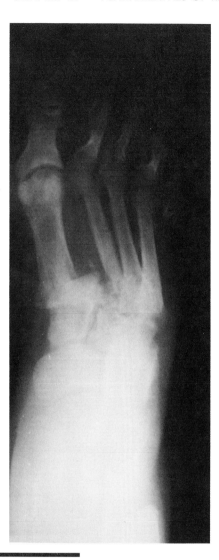

**FIGURE 12-81** ■ Foot of a patient with complications of diabetes. Note amputation of the fifth metatarsal and subluxations and dislocations of the first four metatarsals. (Courtesy of North Hills Passavant Hospital, Pittsburgh, PA.)

## LIMITATIONS OF PLAIN FILM RADIOGRAPHY

Plain film radiography, as stated, is generally the first-order diagnostic test in evaluation of the musculoskeletal system. Almost every patient the physical therapist evaluates has had a series of plain film studies before being referred to physical therapy. The goal of this chapter is to provide the physical therapist with a fundamental understanding of radiographic findings, which should become an integral part of the physical therapist's history taking, evaluation, and treatment plan.

Of equal importance is an understanding of the limitations of plain film radiography. Orthopaedic physical therapy commonly involves extensive evaluation and treatment of soft tissue pain and dysfunction. The patient with myositis ossificans of the biceps illustrated in Figure 12–28A and B is an example of a patient who experiences severe pain but presents with a series of normal films. Plain film radiography could not pick up the soft tissue calcification until several weeks after the process began. A thorough history and evaluation of this patient would lead a clinician to suspect hemorrhage within the muscle belly, and conservative measures might prevail until further diagnostic studies confirmed the condition in its early stages. Early soft tissue calcifications, whether located in muscle, bursae, or tendons, are not seen on plain films. Plain films also have limitations in detecting obscure or minute fractures. Early stages of tumor growth, metastatic disease, infection, and avascular necrosis are generally not detectable on plain films. Irritations of bursae or tendons, easily reproducible on clinical examination, are not readily detectable on plain films. Some ligamentous tears and ligamentous laxity are not detectable. Early spur formation may not be detectable.

The fact that a patient has confirmed normal films does not rule out fracture or pathology. The physical therapist should always obtain a thorough history and appropriate clinical evaluation. If the reported mechanism of injury raises suspicion of fracture or if the pain pattern is not congruous with what is expected in musculoskeletal dysfunction, the patient should be referred back to the physician for further diagnostic study or evaluation. The role of the physical therapist is not to make a differential diagnosis but to have the competence to recognize what evaluation findings fall outside the scope of physical

projection. Compare the clean lines of the bony cortices and well-preserved joint spaces with the older hand in Figure 12–92. Note the severe osteoarthritis of the first carpometacarpal joint.

Figures 12–93 and 12–94 demonstrate a fractured fifth metacarpal at evaluation and after reduction with casting. This fracture has commonly been called a boxer's fracture but is unrelated to the typical hand fractures of modern boxing. Rather, the mechanism of this injury is more likely a wild punch thrown in a street fight or at a wall.

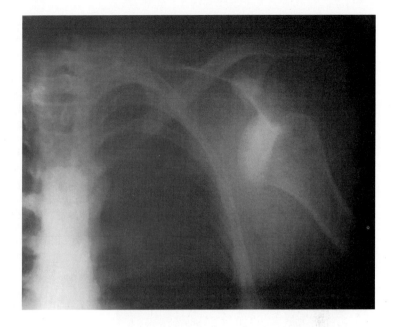

**FIGURE 12–82** ■ Traumatic and recurrent anterior glenohumeral dislocation in a 25-year-old man. (Courtesy of North Hills Passavant Hospital, Pittsburgh, PA.)

therapy treatment of musculoskeletal dysfunction.

## OVERVIEW OF COMMON IMAGING STUDIES

The clinical sciences involved in medical diagnostic studies vary widely in factors such as tissue-specific sensitivity, structural clarity and definition, radiation exposure, invasiveness, risk, and cost. As progress in medical technology con-

tinues, determination of the best diagnostic study for an individual patient is increasingly complex. Physicians from different disciplines of medicine turn to the radiologist as the imaging specialist for assistance in planning efficient and comprehensive diagnostic investigation.

Determining the best choice or choices of diagnostic study does not always unveil the whole truth. If the results of any diagnostic study do not fit the clinical findings, further clinical and diagnostic investigation is warranted. No matter how sophisticated technology be-

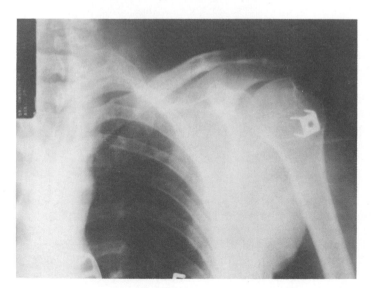

**FIGURE 12–83** ■ Chronically anteriorly dislocating glenohumeral joint after reduction and internal fixation. Note the Hill-Sachs lesion on the posterolateral aspect of the humeral head. This "dent" is the result of an impaction fracture sustained during dislocations. The presence of this lesion is a clinical sign of recurrent anterior dislocation. The lesion itself contributes to more frequent dislocation with less precipitating force, as the dented humeral head slips more easily under the anterior glenoid margins. (Courtesy of North Hills Passavant Hospital, Pittsburgh, PA.)

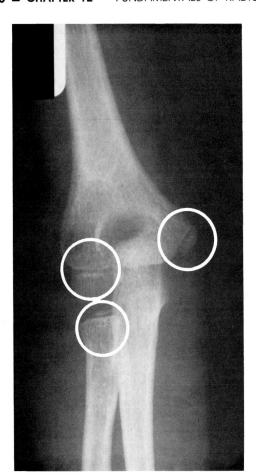

FIGURE 12–84 ■ Normal radiographic appearance of the elbow of a 5-year-old girl. Note developing secondary centers of ossification and epiphyseal plates at the humeral condyles and radial head. (Courtesy of Slippery Rock University School of Physical Therapy, Slippery Rock, PA.)

ence is that in tomography the film and the x-ray source move synchronously in opposite directions. As the x-ray beam penetrates the body, the focal plane of the image is at the level of the axis of rotation or fulcrum. Structures in the focal plane are in focus, and structures in all other planes are blurred by motion. Various depths of planes are chosen to be imaged by preadjusting the fulcrum or by maintaining a fixed fulcrum and adjusting the height of the table on which the patient lies.

Tomography is used most effectively in areas of high contrast, including bone and lungs. It can be of value in making a diagnosis that is not clear from conventional radiography. When evaluating bone lesions, conventional radiography can often confirm a pathologic process but to-

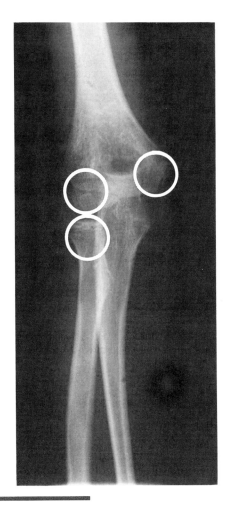

FIGURE 12–85 ■ Normal radiographic appearance of the elbow of a 10-year-old boy. Compare growth maturity of ossification centers (circles) to that of the 5-year-old in Figure 12–84. (Courtesy of Slippery Rock University School of Physical Therapy, Slippery Rock, PA.)

comes, false-positives and false-negatives happen. Diagnostic imaging studies are an adjunct to clinical and laboratory findings, not the entire answer.

An explanation of the capabilities and limitations of diagnostic studies commonly associated with evaluation of the musculoskeletal system follows.

## Tomography

Tomography is a technique of radiography that focuses on one predetermined plane of the body, blurring out structures above or below that plane of interest. Tomography requires the same basic tools as conventional plain film radiography: an x-ray source, the object, and the film. The differ-

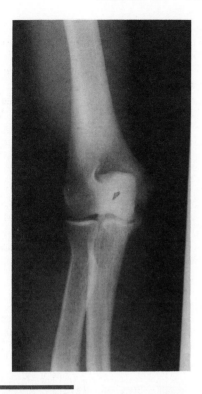

**FIGURE 12–86** ■ Normal radiographic appearance of the elbow of a 30-year-old man. (Courtesy of Slippery Rock University School of Physical Therapy, Slippery Rock, PA.)

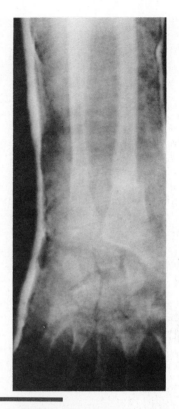

**FIGURE 12–87** ■ Transverse fractures at the distal third of the shafts of the radius and ulna, radiographed in dorsoplanar (PA) projection through plaster. (Courtesy of Slippery Rock University School of Physical Therapy, Slippery Rock, PA.)

mography may be needed to define the true extent of involvement.

A major clinical application of tomography is in evaluating fractures. Fractures of bones of irregular shape are often difficult to visualize on conventional films. Occult fractures of the tibial plateau, skull, and cervical spine are often well defined by tomography (Fig. 12–95). Known fractures on conventional films may be obscured by superimposition of images, and tomography aids in determining the characteristics of the

**FIGURE 12–88** ■ Lateral projection through plaster of radial and ulnar shaft fractures. Note the amount of displacement not evident on the PA view in Figure 12–87. The distal fragments are offset dorsally relative to the proximal shafts. Apposition of fragments is sufficient to promote fracture healing and remodeling. (Courtesy of Slippery Rock University School of Physical Therapy, Slippery Rock, PA.)

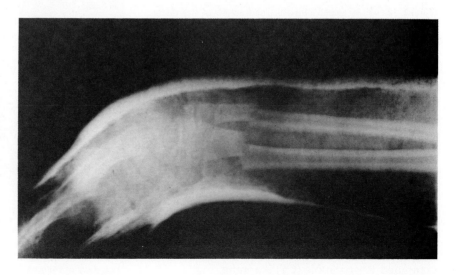

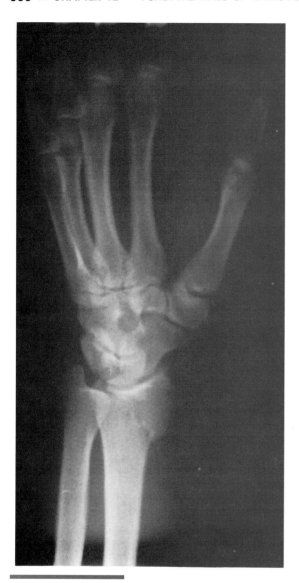

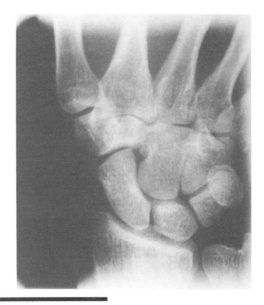

**FIGURE 12–90** ■ This dorsoplanar (PA) projection of the hand with a ulnar deviation best visualizes the scaphoid bone. (Courtesy of Slippery Rock University School of Physical Therapy, Slippery Rock, PA.)

**FIGURE 12–89** ■ Linear intra-articular fracture of the distal radius. (Courtesy of Slippery Rock University School of Physical Therapy, Slippery Rock, PA.)

fracture site. Assessment of healing is often compromised on conventional films by fixation devices or callus formation. Tomography is useful in these cases to evaluate the healing process.

Tomography does not, however, enhance detail. It is a process of "controlled blurring." Motion of the patient and equipment variables can easily alter the quality of a tomogram. Other disadvantages of tomography include insufficient soft tissue detail and difficulty in positioning a traumatized patient for the various angles of projection. For these reasons, tomography has, in some areas of clinical practice, been replaced by computed tomographic (CT) scanning.

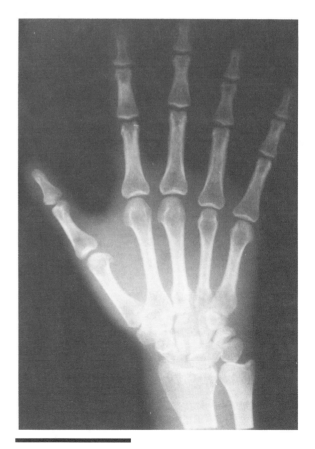

**FIGURE 12–91** ■ Dorsoplanar, or (PA), projection of a radiographically normal hand. (Courtesy of Slippery Rock University School of Physical Therapy, Slippery Rock, PA.)

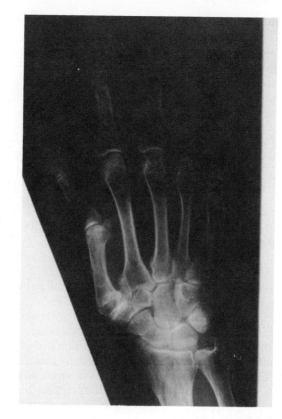

FIGURE 12-92 ■ Degenerative osteoarthritis of the first carpometacarpal joint. (Courtesy of Slippery Rock University School of Physical Therapy, Slippery Rock, PA.)

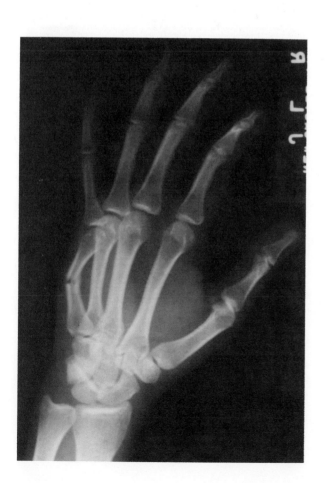

FIGURE 12-93 ■ Incomplete transverse fracture of midshaft of fifth metacarpal. Projection is dorsoplanar oblique. (Courtesy of Slippery Rock University School of Physical Therapy, Slippery Rock, PA.)

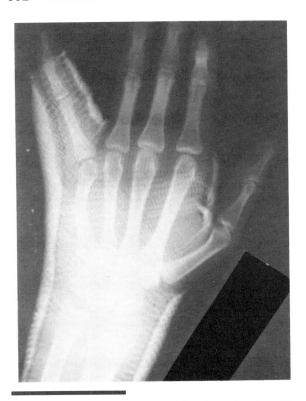

FIGURE 12–94 ■ Postreduction PA radiograph of a fifth metacarpal shaft fracture taken through plaster. (Courtesy of Slippery Rock University School of Physical Therapy, Slippery Rock, PA.)

## Contrast Media in Radiography

Details not evident on plain film radiography may be demonstrated through the administration of contrast media. The substances are given orally, rectally, or by injection. Barium sulfate is a radiopaque medium commonly used in gastrointestinal studies. Radiopaque organic iodides are used for study of the kidney, liver, blood vessels, bladder, and urethra. Radiolucent gases, such as oxygen, helium, carbon dioxide, nitrous oxide, nitrogen, and air, are used to visualize the brain, subarachnoid space, pleural space, peritoneal cavity, pericardial space, and some joints.

Myelography is the study of the spinal cord, nerve roots, and dura mater using radiographic contrast media. Different myelographic methods include positive contrast myelography using water-soluble iodine or iodized oils and negative contrast myelography using air. After injection of the contrast medium into the subarachnoid space, the fluoroscopic table on which the patient is positioned is tilted until the contrast me-

dium reaches the spinal level to be evaluated. Plain films are then taken (Fig. 12–96). Computed tomography may also be used at this time to visualize more anatomic detail. When CT scanning is used in conjunction with myelography, the image is referred to as a CT myelogram. Abnormal results on a myelogram may reveal a ruptured intervertebral disc, spinal cord compression, stenosis, intravertebral tumor, obstructions in the spinal canal, or nerve root injury.

Arthrography is the study of structures in an encapsulated joint using radiographic contrast media. Contrast medium is injected directly into (Fig. 12–97) the joint space, distending the capsule and outlining internal structures. Arthrography has commonly been used in evaluating the knee and shoulder joints. Indications for arthrography at the knee include suspected meniscal tears, synovial abnormalities, ligamentous tears, osteochondral fractures, osteochondritis dissecans, and joint capsule abnormalities. Evaluation of the shoulder by arthrography can determine the presence of adhesive capsulitis, rotator cuff tears, and bicipital tendinitis or tears.

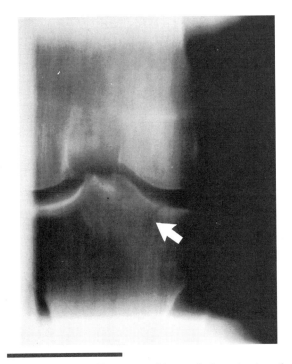

FIGURE 12–95 ■ Tomogram of intra-articular extension of a tibial plateau fracture. The depth of the plane of focus is recorded on the film in centimeters. This was an AP projection at 12.5-cm depth. (Courtesy of Slippery Rock University School of Physical Therapy, Slippery Rock, PA.)

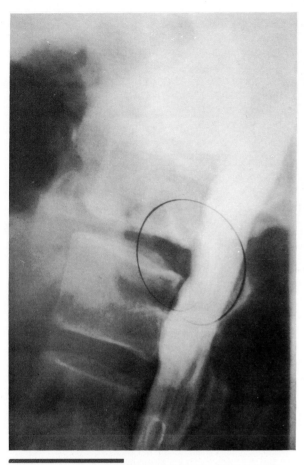

**FIGURE 12–96 ■** Positive contrast myelogram of the lumbar spine. Diagnosis of herniated nucleus pulposus at L-4 to L-5 was later confirmed at surgery. (Courtesy of North Hills Suburban MRI, Pittsburgh, PA.)

## Nuclear Medicine

Nuclear medicine is a clinical science involving the diagnostic use of radioactive materials or isotopes. Radiopharmaceuticals are tissue-specific radioactive materials administered orally or intravenously. Concentrations of these substances are different in abnormal tissues and normal surrounding tissues. Scintillation cameras are used to image the unequal distribution of the radiopharmaceuticals. Images are recorded on x-ray film. Two types of imaging, referred to as "hot spot" and "cold spot" imaging, designate tissue areas of hyperfunction and hypofunction, respectively. Bone scans and brain scans are examples of hot spot imaging. Lesions in these tissues appear darker than the body background. Liver and lung scans are examples of cold spot

imaging. Lesions in these areas appear lighter than the background.

Bone scanning can best be described as a sensitivity test. The primary advantage of bone scanning is that it can reveal early bone disease or bone healing (Fig. 12–98A and B). It is not specific in differential diagnosis of disease. Findings on bone scans are used in conjunction with other laboratory, imaging, and clinical tests.

Indications for bone scanning include detection of fractures, assessment of normal or abnormal fracture healing, and detection of metastatic disease, benign bone tumors, arthritis, osteomyelitis, avascular necrosis, or Paget's disease. Bone scanning is often utilized to assess unexplained bone pain. Osteoblastic activity around the margins of the temporomandibular joint secondary to disc displacement or bite abnormalities may be seen on a bone scan.

## Computed Tomography

Computed tomography was produced in England in 1967 by Electric Music Industries and first bore the name EMI scanning. It has also been called computerized axial tomography (CAT) and computerized transaxial tomography (CTI). The preferred term at this time is CT.

CT is a merging of x-ray technology with computers to create cross-sectional axial images of any part of the body. The process begins when an x-ray source rotates around the supine patient and x-rays penetrate the body from numerous angles. Detectors in the surrounding scanner measure tissue x-ray attenuation and transmit this information to a computer. The computer then reconstructs the body image using these measurements taken at the periphery of the axial slice of body being scanned (Fig. 12–99). The image is seen on a screen, photographed, and stored on x-ray film. By viewing a consecutive series of axial slices, a three-dimensional image can be constructed.

Radiologists evaluate CT scans by analyzing shape, symmetry, position, and density contrast of body structures. Space-occupying lesions deform or displace adjacent structures. Increased tissue density is characteristic of some neoplasms, aneurysms, infections, and degenerative tissues. Hemorrhage and hematomas also become more dense after clotting has occurred. Decreased tissue density may be due to infarctions, necrotic malignant tumors, benign tumors, cysts,

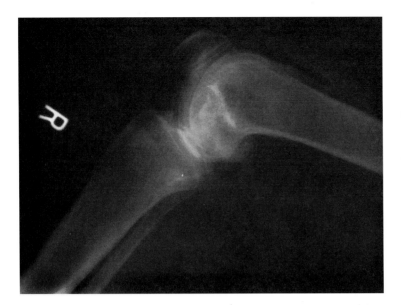

**FIGURE 12-97** ■ Arthrographic study of the knee. The contrast medium distends the joint capsule, outlining its proximal expanse suprapatellarly and its posterior expanse at the politeal space. (Courtesy of North Hills Passavant Hospital, Pittsburgh, PA.)

or infections. Some lesions are similar in density to surrounding tissue and require contrast media for differentiation. Contrast enhancement is often indicated for suspected vascular abnormalities or aneurysms. In CT myelography, contrast media are used to enhance detail of spinal structures.

CT can be described as an anatomic technique.

It shows the "geography" of body structures with 100 times more sensitivity than conventional radiography. CT is limited in that it can measure only tissue attenuation of x-rays; it cannot show tissue perfusion, metabolism, or blood vessel flow. Thus, CT is not the best imaging study for subdural hematoma or early ischemic disease of the brain.

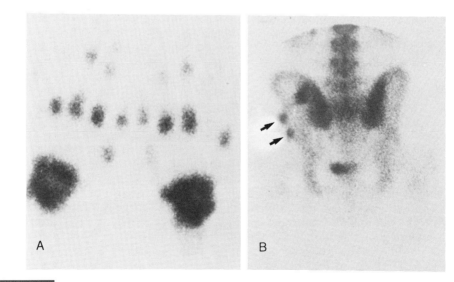

A    B

**FIGURE 12-98** ■ (A) Bone scan of hands with early changes of rheumatoid arthritis. The radiopharmaceutical technetium was injected 2 hours before the scan. Marked uptake of technetium is seen in both wrists and most of the metacarpophalangeal joints. Increased uptake is present in the interphalangeal joints of the thumb, middle fingers, and left index finger. The minimal increase in uptake of the remaining joints is normal. (B) Technetium bone scan at pelvis. Abnormal uptake is noted in two circular areas at the location of the gluteus medius muscle (arrows). On the basis of these results and clinical findings, a diagnosis of early stage myositis ossificans was made. The initial injury was a contusion of the muscle. (Courtesy of North Hills Passavant Hospital, Pittsburgh, PA.)

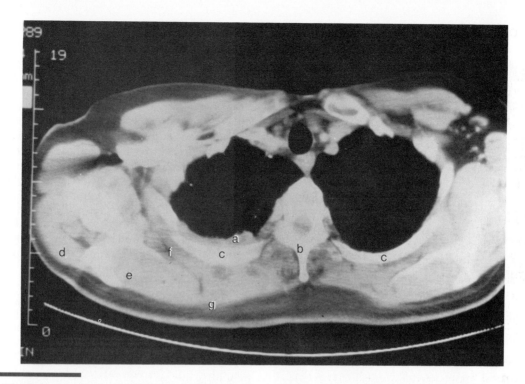

**FIGURE 12-99** ■ Transverse axial CT image at the level of the thoracic inlet. The patient was a retired coal miner. Note pleural thickening caused by occupational hazards in the left lung (a). The patient's chief complaint was left scapular and radiating left upper extremity pain. This CT evaluation is negative for pathologic disease. See Figure 12-100 for further evaluation results. Note vertebral body (b), ribs (c), Infraspinatus (d), supraspinatus (e), subscapularis (f), and trapezius (g). (Courtesy of North Hills Suburban MRI, Pittsburgh, PA.)

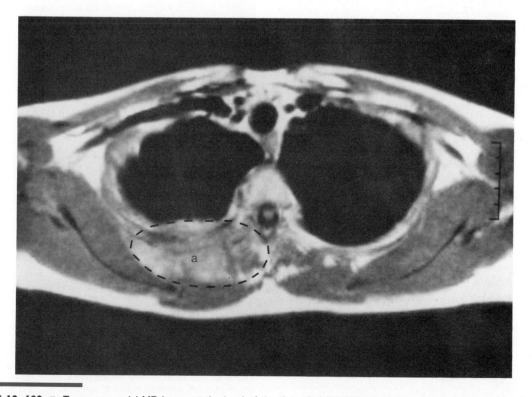

**FIGURE 12-100** ■ Transverse axial MR image at the level of the thoracic inlet. Note the large expanse of lung tumor invading subscapularis muscle (a). This tumor is not detectable on the CT scan in Figure 12-99. (Courtesy of North Hills Suburban MRI, Pittsburgh, PA.)

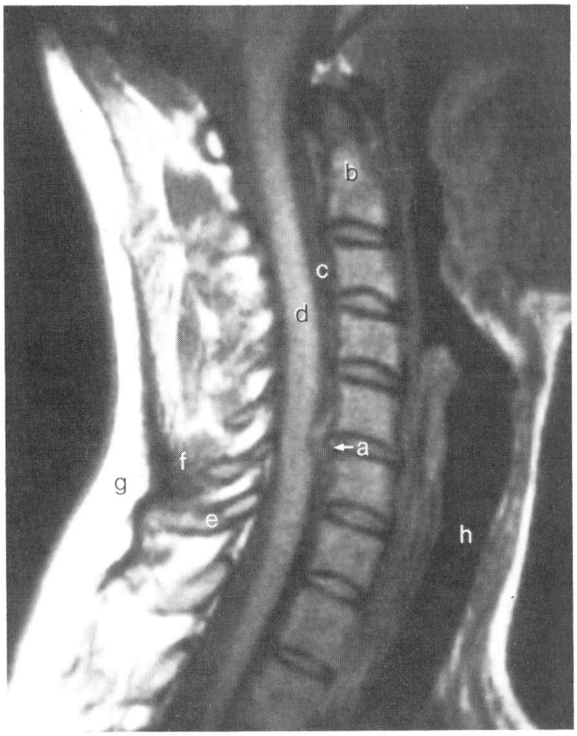

**FIGURE 12–101** ■ Sagittal MR image of the cervical spine. Note posterior intervertebral disc herniation at C-5 to C-6 (a). Other structures are odontoid process of C-2 (b), cerebrospinal fluid (c), spinal cord (d), spinous process of C-6 (e), muscle (f), skin and fat (g), and trachea (h). (Courtesy of North Hills Suburban MRI, Pittsburgh, PA.)

## Magnetic Resonance Imaging

Properties of magnetic resonance imaging (MRI) were discovered in the 1940s and development of this clinical science expanded rapidly into the 1980s, when it was introduced for tissue visualization. MR imaging provides anatomic and physiologic information noninvasively. MR imaging does not involve ionizing radiation; it gathers information produced by the interaction of tissue with electromagnetic forces.

Briefly, the process begins when a patient is placed inside a scanner containing magnetic field coils and radio transmitters and receivers. Most atomic nuclei in the body have magnetic properties. When the patient is exposed to a strong magnetic field, the previously random nuclei line up in the direction of the field. These nuclei are not static but rotate, like spinning tops, about an axis roughly parallel to the field. This spinning motion of nuclei is called precession and occurs at specific frequencies. Radio waves are then

pulsed to the patient at this frequency, and precessing nuclei absorb this energy through the process of resonance. The radio waves are then turned off, and as the nuclei relax into their random patterns, the absorbed energy is released in the form of radio waves. Radio receivers in the scanner amplify these waves and transmit them to a computer. Through complex calculations, an electronic image is constructed and displayed on a screen. Images are photographed and recorded on x-ray film. Tissue images are differentiated by their radio signal strength. Strong signals appear whiter, weak signals blacker. Signal strength of a particular tissue is determined by the number of precessing nuclei per volume of tissue and the rate of relaxation of the nuclei. In MRI, soft tissues and bone marrow give strong signals. Air and cortical bone give weak signals. An advantage of MRI is that cross-sectional images can be

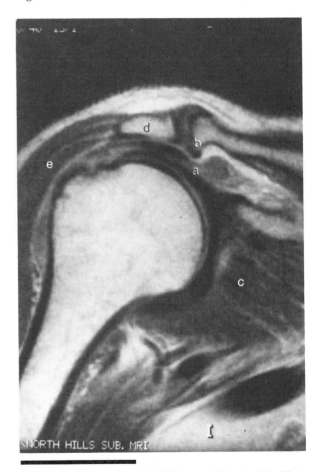

**FIGURE 12–102** ■ Coronal MR image of the shoulder. Note impingement of supraspinatus muscle (a) secondary to clavicular spur and enlargement of acromiclavicular joint (b). Other structures are subscapularis (c), acromion (d), and deltoid (e). I indicates interior orientation. (Courtesy of North Hills Suburban MRI, Pittsburgh, PA.)

displayed on screen from multiple planes without repositioning the patient.

In neurologic evaluation, MRI is superior to CT in imaging the cerebellum and the brain stem. These areas are often obscured on CT scans by dense surrounding bone. MRI differentiates gray and white brain tissue with more contrast than CT and is better for detecting white matter diseases such as multiple sclerosis. Gadolinium is a paramagnetic contrast agent used in evaluation of the central nervous system and has improved the ability of MRI to detect brain meningiomas. Metastatic and primary brain tumors are generally detected better by MRI than CT (Fig. 12–100). The spinal cord and contents of the neural canal can be evaluated without the contrast necessary in CT myelography. MRI is useful in evaluating disc herniations (Fig. 12–101). Its advantage is less in imaging calcified structures; calcification in some kinds of tumors is more easily detected by CT scanning.

In orthopaedic evaluation, the multiplanar capabilities of MRI have expanded its role in examination of joints. It is gradually replacing arthrography and arthroscopy in evaluation of the knee joint (Fig. 12–102). Excellent soft tissue and bone marrow contrast has led to the early detection of soft tissue and bone tumors. Avascular necrosis can also be detected in its early stages by MRI.

## SUMMARY

Plain film radiography is the most common first-order diagnostic screening procedure in the evaluation of musculoskeletal disease or dysfunction. The results of plain films are correlated with clinical findings to form the basis for treatment or to direct further diagnostic study.

Physical therapists need a working knowledge of radiologic fundamentals and radiologic terminology to interpret the radiologist's descriptive assessment of the patient. Pertinent information from the radiologist's report is required to complete a thorough history and physical therapy evaluation of the patient. Familiarity with radiologic vocabulary assists in communication with other medical personnel and augments the process of educating the patient.

Physical therapists need to appreciate both the capabilities and limitations of plain film radiography. They should also understand that, like all other diagnostic procedures, radiology can produce false-positives and false-negatives. The clinical value of comprehensive history taking and physical therapy evaluation should not be underestimated. The responsibility of the physical therapist is not to make the differential diagnosis but to have the competence to recognize what evaluation findings are or are not within the scope of physical therapy treatment. A basic understanding of radiology helps the physical therapist in gaining this competence.

## References

1. Brashear HR, Raney RB: Shand's Handbook of Orthopedic Surgery. St. Louis: Mosby Year Book, 1986.
2. Salter RB: Textbook of Disorders and Injuries of the Musculoskeletal System. Baltimore: Williams & Wilkins, 1983.
3. Gozna ER, Harrington IJ: Biomechanics of Musculoskeletal Injury. Baltimore: Williams & Wilkins, 1982.
4. Gustilo RB: The Fracture Classification Manual. St. Louis: Mosby Year Book, 1991.

## Bibliography

Ballinger PW: Merrill's Atlas of Radiographic Positions and Radiologic Procedures. St. Louis: Mosby Year Book, 1991.

Eastman Kodak Company, Health Sciences Markets Division: The Fundamentals of Radiology. Rochester, NY: Author, 1980.

Fischbach FT: A Manual of Laboratory Diagnostic Tests. Philadelphia: JB Lippincott, 1988.

Fodor J, Malott JC: The Art and Science of Medical Radiology. St. Louis: Catholic Health Association of the United States, 1987.

Gurley LT, Callaway WJ: Introduction to Radiologic Technology. St. Louis: Mosby Year Book, 1986.

Hole JW: Human Anatomy and Physiology. Dubuque, IA: Wm. C. Brown Publishers, 1987.

Jacobs ER: Medical Imaging; a Concise Text. New York: Igaku-Shoin, 1987.

Kaltenborn FM, Evjenth O: Manual Mobilization of the Extremity Joints. Oslo, Norway: Olaf Norlis Bokhandel, 1989.

Kee JL: Laboratory and Diagnostic Tests with Nursing Implications. Norwalk, CT: Appleton & Lange, 1991.

Keim HA: Clinical Symposia; Scoliosis. Summit, NJ: CIBA Pharmaceutical Company, 1978.

Meschan I: Anatomy Basic to Radiology. Philadelphia: WB Saunder, 1975.

Squire LF, Novelline RA: Fundamentals of Radiology. Cambridge, MA: Harvard University Press, 1988.

# *Thirteen*

# Education of Patients

## Z. ANNETTE IGLARSH

INTRODUCTION
PHYSICAL THERAPIST AS AN
EDUCATOR
METHODS OF EDUCATING
PATIENTS

LEARNING ENVIRONMENT
EXERCISE INSTRUCTION
TEACHING STYLE

## INTRODUCTION

The effective physical therapist acquires a comprehensive knowledge base of anatomy, biomechanics, and pathokinematics. A structured, objective examination is built onto this knowledge base. By analyzing the patient from this perspective, the therapist uses the hypothesis-oriented algorithm (see Fig. 9–21) and sorts through the differential diagnosis using branched problem solving. Objective, functional treatment goals are established and symptom-specific treatment regimens are developed. Unfortunately, the physical therapist using this approach is performing all the correct actions but the treatment may not be effective. This therapist left out the most important component of the patient's care — the patient.

The patient is both the best source of medical information and the most appropriate copractitioner. If the therapist establishes good rapport with the patient at the beginning of the treatment series, the patient can provide the therapist with important information related to the evaluation and differential diagnosis. The patient can also contribute to the rehabilitation by performing exercises at home in the time between office visits. Thus, patients can be active participants in their care; however, patients must be guided in this active participation and become educated in their physical status to best perform self-care.

## PHYSICAL THERAPIST AS AN EDUCATOR

The effective therapist must be an effective educator, as well as a competent clinician. Physical therapy protocols are parallel in design to education protocols. The educator identifies objective goals that are measurable and selects methods of dispensing information to meet these goals.

As an educator-guide, the therapist must initially establish goals for teaching the patient. An objective approach enables the therapist to set the anticipated goals and then back up to establish the steps required to achieve the stated short or intermediate goals. Once the therapist establishes these goals, goal achievement must be approached from two perspectives: the factors that determine the most effective teaching approach *and* the methods that maximize the positive impact of these factors while minimizing the negative impact:

The Patient
    Knowledge of the diagnosis
    Effective learning style
        Auditory
        Visual
        Manipulative/experiential
    Effective learning approach
        Whole to part
        Part to whole
        Branched algorithm
        Rote memorization
    Intellectual level
    English vocabulary level
    Social/family support
The Therapist
    Knowledge of the diagnosis
    Knowledge of treatments proposed
    Knowledge of teaching styles
        Passive teaching
        Active teaching
    Experience/ability in using teaching styles
        Availability of teaching materials
        Appropriateness of teaching environment

Patients should be educated consumers; they should be aware of the basic characteristics of their diagnosis and prognosis. This information orients them to the importance of their input: presenting significant symptoms, describing their response to treatment, and noting the changes in their symptoms over time in response to treatment. Often a clear understanding makes a patient more motivated to participate in office treatment regimens and home treatment programs.

## METHODS OF EDUCATING PATIENTS

People learn better by some methods than others. In addition, some types of information are more effectively presented in styles ranging from auditory to visual to manipulative. Concepts, philosophy, or overviews of illness or treatment approaches are most effectively taught by lecture. Function or pathology is most effectively presented in diagram or chart form. Exercise and functional re-education are best understood and retained in active, participatory learning experiences.

The first two styles, lecture and diagrams, are passive types of teaching styles. These can be made more active, and thus more effective, by encouraging the patient to ask questions and participate in discussions and to color or label the diagrams appropriately. The third method, manipulative or experimental, is active participatory learning and is more effective if the patient sees the exercise demonstrated and is given visual descriptions, performs the exercises with guidance, and performs the exercises alone while writing down any needed clues or details to exercise diagram handouts.

Information can be delivered to the patient in different forms. In "whole to part" orientations a concept is presented and then broken down into each component for explanation. "Part to whole" orientation is a building process of learning. Each part of the whole concept is taught and built on to reach the whole. The branched algorithm (see Fig. 9–21) is a problem-solving process of deductive reasoning. That is, the patient chooses between two alternative responses, and each choice leads to a series of sequential alternatives and final concept. The process of memorization is the least interactive but permits retention of a large amount of material.

The therapist should assess the patient's intellectual level. However, jargon should be avoided, despite the patient's intellectual level, because it impedes communication. A person with a low intellectual level learns better if extensive illustrations and demonstrations are used. Even a patient with high intellect may not have good body awareness. Generally, athletes, dancers, and physical therapists have good body awareness and learn exercises and functional re-education activities easily. A patient with poor body awareness may need multiple visual examples and may learn activities more slowly. A patient with poor knowledge of English may need a translator, or the therapist can use key words in the patient's own language or charts and nonverbal demonstration.

The therapist has not effectively explained the patient's physical condition or taught an exercise program unless the patient can go home and repeat the lesson to his or her family, spouse, or companion. A patient who has difficulty explaining the lesson should invite a family member, spouse, or companion to attend the next therapy session. This session should be designed to repeat the instruction for the patient and allow the guest to ask questions. If this is not possible because of the clinic's location or availability of the support person, the therapist may arrange to videotape the next session.

Therapists must also analyze their own characteristics to be effective teachers. They should have an extensive knowledge of the proposed treatment's indications, contraindications, assumed outcome, and mode of operation. All of these factors should be translated into lay terminology. The therapist should also be able to describe what the patient should feel when the procedure is applied. This decreases the patient's anxiety and increases the patient's confidence in the therapist.

Therapists must be aware of and be effective in the several teaching styles previously mentioned. They must select passive and active teaching methods based on the projected learning style of the patient and the nature of the material to be taught.

Effective teaching requires establishment or enhancement of the patient's motivation. People learn best if they know why it is important to learn the material. Some are motivated if they learn that they can help themselves feel better, if they realize that they are the copractitioner in their case, or if they can make better decisions about their health care as an active participant and an educated consumer.

Therapists should try to gain experience and expertise in a variety of learning styles. They may have been given courses in their professional education programs or in their clinical affiliations. They may apply teaching styles they have seen in nontherapy or nonhealth-care settings. Peers often use techniques the therapist may want to emulate. The therapist should try these styles when teaching patients and small groups to identify the most effective styles.

An effective teacher uses a wide variety of educational material. Pamphlets, exercise forms, videotapes, and audiotapes may be used, depending on the material to be presented and the patient's learning style. Pamphlets should be easy to read in terms of print, diagrams, and reading level. Depending on the population of patients, the therapist may store multilingual print materials. Exercise forms should have clear diagrams and simple explanations. Patients should be encouraged to add their own clues to the form.

Videotapes can be "homemade" but should be simple and easy to follow. Patients may simply choose to tape their own therapy session. Audiotapes may enable the patient to perform the exercises using repeated instructions by the therapist. Audio instruction should be given in great detail to compensate for the absence of visual clues.

## LEARNING ENVIRONMENT

Securing an appropriate teaching environment is often the factor forgotten by the therapist. To enhance concentration, the patient should feel comfortable in the environment. Both the patient and the therapist should be shielded from interruption. The environment should be well lighted, ventilated, and as free from distractions as possible. A patient who is easily distracted should be taught in a more isolated part of the clinic. The environment should also make guests feel comfortable if they are to assist in the performance of the home protocols.

## EXERCISE INSTRUCTION

Patients should be guided toward a reasonable home exercise regimen that takes into consideration time to perform the program and the length of the regimen. A short sequence of exercises done more frequently during the day is effective in functional re-education programs or for a patient who has poor endurance. A longer program done less frequently can build strength or endurance. Initially, the therapist should teach the patient only two or three exercises. When the patient performs these exercises appropriately, one or two new exercises can be added in each session. The therapist should review the exercise regimen in each session to offer corrections as needed. The therapist may elect to give the compliant patient the parameters within which the exercises can be progressed in the interval between office visits.

## TEACHING STYLE

Therapists increase their effectiveness as teachers and guides by evaluating the learning-teaching characteristics during the subjective portion of the initial evaluation. The therapist can ask questions to determine the patient's knowledge of the diagnosis, but it is more difficult to determine the patient's learning style or most effective learning approach. In some cases the therapist can assess how the patient follows the questioning portion of the subjective evaluation to project the patient's best learning style and approach. However, because these are only assumptions, the style and approach may have to be altered during the instructional process if they prove to be ineffective. Intellectual level of the patient can be related to the patient's academic achievement, occupation/profession, or reasoning during the evaluation. Verbal language skill can also be determined during the subjective interview. Family support is also determined during subjective questioning or by interviewing family members.

Therapists should try several styles of teaching to determine their most comfortable and effective style. They should research the diagnosis and treatment protocols and determine whether the material would best be presented in active or passive teaching formats. Time should also be allotted to prepare effective teaching materials and secure the appropriate learning environment.

## SUMMARY

This text has provided the reader with a comprehensive clinical approach to orthopaedic physical therapy by presenting a foundation in anatomic and movement sciences, objective evaluations, differential diagnoses, structured treatment plans, and clinical applications in case studies. This final chapter on education of patients identifies the patient as a copractitioner and teaches the therapist how to be an effective guide to promote the patient in this role. Even very knowledgeable therapists are not successful practitioners unless they can effectively share their knowledge with their patients.

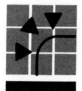

# Index

Page numbers in *italics* refer to illustrations; page numbers followed by t refer to tables.

Note: Specific musculoskeletal structures can be found under *Bone(s), Ligament(s), Muscle(s),* etc.

ISBN 0-7216-3257-2

9 780721 632575

90069